Geriatrics & Gerontology of the Dog and Cat

2nd Edition

Geriatrics & Gerontology of the Dog and Cat

Johnny D. Hoskins, DVM, PhD, DACVIM
Professor Emeritus
Department of Veterinary Clinical Sciences
School of Veterinary Medicine
Louisiana State University
Baton Rouge, Louisiana

SAUNDERS
An Imprint of Elsevier

SAUNDERS
An Imprint of Elsevier

11830 Westline Industrial Drive
St. Louis, Missouri 63146

GERIATRICS AND GERONTOLOGY OF THE DOG AND CAT 0-7216-8799-7

NOTICE

Veterinary medicine is an ever-changing field. Standard safety precautions must be followed, but as new research and clinical experience broaden our knowledge, changes in treatment and drug therapy may become necessary or appropriate. Readers are advised to check the most current product information provided by the manufacturer of each drug to be administered to verify the recommended dose, the method and duration of administration, and contraindications. It is the responsibility of the licensed prescriber, relying on experience and knowledge of the patient, to determine dosages and the best treatment for each individual patient. Neither the publisher nor the author assumes any liability for any injury and/or damage to persons or property arising from this publication.

Previous edition copyrighted 1995

International Standard Book Number 0-7216-8799-7

Acquisitions Editor: Liz Fathman
Developmental Editor: Jolynn Gower
Publishing Services Manager: Patricia Tannian
Project Manager: Sarah Wunderly
Design Manager: William Drone

Printed in the United States

Last digit is the print number: 9 8 7 6 5 4 3 2 1

Contributors

Anthony P. Carr, Dr. med. vet., DACVIM
Small Animal Clinical Sciences
Western College of Veterinary Medicine
Saskatoon, Saskatchewan, Canada

Claud B. Chastain, DVM, MS, DACVIM
Associate Dean for Academic Affairs and Professor
College of Veterinary Medicine
University of Missouri
Columbia, Missouri

David A. Dzanis, DVM, PhD, DACVN
Dzanis Consulting & Collaborations
Santa Clarita, California

Tina R. Ellenbogen, DVM
Mobile Veterinary Services and Animal HomeCare and Hospice
Bothell, Washington

William D. Fortney, DVM
Head of Small Animal Medicine
Clinical Sciences
College of Veterinary Medicine
Kansas State University
Manhattan, Kansas

Clenric Guy Hancock, DVM, MEd
Program Director
Veterinary Technology Department
St. Petersburg College
St. Petersburg, Florida

Elizabeth Head, BSc, MA, PhD
Assistant Professional Researcher
Institute for Brain Aging and Dementia
University of California at Irvine
Irvine, California

Johnny D. Hoskins, DVM, PhD, DACVIM
Professor Emeritus
Department of Veterinary Clinical Sciences
School of Veterinary Medicine
Louisiana State University
Baton Rouge, Louisiana

Gary M. Landsberg, BSc, DVM, DACVB
Clinician/Veterinary Behaviorist
Doncaster Animal Clinic
Thornhill, Ontario, Canada

Franklin D. McMillan, DVM, DACVIM
Medical Director
VCA Miller—Robertson Animal Hospital
Los Angeles, California

Steven A. Melman, VMD
Founder, DermaPet
Potomac, Maryland

Sandra R. Merchant, DVM, DACVD
Professor of Dermatology
Veterinary Clinical Sciences
School of Veterinary Medicine
Louisiana State University
Baton Rouge, Louisiana

Reto Neiger, Dr. med. vet., PhD, DACVIM, DECVIM-CA
Lecturer, Small Animal Internal Medicine
Veterinary Clinical Sciences
Royal Veterinary College
London, United Kingdom

Robert R. Paddleford, DVM
Associate Professor and Director of Anesthesiology (Retired)
Director of Anesthesia and Intensive Care
College of Veterinary Medicine
University of Tennessee
Knoxville, Tennessee

Janet E. Steiss, DVM, PhD, PT
Associate Professor
Department of Biomedical Sciences
College of Veterinary Medicine,
Nursing & Allied Health
Tuskegee University
Tuskegee, Alabama

Joseph Taboada, DVM, DACVIM (Small Animal Internal Medicine)
Professor, Small Animal Internal Medicine
Associate Dean; Student and Academic Affairs
School of Veterinary Medicine
Louisiana State University
Baton Rouge, Louisiana

Don R. Waldron, DVM, DAVCS
Professor of Surgery
Small Animal Clinical Sciences
Virginia-Maryland Regional College of Veterinary Medicine
Blacksburg, Virginia

Preface

Geriatric medicine is currently a major area of growth in veterinary practice and continues to emerge in importance for older dogs and cats as well as for their owners. As the population of older dogs and cats increases, the veterinary practice community is being more active and more sophisticated in ways to monitor and manage older dogs and cats. This edition of *Geriatrics and Gerontology of the Dogs and Cats* reviews some of the most common and best recognized geriatric diseases and provides an update of selected aspects of some of the most recently recognized disorders in geriatric dogs and cats. I am delighted to have collected contributors who have worked in their respective topics for some time and with distinction. I have chosen the contributors based on their knowledge and, in part, because they are familiar to me and may be familiar to the reader.

I am pleased with the eclectic composition of this book, which encompasses discussion of the oldest and newest aspects of geriatric medicine. In addition to the authors, this work was ultimately brought to you by the large, talented editorial staff of Elsevier. I hope that clinicians and veterinary technicians will share my enthusiasm about this book.

Johnny D. Hoskins, DVM, PhD

Contents

CHAPTER 1

Geriatrics and Aging

WILLIAM D. FORTNEY

Geriatrics is that branch of medicine and surgery that treats problems peculiar to old age. Aging is the accumulation of progressive body changes associated with or responsible for disease, decreased physiologic function, and death.[1] Aging itself is not a disease. Life span and life expectancy differ among species and among individual members of a species, and this variability suggests that a genetic component is responsible for the normal aging process. Discounting genetic factors, the variations may be attributed to acquired diseases and environmental stressors.

Aging in a dog or cat is associated with gradual deterioration in the delicate interrelationships among the body systems, which predisposes the dog or cat to acquired disease. Some diseases cause death indirectly, through their effects on cells, tissues, and organs (e.g., ischemic heart disease and diabetes mellitus). However, death is frequently assumed to be the result of the normal aging process. If a dog or cat dies of natural causes at a young age, it is usually the direct result of an underlying disease. If a dog or cat dies at a senile age, it is attributed to disease or age or both. The dichotomy between age and disease in this circumstance is ambiguous. Death is a well-defined event with a strong correlation with age.

THEORIES OF AGING

Many theories attempt to explain the aging process. In a recent review of 24 different theories of aging, Morse and Rabinowitz proposed a unified theory that essentially states that an organism's (animal's) biologic progress is genetically determined, is set in motion at conception, and lasts for the duration of life.[2] The speed at which aging occurs is secondary to influences from many environmental forces and stressors that occur within the organism (animal) and are genetically programmed. The balance among these influences ultimately determines the effects of aging.

EFFECT OF AGING ON ANIMALS' BODY SYSTEMS

A common characteristic of aging body systems is progressive and irreversible change. The effects of disease, stress, malnutrition, lack of exercise, genetics, and environment may hasten this change. Elderly animals seldom have a single disease, but instead have a unique combination of multiple organ disease with varying levels of dysfunction. Veterinarians should not accept that poor health and old age are synonymous. Knowledge of the common pathologic changes associated with age and their effect on function allows the veterinarian to plan and manage more effective health care programs for aged dogs and cats.[1] Box 1-1 outlines the common effects of aging.

CHALLENGES OF HEALTH CARE

An aging dog or cat presents major challenges to the owner and veterinarian. Care for such animals involves a proactive, comprehensive health care program that addresses the older animal's special needs.[3] This specialized medical

Box 1-1 Effects of Aging

Metabolic Effects

Decreased metabolic rate plus lack of activity decreases caloric needs by 30% to 40%.
Immune competence decreases, despite normal numbers of lymphocytes.
Phagocytosis and chemotaxis decrease, and older animals are less able to ward off infections.
Autoantibodies and immune-mediated diseases develop.

Physical Effects

Percentage of body weight represented by fat increases.
Skin becomes thickened, hyperpigmented, and inelastic.
Footpads hyperkeratinize, and claws become brittle.
Muscle, bone, and cartilage mass are lost, with subsequent development of osteoarthritis.
Dental calculus results in tooth loss and gingival hyperplasia.
Periodontitis results in gingival retraction and atrophy.
Gastric mucosa becomes atrophic and fibrotic.
Hepatocyte numbers decrease, and hepatic fibrosis occurs.
Pancreatic enzyme secretion diminishes.
Lungs lose elasticity, fibrosis occurs, and pulmonary secretions become more viscous. Vital capacity decreases.
Cough reflex and expiratory capacity decrease.
Kidney weight decreases, glomerular filtration rate decreases, and tubules atrophy.
Urinary incontinence frequently develops.
Prostate gland enlarges, testes atrophy, and prepuce becomes pendulous.
Ovaries enlarge, and mammary glands become fibrocystic or neoplastic.
Cardiac output decreases, and valvular fibrosis and intramural coronary arteriosclerosis develop.
Bone marrow becomes fatty and hypoplastic, and nonregenerative anemia develops.
The number of cells in the nervous system decreases. Senility causes loss of house training.

service is based on the following premises: first, that there are fundamental differences in specific diseases, behavior traits, and nutritional needs of older animals compared with younger ones; second, that prevention of, early detection of, and timely intervention for medical problems can have a significant impact on the life span and quality of life of an older dog or cat.

Care for older dogs and cats should focus on owner education, disease prevention strategies, and detection of medical and behavioral problems at the earliest possible stage—when the prognosis is better, and numerous treatment options still exist. The term *senior* or *geriatric* describes that life stage of progressive decline in physical condition, organ function, sensory function, mental function, and immunity. Although it is generally accepted that the senior life stage begins around 7 years of age for the average dog or cat, several interrelated factors, including size and individual genetics, affect the onset and rate of the progressive decline.

Care for older animals begins at the first examination of the new puppy or kitten, when the animal's entire life-stage health program is outlined to the owner, and the program is implemented when the animal reaches 7 years of age. Senior care promotes routine examinations of healthy animals on a twice-a-year basis starting at 7 years of age and advocates routine diagnostic screening for developing diseases. Apparently healthy animals make up just one component of the group targeted for senior care. Another component consists of older dogs and cats that are asymptomatic or exhibiting early signs of a problem, but whose owners either do not recognize the signs or just attribute them to "old age" and fail to seek veterinary care.

ESTABLISHING NEW APPROACHES

Historically, veterinarians have reacted to existing problems in older animals. Veterinarians wait until owners elect to seek professional help for their animals, once the disease signs are blatantly obvious or no longer tolerable. When owners are not adequately educated regarding the early warning signs of disease, or healthy animals are not regularly screened for age-related diseases, veterinarians are presented with animals that have moderate to advanced diseases. As a result considerable time and resources are dedicated to managing these diseases effectively, and th

Box 1-2 Developing a Health Care Program

Although success is never guaranteed, the following steps may help to implement a successful senior care program. Using all the tools developed for senior care can greatly simplify the implementation process and increase the opportunity for program success.

1. Convince personnel that a senior health care program can become a significant asset to the veterinary practice before investing the time, energy, training, and resources necessary to develop and maintain the program. Remember that this program may not be for every veterinary practice or for every animal owner. Ultimately, senior care is a long-term investment in the growth of the veterinary practice, so start slow and let the program evolve. Insist that every member of the hospital staff be program proficient and knowledgeable.
2. Convince the hospital staff of the significant health benefits the program offers the senior dog and cat. Critical to the success or failure of senior care is program ownership by every staff member. It is recommended that the entire staff help in the initial program development and that a specific staff member be empowered as the practice's senior care coordinator.
3. Review the existing senior care educational tools to create a very specific and detailed program for the veterinary practice. Important program decisions include:
   - Determining the age at which to initiate senior care
   - Establishing the frequency of senior care visits
   - Scheduling senior care periods that least affect regular office appointments
   - Calculating fees associated with the senior care service
   - Compiling a library of owner educational materials
   - Developing a program marketing strategy
4. Convince the owners of the significant health benefits the senior care program offers their aging dog or cat, by means of a mailing marketing strategy or while the owners are in the examination room. Although a percentage of owners will readily accept the senior care program on your recommendation alone, the rest will need convincing. Increased owner knowledge usually equates to increased owner acceptance and compliance. Early and persistent owner education is a long-term investment in senior care.
5. Remember that a well-designed marketing strategy correlates with success. Use newsletters, reminder cards, invoices, the telephone book, and the media to educate owners and prospective owners on age-related problems and the ways in which senior care can benefit the older animal. Emphasize the state-of-the-art advances in diagnostic testing, anesthesia, and anesthetic monitoring equipment; behavior-modifying drugs; osteoarthritis therapies; cancer chemotherapy; cardiac medications; dental care; and specialized nutrition as part of senior care.
6. Bundle the service fee structure so the owner can realize a financial benefit by having the entire senior care evaluation, as opposed to paying for tests on an individual basis.
7. Start the program slowly and be patient; the senior care program will continue to grow. Be willing to fine-tune the program based on feedback from owners and hospital staff.
8. Keep in mind that periodic program review by the owners and hospital staff is critical in senior care success and in maintaining the consistently high standard of care that has been established for the senior animals. Every year add new diagnostic tests or screening procedures, new treatment options, and updated owner educational materials to reflect medical and technologic advances.

available treatment options are often limited. Veterinarians should take a more proactive approach to common age-related problems.

Senior care is a proactive health care program that changes the way veterinarians traditionally approach the older animal (Box 1-2). This health care program has some distinct advantages over geriatric health care programs. Marketing surveys have shown that the term *senior* is more "owner friendly" than the term *geriatric.* Senior care is also a more inclusive health care program that starts at 7 years of age and includes twice-yearly examinations and regular health screening. However, the major benefit of senior care is that various commercial companies continue to support such programs by developing and providing all the marketing and implementation tools necessary to make senior care successful in the veterinary practice.[4] Tools for owner education, tools for gathering and reporting health data, and tips for program implementation are currently provided. These companies also help raise owner awareness of age-related health issues by sponsoring a special Senior Health Month.

HEALTH CARE FOR OLDER DOGS AND CATS

Why build a senior care program in the veterinary practice? By advocating more comprehensive case histories, performing thorough physical examinations, and recommending more diagnostic testing of older animals, the veterinarian is providing higher quality veterinary medicine for the senior animal. A great deal of professional satisfaction for the veterinarian and hospital staff comes from helping those long-established senior animals live longer, healthier lives; in addition, managing most age-related diseases in their early phases is far more rewarding than in the end stage. The availability of medical information on television and the Internet has made interested animal owners much more aware of the health needs of their senior animals and the various diagnostic and treatment options available. Because owners of older dogs and cats have long-standing bonds with their animals, many of these owners are demanding and willing to pay for high-quality health care. The continued advancement of medical knowledge—manifested in the availability of more sophisticated diagnostic testing, advances in specialized nutrition, and newer therapeutic options—has better positioned veterinarians to treat age-related problems and provide the high-quality health care these owners are demanding. The more progressive veterinary practices are using senior care as a platform to address the growing demand for high-quality health care. Further details in how to construct comprehensive health care programs for older dogs and cats are provided in Chapter 2.

PRACTICAL BENEFITS

Senior care can be a major profit center for the veterinary practice. With more than 39% of the dog and cat population considered seniors, tremendous financial opportunities exist. The veterinary profession has been very successful at providing comprehensive health care programs for puppies and kittens, but there are about 2.25 times as many senior dogs and cats as puppies and kittens, and dogs are puppies for 1 year but are seniors for 4 to 10 years.

By eliciting a more detailed history for the senior dog or cat, performing thorough physical examinations, and performing more diagnostic tests, not only does the veterinarian increase the standard of care provided to the senior animals, but in addition about 40% of those animals will require additional diagnostic testing or medications. Ultimately, a properly implemented senior care program can represent 35% or more of the hospital's gross annual income.

How will the local veterinary practice grow during the next 5 years, as veterinary competition increases, as the pet population stabilizes, as vaccine income decreases in response to changes in recommended vaccine protocols, as more flea and tick products become available over the counter, and as Internet prescription buying becomes routine? Better-managed senior care may be the answer. The goal of senior care is to optimize the quality of life for the healthy and sick senior animal by using preventive health strategies combined with a comprehensive health assessment, state-of-the-art veterinary diagnostics, and the various treatment options available.

References

1. Mosier JE: Effect of aging on body systems of the dog. *Vet Clin North Am* 19:1, 1989.
2. Morse DR, Rabinowitz H: A unified theory of aging. *Int J Psychosom* 37:5, 1990.
3. Hoskins JD: Annual evaluation of senior and geriatric dogs. *Vet Forum* 17:42, 2000.
4. Turnwald GH, Baskett JJ: Effective communication with older owners. *J Am Vet Med Assoc* 209:725, 1996.

CHAPTER 2

Owner Services and Hospice Care

CLENRIC GUY HANCOCK, FRANKLIN D. MCMILLAN, and TINA R. ELLENBOGEN

Owners of geriatric dogs and cats, whether the animals are in their "golden years" or nearing the ends of their lives, have a need for and a potential to benefit from many special services. Owners seldom articulate or even recognize these needs and cannot obtain the services to meet these needs through many veterinary practices. Veterinary practices may need to adopt a new model of delivery to make the full range of needed services available to animal owners. Demographics suggest that more and more owners will, as a result of experience with human hospice, demand and be attracted to veterinary practices that offer these services.

The model of care that seems best suited to making the necessary services widely available to animal owners is the one developed by the modern hospice movement. Veterinary practices that adopt this model will serve owners better, in addition to gaining many other benefits. It is compelling that the hospice model's attributes match well with the findings of the Brakke study and the megastudy of the National Commission on Veterinary Economic Issues. The changes dictated by these studies include effective delegation of tasks, use of team approach to care, a defined scope of practice for each team member, and a holistic, nursing-centered perspective.

NURSE-CENTRIC MODEL

In an efficiently run veterinary practice the team members all spend a maximum amount of time doing tasks that only they can do and that cannot be delegated to unlicensed team members or those with fewer credentials. The veterinarians do not perform tasks that can be performed by credentialed veterinary technicians. Technicians, in turn, do not routinely perform tasks that can be performed by technician assistants.

A staffing model considered optimum in many well-managed veterinary practices, as well as in many dental offices, assigns two veterinary technicians to each veterinarian and two technician assistants to each veterinary technician. Each person on the team has a well-defined scope of practice and responsibility, respecting the familiar hierarchical chain of authority. If one examines this model by counting worker-hours, there are 6 man-hours of income-producing work in nursing care for each hour of veterinary work. Even though nonveterinarian team members work at lower hourly pay rates, the nursing care team generates far more income than the veterinarian. Therefore, in spite of the veterinarian's position at the top of the hierarchy, the term *nurse-centric* better describes the health care services being delivered as well as the source of practice revenue. Veterinary care is nurse-centric already but has not been perceived as such because veterinarians quite naturally focus on their position in the hierarchy and ownership of practices. Adopting a nurse-centric perspective of veterinary care will help members of the profession visualize many new opportunities to better serve owners whose animals are in the geriatric or golden phase of their lives.

QUALITY OF LIFE

The goal of all animal care, at all stages of the animal's life, is to protect and maximize quality of life. This goal is the same for the animal owner and veterinarian and is best achieved when all human caregivers work together as a team. The special problems experienced by animals in their golden years present additional challenges to all caregivers attempting to maximize the animal's quality of life. These special problems and challenges also make quality-of-life concerns in the older animal the most important of the animal's life.

What is quality of life? The intuitive belief that we understand what quality of life is belies its truly elusive nature. In the broadest sense, quality of life is the way an individual feels about his or her life overall—the level of satisfaction one has with one's own life. Quality of life is closely related to a number of other concepts, such as well-being, contentment, and happiness. In the veterinary medical literature, quality of life is routinely equated to health status. Because many factors unrelated to health, such as social relationships and play, also contribute to quality of life, this view is now known to be incomplete. Quality of life entails a wide scope of factors, and health status is only one of these.

For sensitive animals—both human and nonhuman—feelings (or *affect*) contribute pleasantness or unpleasantness on a continual basis to personal experience. When people evaluate their well-being, the ratio of their affective pleasantness to unpleasantness over time plays a central role, and emotional pleasantness is one of the strongest predictors of life satisfaction. In this way, the concept of emotional pleasantness appears to play the primary role in quality of life. Specifically, quality of life refers to the level of pleasant and unpleasant feelings in one's life over time.

Feelings are pleasant and unpleasant, and of physical and emotional origin. Unpleasant feelings of physical origin include such conditions as weakness, nausea, pain, pruritus, hypoxia, thirst, hunger, constipation, and temperature extremes. Those of emotional origin include fear, anxiety, boredom, frustration, loneliness, separation distress, depression, hopelessness, and helplessness. Pleasant feelings of physical origin include such things as physical contact and gustatory (taste) pleasures. Those of emotional origin include social companionship, play, and mental stimulation.

Feelings appear to play such a central role in quality of life that feeling states can be regarded as the single common denominator for all factors that influence quality of life. That is, it is through feelings that anything influences quality of life, and any factor that does not have an influence on feelings is not a factor in quality of life. For instance, disease influences quality of life because of its associated unpleasant feelings of discomfort. Social isolation influences quality of life because of its association with unpleasant feelings of loneliness. Physical impairments and disabilities influence quality of life by creating unpleasant feelings or impairing the opportunities to experience pleasant feelings, for example, when paralysis prevents a dog from playing in the way he or she has enjoyed previously.

One convenient conceptualization of quality of life is a scale with pleasant feelings on one side and unpleasant feelings on the other. The entire array of feelings, both physical and emotional in origin, are included on the "feelings scale." Quality of life is the state of balance between the pleasant and unpleasant feelings. Anything that tips the scale one way or the other is an influence on quality of life; anything that doesn't tip the scale is irrelevant to quality of life. How much any factor tips the scale represents the degree of its importance to quality of life. When the veterinarian advises an animal owner regarding how a medical condition or procedure will affect the animal's quality of life, the determination is ultimately based on whether the feelings scale is tipped, and how much. For example, the basis for telling an owner that a lipoma, a toe amputation, or a loss of hearing in one ear will not affect quality of life is that these conditions presumably will not tip the feelings scale one way or the other. Conversely, the reason for advising an owner that scabies, glaucoma, osteoarthritis, or deprivation of social interaction will affect quality of life is that all will tip the feelings scale. Likewise, adding pleasurable experiences to an animal's life, such as trips to the dog park and food treats, will tip the scales and thereby influence quality of life.

The intensity of feelings is a critical factor in the balance of the quality-of-life scale. If a single unpleasant feeling, such as pain or nausea or fear, were intense enough, it would tip the scale and by itself make quality of life very low. As disease states progress, the unpleasant feelings grow more intense, and the pleasant feelings (enjoyment of play, social interaction, eating) grow less intense. Eventually, the scale tips so strongly toward the unpleasant side that quality of life is unmistakably judged to be poor. Currently, there is no numeric scale that allows the quality-of-life balance to be precisely quantified in clearly defined units of measurement, and the quality-of-life balance includes a large "gray area" in which it is hard for us to be sure if the animal's quality of life is such that life is predominantly enjoyable rather than predominantly full of misery, discomfort, and suffering. It is important to note that there are no clear-cut demarcations or recognizable cutoff points on the balance continuum, above which quality of life is "satisfactory" (or "acceptable," "reasonable," or "good") or below which quality of life is "unacceptable."

Consistent with the preceding analysis, quality of life in animals may be defined as follows: Quality of life is a multidimensional, experiential continuum. It involves an array of feeling (affective) states, broadly classifiable as unpleasant or pleasant feelings. The greater the pleasant feelings are, and the lesser the unpleasant feelings, the higher the quality of life.

The paramount objective in animal care—medical and nonmedical—is to maximize quality of life. This goal is accomplished by the dual effort of decreasing unpleasant and increasing pleasant feelings. As much as possible, all unpleasant and pleasant feelings must be assessed and factored into the balance of the individual's overall subjective experience. Ultimately, quality of life is determined by how the feelings scale tips.

CARE DURING THE GOLDEN YEARS

The goal of animal owner services during the golden years and at the end of life should be to maximize the enjoyable and meaningful interaction between the owner and the animal. Achieving this goal has the benefit of improving the quality of life for both. The animal should not suffer for the sake of the owner's quality of life, nor should the owner suffer needlessly in preserving the animal's quality of life. In most instances, the gains are mutual rather than competitive. Veterinarians are pledged to serve the animal, but this must usually be done through the client. The hospice and nurse-centric models of care allow and oblige veterinarians to be proactive in improving both the animal's and the owner's quality of life.

There are three realms of care that should be addressed when one provides comprehensive care to geriatric animals, and especially those coming to the end of their lives. The realms are physical, psychosocial, and spiritual care.

Physical Care

High-quality nursing is the foundation of care for animals when there is no longer an expectation of achieving a cure. The major goals are maintaining maximum physical comfort, including assistance with the animal's bodily functions and activities of daily living, minimizing any complications and side effects, and preventing or relieving pain and all other physical discomforts (e.g., nausea, hunger, pruritus, and constipation).

Psychosocial Care

The responsibilities in psychosocial care involve both the animal and the family or household. The animal's attitude, responsiveness, and enthusiasm for interactions with the family must be assessed regularly. When the animal's psychosocial condition declines, it is important to reassess the nursing interventions, methods of pain relief, and owner activities to make adjustments that may restore the quality of life. In-home environmental assessments and enhancements (much as a visiting nurse or occupational therapist would do) may influence whether nursing care will succeed. A behaviorist or trainer can be invaluable in helping people cope with behavioral changes and understand their animal's behavior. Psychosocial care includes professional evaluation and assistance for the family members in dealing with conflicts exacerbated by the animal's condition, anticipatory grief, burden of caring for the animal, exhaustion, and other difficulties. Because veterinarians are not qualified to provide psychosocial services to people, a suitably credentialed counselor must be on retainer or available to take referrals.

Spiritual Care

For many animal owners, spiritual support may be an important service. Spiritual care needs affect only the owners and family members, but just as with psychosocial services, veterinarians need to have spiritual counselors available through retainer or referral. It is very important that the spiritual counselors accept their roles as nondenominational caregivers and not try to promote their own religious beliefs. The death of an animal may prompt a spiritual crisis, especially if owners are experiencing internal conflicts over belief systems or if there are conflicting beliefs within the family or household. Owners may need or appreciate help in talking through the questions and conflicts they are experiencing because of their animal's serious illness or death.

HOSPICE PHILOSOPHY

It is important to examine human hospice care, because so much about hospice is applicable to helping families faced with the approaching death of an animal companion. The term *hospice* is derived from the same root word used for hospital, hotel, hostel, and hospitality. In more ancient times it referred to a place where a traveler could find rest, refreshment, and safety. A Greek hospital in 1134 BC is described as having hot and cold baths; gymnasiotherapy; an amphitheater for entertainment; sunshine and fresh air, combined with pleasant vistas; libraries; and rooms for visitors.[1]

The modern hospice movement in the United States began in the early 1970s. The National Hospice and Palliative Care Organization Web site indicates that approximately 3,368 hospices were in operation in the United States in 1999, serving 700,000 patients, or one in every four deaths. The development of these hospices was precipitated by the belief that dying patients and their families were not being served very well by the medical care system. "There is a difference between prolonging life and prolonging the act of dying until the patient lives a travesty of life." says Sandol Stoddard in her book, *The Hospice Movement*.[1] Although modern hospitals are capable of amazing accomplishments in curing and saving patients, their focus is on treating and curing illness. When the patient is not curable, however, to persist in applying inappropriate care as if a cure were possible is pointless. This practice subjects patients to many indignities and discomforts and isolates them from many things that are important. Dame Cicely Saunders, a physician and the founder of St. Christopher's hospice in England, said that "a patient should no more undergo aggressive treatment, which not only offers no hope of being effective, but which may isolate him from all true contact with those around him, than he should merely be relieved of symptoms when the underlying cause is still treatable or has once again become so."[1]

The National Hospice and Palliative Care Organization defines hospice as "... a medically directed, nurse coordinated program providing a continuum of home and inpatient care for the terminally ill patient and family. [It provides] ... palliative and supportive care to meet the special needs arising out of the physical, emotional and spiritual, and social and economic stresses experienced during the final stages of illness, and during dying and bereavement. This care is available 24 hours per day, 7 days per week and is provided on the basis of need, not ability to pay."[2] Hospice is characterized by palliation of symptoms, a caring environment, sustained expert care, and the pledge that families and patients will not be abandoned.

In the hospital environment, the patient and immediate family are often helpless to stop procedures and practices that none of them desire. Life may be prolonged, but so is suffering, and therefore such care may actually diminish rather than improve quality of life. Use of the hospice concept maximizes the quality of life for terminal patients by supporting them with psychosocial services, providing respite care to relieve primary caregivers, and maintaining most patients in their homes. More than 62% of hospice patients die at home, unlike nonhospice patients, of whom 75% die in hospitals.

Hospice is team care provided by teams that include an administrator, medical director, nurse, home health aide, social worker, pastor, and volunteers. It combines skilled medical care with social, psychological, and spiritual support for the patient and family group. After the patient's death the survivors receive bereavement assistance through support groups and volunteers.

Hospice Services

Patients are frequently referred to hospice when their primary physician recognizes that their life expectancy is less than 6 months. The hospice philosophy involves assisting the patient and family to acknowledge the imminence of death. The patient and family then begin to make realistic plans for maintaining the highest quality of life for whatever time remains.

Other key concepts of hospice philosophy are very important. The first is expert medical care. The physician and nurse use every resource to keep the patient free of pain and to minimize symptoms. Another concept is that the unit of care is the family. Psychosocial counseling and support are an important element of hospice care, and this care for the family continues for up to 1 year after the patient's death. A hospice may include a physical building with inpatient beds, but many hospices have only an office building, with patients being served primarily in their homes and in nursing homes and hospitals as needed. Seventy-three percent of hospices are nonprofit organizations and serve everyone, regardless of ability to pay. Medicare and Medicaid reimbursement are the most important source of funds for patient care. The patients served by hospices are under care for a median length of stay of 25 days. By diagnosis, 64% have cancer, 8% have heart disease, 5% have respiratory disease, and 23% have other conditions.

The Hospice Concept for Dogs and Cats

There are many parts of the hospice concept that are applicable to veterinary medicine, yet some major differences from human medicine deserve discussion. In dogs and cats it may be even more difficult than in people to know when the patient has 6 months or less to live, as fewer statistics are available regarding animal life spans following any particular diagnosis. Also, 6 months is a much larger proportion of life span in dogs and cats than in humans.

Another difference is that an animal's primary caregiver makes the decisions regarding treatment, not the animal. This corresponds more closely to pediatric hospice care.

The third difference is that in human medicine, a patient's physician refers him or her to hospice, where physicians more experienced in palliative care may consult or participate in treatment. However, for veterinarians there is currently no hospice to which to make a referral. The veterinarian has to make the transition from the "cure" state of mind to the "care" approach. This is not an easy transition, because the veterinarian has to face a loss just as the members of the animal's household do.[3] The goal for the afflicted animal is always comfort (or eliminating discomfort). For curable diseases, the method for restoring comfort is to eliminate (cure) the disease. For noncurable but treatable diseases, comfort is restored through medical, surgical, or supportive treatment.

For untreatable disease, comfort remains the primary goal, because the veterinarian can no longer use the elimination or treatment of the disease as the foremost tool to restore comfort. Instead, the veterinarian aims to achieve comfort using every means other than elimination of disease. The phrase *transition from "cure" to "care"* implies that the medical care is moving in a different direction. However, it is not; rather, caretakers are resorting to different means to achieve the same ultimate goal. Although the veterinarian and staff may have this philosophy or perspective, they still experience grief over the death of animals. The first stage of grief is denial. Being in denial about the animal's approaching death can lead to recommending treatments that decrease rather than increase the animal's comfort.

One physician offered the following words[4]:

> The basic aim in this hospital is to get people cured and out of the hospital as soon as possible. We are not running a luxury hotel devoted to making patients happy, but we are organized for efficiency to mobilize all possible resources for cure. The dying person who lingers in such a hospital is seen by the medical staff as one of their failures. And scientists do not wish to fail—even when there is no further chance of sustaining a meaningful and happy life, the tempo of efficiency is maintained or even increased with more discomfort, pain, machines, more needles stuck in veins, more impossible expense—and all for nothing in so many cases. As the clergy and psychiatrists seek to relieve anxieties, they are being increasingly frustrated as to how to help families that are caught up in the misery of such prolonged deaths.

Veterinarians want to use all their talents, knowledge, and technology to save animals. However, there are many cases in which a cure cannot be achieved; the reasons vary from lack of understanding of illness to the owner's lack of funds. In every case and for whatever reason, a crossroad will be reached at which it is imperative to reassess what is best for the animal: continued attempts to cure or a new primary emphasis on palliative care.

It is not easy to recognize when an animal's prognosis has become certain, nor is it easy to face the owner with this news and recommend a change of approach from cure to care. Yet in serving the animal and the family, veterinarians have to make this difficult transition and help those last days to be counted among the best. The benefits to animals are extended quality of life and reduced suffering and pain.[5] The benefits to owners include more time to adjust to the impending death of the animal and possibly the ability to avoid facing the euthanasia decision.

The fourth, and most important, difference between hospice care in animals and people is that medical care for animals contains the therapeutic option of euthanasia. The concept of hospice care centers is to optimize quality of life as disease continues its progressive course. Euthanasia is the last tool available to end the discomforts of illness and is used when such discomforts diminish the quality of life to a level of misery versus pleasure.[2,6,7] Owners and veterinarians both have the same duty to animals to protect them against discomfort and maximize quality of life. As quality of life declines in progressive illness, hospice care serves the animal by restoring certain comforts. As the disease progresses, however, the discomforts of the illness eventually exceed even the most diligent hospice care. It is at this point that euthanasia sharply differs from the future care of people versus animals. For people, continued hospice care is the only available option. For animals, the use of euthanasia as protection against discomfort, suffering, and poor quality of life is a compassionate course of action.

APPLICATIONS IN VETERINARY MEDICINE

Presuming both a desire to offer hospice care and the ability to make the philosophic transition, examining the human hospice helps to identify services and techniques adaptable to veterinary medicine. Presentations given by the authors and others at Delta Society Annual Conferences, American Veterinary Medical Association conventions, North American Veterinary Conferences, Western Veterinary Conferences, and many state veterinary meetings have conveyed insights and experiences regarding the concept of hospice care for animals.[8]

As a first step the veterinary staff can inform owners that hospice care—terminal life care—exists as an alternative to immediate euthanasia. Presenting hospice care as an alternative rather than a supplement to euthanasia may not, however, be in the animal's best interest. The choice to euthanize an animal is ultimately the owner's decision; however, it is important to note that veterinarians, by virtue of their professional oath, have an obligation to protect the animal from suffering. In virtually all cases of progressive incurable illness the animal reaches a point at which suffering is simply not necessary or fair. If hospice care is perceived solely as an alternative to suffering then certain owners, eager to find any reason to avoid euthanasia, will happily grasp this as a guilt-free means to reject the euthanasia option.

When the hospice option is selected, the care involves providing continuous relief of pain and all other discomforts. For the specific discomfort of pain, this would be achieved through the regular use of analgesic agents. Whenever possible, this should be achieved by preventing, not treating, the discomfort. In some cases, adequate relief of pain results in sedation or even more profound depression of consciousness. The animal's death may, in fact, be hastened, but the animal dies naturally instead of by euthanasia. The veterinarian may prefer euthanasia but cannot expect all owners to agree.

Second, maximize the pleasurable feelings the animal can experience. In ailing people, for example, the increased social companionship from caring individuals can greatly offset the unpleasant physical feelings associated with the disease, such that quality of life is substantially benefited. For the ill animal, providing pleasures such as social interaction and companionship, tasty foods, mentally stimulating activities (such as play, walks, or any other exciting activities permitted by the animal's physical and mental condition), and human contact (petting, massaging) can be greatly beneficial to the animal's quality of life. Additionally, many of the services provided in human hospices can be provided using veterinary hospital staff. Skilled nursing care in the animal's home can be arranged by having veterinary technicians and other staff make house calls on the way to work, during the lunch hour, or after work, as needed. Fixed-facility practices can also refer to and collaborate with house-call veterinarians for delivery of in-home services.

The third component of hospice care is psychosocial services for the animal's family. The resources to provide this support are not typically available at veterinary hospitals and may be found elsewhere. Current and former human hospice employees may be willing to serve in a part-time or volunteer capacity. Local psychologists and social workers in private practice may be willing to take these cases on a fee basis or as volunteers. Hospital bereavement counselors may also be prospects. If these people have not had hospice experience or training, it will be valuable for them to obtain such training. The local hospice is the best resource to obtain guidance, training, or educational materials.

The fourth component is volunteers, which most veterinary hospitals seldom use. Perhaps an untapped opportunity exists to better use volunteers in many areas of the veterinary hospital, including in hospice care. Hospice volunteers provide support to the family and animal by running errands, allowing owners to take a break from animal care, and spending time with the family. They continue this support for up to a year after the animal has died. Most of the hospice volunteers are friends, relatives, and family members previously served by the hospice during the death of a loved one.

The volunteers should be well trained before they have animal contact as part of the hospice team. The greatest difficulties anticipated for veterinary hospitals are providing volunteer training and operating as a team. Perhaps the local hospice can include veterinary volunteers in

TABLE 2-1. TIMELINE PHASES OF TERMINAL CARE*

	SIX MONTHS BEFORE DEATH	LAST MONTH BEFORE DEATH	AFTER DEATH
Patient signs	Ambulatory; coherent; some side effects from medication; initial stages of grief, anger, and denial	End-stage pronounced withdrawal; requires total care; intensive management of symptoms and pain; no appetite	
Medical director	Performs initial examination of patient; develops plan of care	Monitors symptoms and assesses plan of care; addresses increased need for medication changes to manage symptoms and control pain	May have further communications with the family
Nurse case manager	Assesses hospice conference with family; confers with physician; develops plan of care; orders medications; orders durable medical equipment; trains and instructs primary caregivers	Oversees daily monitoring of end-stage process, side effects of medication, symptoms manifested, and pain management; coordinates preparation for death with other team members; provides increasing support for both family and patient	Calls and/or visits family; assesses special bereavement needs; may attend funeral; completes discharge charting
Social services	Assesses patient and family psychosocial and bereavement needs to develop plan of care; establishes trusting relationships with patient and family	Continues monitoring of approved plan of care; assists patient and family in resolution and closure; ensures final arrangements; facilitates support systems	Calls and/or visits family; may attend funeral; begins bereavement follow-up, identifies dysfunctional grieving, and initiates appropriate intervention
Volunteers	Confer with hospice team for direction; learn interest of patient; make initial visitations	Provide respite periods for family; provide patient with emotional support	Provide bereavement support to family and significant others; maintain regular contact for up to 12 months

From Timeline Phases of Terminal Care. *Progressive changes in physical and psychologic conditions: six-month hospice plan of care,* Arlington, Va, National Hospice & Palliative Care Organization (1901 N. Moore St., Suite l, Arlington, VA 22209).
*This table is excerpted from a National Hospice Organization publication. The original has columns for each month from 6 months before death up to the last month, and rows for additional personnel. Some of the items that are more applicable to veterinary medicine are shown.

their training classes. The team concept requires meetings and communication among team members. Being a human hospice volunteer may be the best way to understand the concepts and learn techniques that can be applied in the veterinary setting. Specific tasks and assignments of various team members are presented in Table 2-1.

A final area of concern in hospice care is record keeping or charting. This is a consistent, well-structured, and closely monitored process in human medicine. Veterinary records do not usually contain any significant information about the human-animal bonds and relationships within the household. Unless this information is recorded routinely, it will not be there when needed by the hospital or hospice team.

Dr. Al Marshall of Largo, Florida,[9] has suggested a simple way to record this information in the veterinary record. He envisions a chart with animals in one column and household members across the top (Figure 2-1). In each box can be recorded the significant activities in which each person participates with a particular animal. Dr. Marshall believes this will be useful for managing medical cases and obtaining accurate histories, as well as for managing bereavement and hospice issues.

A tool like the one in Figure 2-1 will help all of the veterinary staff keep in mind how various members of the household may be affected by the terminal illness or loss of a particular animal. It serves as a basis for discussion and further record keeping by the hospice team. It is also recommended that information about owners—any illnesses, losses of animals, friends, family, job, whether they live alone, and whether they appear to be extremely attached to the animal—be kept in the records. All of these factors can predispose owners to increased loneliness, more dependence on the relationship with the animal, and increased grief should the animal die. These are risk factors, not guarantees that the grief will be more intense or last longer. Having the information simply makes veterinarians more aware of the grief potential and more sensitive to the needs of the owners. This information should be recorded in new veterinary records and updated by the staff at each visit and as it is volunteered by the owner. It will then be available to everyone as needed.

Name	James					Doris					Heather					Richard					Arthur				
Relationship	Spouse					Spouse					Daughter, 8 yrs					Son, 10 yrs					Father-in-law				
	P	F	W	I	B	P	F	W	I	B	P	F	W	I	B	P	F	W	I	B	P	F	W	I	B
Snoopy	X				X		X			X				X	X				X	X			X		X
Garfield						X	X			X						X			X	X				X	X

Figure 2-1. Human-animal interactions and relationships. *P,* Primary (pet "belongs to this person"); *F,* feeds pet daily; *W,* walks pet daily; *I,* interacts regularly (plays with, talks to, trains); *B,* highly bonded.

DEATH AND THE GRIEF REACTION

The grief reaction may occur any time there is a perceived loss. The reaction to animal loss has been noted for its intensity and duration. Studies point out the similarity between people's relations to children and to animals, and how people tend to prefer childlike physical features in animals, such as proportionally larger heads and eyes. In addition, people's emotional relationships with animals are more like their relationships with children than with adults. The death of a child is widely recognized as being extremely stressful because of the perceived innocence and purity of the adult-child relationship. It follows that because of the similarities in relationships with children and animals, animal death could be expected to induce strong feelings.

After a loss, people experience many emotions including denial, anger, guilt, and depression. These emotions continue to recur with gradually less intensity until resolution is complete. People progress toward resolution by talking about their feelings. It is important for sympathetic, active listeners to be available so that people feel safe enough to express their feelings.

However, the resolution of animal loss grief is complicated by two special difficulties not associated with other losses. First, people lack widely accepted social customs such as funerals and burials to provide opportunities for expression of grief. Second, there is a relative lack of social support systems in the event of animal death. The person who grieves over the loss of their animal not only experiences a lack of support from others, but may in fact encounter a negative reaction to their personal grief. This is known in the bereavement field as disenfranchised loss. Rather than risk derision or unhelpful comments, such as "It was only a dog," people keep their emotions bottled up inside. They avoid the immediate hurt by being silent, with the consequence that grief is prolonged because they are unable to deal with or express their feelings.

Many veterinary hospital staff members may not realize that they, too, often suffer a loss and experience grief when an animal dies. Their first reaction may be denial ("I can't believe that dog is dead!") followed by anger over losing an animal. If this anger is directed at the owner, it may relieve the staff at the expense of serving the owner. This is followed by guilt and depression, for example, "If only I had noticed [this] or done [that], he might still be with us." The significance of the loss and, therefore, the intensity of the grief vary from case to case, of course. The average veterinarian may lose as many as six patients a week, based on a caseload of 3,000 dogs and cats with an average life span of 10 years. However, veterinarians are spared somewhat because not all of these patients die in the hospital or during veterinary care. Despite this, the fact remains that veterinarians face a significant incidence of animal loss owing to the shorter natural lives of the animals when compared with people.

USEFUL TECHNIQUES FOR VETERINARIANS AND HOSPITAL STAFF

Preparation of Owners for Animal Loss

American society has been described as worshipping youth and denying death. There are some widely accepted rituals that help people to cope with the death of a loved one, but there are no generally accepted traditions, customs, or rituals for dealing with animal deaths. The person coping with an animal's death does not usually attend a memorial service, a funeral, or a cemetery internment. Without these rituals, there is little opportunity to express one's feelings and share them with sympathetic friends. As previously mentioned, the support group of friends, relatives, and others is mostly lacking in reference to animal loss.

It is important for veterinarians to become proactive in preparing owners for an animal's death, beginning several years in advance. A mention of realistic life expectancy for the species and breed presented for examination on the first visit is appropriate. If owners work through the process of planning some of the details of their animal's last days and disposition of the body, they can avoid making poor decisions during the most emotional time of their grief. Poor decisions made under emotional strain may prolong the grief recovery of one or more members of the animal's household.

One technique that may be borrowed from human medicine, with appropriate modifications, is the concept of advance directives. These directives were part of the Federal Omnibus Budget Reconciliation Act of 1990 and went into effect on December 1, 1991. The Act requires hospitals and other health care providers to give information to patients about their rights to make personal health care decisions, including accepting or refusing medical treatment. Advance directives allow the patient to specify in advance whether he or she wants, or wishes to avoid, resuscitation, maintenance on feeding tubes, and other procedures.

Modified veterinary advance directives offer the potential to help owners make decisions and prepare for the inevitable death of their animals (Figure 2-2). By asking owners to complete an advance directive questionnaire, the veterinarian can help everyone in the household begin to consider the elements of their animal's quality of life, how to decide on euthanasia if it should be needed, and what should be done with the animal's remains. Some questions that can be asked in the advance directive are as follows:

- How would you wish to have your animal spend its last hours: at home or in the veterinary hospital?
- What activities are most important to your animal?
- Rate each of the following on a 5-point scale from not very important (1 point) to very important (5 points):
    - Regular meals
    - Getting snacks and treats
    - Walks with you
    - Being outside
    - Playing games such as Frisbee or fetch
    - Sitting with you for meals, watching TV, etc.
    - Watching household activities
    - Going with you in the car
    - Swimming
    - Other activities that your animal enjoys

The answers on the scale are essential keys to determining the animal's quality of life. At the end of life, the animal may not be able to do all of the activities or may not have the stamina to do them as long as usual. The owner should discuss these items regularly with the household and the veterinarian and hospital staff to ensure that the highest possible quality of life is maintained until death occurs naturally or through euthanasia.

- Euthanasia is used in animals as a means to compassionately end the discomfort and suffering caused by a disease that cannot be effectively treated.
- Do you agree with this principle and would you consider euthanasia of a very ill animal?
- Would you consider euthanasia if you determine that your animal's quality of life is very poor in spite of the best supportive care and pain relief?

These questions about euthanasia should be worded carefully so as not to unnecessarily frighten owners or lead them to think that owning an animal is not a pleasurable experience. The question can be presented as one way for owners to provide optimal care for their animals by thinking ahead about how they can best meet their animal's needs.

A companion document called the Advance Care Plan deals with how the owners wish the medical care to be performed under various conditions. Project Grace, at *http://www.p-grace.org*, provides a one-page advance care plan and advocates that everyone complete it and distribute copies to family members and physicians. Project Grace advocates this plan for every adult, not just those facing a terminal illness. A proposed Advance Care Plan for a dog or cat is shown in Box 2-1.

OPPORTUNITIES TO PROVIDE SERVICE

Acknowledging Grief

Astute veterinarians and practice management consultants have recommended a variety of ways to provide better service to grieving owners. The first is attempting to schedule euthanasia conferences or euthanasia appointments at the beginning or end of the day to avoid the busy times. This allows the veterinarian to spend more time with the owners at this critical time in their animal's life and spares them the embarrassment

1. Who will participate in discussions and decisions about the patient's care?

Name	Relation	Phone	Scale of attachment
______	______	______	Low 1 2 3 4 High
______	______	______	Low 1 2 3 4 High
______	______	______	Low 1 2 3 4 High

Who will not participate?

______	______	______	Low 1 2 3 4 High
______	______	______	Low 1 2 3 4 High

2. Who, if anyone, is the primary caregiver of the patient?

3. If the patient's condition becomes terminal, who wants to be sure to visit and have a last opportunity to say goodbye?

4. How important are the following factors in causing you to consider euthanasia?

Scale: Euthanasia is not a consideration	1	2	3	4	5	Euthanasia highly desirable
Reduced mobility..........................	____	____	____	____	____	
Poor appetite	____	____	____	____	____	
Weight loss.................................	____	____	____	____	____	
Need medication 3 times daily........	____	____	____	____	____	
Need increasing nursing care.........	____	____	____	____	____	
Chronic pain	____	____	____	____	____	
Loss of eyesight	____	____	____	____	____	
Loss of bowel control	____	____	____	____	____	
Loss of urinary control	____	____	____	____	____	

Note: These items should be discussed among all the caregivers in the household, or separate forms should be completed by each member.

5. If you were forced to choose euthanasia, who among the family would want to be present?

____ All caregivers ____ Only the primary caregiver
____ None of the caregivers ____ Other (list) ______________________

6. What is your preference in caring for the remains?

____ Burial in a common grave ____ Burial at home
____ Burial in a marked grave ____ Freeze drying
____ Cremation and mass burial ____ Cremation, return ashes
____ Other ______________________

7. Which of the following, if any, would you consider doing in memory of your special relationship with this pet?

____ Pet cemetery memorial service
____ Memorial service at home
____ Hang a special picture
____ Plant a tree or living memorial
____ Make a donation to an animal organization
____ Make a donation to a veterinary/veterinary technology college

8. How would you direct close friends to acknowledge their sympathy?

____ Cards ____ Flowers
____ Telephone call ____ Donation to ______________________

Figure 2-2. Sample of veterinary advance directives form.

Box 2-1 Advance Care Plan (after Project Grace)

I _______________ want to choose how (animal's name) will be treated by the veterinary care team during the days and months of his life. I want medical care for my dog/cat that is beneficial to his/her emotional well-being as well as his/her physical well-being. I want treatments for my dog/cat that have, on balance, a net benefit to his/her quality of life. My choices about treatments that would have little chance of making his condition better are below. Checking "no" means that I do not want the treatment.

Illness or Condition	CPR	Surgery	Fluids or Blood	Tube Feeding
Coma	Yes ___ No ___	Yes ___ No ___	Yes ___ No ___	Yes ___ No ___
Irreversible disorientation or dementia	Yes ___ No ___	Yes ___ No ___	Yes ___ No ___	Yes ___ No ___
Impending death	Yes ___ No ___	Yes ___ No ___	Yes ___ No ___	Yes ___ No ___

of having a waiting room full of strangers witnessing their grief. A second step is preparing owners by explaining the process and what to expect at each step. It is helpful to answer questions about what the animal will experience as well as any other questions. The further this can be done in advance, the better, as it preconditions owners for the approach of the end of their animal's life. Finally, a sensitive way to handle billing is to meet with the owners beforehand or to mail a bill afterward.

For a number of years it has been recommended to send a card, sympathy note, or some remembrance to the family soon after an animal's death. Some veterinarians have a personal preference for handwritten sympathy notes; veterinarians often write personal notes to reassure owners that they (the owners) are not responsible for their animal's death. Hospital staff members should sign the letter if they had much interaction with the animal or the family. These expressions of sympathy are greatly appreciated.

Another well-received follow-up is a donation in the name of the deceased animal to a charity, which then sends a letter stating that a donation has been received from the veterinarian. This is a good idea, but the processing of the donation and the sending of the follow-up letter are not under the veterinarian's control and may not occur in as timely a fashion as the veterinarian would like. A note from the veterinary hospital and staff is worthwhile even when a donation is made.

Caring for the Remains

The disposition of the remains is an important issue that is best decided far in advance of the necessity. The veterinarian should use terminology that implies that the body of the deceased animal is an object worthy of respect in proportion to the respect accorded the animal during its life. The phrase *"dispose of the body"* implies that the body is a waste object and not of value. Such words as "care," "treat," "tend to," "prepare," or even "handle" do not have the negative connotation of "dispose."

It is important to be knowledgeable and helpful to the owner, as well as nonjudgmental about the owner's wishes or choice in the matter. Products such as urns and cardboard animal caskets are available and should be considered as a way to add dignity to the handling of an animal's remains. Veterinarians who are proactive in helping families face the issue of what to do with the remains will obtain information about animal cemeteries, cremations, and local laws to give to owners. Owners can be encouraged to consider the options long before the actual need occurs through the use of advance directives. Some human cemeteries allow burial of animals with people, some have a special animal area, and others refuse animals. Some animal cemeteries accept human remains so that family members can be interred with their animals.

During the difficult time surrounding an animal's death, the best service is to minimize the burden and ease the stress on the grieving survivors by "taking care of all the arrangements" for them. This is a service currently offered extensively by human funeral homes and one that is gratefully accepted by grief-stricken relatives and loved ones. In veterinary medicine, the ideal, once the owner has expressed his or her wishes regarding care of the animal's body, is to make the arrangements for tending to the disposition of the animal's body—including all arrangements for cremation, burial, or any other funeral procedure—for the owner. The less left to the owner, the more the veterinarian's services will be appreciated. Having the owner's wishes regarding these arrangements recorded in the animal's records far in advance of death is of great benefit.

Memorialization

In the foreword to *Rituals of Living and Dying*, Stanley Kippner states, "Mary Chadwick, a psychoanalyst, has described the fear of death as the western individual's most fundamental anxiety." Kippner further quotes Dr. Chadwick as follows: "Rituals build community, creating a meeting ground where people can share deep feelings, positive and negative. Rituals and rites of passage are traditionally among the most powerful culturally sanctioned vehicles available for exerting this influence. They are social inventions for instructing the human spirit on its journey into the world."[10] People use rituals to deal with significant events in their lives.

In *Rituals of Living and Dying*, Feinstein and Mayo state that rituals, like myths, address the following:

- Our urge to comprehend our existence in a meaningful way
- Our search for a marked pathway as we move from one stage of our lives to the next
- Our need to establish secure and fulfilling relationships within a human community
- Our longing to know our part in the vast wonder and mystery of the cosmos

The guidance the culture's mythology has to offer is etched into the mind and body of every person participating in the ritual. In this manner, rituals, family ceremonies, community celebrations, church liturgies, and the sacraments of baptism, marriage, and burial help to form the individual's personal mythology and continue to shape it with each life passage.

Memorialization is a technique for creating personal rituals, where none exist, to add meaning to the life shock of an animal's death. Memorialization is a way to recognize the significance of the animal's role in an owner's life and the uniqueness of that animal. It is also a way to create opportunities in which it is permissible to express grief. Because memorialization is very important, both in affirming the value of an individual animal and in helping resolve grief over the loss, it should not be left to chance. Veterinarians should take the initiative to be proactive in helping owners consider ways to memorialize the animals they have lost.

Bereavement Services

Bereavement services can be characterized as crisis intervention, support groups, and counseling. Animal loss crisis intervention hotlines are available at the University of California at Davis, the University of Florida, and other colleges of veterinary medicine. The first hotline was founded by Mader and Hart (Human-Animal Bond Program, University of California at Davis), who solicited volunteers from the veterinary students. The students undergo crisis intervention training and then answer calls on a rotating basis under the supervision of Mader. The service is modeled after community crisis intervention hotlines that deal with suicide prevention and similar problems.

Animal loss support groups offer a complementary service to crisis intervention. The support group is a safe place for self-disclosure of grief. Talking about the strong feelings accompanying a loss is therapeutic. Hearing others who are at different stages in the process talk about their grief is reassuring. It shows that progress toward resolution is possible and that a person is not alone in having very strong feelings about an animal's death. These groups are usually provided free or for a minimal fee. However, they should be facilitated or led by an experienced bereavement counselor with the proper credentials to provide mental health counseling. Veterinary associations or individual practices may sponsor animal loss support groups, but one of the greatest difficulties is maintaining steady attendance, as many people attend only once. It may be necessary to put regular notices in the newspaper, send cards to owners who lose animals, and distribute brochures in veterinary facilities and animal cemeteries to keep reaching people currently in need. Although many people attend the group only one time, receiving enough benefit that further visits seem unnecessary to them, others attend regularly for many months.

SUMMARY

Veterinarians can apply knowledge about grief responses, advance directives, memorialization, and hospice care concepts to assist owners with geriatric dogs and cats through the inevitable loss they will endure. The results will be more and welcomed opportunities for expanded levels of veterinary care, improved client relations and bonding with clients, and more satisfactory closures to special human-animal relations.

References

1. Stoddard S: *The hospice movement: a better way of caring for the dying,* New York, 1991, Vintage Books.
2. Cohen K: *Hospice: prescription for terminal care,* Germantown, Md, 1979, Aspen Systems.
3. McMillan FD: Comfort as the primary goal in veterinary medical practice, *J Am Vet Med Assoc* 212:1370, 1998.
4. Rossman P: *Hospice: creating new models of care for the terminally ill,* New York, 1977, Association Press.
5. Max MB: Improving outcomes of analgesic treatment: is education enough? *Ann Intern Med* 113:885, 1990.
6. McMillan FD: Quality of life in animals, *J Am Vet Med Assoc* 216:1904, 2000.
7. McMillan FD: Rethinking euthanasia: death as an unintentional outcome, *J Am Vet Med Assoc* 219:1204, 2001.
8. Harris, JM, Hancock G, Mader B: 10th Annual Delta Society Conference, Portland, Ore, Oct 10-12, 1991.
9. Marshall, A. Unpublished.
10. Feinstein D, Mayo PE: *Rituals for living and dying: how we can turn loss and the fear of death into an affirmation of life,* San Francisco, 1990, Harper San Francisco.

Supplemental Readings

National Hospice & Palliative Care Organization Web site: Available at: http://www.nhpco.org, Stats/Research/Resources, 2001.

Short CE, Van Poznak A: *Animal pain,* New York, 1991, Churchill Livingstone.

CHAPTER 3

Nutritional Requirements and Dietary Management

DAVID A. DZANIS

The practice of feeding dogs and cats according to their physiologic state, that is, "life-stage" nutrition, is a relatively new concept. The Ralston Purina Company may have been among the first to partially explore this concept with the introduction of Puppy Chow to augment its Dog Chow product. Hill's Pet Nutrition may have also been one of the pioneers in promotion of this practice with its Science Diet and Prescription Diet lines of products. However, it probably wasn't until Quaker Oats introduced the Cycle product line of dog foods in the 1970s that the principle of varying the nutrient content of food based on an animal's age and other physiologic factors became widely presented to the public. Most notable for purposes of this discussion was the introduction of Cycle 4, a product expressly intended to serve the nutritional needs of the older adult animal. Since that time, more and more companies have embraced the concept of life-stage nutrition and offer a variety of formulas for adults and juveniles, animals of specific sizes and breeds, animals with specific performance needs, and less active pets. Probably a majority of these firms also market a "senior" diet as part of their life-stage product lines.

Despite the apparent popularity of diets specifically intended for geriatric dogs and cats, there is a lack of consensus among experts as to the true nutritional requirements of the older animal. Evidence to support this fact is the lack of any officially recognized criteria against which the nutritional adequacy of a geriatric diet can be judged. The Association of American Feed Control Officials (AAFCO), an organization that develops model feed laws and regulations for adoption by state regulatory agencies, has established both the AAFCO Dog and Cat Food Nutrient Profiles and minimum feeding trial protocols for the purpose of substantiating nutritional adequacy of products.[1] Except for a conditional exemption for members of a pet food "product family," all "complete and balanced" dog and cat foods marketed in the United States must be assessed according to one of these two methods. However, the only life stages addressed by these methods are adult maintenance, growth, and gestation and lactation. Similarly, neither of the publications on nutrient requirements of dogs and cats as recommended by the National Research Council attempt to address the needs of the older animal.[2,3]

The reason for this is simple. The body of scientific study on the nutritional needs of the geriatric dog and cat compared with those of animals in other life stages is almost nonexistent. Most work has been done in growing animals, because the high nutrient demands during this brief period of life make the identification and study of nutritional deficiencies relatively easy. For similar reasons, study of the nutritional requirements of female animals during gestation and lactation is not uncommon, although the process is definitely more complex than it is for a growth study. Still, it is often less costly and definitely more productive to conduct studies on these life stages than on animals at maintenance, which by definition is characterized by a relative absence of nutritional stressors. Animals at maintenance are less likely to demonstrate clear signs of deficiency, and any signs that may be observable may take extended periods of time to become readily apparent. The problem may be compounded when dealing with older animals versus young adults.

Another problem is the availability of suitable subjects for geriatric nutrition studies. Although young and breeding animals can be easily obtained from purpose-bred facilities, sufficient numbers of older animals are more difficult to procure, with the degree of difficulty increasing proportionately with age. A sizable number of client-owned animals could be used, but the problems inherent to a clinical trial compared with more controlled experimental conditions (e.g., variability among subjects, owner compliance) limit the extent and strength of the data that could be derived by this means.

Finally, it is difficult to do work on geriatric nutrition when there is a lack of consensus regarding when an animal becomes a "senior." Several sources have provided chronologic estimates of when a dog or cat becomes "old."[4,5] Many pet food products intended for the older animal also give age-specific indications for use (e.g., "for dogs over 7 years of age"). However, as any veterinary practitioner can testify, the health and vitality of pets at a given age can be quite variable. While one 10-year-old dog can show easily demonstrable signs of age-related changes, another of the same age and breed may be far from reaching its golden years. Some generalizations can be made, such as the fact that the larger breed dogs tend to age faster than smaller breeds. Still, aging is an individualized event, and any nutritional assessment or intervention should be done on the basis of true need and not solely on chronology.

NUTRIENT REQUIREMENTS

As a rule, the nutrient requirements for adult maintenance are presumed to be adequate for the geriatric dog or cat. The minimum nutrient profiles for pet foods intended to meet the requirements for maintenance are found in Table 3-1. That said, there are numerous changes that can occur with aging that can affect the ability of the older animal to procure, consume, digest, and use nutrients. Some of the structural and metabolic changes associated with aging are provided in Box 3-1.

Energy

Advancing age is characterized by a decline in lean body mass and metabolic rate. Physical activity may also decrease over time. These changes suggest that the dietary energy needs of the older animal are less than those of a young adult at maintenance. It has been estimated that a dog over 8 years of age requires approximately 20% fewer calories to maintain weight compared with a 1- to 2-year-old adult of comparable body weight.[5] These findings are similar to those found in humans. On the other hand, the energy requirements of cats do not appear to decline with age, perhaps because the difference in levels of activity between young and old cats is not as pronounced as it is in dogs and people.

Because energy needs are presumed to be reduced in older animals, most commercial diets intended for seniors are lower in caloric density than their adult maintenance counterparts. However, there is great variability among commercial product lines, and one firm's senior food may contain more calories per given weight than another's maintenance product. Still, this trend does not account for the fact that for many older animals, other age-related changes may make it more difficult to consume enough food to meet caloric needs. Such changes may include locomotive or dental conditions that preclude getting to and eating the food. Competition for food from younger housemates may also play a role. Even if food is readily available, a decrease in digestive and absorptive efficiency may limit the ability of the animal to utilize the food to the same extent. Digestive efficiency, especially for fat, tends to decrease in cats with age.[5] Thus, the same amount of the same food may not maintain an older cat as well as it did when the cat was younger.

Evidence against the premise that older dogs and cats should be offered a lower caloric density food than that offered young adults is the prevalence of obesity in various age groups. The highest proportion of overweight dogs and cats is in the middle-aged population; this proportion decreases after 8 to 10 years of age.[5] Part of the explanation may be that the obese animals suffer a higher mortality before reaching old age. Regardless, the proportion of underweight animals is higher in the older animal populations than in younger populations. This suggests that the risks associated with excessive caloric intake—and therefore the need for reduced calorie diets for senior dogs and cats—may have been overrated.

Protein

Protein contents of commercial senior pet foods are also generally lower than their maintenance product counterparts. If anything, the

TABLE 3-1. AAFCO DOG AND CAT FOOD NUTRIENT PROFILES FOR ADULT MAINTENANCE[a]

		DOG		CAT	
NUTRIENT	UNITS (DRY MATTER)	MIN	MAX	MIN	MAX
Protein	%	18		26	
Arginine	%	0.51		1.04	
Histidine	%	0.18		0.31	
Isoleucine	%	0.37		0.52	
Leucine	%	0.59		1.25	
Lysine	%	0.63		0.83	
Methionine-cystine	%	0.43		1.10	
Methionine	%			0.62	1.5
Phenylalanine-tyrosine	%	0.73		0.88	
Phenylalanine	%			0.42	
Threonine	%	0.48		0.73	
Tryptophan	%	0.16		0.16	
Valine	%	0.39		0.62	
Fat[b]	%	5		9	
Linoleic acid	%	1		0.5	
Arachidonic acid	%			0.02	
Minerals					
Calcium	%	0.6	2.5	0.6	
Phosphorus	%	0.5	1.6	0.5	
Ca:P		1:1	2:1		
Potassium	%	0.6		0.6	
Sodium	%	0.06		0.2	
Chloride	%	0.09		0.3	
Magnesium[c]	%	0.04	0.3	0.04	
Iron[d]	mg/kg	80	3000	80	
Copper[e]	mg/kg	7.3	250	5	
Manganese	mg/kg	5		7.5	
Zinc	mg/kg	120	1000	75	2000
Iodine	mg/kg	1.5	50	0.35	
Selenium	mg/kg	0.11	2	0.1	
Vitamins and Others					
Vitamin A	IU/kg	5000	250,000	5000	750,000
Vitamin D	IU/kg	500	5000	500	10,000
Vitamin E[f]	IU/kg	50	1000	30	
Vitamin K[g]	mg/kg			0.1	
Thiamine[h]	mg/kg	1		5	
Riboflavin	mg/kg	2.2		4	
Pantothenic acid	mg/kg	10		5	
Niacin	mg/kg	11.4		60	
Pyridoxine	mg/kg	1		4	
Folic Acid	mg/kg	0.18		0.8	
Biotin[i]	mg/kg			0.07	
Vitamin B_{12}	mg/kg	0.022		0.02	
Choline[j]	mg/kg	1200		2400	
Taurine (extruded)	%			0.10	
Taurine (canned)	%			0.20	

Modified with permission from Association of American Feed Control Officials: *Official publication*, Oxford, Indiana, 2003, AAFCO, pp 125-140. Order forms for the publication are available at *www.aafco.org*.

[a]Presumes an energy density of 3.5 kcal/g ME for dog food and 4 kcal/g for cat food, based on the "modified Atwater" values of 3.5, 8.5, and 3.5 kcal/g for protein, fat, and carbohydrate (nitrogen-free extract [NFE]), respectively. Rations greater than 4 kcal/g (dog food) and 4.5 kcal/g (cat food) should be corrected for energy density; rations less than these amounts should *not* be corrected for energy.

[b]Although a true requirement for fat per se has not been established, the minimum level was based on recognition of fat as a source of essential fatty acids, as a carrier of fat-soluble vitamins, as an enhancer of palatability, and as a means of supplying an adequate caloric density.

[c]If the mean urine pH of cats fed ad libitum is not below 6.4, the risk of struvite urolithiasis increases as the magnesium content of the diet increases.

[d]Because of very poor bioavailability, iron from carbonate or oxide sources that are added to the diet should not be considered in determining the minimum nutrient level.

[e]Because of very poor bioavailability, copper from oxide sources that are added to the diet should not be considered in determining the minimum nutrient level.

[f]Add 10 IU vitamin E above minimum level per gram of fish oil per kilogram of diet (cat foods only).

[g]Vitamin K does not need to be added unless diet contains greater than 25% fish on a dry matter basis (cat foods only).

[h]Because processing may destroy up to 90% of the thiamine in the diet, allowances in formulation should be made to ensure the minimum nutrient level is met after processing.

[i]Biotin does not need to be added unless diet contains antimicrobial or antivitamin compounds (cat foods only).

[j]Methionine may be used to substitute for choline as a methyl donor at a rate of 3.75 parts for 1 part choline by weight when methionine exceeds 0.62% (cat foods only).

BOX 3-1 Structural and Metabolic Changes Associated with Aging

Oral cavity	Dental calculus, periodontal disease, loss of teeth, oral ulcers, gingival hyperplasia
Digestive system	Altered liver and pancreatic functions; altered intestinal digestion and absorption; altered esophagus, stomach, and colon motility
Endocrine system	Decreased function of thyroid glands or pancreatic islet cells; hyperplasia or tumors of pituitary or adrenal glands; neoplasia of pancreatic islet cells
Integument	Loss of elasticity; thickened skin; dry, thin haircoat; altered function of sebaceous glands; graying of muzzle; brittle nails; hypersensitivity
Cardiovascular system	Structural alterations in the heart and blood vessels
Genitourinary system	Reduced renal function, blood flow, and glomerular filtration rate; prostate gland hypertrophy; hyperplasia; squamous metaplasia; cysts; neoplasia
Musculoskeletal system	Loss of muscle mass and tone; brittle bones; degenerative joint disease; disturbed gait
Nervous system and special senses	Reduced reactivity to stimuli; altered memory; diminished visual acuity, hearing, taste perception, and smell
Metabolism	Reduced sensitivity to thirst; reduced thermoregulation, physical activity, and rate of metabolism

ability of older dogs and cats to digest and utilize protein is probably diminished because of decreased gastrointestinal efficiency. Relevant studies in cats have provided mixed results but certainly do not suggest that the requirements for protein are reduced with age. The reason senior pet foods tend to be lower in protein despite the lack of evidence to suggest lower requirements is likely based on attempts to ameliorate the progression of subclinical chronic renal disease presumed to be present in older animals.

Work in laboratory animals suggests that a high intake of protein increases intrarenal pressures in renally compromised individuals, which subsequently damages the nephrons and exacerbates loss of function. However, this hypothesis has yet to be proved true for dogs and cats.[6] Although renal hypertension may be observed in renally compromised dogs on high protein diets, this does not appear at this time to translate into an increased rate of renal dysfunction or mortality. Also, in dogs that do have renal hypertension, the degree of protein restriction usually employed does not return these values to normal. For dogs and cats with clinical or biochemical signs of renal insufficiency (including those revealed by some of the early detection methods that exist today), protein restriction as needed to ameliorate these signs may be warranted. However, few data suggest that protein restriction before this point will have a profound effect on lowering the rate of progression of renal disease or longevity.

On the other hand, restriction of protein intake to a level below what is considered adequate for adult maintenance can be detrimental. As with younger adult dogs and cats, sufficient intake is still required for tissue replacement and repair, production of hormones and enzymes, and a host of other functions. Part of the aging process includes a decline in lean tissue mass. Less than adequate intake of protein can only serve to exacerbate the rate of loss. Older animals are also less capable of initiating an effective immune response, which may leave them less able to respond to infections and other bodily insults. Because protein is required for production of both immune system cells and humoral antibodies, protein restriction can only compound the potential for problems.

Although most commercial senior diets are lower in protein than adult maintenance products, they generally still meet the minimum allowances established by the AAFCO Dog and Cat Food Nutrient Profiles for maintenance (18% dry matter for dogs, 26% dry matter for cats). These allowances provide safety factors to account for potential variability in bioavailability of ingredients and individual animal needs. However, products that are substantiated for nutritional adequacy solely by virtue of passage of an AAFCO feeding trial for adult maintenance (which is conducted on younger adults), or products intended for the dietary management of a clinical condition, may contain protein levels below the AAFCO allowances and may not necessarily contain adequate protein to meet the needs of the normal geriatric animal.

Macrominerals

Phosphorus levels may be restricted in senior diets, primarily for the same reason that protein is restricted. A reduction in renal function may result in an increase in the serum phosphate level, which subsequently results in a depression of serum ionized calcium. In response, the parathyroid glands are stimulated to increase synthesis and release of parathormone, which through various actions (mobilization of bone, increased intestinal absorption and renal resorption of calcium) serves to return serum calcium and subsequently phosphorus levels to normal. However, this occurs at the expense of a higher circulating level of parathormone. This hormone is thought to be responsible in part for the adverse effects of renal disease on the body and may perpetuate existing damage.

This process occurs at any stage of renal disease, even before clinical signs may become evident. Restriction of phosphorus intake concomitant with the degree of renal impairment should theoretically hinder the rise in circulating parathormone and delay progression of the renal dysfunction. Work in 15 of 16 nephrectomized dogs has shown an increase in kidney deterioration and mortality in dogs on a high (1.5% dry matter) versus a low (0.44% dry matter) phosphorus diet over a 2-year period.[7] However, these dogs were already compromised to the point that clinical or biochemical signs of renal disease were evident and the level of parathormone necessary to maintain calcium-phosphorus homeostasis was higher. What this means to older animals with presumed but undetectable renal insufficiency is unclear. The rate of disease progression probably accelerates as function declines. Thus, at higher levels of function, where parathormone levels may be only slightly elevated, phosphorus restriction is less likely to have a profound effect on the rate of dysfunction. It could take many years for any protective effect to be significant, and for many senior pets, death from other causes may preclude any benefit.

Clearly, phosphorus supplementation is contraindicated in the older dog or cat. Also, levels of intake approaching the minimum maintenance requirement appear prudent (0.5% dry matter for dogs and cats). Few commercial diets contain phosphorus levels as high as the upper level in the above study, especially diets intended for maintenance. Most diets likely contain less than 1% dry matter, which should be adequately restrictive for animals not showing evidence of renal insufficiency. Although dogs in the low-phosphorus group in the above study were given phosphorus at levels below the AAFCO minimum, there is no indication that that degree of restriction is warranted or desirable in the older pet that is not showing clinical or biochemical signs of renal insufficiency.

Calcium levels may also be restricted in diets formulated to be low in phosphorus, presumably to maintain a desirable calcium-to-phosphorus ratio (typically assumed to be 1.2:1 to 1.4:1). However, because the requirements for calcium most likely are the same as for maintenance (if anything, they may be higher in the renally compromised animal with lower 1,25-dihydroxycholecalciferol synthesis or in the older animal with less efficient absorption capabilities), the rationale for this restriction is unclear.

Salt concentrations may be restricted in many senior diets, compared with salt concentrations in adult maintenance products. The nutritional requirement for sodium in the adult is very low, and because of the ubiquitous distribution of sodium in typical ingredients it is probably close to impossible to formulate a practical ration that would fail to meet minimum requirements, especially in the case of dog foods. However, salt also enhances palatability, so undue restriction may have adverse consequences on consumption, especially if the animal's taste acuities are in decline.

Other Nutrients

Few data exist regarding the micromineral and vitamin requirements of the geriatric dog or cat. Amounts necessary for adult maintenance are presumed to be adequate.

Many manufacturers of senior diets tout the addition of antioxidants in their formulas. Antioxidants help control formation of and damage caused by free radicals, which are thought to be a major factor in cancer formation, the development of debilitating diseases such as osteoarthritis, and even the aging process itself. Many of these substances are recognized essential nutrients (vitamin E) or components of antioxidant enzymes (e.g., selenium, copper, iron, manganese). Others are not recognized as dietary essential nutrients at this time (e.g., vitamin C, beta-carotene, lutein).

Research has shown that the addition of various "cocktails" of antioxidants can be of benefit to immune function and cognitive ability in older dogs.[8,9] Unfortunately, because the effects of individual antioxidant components were not isolated in these studies, it is difficult to make any recommendations beyond the amounts of essential nutrients that are already recognized as adequate for all adult maintenance dog and cat foods. Further, it must be recognized that antioxidants delay, but do not wholly reverse, oxidative damage caused by free radicals. Therefore, for optimum effect, antioxidants must be

TABLE 3-2. BODY CONDITION SCORING OF DOGS AND CATS

SCORE	BODY CONDITION	CLINICAL SIGNS
Dogs		
1	Emaciated	Ribs, lumbar vertebrae, pelvic bones, and all bony prominences are evident from a distance. No body fat is discernible, and obvious loss of muscle mass exists.
2	Very thin	Ribs, lumbar vertebrae, and pelvic bones are easily visible. No fat is palpable, some evidence of other bony prominences exists, and animal exhibits minimal loss of muscle mass.
3	Thin	Ribs are easily palpated and may be visible with no palpable fat. Tops of lumbar vertebrae are visible. Pelvic bones are becoming prominent. Waist and abdominal tuck are obvious.
4	Underweight	Ribs are easily palpable, with minimal fat covering. Waist is easily noted, viewed from above. Abdominal tuck is evident.
5	Ideal	Ribs are palpable without excess fat covering. Waist is observed behind ribs when viewed from above. Abdomen is tucked up when viewed from side.
6	Overweight	Ribs are palpable with slight excess fat covering. Waist is discernible when viewed from above but is not prominent. Abdominal tuck is apparent.
7	Heavy	Ribs are palpable with difficulty, with heavy fat cover. There are noticeable fat deposits over lumbar area and base of tail. Waist is absent or barely visible. Abdominal tuck may be absent.
8	Obese	Ribs are not palpable under very heavy fat cover or are palpable only with significant pressure. Heavy fat deposits are evident over lumbar area and base of tail. Waist is absent. No abdominal tuck exists. Obvious abdominal distention may be present.
9	Grossly obese	Massive fat deposits are present over thorax, spine, and base of tail. Waist and abdominal tuck are absent. Fat deposits are present on neck and limbs, with obvious abdominal distention.

Adapted from Laflamme DP: Body condition scoring and weight maintenance. In *Proceedings of the North American Veterinary Conference*, Orlando, FLa, 1993, Eastern States Veterinary Association; Laflamme DP, Kealy RD, Schmidt DA: Estimation of body fat by body condition score, *J Vet Intern Med* 8:154, 1994; and Laflamme DP, Kuhlman G, Lawlor DF et al: Obesity management in dogs, *J Vet Clin Nutr* 1:59, 1994.

provided early in the animal's life, not just during the senior years.

Chondroprotective agents such as glucosamine and chondroitin sulfate are routinely added to senior diets. The premise behind their inclusion is that supplementation may augment endogenous production of these substances in the cartilage and joint fluid of animals, alleviating signs of osteoarthritis. Studies have suggested benefit in affected animals (especially dogs), although not necessarily in seniors.[10-12] Definitive long-term evaluation of safety with routine consumption of these substances by dogs or cats has not been reported. Therefore, although supplementation to address an existing clinical condition may be warranted, insufficient evidence supports the recommendation of routine supplementation for nonarthritic older animals at this time.

FEEDING MANAGEMENT

Because of the high variability in the effects of age on dogs and cats, feeding management of the older pet must be highly individualized. However, it is still helpful to categorize the geriatric population into subsections in which some commonality in nutrient needs may be seen. Two sources have independently classified older pets into four groups: animals that have maintained weight and good condition (physiologically young); those with a propensity to gain weight (metabolically efficient); those with a propensity to lose weight (metabolically inefficient); and animals with clinical disease (true geriatric).[5,13] For animals within each group the same nutritional goals apply.

To determine the appropriate grouping of an individual, a full assessment of the health of the animal is needed. Along with a physical examination and appropriate laboratory analyses, a determination of body condition score (BCS) is helpful. There are a number of different scoring systems that may be used. However, a nine-point (versus a five-point) scale allows for more interpolation. A suggested BCS scale is provided in Table 3-2. It must be noted, however, that the criteria are probably not based on the body composition of older animals. This may be problematic only for animals above optimal condition, where an excess of fat may disguise the loss of lean tissue.

Food Type

For animals that have maintained ideal weight and body condition and show little if any evidence of age-related changes, no change in the current

TABLE 3-2. BODY CONDITION SCORING OF DOGS AND CATS—cont'd

SCORE	BODY CONDITION	CLINICAL SIGNS
Cats		
1	Emaciated	Ribs are visible on shorthaired cats. There is no palpable fat. Severe abdominal tuck is evident. Lumbar vertebrae and wings of ilia are easily palpated.
2	Very thin	Signs include shared characteristics of BCS 1 and 3.
3	Thin	Ribs are easily palpable with minimal fat covering. Lumbar vertebrae are obvious. There is an obvious waist behind ribs, and minimal abdominal fat.
4	Underweight	Signs include shared characteristics of BCS 3 and 5.
5	Ideal	Animal is well proportioned. Waist is observed behind ribs. Ribs are palpable with slight fat covering. Abdominal fat pad is minimal.
6	Overweight	Signs include shared characteristics of BCS 5 and 7.
7	Heavy	Ribs are not easily palpated with moderate fat covering. Waist is poorly discernible. There is an obvious rounding of abdomen with a moderate abdominal fat pad.
8	Obese	Signs include shared characteristics of BCS 7 and 9.
9	Grossly obese	Ribs are not palpable under heavy fat cover. There are heavy fat deposits over lumbar area, face and limbs. There is distention of abdomen with no waist. Extensive abdominal fat deposits are evident.

diet may be necessary. The diet history should still be documented, however, including diet type, amounts offered and consumed, use of supplements, and so on. This is helpful in case the body weight or health status changes in the future. It also helps uncover any potentially harmful practices, such as excessive reliance on treats, human food, or supplements. Although younger animals may be able to tolerate dietary extremes for extended periods of times, the same may not be true for the older dog or cat.

Animals that tend to carry excess body weight (BCS >6) but are otherwise in reasonable health may need to go on a calorie-restricted diet to help reduce body weight or prevent further weight gain. If the animal is currently offered a maintenance or all-life-stages product, switching to a slightly less calorie-dense senior pet food may be indicated (Table 3-3). Alternatively, smaller portions of the currently fed product may suffice. In either case, portion control will likely need to be initiated. Details on methods to achieve effective weight loss in pets are described elsewhere.[14] The degree of restriction should not be extreme. The rate of weight loss considered to be safe in obese animals is between 0.5% and 2% of initial body weight per week. Because restriction of calorie intake inexorably results in loss of lean body mass as well as fat, extreme caution must be taken with the senior pet, since the aging process itself already results in some lean tissue loss. Therefore, weight loss at rates approaching the lower end of the acceptable range appears prudent.

TABLE 3-3. AAFCO MAXIMUM CALORIE CONTENT FOR "LITE" PRODUCTS (KCAL METABOLIZABLE ENERGY PER KG AS FED)

CATEGORY (% MOISTURE)	DOG FOOD	CAT FOOD
Dry (<20%)	3100	3250
Semimoist (≥20%, <65%)	2500	2650
Canned (≥65%)	900	950

Reproduced with permission from Dzanis DA: Disorders of nutritional excess. In Morgan RV, Bright RM, Swartout MS, eds: *Handbook of small animal practice,* ed 4, Philadelphia, 2003, Elsevier Science, p 1190.

On the other hand, animals that tend to be thin or have trouble maintaining weight may need higher caloric density foods than the one they currently are fed. The problem is that although calorie content information of pet foods is required if the label carries the words *lite, low calorie*, or something similar, the same information is not mandatory on food labels without those

TABLE 3-4. ESTIMATING CALORIE CONTENT OF A PET FOOD FROM THE LABEL "GUARANTEED ANALYSIS" VALUES

Step 1	Multiply the percent crude protein × 3.5.
Step 2	Multiply the percent crude fat × 8.5.
Step 3	Add the percentages of crude protein, crude fat, crude fiber, moisture, and ash, and subtract the total from 100. This provides the percent nitrogen-free extract (NFE), which is the carbohydrate portion.
Step 4	Multiply the percent NFE from Step 3 × 3.5.
Step 5	Add the results from Steps 1, 2, and 4, and multiply the total × 10. The result is the calorie content in kcal metabolizable energy (ME) per kg "as fed" (AF).
Step 6	To determine calories on a dry matter (DM) basis, divide the result from Step 5 by the proportion of DM in the product [(100-% moisture)/100].

Example:
Step 1: Crude protein 24% × 3.5 = 84
Step 2: Crude fat 10% × 8.5 = 85
Crude fiber 3%
Moisture 10%
Ash 5%
Step 3: 24% + 10% + 3% + 10% + 5% = 52%
NFE = 100-52 = 48
Step 4: NFE × 3.5 = 48% × 3.5 = 168
Step 5: (84 + 85 + 168) × 10 = 337 × 10 = **3370 kcal ME/kg AF**
Step 6: 3370/(100-10/100) = **3744 kcal ME/kg DM**

Reproduced with permission from Dzanis DA: Nutrition through the life cycle. In Morgan RV, Bright RM, Swartout MS, eds: *Handbook of small animal practice,* ed 4, Philadelphia, 2003, Elsevier Science, p 1173.

words, and hence often is absent. If the information is not provided on the label, there are methods to calculate the metabolizable energy content using the values given in the guaranteed analysis (Table 3-4). However, this method may not be sufficiently accurate for many products. The calculation tends to overestimate the true calorie content of poor quality, less digestible foods and underestimate a premium, highly digestible food by up to 20%. Comparisons may also be made by judging the relative nutrient content of two products. The higher in fat a food is, typically the higher it is in calories. Conversely, higher crude fiber content usually translates to lower calorie density. Extra caution should be taken when comparing canned products. Even a few percentage points difference in moisture content can have a large effect on overall caloric density. Comparison of products of different processing types (e.g., canned versus dry) is possible by conversion of all nutrients to a dry matter basis, but it is far easier to keep comparisons between foods within the same processing type. This method is even less accurate than the aforementioned calculation process. Therefore, it may be best to confirm any comparisons by requesting calorie content information directly from the manufacturer.

The nutritional considerations of the clinically ill animal are similar whether the animal is young or old. Conditions that respond to dietary modifications, such as renal, hepatic, or cardiovascular disease, should be treated accordingly. Some common medical conditions and basic approaches to dietary management are given in Table 3-5. In some cases, the degree of nutrient restriction may be below what is considered adequate for adult maintenance. In extreme cases, enteral or parenteral nutritional support may be required. The basics for providing these modes of nutrient delivery to the older animal are not different from those for other life stages.

Amount, Frequency, and Other Considerations

The amount of food to be offered is dependent on the individual's needs and the type of food being offered. An estimate of current calorie intake can be performed based on determination of the calorie content of the food and amount of the current daily allotment. If the current food is to be continued, a proportional increase or decrease may be needed depending on whether the animal needs to gain or lose weight, respectively. However, if the type of food is also changed, further consideration has to be given to the difference in caloric density between the two products. In any case, the amounts offered should be

TABLE 3-5. DIETARY MANAGEMENT OF ORGAN SYSTEM DYSFUNCTION IN THE AGING DOG OR CAT

DIET TYPE	DISORDER OR CLINICAL SIGN REQUIRING FEEDING MANAGEMENT
Low protein	Uremic renal failure Oxalate and urate urolithiasis Hepatic encephalopathy
Low fat	Obesity Chylothorax Hyperlipidemia Hyperlipoproteinemia Hypothyroidism Small bowel disease
Low mineral	Urolithiasis Feline urologic syndrome Chronic renal failure
Restricted protein source	Food-induced allergy Flatulence
Low copper	Copper-associated hepatopathy Chronic active hepatitis
Gluten free	Gluten-induced enteropathy
Low fiber, moderate fat	Chronic liver disease Gastrointestinal surgery Gastric dilatation or volvulus Flatulence Hyperadrenocorticism
High fat, high protein	Soft-tissue wounds Hypoglycemia Fractures Fever Stress, environmental or psychological disorders Cachexia or starvation Anorexia Anemia Hepatic lipidosis Hyperthyroidism
Maintenance	Renal disease, nonuremic Steatitis Advanced age with reduced calorie requirements Obesity
Low fat, high fiber	Hyperlipoproteinemia Obesity Diabetes mellitus (also high protein, low carbohydrate)
Moderate fat, moderate fiber	Large bowel disease Constipation
Reduced sodium	Heart failure Hypertension Chronic renal failure Chronic liver disease with ascites or edema

continuously altered, with the goal of achieving an ideal BCS. In fact, research has shown that dogs fed amounts appropriate to maintain a BCS closer to the ideal had a longer median life span and suffered less from the onset of osteoarthritis and other debilitating diseases in their old age.[15,16] Therefore, any initial suggestions on amounts to feed should be regarded only as rough estimates and are to be freely amenable to modification.

The frequency of feeding also depends on the individual's needs and history. Cats offered dry food are often allowed free access, and if weight can be maintained with this regimen there is little reason to change it. On the other hand, many dogs are typically fed once daily. However, conditions that may compromise the animal's ability to consume large quantities at one sitting may require more frequent meals. Also, the obese animal may benefit from more frequent feedings to alleviate boredom.

If the animal's ability to eat is compromised by dental problems or other conditions, moistening the food with water prior to feeding may be necessary. In some cases, a gruel may be needed to accomplish adequate intake. Alternatively, switching from a dry to a canned food may be indicated. However, care must be taken to ensure that the nutrient contents of the two are equivalent.

SUMMARY

For all practical purposes, the nutritional requirements of the geriatric dog or cat are not significantly different from those of the younger adult. Except for animals with clinical disease responsive to dietary modifications, there is little evidence at this time to suggest that use of special formulas that deviate from maintenance requirements will significantly improve health or longevity. However, this does not mean that the nutritional needs of the geriatric pet can be ignored. A good assessment of the diet and feeding practices is needed, with changes tailored to the individual and implemented appropriately. Feeding older dogs and cats to maintain an ideal BCS appears a very prudent course of action.

References

1. Association of American Feed Control Officials: *Official publication*, Oxford, Ind, 2003, AAFCO.
2. National Research Council: *Nutrient requirements of dogs,* revised 1985, Washington, DC, 1985, National Academy Press.
3. National Research Council: *Nutrient requirements of cats,* revised 1986, Washington, DC, 1986, National Academy Press.
4. Goldston RT: Geriatrics and gerontology, *Vet Clin North Am Small Anim Pract* 19:1, 1989.
5. Burkholder WJ: Age-related changes to nutritional requirements and digestive function in adult dogs and cats, *J Am Vet Med Assoc* 215:625, 1999.
6. Brown S: *The protein debate*. Proceedings of Focus on Geriatric Nutrition, Chicago, 1996, Watt Publishing.
7. Finco DR, Brown SA, Crowell WA: Effects of dietary protein and phosphorus on the kidneys of dogs. In Carey DP, Norton SA, Bolser SM, eds: *Recent advances in canine and feline nutritional research,* Proceedings of the 1996 Iams International Nutrition Symposium, Wilmington, Ohio, 1996, Orange Frazer Press.
8. Devlin P, Koelsch S, Heaton P et al: The maintenance of a vaccine-induced immune response in adult and senior dogs fed an antioxidant-supplemented diet, *Compend Contin Educ Pract Vet* 23(suppl 9A):96, 2001.
9. Milgram NW, Zicker SC, Head E et al: Dietary enrichment counteracts age-associated cognitive dysfunction in canines, *Neurobiol Aging* 82:375, 2002.
10. Lipiello L, Idouraine A, McNamara PS et al: Cartilage stimulatory and antiproteolytic activity is present in sera of dogs treated with a chondroprotective agent, *Canine Pract* 23:10, 1998.
11. Anderson MA, Slater MR, Hammand TA: Results of a survey of small animal practitioners on the perceived clinical efficacy and safety of an oral nutraceutical, *Prev Vet Med* 38:65, 1999.
12. Canapp SO, McLaughlin RM, Hosknson JJ et al: Scintigraphic evaluation of dogs with acute synovitis after treatment with glucosamine hydrochloride and chondroitin sulfate, *Am J Vet Res* 60:1552, 1999.
13. Dzanis DA: Nutrition through the life cycle. In Morgan RV, Bright RM, Swartout MS, eds: *Handbook of small animal practice,* ed 4, Philadelphia, 2003, Elsevier Science.
14. Burkholder WJ, Bauer JE: Foods and techniques for managing obesity in companion animals, *J Am Vet Med Assoc* 212:658, 1998.
15. Kealy RD, Lawler DF, Ballam JM et al: Effects of diet restriction on life span and age-related changes in dogs, *J Am Vet Med Assoc* 220:1315, 2002.
16. Kealy RD, Lawler DF, Larson BT et al: *Estimated body composition values of control-fed versus restricted-fed Labrador retrievers in a life span study*, Proceedings of the Purina Pet Institute Symposium, St Louis, 2002, Nestlé Purina Pet Care.

CHAPTER 4

Aging and Effects on Behavior

GARY M. LANDSBERG and ELIZABETH HEAD

The effects of aging on the brain can be subtle and slowly progressive. Aging dogs and cats often suffer a decline in cognitive brain function (memory, learning, perception, awareness). Cognitive dysfunction may manifest itself as disorientation; forgetting of previously learned behaviors such as house-training; a decrease in interactions with people; the onset of new fears and anxiety; decreased recognition of people, places, or pets; and other signs of deteriorating memory and learning ability.[1,2] These behavioral signs can also be caused by medical problems, which will need to be differentiated from cognitive dysfunction.

EVALUATION OF BEHAVIORAL CHANGES

Older dogs and cats may exhibit a variety of behavioral changes, with severe signs, such as destructiveness, anxiety and phobias, repetitive or compulsive disorders, night waking, house-soiling, and increased vocalization and aggression, to more subtle signs, such as a decrease in responsiveness to the owner or decreased activity levels (Box 4-1).[3] When the older dog or cat exhibits any medical or behavioral sign, the veterinarian should diagnose the underlying cause of the abnormality so that an appropriate treatment program can be implemented.

The age of onset can be important for ruling in or ruling out certain diagnoses. In some cases, perhaps owing to changes in intensity or frequency of the problem or changes in the household that preclude living with the problem any longer, the owner may be seeking guidance only now for a behavioral problem that began when the animal was younger. A critical but often overlooked part of obtaining a case history is to determine the age at which the problem began to emerge and, if it is long standing, why the owners have waited until this time to seek assistance.

A minimum clinical evaluation might include a thorough physical examination, complete neurologic examination, ocular evaluation (including Schirmer tear test, measurements of intraocular pressure, and retinal examination), complete blood count, serum chemistry profile, urinalysis, blood pressure determinations, liver function tests, and endocrine screening tests (e.g., thyroid and adrenal function testing).

NATURE OF BEHAVIORAL PROBLEMS

Incidence studies on behavioral problems in older dogs and cats may be misleading with respect to the type of behavioral problems that are most commonly seen in a clinical practice. Most studies refer only to those cases seen at specific behavior referral practices. Although the cases seen by behavioral consultants may be indicative of more serious or complex problems, they often represent only a small fraction of the behavioral problems that might be observed by the owners. In a recent study of 103 dogs older than 7 years referred to a St. Louis area behavior referral practice, separation anxiety (30%) was the most common reason for referral, with other reasons ranked as follows: aggression toward people, 27%; aggression toward animals, 17%; compulsive

BOX 4-1 Sample Behavior Evaluation Form

Owner observations are an important aspect of health care for all dogs and cats but are especially important in the senior animal. Please complete this questionnaire and return it to our receptionist before you see the doctor. It helps us to ensure that nothing is overlooked and tells us about some of the signs that might not be evident on a standard physical examination.

Owner's Name: **Type of Pet: Dog** ______ **Cat** ______

Animal's Name: **Age:** **Date:**

Key: 0—normal; 1—mild; 2—moderate; 3—severe	**0**	**1**	**2**	**3**	**When began?**
Weight gain ___ Weight loss ___					
Appetite increase ___ Appetite decrease ___					
Vomiting ___					
Diarrhea ___ Colitis (stool with mucus or blood) ___					
Constipation or difficulty with defecation ___					
Increased drinking ___ Increased urination ___					
Coughing ___ Weakness after exercise ___					
Panting ___ Lumps or tumors ___					
Skin problems ___					
Describe: ______________________ ______________________					
Bad breath/sore gums/difficulty chewing ___					
Muscle tremors or shaking ___					
Weakness/incoordination ___					
Difficulty climbing stairs/increased stiffness ___					
Diminished vision ___					
Diminished hearing ___					
House-Soiling					
Urine: ___ Horizontal surface ___ Vertical surface ___					
Incontinence ___ Bowel movement ___					
Indoor elimination in view of owners ___					
Goes outdoors and eliminates indoors on return ___					
Elimination in crate or sleeping area ___					
Impaired Learning or Memory					
Decreased ability to work ___					
Forgets previously learned tasks/commands/name ___					
Decreased recognition of familiar people/animals ___					
Social					
Decreased interest in petting/affection ___					
Decreased tolerance of handling ___					
More possessive ___					
Increased need or demand for affection/attention ___					
Problems with social relationships with other pets ___					

BOX 4-1—cont'd

	0	1	2	3	When began?
Disorientation					
Gets lost ___ Goes to wrong side of door ___					
Confused ___ Can't maneuver over obstacles ___					
Anxiety					
Decreased tolerance of being left alone ___					
Increased irritability ___ Restless or agitated ___					
Anxiety ___ Fear ___					
Phobias ___ Aggression ___					
Describe: ______________________________					
Purposeless or Repetitive Activity					
Vocalizing or whining ___ Pacing ___					
Circling ___ Licking ___					
Stares into space ___ Self-trauma ___					
Sucking ___ Hallucinates ___					
Describe: ______________________________					
Sleep-Wake Cycle					
Wakes at night/restless sleep ___					
Decreased activity/sleeps more ___					
Apathy or Depression					
Less reactive to stimuli ___ Listless ___					
Decreased interest in food ___					
Decreased grooming or hygiene ___					

Other problems or concerns (or use this space to describe any of the above in more detail):

____

____

Is your dog or cat presently on any medications?

Describe: ______________________________

____

Has your dog or cat been previously diagnosed as having any medical problems?

Describe: ______________________________

____

disorders, 8%; cognitive dysfunction, 7%; phobias, 5%; anxiety, 4%; house-soiling, 3%; and vocalization, 1%.[4] The author (GL) has recently collated data for cats aged 11 and over at three behavior referral practices and out of 83 cats, the reasons for referral were ranked as follows: inappropriate elimination, 73%; intraspecies aggression, 10%; aggression to people, 6%; excessive vocalization and night waking, 6%; overgrooming, 4%; and fear and scratching, 1% each.

Both medical conditions and primary behavioral problems can be responsible for these behavioral signs. It is important to remember that the older dog and cat may be subjected to many of the same stressors that lead to problems in younger pets (moving, schedule change, new members of the family through birth or marriage, family members leaving the home through divorce or marriage). Yet because of the effects of learning, brain aging, and other age-related medical problems, older dogs and cats may be more resistant to change and more difficult to retrain. The potential causes of and factors that contribute to these behavioral problems are discussed in the next section.

CAUSES OF BEHAVIORAL PROBLEMS

Aging can have an effect on virtually every body system, which may in turn have a direct or indirect effect on the behavior of a dog or cat. Aging changes are generally progressive and irreversible. Disease, stress, nutrition, exercise, genetics, environment, and effects of oxidative damage all have an impact on the natural aging process. In general, behavioral signs may arise as a result of a disease process, they may be related to the effects of age on the body systems including the brain, they may be primary behavioral problems, or they may be some combination of any of these factors. For example, it would not be unusual for an older dog or cat with hearing and visual deficits to also have arthritis and/or cognitive dysfunction. Therefore, it might be difficult to determine which medical condition is most responsible for a specific behavioral change such as decreased interaction with the owner. In some cases, a therapeutic trial (i.e., response to medical therapy) might be the most practical means of determining which medical signs are attributable to which medical problems.

MEDICAL AND PHYSICAL HEALTH AND ITS EFFECTS ON BEHAVIOR

The natural aging process is associated with progressive and irreversible changes in the body systems that could affect the dog's or cat's behavior. Medical changes associated with aging may have an impact on behavior if they directly or indirectly affect the central nervous system, lead to an alteration in sensory function, affect stool or urine output, or lead to pain or neurologic deficits.[5] In general in the older animal, immune competence declines, tumor production increases, rapid eye movement (REM) sleep decreases, tissue dehydration and tissue hypoxia occur, and organ function degenerates.

Behavioral changes ranging from lethargy to aggression may occur in hypothyroid dogs,[6] whereas dogs with adrenal dysfunction may exhibit altered sleep-wake cycles, lethargy, house-soiling, panting, and polyphagia. Respiratory capacity may decline, and anemia, cardiac disease, and decreased organ perfusion increasingly occur. Endocrine imbalances may arise, leading to increasing cortisol output, an increase or decrease in reproductive hormones, or an increase or decline in thyroid hormones.

Arthritis, decrease in bone and muscle mass, and neuromuscular deterioration can lead to chronic pain and affect locomotion. Any medical condition that is associated with chronic pain or discomfort (e.g., arthritis, dental disease) can lead to increased irritability or fear of being handled. If mobility is affected, the dog or cat may become increasingly aggressive rather than retreating. A decrease in mobility can reduce the animal's ability to access its elimination area. Special senses can also be affected by age with a decline in hearing, sight, and smell perhaps having the greatest effects on behavior. Dogs with impaired sight or hearing may be either less responsive or more reactive to stimuli.

Changes in the animal's environment may also contribute to the emergence of behavioral problems. Schedule changes, a new member of the household (e.g., baby, spouse), a new pet, or moving can have a dramatic impact on an animal's behavior. Medical or degenerative changes associated with aging may cause the dog or cat to be more sensitive or less adaptable to change. Many owners then inadvertently reward the undesirable behavior or become anxious or disturbed about the behavioral problem, which adds further to the animal's anxiety. The owners may also attempt to punish the animal for undesirable behavior, which may lead to further anxiety and conflict on the part of the animal. Of course, concurrent medical, physical, and cognitive changes would have a further impact on an animal's behavior.

AGING AND ITS EFFECT ON THE BRAIN

A number of degenerative changes in the brains of older dogs and cats may be associated with behavioral signs of cognitive dysfunction. In the older dog, there can be a reduction in overall brain mass including cerebral and basal ganglia atrophy, increase in ventricular size, narrowing and retraction of the gyri, widening of the sulci, leptomeningeal thickening in the cerebral hemispheres, demyelination, glial changes involving an increase in the size and number of astrocytes, and reduction in neurons.[7,8] In one study, an 18.5% reduction in neurons was found in dogs older than 19 years in comparison with younger dogs.[9] Other neuronal changes in older dogs include increasing amounts of lipofuscin and neuroaxonal degeneration. Accumulation of diffuse beta-amyloid plaques with perivascular infiltrates also increases.[7]

Although the role of beta-amyloid accumulation in the development of cognitive dysfunction is yet to be determined, it is neurotoxic, correlates with the severity of cognitive dysfunction in laboratory tests, and can lead to compromised neuronal function, degeneration of synapses, apoptosis-induced neuronal loss, and a depletion of neurotransmitters. Studies have shown that beta-amyloid is undetectable in young dogs, is most extensive in the oldest dogs, and that the greater the beta-amyloid accumulation, the greater the cognitive impairment.[10,11] In dogs, errors in learning tests, including measurements of discrimination, reversal, and spatial learning, were strongly associated with increased amounts of beta-amyloid deposition.

Although atherosclerosis, cerebral ischemia, and cerebral hemorrhage are uncommon in dogs and cats, numerous vascular and perivascular changes have been identified in older dogs, including occasional cases of microsized hemorrhage or infarcts in periventricular vessels. Arteriosclerosis of the nonlipid variety may be commonly seen in the older dog (because of fibrosis of vessel walls, endothelial proliferation, hyalinization, mineralization, and beta-amyloid deposition). The angiopathy present within some aged dogs may compromise blood flow and glucose use.

In addition, the brain of the older dog or cat may be subjected to further hypoxia because of decreased cardiac output, anemia, and conditions that lead to hypertension (diabetes mellitus, hyperthyroidism, hyperadrenocorticism, chronic renal disease, and cardiac or respiratory insufficiency). Decreased physical activity and sensory orientation, personality changes, soiling and incontinence, decreased responsiveness, and decreased ability to perform learned tasks may be related to the hypoxia created by decreased cardiac output, anemia, and hypertension. Although a great deal of speculation exists regarding the mechanisms that contribute to the onset of these signs, there seems to be sufficient information to indicate that alterations in neurotransmitter function and increasing beta-amyloid accumulation are at least in part responsible.[12,13]

There are a number of parallels among canine aging, human aging, and Alzheimer's disease. Dogs and humans both develop cognitive impairments with age, and a subset of each group develops severe impairments, although some dogs and people show no impairment whatsoever. There are also similarities in the neuropathology of dogs with cognitive dysfunction. Diffuse beta-amyloid plaques within the cerebrum and hippocampus as well as beta-amyloid angiopathy have been identified in geriatric humans, dogs, and cats with signs consistent with cognitive dysfunction.[14,15] Numerous cerebrovascular beta-amyloid deposits have been shown to occur in the three species. In both dogs and humans, severe cognitive impairment is associated with more extensive plaque formation. Genetics may be a contributing factor in the extent or age of onset of beta-amyloid distribution, as some dog breeds develop beta-amyloid at an earlier age than others, and there is a high concordance rate within litters in the extent of beta-amyloid.[16]

Functional changes that may occur in the aging brain include depletion of catecholamine neurotransmitters (norepinephrine, serotonin, dopamine),[17,18] increased monoamine oxidase B activity,[19] a decline in cholinergic activity,[20] and an increase in free radical production.[21] With age, mitochondrial function declines so that energy production is less efficient and the production of free radicals, which damage cell membranes, is increased. The role of vascular insufficiency (decreased cardiac output, anemia, arteriosclerosis, blood viscosity changes, vasospasm) in enhancing the neurodegenerative process is unknown, but there may be a link between hypoxia and cognitive dysfunction.

Although oxygen is required for survival, a small amount of oxygen that is used by the mitochondria for normal, aerobic energy production is converted to reactive oxygen species (also known as free radicals), such as hydrogen peroxide, superoxide, and nitric oxide, within the mitochondria. As mitochondria age, they become less efficient and produce relatively more free radicals and less energy than do young mitochondria.[22,23] In addition, neutrophils and macrophages respond to infection and inflammation by increasing amounts of free radicals. The normal body's antioxidant defenses are enzymes, such as superoxide dismutase, catalase, and glutathione peroxidase, and free radical scavengers, such as vitamins A, C, and E, which eliminate free radicals as they are produced. If free radicals cannot be eliminated by these mechanisms, free radicals may react with DNA, lipids, and proteins, leading to cellular damage, dysfunction, mutation, neoplasia, and even cell death. In the cell this balance of detoxification and production is controlled, and if it is tipped in favor of overproduction, a state of oxidative stress is produced. The brain is particularly susceptible to the adverse effects of free radicals because the brain has high lipid content, a high demand for oxygen, and limited ability for antioxidant defense and repair relative to other tissues. Consistent with this is the observation of a progressive accumulation in oxidative damage to proteins and lipids with age in the canine brain.[24]

Cognitive Dysfunction

When the behavioral signs are due to the effects of neurodegenerative processes in the brain, this generally is referred to as *cognitive dysfunction.* The diagnosis of cognitive dysfunction is made by exclusion. If one or more of the clinical signs shown in the screening checklist are present and no underlying medical cause can be identified on physical examination or diagnostic tests, the owner can then be asked to fill out a more comprehensive checklist to determine all of the signs that might be consistent with cognitive dysfunction (Box 4-2). Primary behavioral conditions are also a possibility, so additional history may be required to rule out any changes in the animal's environment, household, or relationships that might account for the behavioral changes. The cognitive questionnaire can also be use to track response to medical therapy.

Treatment of Cognitive Dysfunction

If cognitive dysfunction is the presumptive diagnosis, then a therapeutic trial should be implemented in an attempt to improve the clinical signs and perhaps slow the progress of the cognitive dysfunction. Although it might be prudent to maintain an older dog or cat on long-term therapy in an attempt to slow the progress of cognitive dysfunction, many owners may not want to continue the treatment unless there is some evidence of improvement in the animal's condition. The cognitive dysfunction checklist can be used as an assessment baseline and then can be filled out after a specified course of treatment to track any improvement or deterioration (see Box 4-2).

Selegiline Therapy. Selegiline is a selective and irreversible inhibitor of monoamine oxidase B (MAOB) in the dog.[25] It is the only drug presently licensed for the treatment of cognitive dysfunction in North America and has been shown to be effective not only in placebo-controlled drug trials in which 69% to 75% of treated dogs showed improvement, but also in a recent field trial of 641 dogs in which there was an overall improvement of 77% at 60 days.[26] Although the mechanisms by which selegiline produces clinical improvement in dogs with cognitive dysfunction are not clearly understood, enhancement of dopamine and perhaps other catecholamines in the cortex and hippocampus is presumed to be an important factor.[27] Selegiline may help to restore dopamine balance through its actions as an MAOB inhibitor. Selegiline appears also to increase 2-phenylethylamine in the dog brain. A neuromodulator that enhances dopamine and catecholamine function, 2-phenylethylamine may itself enhance cognitive function. Selegiline may alleviate cognitive dysfunction through a number of other mechanisms. Release of noradrenaline may be enhanced, and reuptake of noradrenaline may be inhibited. Catecholamine enhancement may lead to improved neuronal impulse transmission. Selegiline metabolites, l-amphetamine and l-methamphetamine may also enhance cognitive function.[28]

Selegiline may contribute to a decrease in free radical load in the brain. Because MAOB is inhibited, fewer toxic free radicals may be produced. Selegiline may directly scavenge free radicals and enhance scavenging enzymes such as catalase and superoxide dismutase. Superoxide dismutase is increased in dogs on selegiline therapy.[29] Selegiline also has neuroprotective effects on dopaminergic, noradrenergic, and cholinergic neurons. For example, it has been shown to protect against the toxic effects of the neurotoxin l-methyl-4-phenyl-1,2,3,6 tetrahydropyridine.[30]

Some dogs improve within the first 2 weeks of receiving selegiline, whereas a few dogs do not show improvement until the second month. For cognitive dysfunction, 0.5 to 1 mg/kg selegiline is administered orally each morning, and if there is not significant improvement in 30 days the dose can be adjusted up to the next tablet size for another month. Gastrointestinal upset is occasionally seen but usually improves if selegiline is discontinued for a few days or a lower starting dose is used. Hyperactivity and restlessness have also occasionally occurred. Toxicity may occur when selegiline is used concurrently with antidepressants, ephedrine, phenylpropanolamine,

Box 4-2 Sample Cognitive Dysfunction Evaluation Form

Owner's Name: **Type of Pet: Dog** ______ **Cat** ______

Animal's Name: **Age:** **Date:**

Key: 0—none; 1—mild; 2—moderate; 3—severe	Date	Date	Date
A: Confusion, Awareness, and Spatial Orientation			
Gets lost in familiar locations	___	___	___
Goes to wrong side of door (e.g., hinge side)	___	___	___
Gets stuck; cannot navigate around or over obstacles	___	___	___
Decreased responsiveness to stimuli	___	___	___
B: Relationships and Social Behavior			
Decreased interest in petting or contact	___	___	___
Decreased greeting behavior	___	___	___
Alterations in or problems with social hierarchy	___	___	___
Need for constant contact; overdependence or clinginess	___	___	___
C: Activity—Increased or Repetitive			
Stares, fixates on, or snaps at objects	___	___	___
Paces ____ Wanders aimlessly___	___	___	___
Licks owners, household objects	___	___	___
Vocalizes	___	___	___
D: Activity—Decreased; Apathy			
Decreased responsiveness to stimuli	___	___	___
Decreased self-care	___	___	___
Appetite—Increased/decreased	___	___	___
E: Anxiety—Increased Irritability			
Restlessness or agitation	___	___	___
Anxiety about being separated from owners	___	___	___
Increased irritability	___	___	___
F: Sleep-Wake Cycles—Reversed Day-Night Schedule			
Restless sleep; waking at night	___	___	___
Increased daytime sleep	___	___	___
G: Learning and Memory—House-Soiling			
Indoor elimination——random sites or in view of owners	___	___	___
Decrease in or loss of signaling	___	___	___
Goes outdoors, eliminates indoors on return	___	___	___
Elimination in crate or sleeping area	___	___	___
Incontinence	___	___	___
H: Learning and Memory—Work, Tasks, Commands			
Impaired working ability	___	___	___
Decreased recognition of familiar people or animals	___	___	___
Decreased response to known commands and tricks	___	___	___
Decreased ability to perform tasks	___	___	___
Inability to learn or slow in learning new tasks (retrain)	___	___	___

Discuss any additional concerns or use this space to describe details of any of the above

____

____

narcotics, or other monoamine oxidase inhibitors (MAOIs), including amitraz tick collars. Therefore, these drug combinations should be avoided in medicated dogs.

Nutritional and Dietary Therapy. The use of antioxidants to decrease free radical damage may slow cognitive decline and improve the behavioral signs associated with cognitive dysfunction. Antioxidants scavenge and minimize production of reactive oxygen species, bind metal ions that might make poorly reactive oxygen species more toxic, and repair damage to target tissues. Vitamin E protects cell membranes from oxidative damage by scavenging radicals within membranes and interrupting lipid peroxidation. Lipoic acid is a mitochondrial cofactor and antioxidant that may slow the progression of behavioral signs related to Alzheimer's disease in humans. Therefore, antioxidants appear to "network," and complex mixtures may be of more benefit than single source additions.

A recent development in canine preventive health care is a senior diet supplemented with antioxidants, mitochondrial cofactors, and essential fatty acids (Hill's b/d), which has been shown to improve dogs' performance of a number of cognitive tasks when compared with the performance of older dogs on a nonsupplemented diet.[31,32] In a laboratory study, 48 dogs older than 7 years were trained on a series of problem-solving tasks in which they had to make correct choices to get a food reward. The dogs were then divided into four groups: one with environmental enrichment (i.e., exercise, novel play toys, and continued testing); one with antioxidant supplementation but no ongoing testing; one with the enriched diet and ongoing testing; and a control group. For 30 months the dogs' performance on a number of tasks was tested, and in each case the dogs on the enriched diet outperformed the dogs on the control diet in their learning ability. At 12 and 24 months, the dogs in the enriched behavioral program were tested against the dogs that had received no enrichment, and dogs that had a combination of the enriched diet and environmental enrichment performed the best.[33] In placebo-controlled home trials, the diet led to improvement in older dogs with disorientation, interaction with the owners or other pets, sleep patterns, house-soiling, and altered activity levels.[34]

In addition to vitamin E, the diet is supplemented with antioxidants including vitamin C (which helps to maintain oxidative protection and helps to regenerate vitamin E and glutathione) and a number of flavonoids and carotenoids from fruit and vegetable components such as spinach flakes, tomato pomace, grape pomace, carrot granules, and citrus pulp (which help to inactivate free radicals). The addition of DL-alpha-lipoic diet and L-carnitine enhances mitochondrial function, and the addition of omega-3 fatty acids helps to promote cell membrane health.[35] Human studies have also found that omega-3 fatty acids may be helpful in the treatment of dementia.[36]

Other Medical Therapies. A number of other medications or supplements are either licensed in other countries for the treatment of cognitive dysfunction in dogs or might be considered for use in dogs based on findings in other species. An α_1- and α_2-adrenergic antagonist, nicergoline, is available in the United Kingdom for the treatment of aging-related behavioral disorders in dogs. Nicergoline may increase cerebral blood flow and have a neuroprotective effect on neural cells. It may also increase dopamine and noradrenaline turnover and inhibit platelet aggregation.[37] Nicergoline is recommended for older dogs with decreased activity, sleep disorders, decreased exercise tolerance, house-soiling (including incontinence), reduced appetite, and decreased awareness. In one open-label trial, there was an overall improvement of 75% over 30 days but this was not compared with placebo.[38] The suggested dose is 0.25 to 0.5 mg/kg daily each morning for 30 days.

Nylidrin hydrochloride, a β-adrenergic agonist, is a vasodilator that may also be useful in improving cerebral blood flow. Its use may be considered in some dogs with cognitive dysfunction. A dose of 3 to 6 mg three times daily for an individual dog has been suggested,[39,40] although there are no published safety or efficacy studies in dogs and cats. Propentofylline is licensed for the treatment of dullness and lethargy in older dogs in a number of European countries including the United Kingdom, Germany, and Spain. It has been advocated to increase oxygen supply to the central nervous system without increasing glucose demand. There is weak evidence that it may also slow the progression of Alzheimer's disease in people.[41] Propentofylline is purported to inhibit platelet aggregation and thrombus formation, make red blood cells more pliable, and increase blood flow. Propentofylline is given at a dose of 3 mg/kg three times daily in dogs.

Drugs that may enhance the noradrenergic system, such as adrafanil and modafinil, might be useful in older dogs to improve alertness and help maintain normal sleep-wake cycles by increasing daytime exploration and activity. In open-field testing in dogs, adrafanil causes increased locomotion without producing stereotypic activity at a dose of 20 mg/kg and higher at both 2 and 10 hours after administration. In a recent comparative study, dogs aged 9 to 16 years were given either adrafanil at 20 mg/kg daily, propentofylline 5 mg/kg twice daily, or nicergoline at 0.5 mg/kg daily for 33 days.[42] Treatment with adrafanil led to a significant increase in locomotion that was unaffected by nicergoline or propentofylline.

There is also some evidence in humans that *Ginkgo* extract at 40 mg/kg three times daily leads to a delay in the progression in Alzheimer's disease and in some cases an improvement.[43] *Ginkgo* extract is licensed in Germany for the treatment of cerebral dysfunction in humans related to vascular insufficiency or depression and early stages of Alzheimer's disease, but there have been no reports of its safety or efficacy in dogs. The mechanisms of action may include reversible MAO inhibition and free radical scavenging.[44,45] Nutritional supplements with phosphatidylserine may also be effective at improving age-associated memory impairment,[46] and drugs that enhance cholinergic transmission, such as those used in humans with Alzheimer's disease, might also be a consideration. Similarly, anticholinergic drugs should be avoided in the elderly.[20] Antiinflammatory drugs and hormone replacement therapy may also be considered. Other homeopathic and natural supplements that have been suggested for calming, reducing anxiety, or inducing sleep include melatonin, valerian, and Bachs flower remedies. Benzodiazepines or buspirone might be useful for treating the clinical signs of anxiety disorders, and benzodiazepines or even sedating antihistamines might be useful for inducing sleep. Clonazepam, oxazepam, and lorazepam would be preferred in the elderly since these drugs have no active intermediate metabolites and therefore decreased potential for hepatic toxicity. Antidepressants such as fluoxetine or paroxetine might also be considered for the treatment of generalized anxiety, and mood and sleep disorders in the elderly pet.

TREATMENT OF SPECIFIC BEHAVIORAL PROBLEMS

Treatment or control of underlying medical problems including cognitive dysfunction may lead to improvement, but those dogs and cats that do not respond entirely may have behavioral factors that need to be assessed and treated. For most behavioral problems, the treatment program (behavioral modification, environmental modification, surgery, and drugs (Table 4-1) will be similar regardless of the animal's age.[1] However, in the older dog and cat it will be increasingly more likely that there are concurrent medical problems that must be addressed. If these medical problems cannot be entirely controlled, then they should be taken into account with respect to behavioral management. For example, in cats and dogs with chronic renal failure, litter box management and access to elimination areas will need to be modified to adjust for the increased volume and frequency of urination. There will likely be an additional need for more frequent cleaning, additional litter boxes, a larger litter box, and perhaps a relocation of the litter boxes to accommodate for the larger volume of urine and more frequent need to eliminate. In dogs with chronic renal failure, more frequent access to elimination areas or a new indoor toilet area may need to be provided. Not only will the animal's health have an impact on the behavioral program, it will also have an impact on the possible results. In addition, any drugs needed to control underlying medical problems may have an impact on behavior. Another important consideration is the selection of drugs for behavioral modification, because some medications have greater potential for adverse effects (e.g., anticholinergic drugs) or may be entirely contraindicated in the presence of certain medical conditions or with other drugs.

Anxiety and Separation Anxiety

Treatment for both dogs and cats involves controlling underlying medical problems and identifying and correcting any owner responses that might be reinforcing or aggravating behaviors that are related to anxiety or separation anxiety.[1] For example, dogs with signs of separation anxiety will need to be taught to settle and relax for progressively longer periods of time away from the owner. However, it may not be possible to leave the older animal alone for very long because of the need for additional opportunities to eliminate, so a midday visit, dog door, or papered indoor elimination area may be needed. For cats, attention on demand should be avoided and the owner should initiate regular and structured play and interaction throughout the day, along with some simple reward-based training for commands. Drugs to reduce anxiety and to improve the animal's cognitive function may also be needed to improve outcome (see Table 4-1).

TABLE 4-1. DRUG DOSAGES FOR BEHAVIOR PROBLEMS

DRUG	DOGS	CATS
Benzodiazepines		
Alprazolam	0.022-0.1 mg/kg tid	0.125-0.25 mg/cat bid or 0.05-0.1 mg/kg tid
Clonazepam	0.1-0.5 mg/kg tid	0.016 mg/kg sid-qid
Clorazepate	0.55-2.2 mg/kg sid-tid	0.55-2.2 mg/kg sid-bid or prn
Diazepam	0.55-2.2 mg/kg prn	1-3 mg/cat sid-bid or 0.5-1 mg/kg (appetite stimulant)
Flurazepam	0.2-0.4 mg/kg for 4-7 days (appetite stimulant)	0.2-0.4 mg/kg for 4 -7 days (appetite stimulant)
Oxazepam	0.2-1 mg/kg sid-bid (appetite stimulant)	0.2-1 mg/kg sid-bid (appetite stimulant)
Azapirones		
Buspirone	2.5-10 mg/dog bid-tid or 1 mg/kg q24h	2.5-7.5 mg/cat or 0.5-1 mg/kg bid
Tricyclic Antidepressants		
Amitriptyline	1-4.4 mg/kg sid-bid	5-10 mg/cat/q24h or 0.5-1 mg/kg q24h
Clomipramine	2-3 mg/kg bid	0.5-1.5 mg/kg q24h
Doxepin	0.5-5 mg/kg bid	
Imipramine	2.2-4.4 mg/kg sid-bid or 0.5-2 mg/kg bid-tid (stereotypy)	2.5-5 mg/cat bid
Selective Serotonin Reuptake Inhibitors		
Fluoxetine	1 mg/kg sid	0.5-1 mg/kg bid
Sertraline	1-3 mg/kg prn	
Paroxetine		1 mg/kg sid
Monoamine Oxidase Inhibitors		
Selegiline	0.5-1 mg/kg q24h	0.5-1 mg/kg q24h
Progestational Hormones		
Megestrol acetate	1.1-4.4 mg/kg sid for 7 days, then one-half dose every 2 weeks	2.5-10 mg/cat for 7 days, then one-half dose every 2 weeks
Medroxyprogesterone acetate	5-11 mg/kg SC or IM q3-4 months	10-20 mg/kg SC or IM or 50 mg/female, 100 mg/male q4 months
Antihistamines		
Chlorpheniramine	4-8 mg bid-tid or 0.5-1 mg/kg bid-tid	2-4 mg bid
Diphenhydramine	2-4 mg/kg tid-qid	2-4 mg/kg tid
Hydroxyzine	2.2 mg/kg tid	10 mg bid
Cyproheptadine	0.3-2 mg/kg q24h	2-4 mg/cat sid-bid
Narcotics and Narcotic Antagonists		
Naltrexone	2.2 mg/kg sid	25-50 mg/cat
Hydrocodone	0.22 mg/kg tid	2.5-5 mg bid-tid (use with caution)

bid, Twice daily; *h,* hours; *sid,* once a day; *IM,* intramuscularly; *prn,* as needed; *q,* every; *qid,* four times daily; *SC,* subcutaneously; *tid,* three times daily.

Excessive Vocalization

In addition to treating underlying medical problems and cognitive dysfunction, treatment generally requires identifying and correcting any owner responses that might be reinforcing or aggravating the excessive vocalization behavior.[1] For dogs, bark control collars and bark control training with or without the aid of a head halter may be useful, whereas cats can be disrupted in the act with sprayed water or compressed air. Nonvocal behavior should then be reinforced. Concurrent drug therapy may also be required if there is an anxiety or cognitive component included with the problem (see Table 4-1).

House-Soiling

Because there may be numerous factors that cause or influence house-soiling, the treatment program will vary according to the diagnosis.[1] Cognitive dysfunction and medical problems should be treated with appropriate drugs or diet (see Table 4-1). However, once the inappropriate elimination or litter avoidance has been established, additional behavioral and environmental management will likely be needed. Addressing any initiating or maintaining factors that still remain should be the first issue. For example, house-soiling caused by to anxiety requires treatment of the underlying issues that are leading to anxiety.

Animals with polyuria will have a need to void more frequently. The frequency of defecation may also increase due to medical problems or a change to higher fiber diet. In cats, more frequent litter box cleaning, additional litter boxes, a larger litter box, and perhaps a relocation of the litter boxes to areas of easy access may be necessary. In dogs that have been trained to eliminate outdoors, the owners may need to change their schedule to accommodate the dog's need for more frequent elimination. Alternately, they may need to provide a dog door or an indoor toileting (paper training) area. Musculoskeletal problems, such as weakness, muscular atrophy, and arthritis, can make it difficult for the dog to get outdoors to eliminate or for the cat to navigate stairs to get to its litterbox. Medication to control pain, carpet runners on stairs for traction, and control of obesity might be helpful. Adjusting the height, size, or location of the litterbox may increase a cat's ability or desire to use its litterbox.

In dogs, once all medical needs have been met, it may also be necessary to reestablish proper training by increasing indoor supervision and immediately taking the dog outdoors if there are any signs that elimination is needed, reestablishing a routine and schedule by taking the dog outdoors as often as necessary, rewarding outdoor elimination, and confining the dog (with or without paper for elimination) away from previously soiled sites. Similarly, cats may need to be supervised to prevent inappropriate elimination and may have to be confined away from previously soiled sites when owner cannot supervise the animals. If there is evidence of cognitive decline, drug or dietary therapy may be useful to improve the success of retraining.

Destructive Behavior

Treatment must first address the underlying cause of the destructive behavior.[1] Treatment of underlying medical problems and cognitive dysfunction may resolve some problems but will not be successful for all cases. Excessive licking and pica may be due to a variety of medical problems, and owner responses to the dog may further reinforce or aggravate the problem. Treatment options include preventing access to sites or objects where inappropriate destruction might occur, using deterrents or "booby traps" to keep animals away from problem areas, using preventive techniques such as confinement, and providing novel and appealing alternatives.

Restlessness and Waking at Nights

If medical problems or cognitive dysfunction are a factor first they must be treated.[1] However, many medical problems in older animals cannot be entirely resolved, and once the altered cycle has been established the owner will need to try and reestablish a normal sleep-wake cycle. Increasing daytime and evening activity and preventing daytime sleep may help to reestablish sleep through the night. Drugs to induce sleep or alternatively to keep the animal more alert and active during the day may be needed to complement this therapy (see Table 4-1). Attention-seeking behavior should be ignored and not reinforced (e.g., the animal should be locked out of the room) or disrupted using a device such as a water gun, compressed air canister, audible alarm, or ultrasonic alarm. Selective serotonin reuptake inhibitors such as fluoxetine might help reestablish normal sleep-wake cycles. Sedating hypnotic benzodiazepines or even an antihistamine such as diphenhydramine might be useful to help induce sleep for a few nights until nighttime sleep can be reestablished. Increased daytime activity and a normalization of circadian rhythms might be reestablished with drugs (such as daily adrafanil), diets, or supplements that enhance cognitive function or that increase daytime activity.

Fears and Phobias

Treatment requires that underlying medical problems and cognitive dysfunction should first be controlled.[1] Because noise phobias in dogs appear to be sometimes related to a decline in hearing, control may be difficult. Housing the animal away from stimuli or masking the stimuli with background music, training the animal to settle in a quiet rest area, using cues to help calm and settle the dog, and administering drugs to help reduce panic and anxiety might be helpful (see Table 4-1). Owners should alter their responses to the animal so that they do not further aggravate or reinforce fearful behavior. In fact, the owner should be a calming influence, with techniques designed to reduce the animal's anxiety (desensitize, counter-condition, response substitution).

Compulsive and Stereotypic Behaviors

Treatment requires the control or resolution of underlying medical problems, including cognitive dysfunction, identification and correction of any source of conflict or anxiety, correction of any owner responses that might be aggravating or reinforcing the problem, introduction of a daily structured regime comprised of increased interactive stimulation, an increase in novel play objects and relaxation times, and administration of drugs to treat the underlying neuropathology.[1] Selective serotonin reuptake inhibitors, or perhaps clomipramine (although this tends to be more anticholinergic), are the primary forms of pharmaceutical intervention, although selegiline might be an alternative if there appears to be an emotional or cognitive component (see Table 4-1).

Aggression

The contribution of medical problems, including pain, and cognitive dysfunction to the perpetuation of aggression may be difficult to assess until treatment has been implemented.[1] Of course, medical problems that cannot be entirely resolved, such as a decline in sensory function, may contribute to limitations in what can be achieved. Prevention by avoiding situations that trigger aggression may be the best option for some of these animals. Aggression in the older animal is often associated with anxiety, so drugs that reduce anxiety or improve serotonergic transmission may prove to be helpful (see Table 4-1). Head halters can provide control and safety and can enhance the owner's ability to immediately and effectively communicate with the animal. Learning will further affect the development and perpetuation of the problem. Therefore, the family's response to the animal's behavior should be assessed to see whether it may be aggravating the problems or reinforcing undesirable behavior.

As the family dog or cat gets older, two types of social problems with other animals may occur. These include problems associated with the addition of a new animal to the home and alterations in the relationship between animals already in the home. The introduction of a new animal may lead to increasing anxiety in the animal already in the home because of the alterations in the attention, play, or exercise the animal receives or because of competition for resources. Generally, if the animal already in the home is sufficiently healthy and has had adequate socialization, there are likely to be few problems. However if the older animal has any medical problems, has been inadequately socialized to other animals, or is fearful or anxious about the introduction of the new animal, aggression (or other behavioral problems such as fear and inappetence) may arise.

If an older dog becomes overly fearful or aggressive when a new puppy is introduced, the dogs should be separated whenever someone is not around to supervise. Before the puppy and the older dog are allowed to interact, the owner should provide enough exercise or play to fatigue the puppy. This will help ensure desirable interactions. The owner should reward all gentle play. The noise of a squeak toy may help distract the puppy from engaging in play attacks. A long lead on the puppy can be used for control and to apply a light correction. A head halter and lead can be very helpful for control. Occasionally, a timely squirt from a water gun or a toy tossed near the puppy will provide the distraction necessary to prevent or stop rough play. As the puppy learns to settle on command and communication skills are further defined, a healthy social relationship should begin to emerge.

Sometimes, aggression between two adult dogs that have lived together for years develops when the older, dominant dog becomes unhealthy, weaker, or less assertive. Medical problems, including pain and sensory decline, cognitive dysfunction, and increasing anxiety, may alter the relationship between young and older dogs. As the older dog ages or as the younger dog matures, the younger dog may begin to challenge the older dog in competitive or social situations. These may include soliciting attention from the owner, greeting visitors, exhibiting territorial displays, and guarding food or toys. The owners may make the situation worse by trying to protect one dog from the challenges of the other, rather than allowing the dogs to work out their relationship on their own. In some cases, muzzles or head halters may be necessary for control and for safety. Treatment involves improving safety with more supervision or separation, controlling the animals' environment and resources, rebuilding the bond between the animals with shared physical activities, obedience training, and leadership exercises with both animals.

The primary social problem between cats occurs when a new cat is introduced into the home. The older cat, especially if it has lived alone for a long period, may be particularly resistant to accepting another member of the same species into the home. An initial separation period, gradual exposure, and counter-conditioning exercises may help. A 7- to 9-week-old, quiet kitten of the opposite sex is most likely to be accepted, although some older cats will not accept another cat in the home no matter what choice is made or what the owner does to try to facilitate the introduction. As the older cat ages and medical problems arise, there may be increasing anxiety or defensiveness toward other cats in the home. As the relationship deteriorates, the younger cat (or cats) may react to the changes in the health or behavior of the older cat with increasing aggression, further aggravating the problem. Although treatment of underlying medical problems, desensitization, counter-conditioning, drug therapy, and use of pheromone product may be effective, it can be difficult to reestablish a healthy social relationship between an aging cat and younger cats once they have been disturbed.

References and Supplemental Readings

1. Landsberg GM, Ruehl WW: Geriatric behavioral problems, *Vet Clin North Am* 27:1537, 1997.
2. Ruehl WW, Hart BL: Canine cognitive dysfunction. In Dodman NH, Shuster L, eds: *Psychopharmacology of animal behavior disorders,* Malden, Mass, 1998, Blackwell Scientific.
3. Landsberg G, Hunthausen W, Ackerman L: *Handbook of behavior problems of the dog and cat,* 2nd ed, WB Saunders, 2003, in press.
4. Horwitz D: Dealing with common behavior problems in senior dogs, *Vet Med* 96:869, 2001.
5. Davies M: The nervous system. In Davies M, ed: *Canine and feline geriatrics,* Oxford, 1996, Blackwell Science.
6. Aronson L: Systemic causes of aggression and their treatment. In Dodman NH, Shuster L, eds: *Psychopharmacology of animal behavior disorders,* Malden, Mass, 1998, Blackwell Scientific.
7. Borras D, Ferrer I, Pumarola M: Age related changes in the brain of the dog, *Vet Pathol* 36:202, 1999.
8. Su MY, Head E, Brooks WM et al: MR imaging of anatomic and vascular characteristics in a canine model of human aging, *Neurobiol Aging* 19:479,1998.
9. Morys J, Narkiewicz O, Maciejewska B et al: Amyloid deposits and loss of neurons in the claustrum of the aged dog, *Neuroreport* 5:1825, 1994.
10. Colle MA, Hauw JJ, Crespau F et al: Vascular and parenchymal beta-amyloid deposition in the aging dog: correlation with behavior, *Neurobiol Aging* 21:695, 2000.
11. Head E, Callahan H, Muggenburg B et al: Visual discrimination learning ability and beta-amyloid accumulation in the dog, *Neurobiol Aging* 19:415, 1998.
12. Ivy GO, Rick JT, Murphy MP, et al: Effects of l-deprenyl on manifestations of aging in the rat and dog, *Ann N Y Acad Sci* 717:45, 1994.
13. Head E, Hartley J, Mehta R et al: The effects of l-deprenyl on spatial short-term memory in young and aged dogs, *Prog Neuropsychopharmacol Biol Psychiatry* 20:515, 1996.
14. Cummings BJ, Su JH, Cotman CW et al: Beta-amyloid accumulation in aged canine brain: a model of early plaque formation in Alzheimer's disease, *Neurobiol Aging* 14:547, 1993.
15. Satou T, Cummings BJ, Head E et al: The progression of beta-amyloid deposition in the frontal cortex of the aged canine, *Brain Res* 774:35, 1997.
16. Bobik M, Thompson T, Russell MJ: Amyloid deposition in various breeds of dogs, *Soc Neurosci Abstr* 20:172, 1994.
17. Arnstein AFT: Catecholamine mechanisms in age-related cognitive decline, *Neurobiol Aging* 14:639, 1993.
18. Milgram NW, Ivy GO, Head E et al: The effect of l-deprenyl on behavior, cognitive function, and biogenic amines in the dog, *Neurochem Res* 18:1211, 1993.
19. Gerlach M, Riederer P, Youdim MBH: Effects of disease and aging on monoamine oxidases A and B. In Lieberman A, Olanow CW, Youdim MBH, Tipton K, eds: *Monoamine oxidase inhibitors in neurological diseases*, 1994, Marcel Dekker.
20. Araujo JA, Chan ADF, Studzinski C et al: Cholinergic disruption age-dependently impairs canine working memory while sparing reference memory and spatial perception, *Society for Neuroscience* 82:4, 2002.
21. Mecocci P, MacGarvey U, Kaufman AE et al: Oxidative damage to mitochondrial DNA shows marked age-dependent increases in human brain, *Ann Neurol* 34:609, 1993.
22. Beckman KB, Ames BN: The free radical theory of aging matures, *Physiol Rev* 78:547, 1998.
23. Shigenaga MK, Hagen TM, Ames BN: Oxidative damage and mitochondrial decay in aging, *Proc Natl Acad Sci U S A* 91:10771, 1994.
24. Head E, Liu J, Hagen TM et al: Oxidative damage increases with age in a canine model of human brain aging, *J Neurochem* 82:375, 2002.
25. Milgram NW, Ivy GO, Murphy MP et al: Effects of chronic oral administration of l-deprenyl in the dog, *Pharmacol Biochem Behav* 51:421, 1995.
26. Campbell S, Trettien A, Kozan B: A non-comparative open label study evaluating the effect of selegiline hydrochloride in a clinical setting, *Vet Ther* 2:24, 2001.
27. Knoll J: l-Deprenyl (selegiline) a catecholaminergic activity enhancer (CAE) substance acting in the brain. *Pharmacol Toxicol* 82:57, 1998.
28. Yasar S, Goldberg JP, Goldberg SR: Are metabolites of l-deprenyl (selegiline) useful or harmful? Indications from preclinical research, *J Neural Transm Suppl* 48:61, 1996.
29. Carillo MC, Ivy GO, Milgram NW et al: Deprenyl increases activity of superoxide dismutase, *Life Sci* 54:1483, 1994.
30. Salo PT, Tatton WG: Deprenyl reduces the death of motoneurons caused by axotomy, *J Neurosci Res* 31:394, 1992.
31. Milgram NW, Estrada J, Ikeda-Douglas C et al: Landmark discrimination learning in aged dogs is improved by treatment with an antioxidant diet, *Soc Neurosci Abstr* 26:531, 2000.
32. Milgram NW, Head E, Cotman CW et al: Age dependent cognitive dysfunction in canines: dietary intervention. In Overall KL, Mills DS, Heath SE, Horwitz D, eds: *Proceedings of the Third International Congress on Veterinary Behavioral Medicine*, Wheathampsead, United Kingdom, 2001, Universities Federation for Animal Welfare.
33. Milgram W: Canine longitudinal study of cognitive aging; an update. Presentation to the 8th Annual Canine Cognition, Aging, and Neuropathology Conference, Albuquerque, New Mexico, 2002.
34. Dodd CE, Zicker SC, Jewell DJ et al: Can a fortified food affect the behavioral manifestations of age-related cognitive decline in dogs? *Veterinary Medicine* 98:396, 2003.

35. Hager K, Marahrens A, Kenklies M et al: Alpha-lipoic acid as a new treatment option for Alzheimer type dementia, *Arch Gerontol Geriatr* 32:275, 2001.
36. Kalmijn S, Launer LJ, Ott A et al: Dietary fat and the risk of incident of dementia in the Rotterdam study, *Ann Neurol* 42:776, 1997.
37. Postal JM: Effectiveness of nicergoline in improving behavioural modification associated with senility in dogs. In *Use of alpha-blocking agent Fitergol in the treatment of behavioural disorders in old dogs,* Pairault, France, 1997, Rhone-Merieux.
38. Penaliggon J: The use of nicergoline in the reversal of behavioural changes due to aging in dogs: a multicentre clinical field trial. *In Proceedings of the First International Conference on Veterinary Behavioural Medicine*, Potter's Bar, United Kingdom, 1997, Universities Federation for Animal Welfare.
39. Luttgen PJ: Diseases of the nervous system in older dogs. Part 1. Central nervous system, *Compend Contin Educ Pract Vet* 12:933, 1990.
40. Mosier JE: Effect of aging on body systems of the dog, *Vet Clin North Am Small Anim Pract* 19:1, 1989.
41. Kittner B, Rossner M, Rother M: Clinical trials in dementia with propentofylline, *Ann N Y Acad Sci* 26:307, 1997.
42. Siwak CT, Muggenburg B, Milgram NW et al: Comparison of the effects of adrafanil, propentofylline, and nicergoline on behavior in aged dogs, *Am J Vet Res* 61:1410, 2000.
43. Lebars PL, Katz MM, Berman N et al: A placebo-controlled, double blinded, randomized trial of an extract of *Ginkgo biloba* for dementia, *JAMA* 278:1327, 1997.
44. Maitra I, Marcooci L, Droy-Lefoix MT et al: Peroxyl radical scavenging activity of *Gingko biloba* extract Egb761, *Biochem Pharmacol* 11:1649, 1995.
45. Whilte HL, Scates PW, Cooper BR: Extracts of *Gingko biloba* leaves inhibit monoamine oxidase, *Life Sci* 58:1315, 1996.
46. Crook TH, Petrie W, Wells C, Massan DC: Effects of phosphatidylserine in Alzheimer's disease, *Psychopharm Bull,* 28(1):61, 1992.

CHAPTER 5

Pharmacologic Principles

JOHNNY D. HOSKINS

Improved medications, surgical techniques, and nutrition, and an apparently increased percentage of animal owners willing to care for their older dogs and cats have contributed to increased numbers of older animals being seen by veterinarians and treated. Although older dogs and cats have long been noted to have different needs than younger animals, much of our working knowledge of veterinary gerontology is extrapolated from human or laboratory animal information. This includes the changes associated with the natural aging process and its effects on drug therapies.

It is clear that there are many changes occurring in the aged dog and cat that can cause multivariable effects on a drug's pharmacokinetics and pharmacodynamics. To sort out these effects and distill them into clinical guidelines is difficult to impossible. Veterinary medicine is further hindered in managing drug therapy for the aged because of the lack of specific information on the topic and because older dogs and cats cannot complain about symptoms caused either by disease or by the drugs used for treatment.

PHARMACOKINETICS AND PHARMACODYNAMICS

Absorption, distribution, biotransformation, and elimination are the parameters that are the major factors in a drug's pharmacokinetic profile.[1] Although significant changes can occur in the gastrointestinal tract of aged mammals, age-related effects on oral absorption appear to be minimal for most drugs in older dogs and cats. Medications administered subcutaneously may be more slowly absorbed in the aged animal. Intramuscular absorptive characteristics may be altered because of a decrease in muscle mass. Thus, the clinical significance of drug absorption and age appears to be overall quite weak.

A drug's distribution characteristics, however, may significantly change with age. As a greater percentage of the body is fat, volumes of distribution of highly lipophilic drugs, such as anesthetic agents, could be significantly increased (and initial plasma levels decreased) as compared with those in a young, adult animal. Conversely, for drugs with high water solubility but low lipid solubility (such as aminoglycoside antimicrobials), volumes of distribution could be decreased (and initial plasma levels increased).

Age effects on hepatic biotransformation appear to be minimal unless severe hepatic compromise is present. Because of reduced hepatic blood flow, drugs exhibiting a high first-pass effect in the liver, such as propranolol, buspirone, diltiazem, omeprazole, chlorpromazine, clomipramine, and selegiline, could potentially require dosage adjustment in older dogs and cats.

Reduced renal function is another important effect of aging with respect to pharmacokinetic alterations. Despite normal renal function tests, reduced renal function can cause clinically significant changes in drug elimination, particularly with drugs having a narrow therapeutic window, such as aminoglycoside antimicrobials, digoxin, and cisplatin.

Pharmacodynamics is defined as the relationship between drug quantity and drug effect. Changes in pharmacodynamics caused by age are not as well understood as pharmacokinetic alterations, and little is known with respect to older dogs and cats. Many drugs have been shown to have a reduced effect in aged animals at a given tissue concentration. It is believed that this change occurs primarily at the molecular level, with reduction in receptor density and receptor function occurring with age. Conversely, certain drugs, especially drugs that have an effect on the central nervous system, can show a particular drug effect at a lower plasma concentration than that seen in the younger animal. In humans, the incidence of adverse drug effects is higher in the elderly. Whether this is caused primarily by alterations in a drug's pharmacokinetic profile or by some other mechanism(s) is not known.

DRUG THERAPY AND TREATMENT PLANS

In an effort to bring some order to the treatment plan for older dogs and cats, it may be useful to review some basic tenets of drug therapy[1]:

- Senior dogs and cats are not geriatric dogs and cats. There is an important difference between senior animals and geriatric animals.
- Identify causative factors involved in the disease process, including ruling out drug toxicity. It should always be remembered that older dogs and cats do not have one disease process occurring at a time but have multiple disease processes occurring at the same time within one or more body systems. Also, the more aged the dog or cat is, the more likely multiple diseases are occurring at the same time. For example, chronic renal failure has been documented in an older cat, but other disease processes may be occurring at the same time—for example, hyperthyroidism, systemic hypertension, inflammatory bowel disease, and diabetes mellitus. The veterinarian needs to avoid making diagnostic as well as therapeutic decisions based on the finding of a single disease process or problem.
- Consider using nondrug treatment plans. This is the least understood part of caring for older dogs and cats, but some alternative medicine approaches may be useful.
- Establish a treatment plan with the owner of the older dog or cat. Because many of the diseases managed in older dogs and cats are chronic and progressive, cures are not attainable —but control, at least for a period of time, *is* attainable.
- Choose initial drugs based on efficacy, cost, and ease of administration; assessment of animal-at-risk profile; matching of side-effect profile to the animal profile; and treatment plan for multiple diseases with one or more drugs.
- Choose initial drug dose based on the aphorism "Start low and go slow."
- Monitor drug therapy for efficacy and adverse effects. Drug therapy in older dogs and cats is often a double-edged sword. In geriatric humans, rates of adverse drug reactions are reported to be two to three times those seen in younger patients. There is no reason to believe that the same thing does not occur in older dogs and cats. Because often more than one disease is being treated and multiple drugs are being used, an increased potential for adverse drug interactions exists. Use therapeutic drug monitoring for drugs with narrow therapeutic windows.
- Determining the appropriate duration of therapy is extremely difficult to impossible. There is no right answer. When in doubt as to how long to treat an animal for a particular disease or diseases, always look to the animal being treated for the answer. Many times, the duration of therapy will be for a lifetime, with no other good choices.
- Avoid polypharmacy—using more drugs than are necessary—in older dogs and cats. Polypharmacy is a problem not only in human medicine but also in veterinary medicine. Polypharmacy may lead to increased morbidity and mortality secondary to drug-drug interactions, it may result in increased adverse effects, or the cost of therapy may lead to premature euthanasia.

ADVERSE DRUG EFFECTS EXPECTED

The goals of any treatment plan for the older dog or cat should be to alleviate pain, suffering, and disability; improve functional capacity; promote quality of life; and prolong life. Meeting these goals starts with selected diagnostic and therapeutic choices. The drug classes for which particular caution is advised when these drugs are used in older dogs and cats include the angiotensin converting enzyme inhibitors; aminoglycosides (aminoglycosides should not be used in older dogs and cats unless other antimicrobial agents are not indicated); antiarrhythmic agents; beta-blocking agents; calcium channel blocking agents; cardiac glycosides (especially digoxin); central nervous system and preanesthetic agents (especially benzodiazepines and opiates); coumarin anticoagulants; histamine-2 antagonists; nonsteroidal antiinflammatory drugs; and oncologic drugs. With the use of these drug classes, an increased potential for adverse drug interactions also exists. Use therapeutic drug monitoring for drugs with narrow therapeutic windows.

GUIDELINES FOR DRUG USE IN OLDER ANIMALS

Beyond the routine clinical management of a specific organ failure in the older dog and cat, the veterinarian should also be aware of specific drug use for the routine clinical management of immune-mediated diseases, acute and chronic pain, and systemic hypertension (see Chapter 10).

Immune-Mediated Disease Strategies

As an animal ages, its immune system may respond by being overreactive or underreactive. When the animal's immune system is overreactive, several different types of immune-mediated disease occur with increased frequency. The tissues and organ systems that react most dramatically in the sensitized animal are the mucous membranes of the mouth and lips, lacrimal gland, thyroid gland, parathyroid gland, esophagus, gastrointestinal tract, anus, liver, erythrocytes, leukocytes, blood platelets, muscles, joints, and nerves. Common examples of immune-mediated diseases in older dogs are keratoconjunctivitis sicca, hypothyroidism, immune-mediated hemolytic anemia, immune-mediated thrombocytopenia, glomerulonephritis, acquired myasthenia gravis, polymyositis, polyneuropathy, perianal fistulas, and immune-mediated skin disease. In addition, it is not unusual for several body systems in the sensitized dog to respond simultaneously with specific or nonspecific signs of immune-mediated disease. Often, a specific body system responds more pronouncedly than another body system. General principles about immune-mediated diseases in older dogs are as follows:

- A general rule in clinical medicine is that any tissue or organ of a sensitized animal can be attacked by the immune system, resulting in signs of immune-mediated disease related to that tissue or organ. No tissue or organ is completely free from immune-mediated disease and its effects in the older animal.
- Multiple immune-mediated diseases may occur simultaneously in older dogs. Many examples exist. Immune-mediated hemolytic anemia and immune-mediated thrombocytopenia often occur simultaneously. Canine hypothyroidism and keratoconjunctivitis sicca often occur simultaneously. Canine perianal fistulas, keratoconjunctivitis sicca, and hypothyroidism often occur simultaneously. Canine hypothyroidism, hypoparathyroidism, and hypoadrenocorticism may occur simultaneously in the older dog.
- When a diagnosis of an immune-mediated disease occurs, the veterinarian should investigate the possibility of a second or third immune-mediated disease occurring at the same time.

Medical management will never completely cure an immune-mediated disease in the dog or cat but will provide medical control and a reasonable quality of life for the animal. A treatment that seems to effect a medical cure may be causing only a brief remission from obvious signs of immune-mediated disease; relapses always occur. Therapies that may be used in the clinical management of immune-mediated diseases of older dogs and cats are presented in Table 5-1.

Infectious Agent Strategies

Most antimicrobial agents currently used in veterinary medicine have wide safety margins, and changes in dosage schedule more often reflect an attempt to save money or make drug delivery more convenient, not an attempt to make drug delivery safer. Most antimicrobial efficacy is correlated with time during which concentration is above the minimum inhibitory concentration of the pathogen. Changes in disposition of most antimicrobial drugs are due to a decrease in renal function, which prolongs the action of these agents and allows a decrease in dosage frequency.

If an animal is showing significant body changes consistent with aging, and renal function is unknown, it is better not to alter the antimicrobial administration schedule. Having available established serum creatinine values for the geriatric animal is very important. Veterinarians should establish baseline values for the dogs and cats before the animals are of geriatric age. A dog or cat that had a serum creatinine level of 1 mg/dl at 10 years of age and currently has a level of 2 mg/dl at 13 years of age has had a 50% reduction in glomerular filtration rate, even though a level of 2 mg/dl is within the normal range. One

TABLE 5-1. THERAPIES FOR IMMUNE-MEDIATED DISEASES

THERAPY	DOSAGE	COMMENTS
Prednisone*	Dog: 2.2-6.6 mg/kg PO; Cat: 4.4-8.8 mg/kg PO; Dosage depends on severity of the disease	Taper dose, and use alternate-day administration once active disease is resolved. Best results when used in conjunction with an additional immunosuppressive agent. Combination therapy may prolong remission and reduce side effects because of high glucocorticoid dosage. Adverse effects include secondary cutaneous and urinary tract infections, demodicosis, diabetes mellitus, gastroduodenal ulcers, leukopenia, hepatopathy, nephropathy, hypertension, electrolyte disturbances, calcinosis cutis (dogs), and skin fragility (cats).
Glucocorticoid pulse therapy	Dog: IV methylprednisolone sodium succinate at 11 mg/kg daily in 250 ml of 5% dextrose and water during a 1-h period for 3 consecutive days	Administer for 3 days in dogs; then, intermediate to low glucocorticoid therapy ± immunosuppressive drugs. Adverse effects include cardiac arrhythmias, pancreatitis, diabetes mellitus, and gastroduodenal ulcers.
Topical glucocorticoids	Dog and cat: hydrocortisone cream; 0.1% betamethasone valerate, flucinolone acetate, or amcinonide	Used for localized lesions and induces cutaneous atrophy.
Azathioprine	Dog: 1.5-2.5 mg/kg every 48 h; contraindicated in cats; used in combination with glucocorticoids	Adverse effects include anemia, leukopenia, thrombocytopenia, hemorrhagic diarrhea, pancreatitis, and hepatotoxicity. Long-term therapy is associated with recurrent skin infections and demodicosis.
Gold therapy or chrysotherapy. Oral form: auranofin Injectable form: aurothioglucose	Dog and cat: Auranofin: 0.12-0.2 mg/kg PO bid; aurothioglucose: 1 mg/kg IM once weekly	Used in combination with glucocorticoids. Adverse effects include bone marrow suppression, nephrotoxicity, and drug eruptions, such as erythema multiforme and toxic epidermal necrolysis.
Chlorambucil	Dog and cat: 0.1-0.2 mg/kg PO every 24 to 48 h	Used in combination with glucocorticoids. Adverse effects include hepatotoxicity and bone marrow suppression.
Cyclophosphamide	Dog and cat: 1-2 mg/kg PO once daily	Always used in combination with glucocorticoids. Stop administration if white blood cell count falls below 500 μL. Adverse effects include bone marrow suppression, teratogenicity, and increased risk of malignancies.
Cyclosporine	Dog and cat: 5-10 mg/kg PO bid for 2 weeks and then adjusted to maintain a therapeutic blood concentration of 400 to 600 ng/ml.	Adverse effects include GI signs, hepatotoxicity, nephrotoxicity, gingival hyperplasia, and papillomatous dermatitis. Drugs that suppress cytochrome P-450 activity may cause potential cyclosporine toxicity.
Dapsone	Dog: 1 mg/kg PO bid-tid	Used in combination with glucocorticoids. Do not use in cats. If agranulocytosis appears, administration should be discontinued. Adverse effects include hemolysis, methemoglobinemia, neuropathies, and hypoalbuminemia.
Tetracycline and niacinamide	Dogs >10 kg: 500 mg of each drug PO tid Dogs <10 kg: 250 mg of each drug PO tid Dogs <5 kg: 100 mg of each drug PO tid	Alternative therapy for milder cases of pemphigus foliaceus and pemphigus erythematosus. Adverse effects include vomiting, diarrhea, anorexia, and increased serum liver enzymes activity.
Mycophenolate mofetil	20-30 mg/kg PO once daily	Usually well tolerated. Adverse effects include bone marrow suppression and GI upset.

bid, Twice daily; *GI,* gastrointestinal; *IM,* intramuscular; *IV,* intravenous; *PO,* orally; *tid,* three times daily.
*Equivalences to 5 mg prednisone: Dexamethasone, 0.5 mg; triamcinolone, 1 mg; methyl prednisone, 4 mg.

recommendation would be to change the administration interval, such as changing to twice daily from three times daily or to once daily from twice daily.

Veterinarians should take more care when determining dosage for aminoglycosides. If the veterinarian is unsure of renal function, once-daily administration at 6 to 8 mg/kg of gentamicin or 10 to 12 mg/kg of amikacin should be used. This dosage strategy is preferable both for improved efficacy and decreased renal toxicity. Aminoglycoside efficacy is correlated with a high serum concentration, and its toxicity is inversely related to frequency of administration.

Antiinflammatory Strategies

As a group, nonsteroidal antiinflammatory drugs are used more often and for longer periods of time in the elderly than in any other age group. These drugs have a high incidence of undesirable side effects, including gastrointestinal upset, ulceration, and prolonged bleeding. Their use in animals with decreased renal function may be associated with worsening of renal function. This association is due to the increased role of prostaglandins in maintaining renal blood flow in the compromised kidney. Nonsteroidal antiinflammatory drugs should be started at the lowest possible dose and dosage regimen. Gradually increase first the frequency and then the amount over weeks. Loss of appetite is a clinical sign of gastrointestinal upset and indicates that treatment should be stopped for 1 day and resumed at one-half the previous dose. An alternative is to combine the nonsteroidal antiinflammatory drugs with misoprostol at 2 to 4 μg/kg twice daily or three times daily as a protectorate. It does not provide any gastrointestinal protection in human patients with chronic renal disease. Therefore, dosing frequency should be reduced in dogs with suspected renal dysfunction. Although many nonsteroidal antiinflammatory drugs do not show alterations in elimination in the elderly, their dynamic effects seem more pronounced. Do not use a cytoprotectorant such as sucralfate in combination with nonsteroidal antiinflammatory drugs, as absorption is greatly impaired and efficacy reduced.

Anesthesia and Analgesic Strategies

Pain is significant in older dogs and cats.[2] Management directed toward pain management should be addressed in each animal requiring medical or surgical care (Tables 5-2 and 5-3).[3] The use of opioid agonists-antagonists or opioid agonists is more commonly done now (Table 5-4). The sedative effects of analgesic drugs may be enhanced in the geriatric animal as a function of age-related changes in pharmacodynamics and alteration of cognitive pathways. It is better to use a smaller amount of a drug more frequently than to try to prolong the action by increasing the dose. Optimizing a dose for oxymorphone involves administering 0.01 mg/kg every 5 to 10 minutes until the animal is quiet and comfortable. The total dose used is determined, and this amount can then be given every 3 to 4 hours as needed. No drugs require as much individualization as pain relievers. There are no standard doses, only standard dose ranges. The more pronounced sedative effect of these agents in the elderly should not deter the veterinarian from using these agents; instead, they should be used with care.

CHRONIC MEDICATION AND INFORMATION CHART

All animals receiving chronic medication should have a physical examination at least annually before any medication prescriptions are refilled (Table 5-5).

TRANSFUSION MEDICINE

Transfusion medicine is another important component in the management of clinical diseases in older dogs and cats.[4]

Individual Components

Fresh whole blood should be administered within 6 hours for maximal effect of coagulation proteins and platelets. Stored whole blood is refrigerated at 4° to 6° C after collection. Packed red blood cells are red blood cells that are separated from plasma using centrifugation, sedimentation, or plasma extraction, and stored at 4° to 6° C. Packed red blood cells should be resuspended with 100 ml 0.9% saline solution prior to administration to prevent sludging. Currently, most blood banks add a red cell nutrient solution to prolong storage and shelf life up to 42 days for most commercially available red cell products. This can also be accomplished in the hospital with use of special collection bags containing this solution. These prepared red blood cells do not need to be resuspended with any additional fluid.

Fresh plasma is plasma extracted from red blood cells within 6 hours and used within 24 hours of collection. Plasma is best extracted using special collection systems and blood bank centrifuge. Gravity sedimentation of red blood cells also allows plasma to be extracted if needed. Fresh frozen plasma is plasma extracted from red blood cells within 6 hours and frozen at −20° C or below (ideal is −70° C) for up to 1 year. After 1 year of storage this product should be relabeled as frozen plasma. Frozen plasma is plasma extracted from red blood cells more than 6 hours after collection

TABLE 5-2. PAIN ASSESSMENT SCALE FOR OLDER DOGS AND CATS

SCORE	ANIMAL BEHAVIOR AND SIGNS	ACTION—RECORD PAIN SCORE AND NOTIFY VETERINARIAN IF 3 OR ABOVE
0 No pain	Bright, bouncy, responsive, self-grooming; normal mobility; dreaming sleep	None
1 Probably no pain	Appears normal; not as clear-cut as above; possible increased heart rate	None
2 Mild discomfort	Eats and sleeps but may not dream; may limp or resist palpation of affected area; increased heart rate and respiration rate may be present	Reassess hourly; if worse give analgesic
3 Mild pain or discomfort	Limps or guards affected area (e.g., tenses abdomen); slightly depressed; restlessness with or without trembling; increased heart rate, respiration rate; cats may still purr; dogs may wag tail	Needs analgesic— 1. NSAID and/or butorphanol (0.1 ml/kg every 6 to 12 h) OR 2. Repeat morphine if wearing off from previous use; do not give butorphanol and morphine
4 Mild to moderate pain	Resists touch of affected area; may look or chew at area; abnormal body position; may not move for hours, with or without trembling, appetite change, increased and shallow respiration rate, and increased heart rate; may give occasional whimper or cry; pupils may be dilated	1. Morphine—dogs, 0.3 mg/kg; cats, 0.1 mg/kg IM or SC 2. Butorphanol (0.15 ml per 5 kg every 4 to 12 h) OR 3. NSAID OR 4. NSAID plus morphine if opioid has already been given
5 Moderate pain	Depressed, trembling, head down, inappetent; may cry or bite if approached or moved or if affected area is touched; marked splinting or prayer position if abdomen is affected; possibly increased heart and respiration rate; animal does not sleep	1. Morphine—dogs, 0.3 to 0.5 mg/kg 2. Butorphanol (0.2 ml per 5 kg every 4 to 8 h; cats, 0.15 mg/kg every 3 to 6 h) 3. NSAID 4. Opioid plus NSAID
6 As above	Animal may cry or whine frequently without provocation; cats may still purr; dogs may wag tail	1. Morphine—dogs, 0.5 mg/kg; cats, 0.2 mg/kg; every 3 to 6 h OR 2. NSAID as appropriate OR 3. Both
7 Moderate to severe pain	As above. Animal is very depressed; will urinate and defecate without moving; will cry if moved, may continually whimper	As above, but higher doses of opioid
8 Severe pain	As above, but with more vocalizing; animal is more depressed and unaware of surroundings; may thrash about intermittently; with traumatic or neurologic pain may scream (especially cats) if approached; usually there is an increased heart rate and increased respiratory rate with increased abdominal effort even if opioids were previously given	1. High dose morphine 2. Plus NSAID as appropriate
9 Severe to excruciating pain	As above, but animal is hyperesthetic, trembles involuntarily if touched close to affected area; neurologic pain or severe inflammation anywhere; this degree of pain can cause death	1. High dose morphine plus NSAID 2. Plus epidural or local analgesic 3. Anesthetic while treating inciting cause
10 Excruciating pain	As above, but animal is screaming or almost comatose; animal is hyperesthetic or hyperalgesic; whole body trembles and animal reacts in pain wherever you touch it; this degree of pain can cause death	Very high doses of opioids do not relieve this pain, but give the following: 1. Morphine—dogs, 1 mg/kg; cats, 0.2 mg/kg or until effective 2. Plus NSAID 3. Plus epidural or nerve blocks OR 4. General anesthesia to treat cause

IM, Intramuscular; *NSAID,* nonsteroidal antiinflammatory drug; *SC,* subcutaneous.
NSAIDs are excellent for treatment of musculoskeletal pain and soft-tissue inflammation. Do not give if animal is bleeding, dehydrated, or hypotensive, or has signs of gastrointestinal tract disease or ulceration or severe pulmonary disease.

TABLE 5-3. SUGGESTED DOSES FOR ANESTHETIC AND ANALGESIC AGENTS

AGENT	DOSAGE	COMMENTS
Anticholinergics		
Atropine	0.02 to 0.04 mg/kg IV, IM, SC	Recommended to offset dominant parasympathetic effects and maintain heart rate, cardiac output, and blood pressure. Also decreases airway secretions.
Glycopyrrolate	0.01 mg/kg IV, IM	Glycopyrrolate does not cross the blood-brain barrier, takes longer to onset of action, and has increased duration compared with atropine.
Tranquilizers and Sedatives		
Diazepam	0.2 to 0.4 mg/kg IV, IM	Propylene glycol carrier makes uptake unpredictable from IM site. Will not mix in same syringe with any drug, except ketamine.
Midazolam	0.1 to 0.2 mg/kg IV, IM, SC	Water-soluble. More potent and shorter acting than diazepam. Mixes with other agents. May cause excitement on recovery in some cats.
Acepromazine	0.025 to 0.05 mg/kg IM, SC	2 mg maximum. Requires hepatic degradation. Potentiates hypotension and hypothermia. Does not provide analgesia and is not reversible. Best to dilute to 1 mg/ml solution.
α_2 Agonists		
Xylazine	1 to 2 mg/kg IM	Requires hepatic degradation and causes marked bradycardia and decreased cardiac output. Reversible.
Medetomidine	20 to 30 g/kg IM	May cause vomiting. Always use with an anticholinergic agent. Medetomidine is more potent and longer acting than xylazine.
Opioids		
Meperidine	1 to 2 mg/kg IM Epidural: 0.5-1.5 mg/kg	Mild analgesia. May cause histamine release if injected IV. Reversible.
Morphine	0.2 to 1 mg/kg IM, SC Epidural: 0.1 mg/kg in 1 ml per 10-lb volume of saline solution	Analgesia with sedation and cardiopulmonary depression. Administer with an anticholinergic. Potentiates hypothermia. Most common agent used for epidural analgesia. Reversible.
Oxymorphone	0.05 to 0.2 mg/kg IV, IM, SC Epidural: 0.1 mg/kg in 1 ml per 10-lb volume of saline solution	4 mg maximum. Analgesia with sedation. Causes panting. Administer with an anticholinergic agent. Commonly combined with acepromazine in animals older than 12 weeks of age for neuroleptanalgesia. Can be used for epidural analgesia. Reversible.
Fentanyl	2 to 4 g/kg IV CRI: 2 to 4 g/kg/h IV Transdermal patch: 2.5 to 10 kg—use 25-g patch (all or part) 10 to 20 kg—use 50-g patch 20 to 30 kg—use 75-g patch Epidural: 1-10 μg/kg in 1 ml per 10-lb volume of saline solution	Very potent analgesic. Rapid onset and short duration of action. Minimal cardiopulmonary effects. Can be delivered by a variety of routes, including epidural. Reversible.
Buprenorphine	0.01 to 0.02 mg/kg IV, IM, SC	30 to 45 minutes to onset of action; long duration due to slow rate of dissociation from receptor; unpredictable reversal with opioid antagonists.
Butorphanol	0.2 to 0.4 mg/kg IV, IM, SC CRI: 0.2 to 0.4 mg/kg/h IV	Agonist-antagonist. Minimal cardiopulmonary depression. Good visceral analgesia. Used to reverse agonist adverse effects and preserve analgesia.
Intravenous Anesthetics		
Thiopental	4 to 6 mg/kg IV, until effective	Ultra–short-acting thiobarbiturate. Termination of action depends on redistribution and hepatic degradation. May cause dysrythmia. Respiratory depression is common, be prepared to intubate and ventilate.
Methohexital	4 to 6 mg/kg IV, until effective	Ultra–short-acting oxybarbiturate. Terminated by redistribution with minimal hepatic metabolism. May cause excitement on induction and recovery. Be prepared to intubate and ventilate.
Propofol	2 to 6 mg/kg IV, until effective CRI: 10 to 12 mg/kg/h IV	Alkyl phenol. Do not bolus; give slowly, over several minutes. Ultra–short-acting; rapid onset, rapid recovery. Noncumulative, can be used as CRI without prolonged recovery. Be prepared to intubate and ventilate.

Continued

TABLE 5-3. SUGGESTED DOSES FOR ANESTHETIC AND ANALGESIC AGENTS—cont'd

AGENT	DOSAGE	COMMENTS
Intravenous Anesthetics—cont'd		
Etomidate	1 to 2 mg/kg IV CRI: 2 to 4 mg/kg/h IV	Nonbarbiturate. No cardiopulmonary effects. May cause nausea, vomiting, myoclonus, excitement on induction and recovery. Noncumulative, can be used as constant rate infusion.
Ketamine	1 to 2 mg/kg IV 11 to 22 mg/kg IM	Dissociative anesthetic. Excessive salivation controlled with anticholinergic agents. Increases intracranial and intraocular pressures. May cause seizures. Elimination depends on renal and hepatic function.
Telazol	1 to 2 mg/kg IV 5 to 13 mg/kg IM	Contains 1:1 tiletamine, a dissociative anesthetic, and zolazepam, a benzodiazepine. Tiletamine is more potent and longer lasting than ketamine. Zolazepam effects may be prolonged in some cats and cause rough recovery.

IV, Intravenous administration; *IM*, intramuscular administration; *SC*, subcutaneous administration; *CRI*, constant rate infusion.

TABLE 5-4. SUGGESTED DOSES FOR TRANQUILIZER AND SEDATIVE ANTAGONIST AGENTS

AGENT	ANTAGONISTIC EFFECTS	DOSE	COMMENTS
Flumazenil	Benzodiazepines	0.1 mg/kg IV to effect	Duration short—1 h in adults; may have agonist effects at high dose
Yohimbine	α_2 receptors	0.25 to 0.5 mg/kg IM; 0.15 mg/kg IV until effective	May cause excitement after IV administration
Atipamazole	α_2 receptors	0.2 to 0.4 mg/kg IM	Most effective reversal agent
Tolazoline	α_1 and α_2 receptors	0.3 mg/kg IV until effective	
Naloxone	Pure narcotic antagonist	0.04 to 0.4 mg IV until effective	Short duration—0.5 to 1.5 h ; animals may renarcotize
Naltrexone	Pure narcotic antagonist	0.04 mg/kg IV	8 to 12 h duration; most effective for reversal of central effects related to epidural opioid administration
Nalmefene	Pure narcotic antagonist	0.1 to 0.2 mg/kg IV or IM	8 to 10 h duration
Butorphanol	Narcotic agonist-antagonist	0.2 mg/kg IV, IM, SC	Used to reverse bradycardia and respiratory depression of agonists while maintaining analgesia
Nalbuphine	Narcotic agonist-antagonist	0.5 to 2 mg/kg IV, IM, SC	Lasts 2 to 4 h; less potent analgesic than butorphanol

IM, Intramuscular administration; *IV*, intravenous administration; *SC*, subcutaneous administration.

and frozen, or fresh frozen plasma that has been stored longer than 1 year or at temperatures greater than –20° C.

Platelet rich plasma and platelet concentrate are concentrated platelet products that are manufactured from successive centrifugation of fresh plasma. The process is complex and requires a blood banking centrifuge. Cryoprecipitate is a concentrated clotting factor product rich in factor VIII and von Willebrand factor, fibrinogen, and fibronectin. It is manufactured by thawing fresh frozen plasma at 1° to 6° C until slushy or until approximately 90% of volume is liquid, then centrifuging at 5 g for 5 minutes or using gravity to extract liquid plasma. Both components (cryoprecipitate and supernatant cryoprecipitate) can be refrozen at –20° C or below (ideal –70° C) for up until 1 year after collection of plasma. If vasopressin is administered to the blood donor at 0.6 μg/kg diluted in 10 ml of sterile saline solution intravenously over 10 minutes approximately 30 minutes before collection, the yield of factor VIII and von Willebrand factor can be improved.

Canine Red Blood Cells

Typing the recipient is strongly encouraged, so that DEA 1.1- and 1.2-positive donors can be used in transfusion programs and so that the blood is correctly directed to positive recipients. Commercial typing cards check only for DEA 1.1. Dogs who are autoagglutinating should always receive negative blood, because the typing cards

(Text continued on p. 56)

TABLE 5-5. CHRONIC MEDICATION AND INFORMATION CHART

DRUG NAME	TESTS NEEDED	TESTING FREQUENCY	REASON FOR TESTING	FAST FOR 8 HOURS BEFORE TESTING	SPECIAL TIMING FOR TESTS	SPECIAL INFORMATION/ OWNER SHOULD CALL IF:
Acepromazine	Serum chemistry profile	Every 12 months	Check for liver dysfunction via serum liver enzymes	Yes	No	Can cause hypotension, especially in animals with preexisting cardiac disease; can cause excessive sedation, seizures
Amitriptyline	Behavioral evaluation	Every 3 months	Monitor for gradual or sudden behavioral changes	No	No	Sedation, dryness of mouth, rapid heart rate, poor grooming
Aspirin	CBC	Every 6 months	Check for anemia	Yes	No	Vomiting, diarrhea, weakness, decreased appetite, increased lethargy, sudden loss of stamina
Atenolol	Serum chemistry profile	Every 6 months	Monitor for liver and kidney dysfunction and electrolyte disorders	Yes	No	Changes in behavior, weakness
	Lead II ECG	Every 6 months	Monitor progression of heart disease and arrhythmias	No	No	
Benazepril	Serum chemistry profile	Every 6 months	Check for azotemia and electrolyte disorder; should use in advancing kidney disease and can cause sodium loss	Yes	No	Give on an empty stomach; vomiting, diarrhea, weakness, decreased appetite, increased lethargy, coughing, sudden loss of stamina
	CBC	Every 12 months	Check for anemia or hemoconcentration	Yes	No	
	Lead II ECG	Every 6 months	Monitor progression of heart disease	No	No	
Buspirone	Behavioral evaluation	Every 3 months	Monitor for gradual or sudden behavioral changes	No	No	Aggression, poor grooming
Captopril	Serum chemistry profile	Every 6 months	Check for azotemia and electrolyte disorder; should use in advancing kidney disease and can cause sodium loss	Yes	No	Give on an empty stomach; vomiting, diarrhea, weakness, decreased appetite, increased lethargy, coughing, sudden loss of stamina
	CBC	Every 12 months	Check for anemia or hemoconcentration	Yes	No	
	Lead II ECG	Every 6 months	Monitor progression of heart disease	No	No	
Carprofen	Serum chemistry profile	Every 3-6 months	Monitor for liver and kidney dysfunction	Yes	No	Vomiting, diarrhea, weakness, decreased appetite, increased lethargy, sudden loss of stamina, seizures, skin eruptions
Chlorpheniramine	CBC and serum chemistry profile	Every 12 months	May cause changes in the liver	Yes	No	May cause transient depression and atropine-like signs
Clomipramine	Behavioral evaluation	Every 3 months	Monitor for gradual or sudden behavioral changes	No	No	Sedation, dryness of mouth, rapid heart rate, poor grooming
Cyclosporine	Ocular pressures and Schirmer tear tests	Every 4-6 months	May not be working properly; may cause eye irritation; may cause increase in serum liver enzymes	No	No eye-drops for last 3-4 h	Owner should avoid contact with medication; medication has to be used regularly as prescribed

CBC, Complete blood count; *ECG*, electrocardiogram.

Continued

TABLE 5-5. CHRONIC MEDICATION AND INFORMATION CHART—cont'd

DRUG NAME	TESTS NEEDED	TESTING FREQUENCY	REASON FOR TESTING	FAST FOR 8 HOURS BEFORE TESTING	SPECIAL TIMING FOR TESTS	SPECIAL INFORMATION/ OWNER SHOULD CALL IF:
Diazepam	Serum chemistry profile	Every 6 months	Check for liver and kidney dysfunction; contraindicated in liver and kidney disease	Yes	No	Scheduled drug—login required; may cause too much sedation and increased appetite; may cause hyperexcitation
	Diazepam serum levels	Every 6 months	Check for adequate therapeutic levels	Yes	4-6 hours after pilling	
Diethylstilbestrol	Serum chemistry profile	Every 6 months	Check for liver or kidney dysfunction	Yes	No	May cause vomiting, diarrhea, lethargy, abnormal bruising or bleeding, polyuria-polydipsia
Digoxin	Serum chemistry profile	Every 6 months	Check for liver and kidney dysfunction and electrolyte disorder	Yes	No	Give on an empty stomach; vomiting, diarrhea, weakness, decreased appetite, increased lethargy, coughing, sudden loss of stamina
	CBC	Every 6 months	Check for anemia or hemoconcentration	Yes	No	
	Digoxin serum level	Every 6 months	Ensure adequate dosage	Yes	8 h after last dose	
	Lead II ECG	Every 6 months	Monitor progression of heart disease and check for ECG signs of toxicity	No	No	
Diltiazam	Serum chemistry profile	Every 6 months	Check for liver dysfunction	Yes	No	Decreased appetite, weakness, increased lethargy, coughing, sudden loss of stamina
	CBC	Every 12 months	Check for anemia or hemoconcentration	Yes	No	
	Lead II ECG	Every 6 months	Monitor progression of heart disease	No	No	
Enalapril	Serum chemistry profile	Every 6 months	Check for azotemia and electrolyte disorder; should use in advancing kidney disease and can cause sodium loss	Yes	No	Vomiting, diarrhea, weakness, decreased appetite, increased lethargy, coughing, sudden loss of stamina
	CBC	Every 12 months	Check for anemia or hemoconcentration	Yes	No	
	Lead II ECG	Every 6 months	Monitor progression of heart disease	No	No	
Fludrocortisone	Serum chemistry profile	Every 3-4 months	Monitor sodium and potassium levels and for liver dysfunction	Yes	No	Vomiting, diarrhea, decreased appetite, increased lethargy
Fluoxetine	Serum chemistry profile	Every 3 months	Monitor for liver and kidney dysfunction	Yes	No	Restlessness, insomnia, weight loss
Furosemide	Serum chemistry profile	Every 6 months	Check for liver and kidney dysfunction and electrolyte disorder; can cause potassium loss	Yes	No	Vomiting, diarrhea, decreased appetite, increased lethargy, polyuria-polydipsia, dehydration
	CBC	Every 12 months	Check for anemia, hemoconcentration, and leukopenia	Yes	No	

TABLE 5-5. CHRONIC MEDICATION AND INFORMATION CHART—cont'd

DRUG NAME	TESTS NEEDED	TESTING FREQUENCY	REASON FOR TESTING	FAST FOR 8 HOURS BEFORE TESTING	SPECIAL TIMING FOR TESTS	SPECIAL INFORMATION/ OWNER SHOULD CALL IF:
Hydralazine	Serum chemistry profile	Every 6 months	Check for kidney dysfunction	Yes	No	Give with food; vomiting, diarrhea, decreased appetite, increased lethargy
	CBC	Every 12 months	Check for anemia, monitor bone marrow function (may cause depression)	Yes	No	
	Lead II ECG	Every 6 months	Monitor progression of heart disease	No	No	
Hydrocodone	Serum chemistry profile	Every 6 months	Monitor for liver and kidney dysfunction	Yes	No	Scheduled drug—login required; sedation, constipation, vomiting, increased coughing
Insulin	Serum chemistry profile	Every 6 months	Monitor for liver and kidney dysfunction	Yes	No	Weakness, lethargy, vomiting, incoordination, disorientation, polyuria-polydipsia
	Blood glucose curve	Every 6 months	Monitor insulin metabolism and effects	No	Give insulin at usual time	
	Urinalysis	Every 6 months	Check for glucose and ketones and for urinary tract infection	No	No	
Methimazole	Serum chemistry profile	Every 3-6 months	Monitor for liver dysfunction	Yes	No	Vomiting, diarrhea, decreased appetite, lethargy, weight loss
	CBC	Every 3-6 months	Monitor for anemia, leukopenia, and thrombocytopenia	Yes	No	
Mitotane	ACTH response test	Every 6 months	Monitor for proper dosage and adrenal gland function	No	Must stay in hospital at least 3 hours	Use with caution in animals with liver or kidney disease; vomiting, diarrhea, decreased appetite, increased lethargy, incoordination, polyuria-polydipsia
	Serum chemistry profile	Every 6 months	Monitor for liver and kidney dysfunction	Yes	No	
	CBC	Every 12 months	Monitor bone marrow function	Yes	No	
	Urinalysis	Every 6 months	Check for urinary tract infection	No	No	
D-Penicillamine	CBC	Every 6 months	Check for anemia and leukopenia	Yes	No	Vomiting, weakness, decreased appetite, increased lethargy, loss of stamina
Phenobarbital	Serum chemistry profile	Every 6 months	Check for liver and kidney dysfunction	Yes	No	Scheduled drug—login required; anxiety or depression, increased appetite, polyuria-polydipsia
	CBC	Every 12 months	Check for anemia	No	No	
	Phenobarbital serum level	Every 12 months or more often if seizures are not adequately controlled	Ensure safe but adequate blood levels being obtained; serum levels should be 15-40 μg/ml	Yes	Before first tablet in morning	
	Fasting and postprandial bile acids	Every 12 months	Monitor for liver dysfunction	Yes	No	

ACTH, Adrenocorticotropic hormone.

Continued

TABLE 5-5. CHRONIC MEDICATION AND INFORMATION CHART—cont'd

DRUG NAME	TESTS NEEDED	TESTING FREQUENCY	REASON FOR TESTING	FAST FOR 8 HOURS BEFORE TESTING	SPECIAL TIMING FOR TESTS	SPECIAL INFORMATION/ OWNER SHOULD CALL IF:
Phenylbutazone	Serum chemistry profile	Every 6 months	Check for liver and kidney dysfunction; can cause toxic changes	Yes	No	Give with food; vomiting, diarrhea, weakness, unusual bleeding or bruising
	CBC	Every 6 months	Can cause changes in the bone marrow	Yes	No	
Phenylpropanolamine	Serum chemistry profile	Every 12 months	Check blood glucose (can cause problems in diabetics) and for liver dysfunction	Yes	No	Restlessness, anxiousness, decreased appetite, urinary incontinence
	Urinalysis	Every 12 months	Monitor for ability to concentrate urine and check for urinary tract infection	No	No	
Piroxicam	CBC	Every month	Monitor for anemia	Yes	No	Give with food; vomiting, diarrhea, weakness, decreased appetite, increased lethargy, sudden loss of stamina
Potassium bromide	Serum chemistry profile	Every 6 months	Monitor for liver and kidney dysfunction	Yes	No	Give with food; can cause sedation, weakness; can take up to 4 months to achieve therapeutic levels
	Potassium bromide serum level	6 weeks after initiation of therapy and then every 6 months	Check adequate or toxic levels of potassium bromide; serum levels should be 1-2 mg/ml (100-200 mg/dl)	Yes	Before first dose in the morning	
Prednisolone or prednisone	Serum chemistry profile	Every 12 months	Monitor for liver dysfunction and electrolyte disorders	Yes	No	Give with food; increased polyuria-polydipsia, hair loss, weakness, significant changes in body weight, panting, behavioral change
	CBC	Every 12 months	Monitor for altered white blood cell levels	Yes	No	
Primidone	Serum chemistry profile	Every 6 months	Check for liver and kidney dysfunction	Yes	No	Scheduled drug—login required; anxiety or depression, increased appetite, polyuria-polydipsia
	CBC	Every 12 months	Check for anemia	No	No	
	Phenobarbital serum level	Every 12 months or more often if seizures are not adequately controlled	Ensure safe but adequate blood levels being obtained; phenobarbital serum levels should be measured to estimate anticonvulsant effect	Yes	Before first tablet in morning	
	Fasting and postprandial bile acids	Every 12 months	Monitor for liver dysfunction	Yes	No	

TABLE 5-5. CHRONIC MEDICATION AND INFORMATION CHART—cont'd

DRUG NAME	TESTS NEEDED	TESTING FREQUENCY	REASON FOR TESTING	FAST FOR 8 HOURS BEFORE TESTING	SPECIAL TIMING FOR TESTS	SPECIAL INFORMATION/ OWNER SHOULD CALL IF:
Propranolol	Serum chemistry profile	Every 6 months	Monitor for liver and kidney dysfunction and electrolyte disorders	Yes	No	Changes in behavior, weakness
	Lead II ECG	Every 6 months	Monitor progression of heart disease and arrhythmias	No	No	
Selegiline (Deprenyl)	Serum chemistry profile	Every 3 months	Check for liver and kidney dysfunction	Yes	No	Vomiting, diarrhea, weakness, depression, decreased appetite
	CBC	Every 3 months	Check for anemia, white blood cell changes, and thrombocytopenia	Yes	No	
Sulfasalazine	Serum chemistry profile	Every 6 months	Check for liver and kidney dysfunction	Yes	No	Eyes are especially sensitive; causes redness or chronic gummy discharge; weakness, depression, decreased appetite
	CBC	Every 6 months	Check for anemia, white blood cell changes, and thrombocytopenia	Yes	No	
	Ocular pressures and Schirmer tear tests	Every 3 months	Check the eyes for normal intraocular pressures and normal tear production	No	No	
Terbutaline	Serum electrolytes	Every month for first 3 months and then every 6 months	Can cause potassium loss	Yes	No	Weakness, depression, decreased appetite
	Lead II ECG	Every 6 months	Monitor for heart disease and arrhythmias	No	No	
Theophylline	Serum chemistry profile	Every 12 months	Monitor for liver and kidney dysfunction	Yes	No	Vomiting, diarrhea, excitement, increased coughing
L-Thyroxine	Serum T_4	Every month for the first 3 months and then every 12 months	Monitor serum T_4 levels for adequate dosing; requirement may change as animal ages	Yes	6-8 h after medication given	Weight gain, extreme weight loss, excitement, restlessness, constant panting
Tylosin	Serum chemistry profile	Every 12 months	Monitor for liver dysfunction	Yes	No	Vomiting, diarrhea, loss of appetite
	CBC	Every 12 months	Monitor red blood cell and white blood cell levels	Yes	No	

are difficult to interpret when autoagglutination is present. Bitches that have whelped and any dog that that has received a transfusion more than 7 days previously should have a cross-match performed prior to transfusion.

Feline Red Blood Cells

Typing felines prior to transfusion is mandatory. Type B blood is rarely stored, but ideally cat type B blood from such breeds as the rex, British shorthair, and Maine coon should be available to the veterinary practice to donate as needed. If type A red cells are given to a type B cat, the results are catastrophic. If autoagglutination is present in the recipient, and interpretation of the card typing results is not clear, then cross-matching is mandatory to attempt to identify incompatibility.

ADMINISTRATION OF RED CELL PRODUCTS

Packed red blood cells that have not been stored in nutrient solutions should be resuspended with sterile saline or non–calcium-containing crystalloid fluids. All red cell products should be administered through a blood administration filter (170 μm) using a nonrotary fluid administration pump (peristaltic flow pumps are acceptable). Before a transfusion is begun, measurements of baseline rectal temperature, pulse rate, respiratory rate, packed cell volume (PCV), and total solids should be obtained. Initial rate of administration should be slow (0.25 ml/kg hourly) for 15 to 20 minutes to monitor for transfusion reaction. Animals should be monitored carefully during transfusion. The calculated dose of red blood cell product should be administered within 4 hours of puncturing the donation bag. The dose of red blood cells to administer to an anemic animal should be calculated as follows:

$$\text{Dose (ml)} = 80 \text{ (Dogs) or } 70 \text{ (Cats)} \times \text{Body weight (kg)} \times \frac{\text{Desired change in PCV}}{\text{PCV transfused blood}}$$

Total daily doses of red blood cell products should not exceed 22 ml/kg/day, unless severe ongoing losses are occurring (do not exceed 22 ml/kg hourly except in the case of massive hemorrhage). If risk of volume overload is present, then maximum administration rate should be 4 ml/kg hourly. In animals with congestive heart failure and anemia the maximum administration rate should be 5 ml/kg/day. Animals that are experiencing severe and rapid blood loss should receive red blood cell products as rapidly as needed to maintain adequate circulating volumes. Slow initial rates of transfusion are usually not used in emergency situations. The packed cell volume and total solids should always be performed within 60 to 90 minutes after completion of the transfusion to determine response.

ADMINISTRATION OF PLASMA PRODUCTS

Typing and cross-matching as discussed above is not relevant to plasma transfusion for either dogs or cats. All plasma products should be thawed at a constant temperature (37° C) and administered through a blood administration filter (170 μm) using a fluid administration pump (peristaltic flow and rotary type pumps are acceptable). The animal's baseline rectal temperature, pulse rate, respiratory rate, PCV, and total solids should be measured before a transfusion is begun. Initial rate of administration should be slow (0.25 ml/kg hourly) for 15 to 20 minutes to monitor for transfusion reaction. Animals should be monitored carefully during transfusion. The calculated dose of plasma product should be administered within 4 hours of puncturing the donation bag. The dose of plasma product to administer should be 6 to 8 ml/kg two to three times per day as required. Cryoprecipitate should be administered at 1 unit per 10 to 20 kg, and the animal should be monitored hourly after transfusion to detect ongoing bleeding or serum activated PTT concentration. Additional transfusions are administered as required to control hemorrhage.

COMPLICATIONS

Acute Intravascular Hemolysis

Acute intravascular hemolysis is the most severe type of transfusion reaction and results in hemoglobinemia and hemoglobinuria. Signs may include restlessness, anxiety, nausea, muscle tremors, urticaria, fever, tachycardia, tachypnea, and seizures. Acute death, thromboembolic disease, or acute renal failure are possible sequelae. The most common situations in which this would occur include those in which type A blood is given to a type B cat, or DEA 1.1/1.2 blood is given to a negative dog previously sensitized to DEA 1.1/1.2-positive blood through previous transfusion or breeding (negative female dog bred to positive male with exposure to positive fetal blood during whelping). Transfusion should be discontinued immediately. Supportive care includes renal diuresis and corticosteroids. Urinary alkalization may assist in removing erythrocytic membrane stroma. Plasmapheresis would be ideal but is not readily available.

Acute Nonhemolytic Reaction

This transfusion reaction is manifested by urticaria, pruritus, fever, or anaphylaxis. Most of the time, the reaction is directed against an incompatible antigen located on the platelet or white blood cell remnants or some plasma protein component. Anaphylaxis should be treated with aggressive fluid resuscitation, corticosteroids, and antihistamines if severe. Epinephrine (0.1 ml/kg or 1:100000 concentration intravenously) may also be necessary if severe bronchoconstriction and cardiovascular collapse are present. Restarting the transfusion is not recommended in this case. If urticaria or fever is the only manifestation, the transfusion should be stopped temporarily, corticosteroids or antihistamines administered, and the transfusion reattempted after 20 to 30 minutes.

Delayed Destruction of Erythrocytes

Typically, DEA 3/5/7 antigen antibody reactions are involved as a result of previous sensitization or naturally occurring antibodies. Rapid drop in PCV within 3 to 7 days and evidence of extravascular hemolysis are the typical signs.

Nonimmunologic Reactions

The most common problems include vascular overload (cough, pulmonary edema, vomiting, urticaria, and serous nasal discharge). In addition, poor component handling can result in hemolysis (physical trauma to red cells during collection or administration, prolonged or inadequate storage, freezing, overheating, and mixing with nonisotonic fluids). If erythrocytic damage is severe, then signs may be similar to acute severe intravascular hemolysis, but more commonly they reflect rapid transfused erythrocytic destruction and extravascular hemolysis. Occasionally a pyogenic substance from the plastic bag or tubing can cause a febrile response. Administration of erythrocytes or plasma products with calcium-containing crystalloid solutions can cause microembolization within the intravenous tubing. Inappropriate plasma product storage or administration can result in poor viability of plasma or clotting proteins and ineffective response. Massive transfusion in severe hemorrhage can result in hypocalcemia or anticoagulant toxicity. Disease transmission can also occur if donors have not been carefully chosen and screened.

AUTOTRANSFUSION

Autotransfusion requires a simple apparatus (metal teat cannula, three-way stopcock, catheter injection port, and blood collection bag) and should be easy to perform. Blood is collected by gravity flow into a collection bag from hemorrhage into the abdomen or thoracic cavity. This technique is indicated in animals with trauma if no ready access to blood supply is available. Its use in other causes of hemoabdomen or hemothorax is not advised because of the potential risk of infusing neoplastic cells or bacteria into the animal. Autotransfused blood does not contain adequate clotting factors or platelets to be helpful in controlling hemorrhage and should be used only as a source of red blood cells and albumin to maintain oxygen-carrying capacity and volume.

RED BLOOD CELL ALTERNATIVES

Oxyglobin solution (Biopure Corporation, Cambridge, Mass.), a hemoglobin glutamer-200 (bovine), is the only commercially available red blood cell substitute available to veterinarians.[5,6] It is expensive, but potential advantages include immediate oxygen unloading capability, ready accessibility and easy storage, and oxygen-carrying capacity that is provided without contributing red cell stroma to animals with immune-mediated hemolysis. In extravascular immune-mediated hemolytic anemia cases, there exists a low risk of contributing to further activation of the immune system as well as suppressing bone marrow response. In intravascular hemolysis, the risk of acute renal failure and thromboembolization is potentially reduced by providing oxygen-carrying capacity without erythrocytic stroma using Oxyglobin instead of using red blood cell products. Some speculate that Oxyglobin can act as a nitric oxide scavenger in the vasculature and can cause or exacerbate pulmonary hypertension. The dose recommended by the manufacturer is 30 ml/kg given no faster than 10 ml/kg hourly (perhaps even more cautiously in normovolemic animals at risk of volume overload). The duration of effect of the product is approximately 24 hours, with 90% elimination by 7 to 10 days. Administration of Oxyglobin does cause tissue discoloration and can interfere with serum chemistry profile and coagulation (depending on instrument type) testing results.

References

1. Plumb DC: Drug considerations in the geriatric patient, *Proc Vet Med Forum* 17:429, 1999.
2. Robertson SA: What is pain? *J Am Vet Med Assoc* 221:202, 2002.
3. Hellyer PW: Treatment of pain in dogs and cats, *J Am Vet Med Assoc* 221:212, 2002.
4. Kristensen AT, Feldman BF: *Canine and feline transfusion medicine,* Philadelphia, 1995, WB Saunders.
5. Rentko VT, Kelly N, Niggemeir A et al: Effects of oxyglobin and packed red blood cells (PRBC) on the erythropoietic response to acute anemia, *J Vet Intern Med* 12:227, 1998.
6. Muir WW, Wellman ML: Hemoglobin solutions and tissue oxygenation, *J Vet Intern Med* 17:127, 2003.

CHAPTER 6

Cancer and Therapeutics*

JOHNNY D. HOSKINS

Increasing age represents the single leading risk factor for the development of cancer.[1] Advancing age is associated with increasing incidence of benign and malignant cancer and higher rates of cancer-associated deaths. The prevalence of cancer is climbing as a result of greater longevity of animals. With longer life span comes the challenge of geriatric medicine, including the treatment of cancer.

AGING AND CANCER

Aging is characterized by progressive impairment of vital functions such as glomerular filtration rate, maximal respiratory capacity, and maximal exercise capacity. The net result of the physiologic changes associated with aging is that the geriatric animal is less resilient and less able to survive physical stress.[2] Aggressive surgery, radiation therapy, and cytotoxic chemotherapy are necessary to treat local and metastatic cancer. The goals of such treatment include cure, decrease in overall tumor burden, prolonged disease-free interval, and improved quality of life for the animal by providing relief of signs associated with cancer. Although animals of all ages afflicted with locally confined malignant disease have a chance of being cured by appropriate surgery or radiotherapy techniques, it is unlikely that animals with disseminated disease will be cured by chemotherapy as it is currently practiced in veterinary medicine, regardless of age.

*Significant portions of this chapter are reprinted as they appeared in the 1st edition, and were written by Barbara E. Kitchell, DVM, PhD, DACVIM.

CANCER SCREENING PROGRAM

Often the single most important prognostic factor for the successful treatment of cancer is early detection. Survival rates for animals diagnosed with extensive disease are much lower than those for animals diagnosed with small tumor burdens and locally confined disease. The stage of cancer at diagnosis is determined by two sets of variables: the biologic behavior of the cancer and the host, and the factors that influence the owner's and veterinarian's behavior in the process of diagnosis. The early detection of cancer in geriatric animals is complicated by the presence of concurrent chronic illnesses that mask early clinical signs of neoplastic disease.[3] Signs that would draw immediate attention and concern in a young animal are often accepted in an older animal as a consequence of aging or a result of other known medical problems.

Cancer screening programs are widely used and are considered very successful for many types of common human cancers. In veterinary medicine, routine cancer screening measures have not been developed and applied, in part because of the lack of consensus on diseases appropriate for such screening, and the difficulty inherent in designing programs that would meet all of the criteria of success outlined above. The feline leukemia virus antigen test might be considered a screening test in wide use clinically, as it allows for the detection of viral infection before the onset of clinical signs and alerts the veterinarian and owner to the potential for further disease consequences with early intervention possible.[4]

A better approach for the veterinary setting may be the institution of earlier detection of problems through owner education. Owners should be made aware of the fact that animals do, in fact, develop cancer. The most common sites of malignant disease in animals include the skin, mammary glands, lymph nodes, and oral cavity. Educated owners may seek medical care sooner for their pets. A list of signs analogous to the American Cancer Society's "Seven Warning Signs of Cancer" has been developed by the Veterinary Cancer Society and is applicable to both dogs and cats (Box 6-1).[4]

CANCER DIAGNOSIS

The primary means of diagnosing malignant disease is through histopathologic or cytologic evaluation of tumor tissue. There is no difference in the techniques applied to either young or old animals. In fact, "even the most clever pathologist cannot determine the age of the animal by microscopic examination of the cancer."[5] Histopathologic evaluation offers the advantage of allowing a pathologic grade of malignancy to be assigned to the cancer lesion. Histopathologic grading is helpful in predicting the degree of aggressiveness of a tumor and the potential for response to therapy. Excisional biopsy specimens are examined for complete excision by evaluation of the tumor tissue margin.

After the diagnosis of malignant disease is completed, the extent of disease in the animal is defined by a staging work-up. Staging is essential for determining appropriate therapy and can include such tests as thoracic and abdominal radiographs, evaluation of regional and distant lymph nodes, and bone marrow examination.

The evaluation of the geriatric animal with cancer is completed by investigating for concurrent age-related illness through a thorough history, physical examination, and clinical laboratory testing. Discovery of underlying chronic diseases, such as renal disease, hepatic disease, or cardiac insufficiency, is crucial to treatment planning and accurate prognostication of potential therapeutic outcomes. Debilitating conditions such as arthritis and dental disease may be addressed to improve the animal's quality of life during therapy.[3]

BOX 6-1 Common Signs of Cancer in Animals*

- Abnormal swellings that persist or continue to grow
- Sores that do not heal
- Weight loss
- Loss of appetite
- Bleeding or discharge from any body opening
- Offensive odor
- Difficulty eating or swallowing
- Hesitation to exercise or loss of stamina
- Persistent lameness or stiffness
- Difficulty breathing, urinating, or defecating

*Developed by the Veterinary Cancer Society.

TREATMENT STRATEGIES

Strategies for treatment of the aging dogs or cats must take into account the impact of concurrent diseases such as cardiac or renal insufficiency on life expectancy and treatment tolerance of the animal. Drug and anesthetic regimens may need to be modified to accommodate concurrent medical problems, and therapies may need to be tailored to individual animals. The *performance status* of the animal, a term referring to the overall quality of the animal's life, must be considered when considering therapy. Animals with higher initial performance status generally have better outcomes.

CANCER STAGING

The staging system for solid tumors is generally based upon the T-N-M staging system.

"T" refers to tumor and generally is determined by the size of the tumor or local invasion or extent (such as invasion of an oral tumor into bone). Neoplasms that have been determined to require precise size determination for prognosis include mammary neoplasia in dogs and cats, oral melanoma in dogs, and oral squamous cell carcinoma in dogs. Veterinarians should use radiography, computed tomography (CT), magnetic resonance imaging (MRI), and ultrasonography to fully define local extent and surrounding tissue involvement for surgical or radiotherapeutic planning. Measurement or description of the primary tumor (local staging) is useful in providing prognostic information for animals with certain tumor types. For example, in cats, for mammary tumors smaller than 2 cm the median survival is 3+ years, and for tumors larger than 3 cm the mean survival is 4 to 9 months; in dogs, the median survival for oral melanoma smaller than 2 cm is 511 days and larger than 2 cm is 164 days; and dogs with thyroid carcinoma less than 20 cc in volume are much less likely to develop metastatic disease than those with tumors of more than 20 cc volume.

"N" refers to regional lymph node involvement and is based on identification of tumor cells in regional lymph nodes. Epithelial and mesenchymal cells are not part of the normal population of lymph nodes. If even a few such cells are identified in a lymph node, they should be considered to be a metastatic population. Histopathologic examination of regional nodes is a very sensitive method of tumor detection. However, cytologic examination is equally or more rewarding in many cases. Fine-needle aspirate cytology of accessible regional lymph nodes, even if the node is normal in size, should be done.

"M" refers to systemic metastatic disease, which includes metastasis to lung, liver, bone, distant lymph nodes, and other organs.

The T-N-M staging system is also designed to further group affected animals into numbered stages. For example, an oral melanoma with characteristics of T1 (tumor size less than 2 cm), N0 (negative nodes), and M0 (negative distant metastasis) is considered stage I, whereas an animal with oral melanoma of stage T1-N0-M1 (positive for distant metastasis) is stage IV. Clinical stage is useful for prognostication in some cases (lung tumors, oral melanoma, mammary carcinoma) but remains merely descriptive or of inconsistent benefit for others (lymphoma, T stage for soft-tissue sarcoma). Veterinarians should remember to consider use of diagnostic tools such as ultrasonography (hepatic or sublumbar node metastatic sites), CT (local extent of oral and intranasal tumors), MRI (hepatic, adrenal tumors, soft-tissue sarcoma of the subcutis), and nuclear scintigraphy (bone scan for osteosarcoma) for clinical staging of veterinary cancer patients.

DIAGNOSTIC TECHNIQUES

Regional Lymph Nodes

Regional lymph node evaluation is recommended for all neoplasms. Palpation of peripheral lymph nodes is the most common method of evaluation for external tumors. Normal to only slightly enlarged nodes are often positive for metastatic disease when evaluated by fine-needle aspirate. Fine-needle aspirate is a more sensitive method of detection of metastatic disease than needle biopsy techniques (Box 6-2).

Thoracic Radiography

When animals are screened for pulmonary metastasis, three radiographic views of the thorax should be obtained. The standard right lateral and ventrodorsal view thoracic radiographs, however, are able to identify the majority of metastatic lesions. The third view is recommended when a radiologist is not available to review the films, or if suspicious lesions are identified on the original two views. The veterinarian may in good conscience eliminate the third view when clinical staging is used to screen for intrathoracic lymph node metastatic sites (lymphoma and mast cell neoplasia).

Ultrasonography

Ultrasonography has become commonplace for identification of intraabdominal parenchymal lesions not detectable by radiography. It also serves as a guide for fine-needle aspirates and needle biopsies of organs. Ultrasound may also be useful for local staging of soft-tissue sarcoma of the subcutis.

Computed Tomography and Magnetic Resonance Imaging

CT and MRI are more sensitive than radiography or ultrasonography for identification of parenchymal lesions. Intrathoracic CT is more sensitive for identifying small pulmonary and lymph node lesions. However, the degree of difference in sensitivity generally does not outweigh the negative aspects of expense, requirement for general anesthesia, and inaccessibility of this technology in some regions of the country. CT and MRI are of much greater value than radiography and even ultrasonography for local staging of, and therapeutic planning for, oral, intranasal, intrathoracic, intraabdominal, and soft-tissue neoplasms.

Nuclear Scintigraphy

Nuclear scintigraphy is used most often for thyroid neoplasms and osseous metastatic sites.

BOX 6-2 Fine-Needle Biopsy Procedure

The first step in performing a fine needle biopsy is determining the necessity for aspiration. Sometimes merely penetrating the tissue with a needle is sufficient to retrieve enough cells for cytology. In other instances, aspiration of cells into the needle by applying a negative pressure to the syringe is necessary. Recommendations are to use the nonaspirate method first to reduce the risk of blood contamination and destroying cells within the lesion. This is often the case when sampling lymph nodes, thyroid gland, or vascular soft-tissue organs.

How a slide is prepared for cytology ultimately determines the quality of laboratory samples and the end results. Preparing slides for semisolid samples requires a somewhat different technique from that used for preparing fluid samples.

Semisolid Samples

Once the specimen is collected, it is imperative to prepare the sample slide as quickly as possible to avoid clotting of the tissue inside the needle.

Place the sample onto a glass slide as quickly as possible after its collection; apply gentle pressure to the syringe if required to expel the aspirated tissue.

Gently lay a second spreader slide on top of the aspirated tissue; allow enough time for the tissue to diffuse into a thin layer.

Move the spreader slide to the opposite end of the sample slide, being careful not to apply excessive downward pressure to the spreader slide; avoid sliding the spreader slide off the end of the sample slide and possibly taking large clumps or pieces of the sample with it.

NOTE: The goal is to smear the sample in such a way that the result is a targetlike appearance, with fluid and blood encircling a central area containing most of the aspirated tissue to be examined.

Fluid Samples

If the sample consists of fluid or blood contamination, spread the fluid on the sample slide using the same technique as that used for preparing peripheral blood smears.

Slide Evaluation

After preparing the slide, stain it and evaluate the following features to determine if the slide is of sufficient quality to provide useful information.

Adequate amount or sample quality—if not sufficient, repeat the fine-needle biopsy; consider using low suction if no suction was used on previous biopsy.

Excess fluid—drain the lesion or swelling and resample any residual mass.

Purulent material—include culture and sensitivity.

Necrotic sample tissue—resample periphery of mass.

Blood—resample.

Stain and evaluate a slide for the presence of diagnostic cells.

Determine the quality and usefulness of the sample slide for achieving the purpose of diagnosis or confirmation of a condition.

Packaging Slides for Mailing

Proper packaging of the slide for mailing as important as its preparation. An inappropriately packaged, well-prepared slide is as useless as a bad slide if it arrives at its destination broken into small pieces or damaged. The same applies to samples in glass blood or serum tubes. The laboratory used by the veterinary hospital for performing tests and reading samples generally supplies or recommends packaging materials and provides guidelines for how samples are to be packed for safe shipping to their facility.

Fix unstained slides for submission to a laboratory in 100% methanol (commonly the first solution in a three-step stain kit) for 2 to 3 minutes to preserve cells and make the most of staining once it reaches the laboratory.

Pack the prepared slides in a Styrofoam specimen mailer (or the laboratory's specified packaging) to guarantee the slide is not broken in transit.

If sending samples in glass blood or serum tubes, use Styrofoam mailers specifically designed for those containers or as directed by the test laboratory.

Dogs with nonfunctional thyroid tumors may have 99m Tc-pertechnetate uptake. However, compared with thoracic radiography, nuclear scintigraphy is of questionable use for identification of pulmonary metastatic disease. There does appear to be correlation between distribution of technetium uptake and capsular invasion, and this technique has been useful in identifying ectopic sites of neoplasia, which may be valuable for surgical planning. Nuclear scintigraphic bone scans are sensitive but not specific methods for identification of osseous metastatic sites. Regions of osteoarthritis and osteomyelitis are also expected to be positive on these scans.

Polymerase Chain Reaction

Polymerase chain reaction is currently being used to identify clonal expansion of neoplastic lymphocytes and plasma cells in dogs. This method is useful for differentiation between antigen-stimulated (reactive) and neoplastic populations of lymphocytes. It may also be useful for identification of systemic foci for lymphoid neoplasms. Polymerase chain reaction technology may be used in the future for detection of minimal residual disease (identification of metastatic cells or residual local neoplastic cells) with markedly improved sensitivity. Another future potential use of polymerase chain reaction will be to differentiate metastatic cells from normal resident cells in regional lymph nodes, blood, or distant organs for neoplasms such as mast cell tumors.

Clinicopathologic Tests

Certain clinicopathologic tests are valuable to provide prognostic information for the animal by assignment of stage or substage. Examples of important clinicopathologic information for staging include serum calcium level for lymphoma and apocrine tumors of the anal sac, complete blood count for evaluation for cytopenias and leukemia for lymphoma, and serum alkaline phosphatase activity for appendicular osteosarcoma. Examples of clinicopathologic information for staging that may become useful in the future for prognostication or identification of minimal residual disease include serum α1-acid glycoprotein in tumor-bearing dogs and cats, telomerase activity in body cavity effusions, matrix metalloproteinase concentrations in tumor-bearing veterinary patients, serum vascular endothelial growth factor concentrations in dogs with hemangiosarcoma, and vascular endothelial growth factor concentrations in body cavity effusions.

COMMON METASTATIC SITES OF SOLID TUMORS

Some common metastatic sites for solid tumors are:

- Mammary tumors—regional lymph nodes and lung
- Perineal or genitourinary tumors—sublumbar lymph nodes, pelvic and caudal lumbar bones, and lung
- Solid intestinal tumors—regional lymph nodes, peritoneal cavity, and liver
- Appendicular osteosarcoma—lung, regional lymph nodes, liver, and secondary osseous sites
- Hemangiosarcoma of the spleen or subcutis—lung, heart, liver, and mesentery
- Primary lung tumors—tracheobronchial lymph nodes and secondary pulmonary sites
- Insulinoma—liver and regional lymph nodes

The following are neoplasms that are rarely overtly metastatic at the time of diagnosis: grade 1 to 2 dermal mast cell tumors of favorable sites; solitary dermal plasmacytoma; low- or intermediate-grade soft-tissue sarcoma of oral cavity or subcutis; carcinoma of the nasal plane, pinnae, or eyelids in cats; and dermal hemangiosarcoma in dogs. This means that if permanent local control can be achieved, the animal is likely to be cured of these neoplasms.

STAGING FOR HEMATOPOIETIC NEOPLASIA

Lymphoma

Staging for lymphoma includes external lymph node, spleen, liver, intrathoracic and intraabdominal lymph node, peripheral blood, and bone marrow evaluation. Evaluation by external lymph node evaluation, complete blood count, thoracic radiography, and abdominal radiography may be all that is necessary for staging of canine multicentric lymphoma before treatment, because confirmation of bone marrow or splenic involvement is of inconsistent prognostic importance. Feline gastrointestinal lymphoma is rarely associated with bone marrow involvement. Of considerable prognostic significance is clinical substage. *Substage* refers to the absence (substage a) or presence (substage b) of clinical signs associated with the neoplasm. Dogs with multicentric lymphoma with substage a have a significantly improved first remission and survival duration as compared with dogs with substage b. In addition, immunophenotype is of great prognostic significance in dogs with multicentric lymphoma.

Multiple Myeloma

Staging and diagnosis of multiple myeloma includes evaluation of lymph nodes, liver, spleen, identification of a solid mass, qualitative (and sometimes quantitative) evaluation of serum and urine globulins, bone lesions, and bone marrow evaluation. Diagnosis of multiple myeloma is generally made after the demonstration of bone marrow plasmacytosis, presence of osteolytic bone lesions, and the demonstration of serum ± urine myeloma component (M-component). It may be difficult to distinguish with certainty multiple myeloma from infectious diseases such as ehrlichiosis in the absence of histopathologic confirmed mass or osteolytic lesions, because some infectious agents may elicit significant plasmacytic organ infiltrate and monoclonal hyperglobulinemia. Identification of osseous lesions is a documented negative prognostic factor for survival in dogs with multiple myeloma following treatment. Clinicians should remember to evaluate serum calcium and renal values in animals with multiple myeloma. Coagulation tests should be considered in animals with multiple myeloma that show any signs of hemorrhage. Solitary dermal extramedullary plasmacytoma is rarely associated with systemic disease.

STAGING FOR DERMAL MAST CELL TUMORS

Traditional staging for dermal mast cell tumors in dogs includes regional lymph nodes, spleen, liver, blood, and bone marrow. Low- to intermediate-grade, nonulcerated, dermal mast cell tumors located in favorable anatomic sites are unlikely to be associated with metastatic disease if resected completely at the time of diagnosis. Complete staging in many of these animals may be unnecessary and misleading, although it is still often performed before the initiation of aggressive treatments such as amputation or expensive treatment such as radiotherapy. Traditional staging for canine mast cell tumors may be misleading for reasons that include the following: 1) there is no difference in cytologic identification between mast cells in liver and splenic tissue from normal dogs and those from tumor-bearing dogs, and 2) identification of mastocytemia (positive buffy coat) is not specific for metastasis of mast cell tumor. Thus, meaningful interpretation of a positive buffy coat smear is difficult. Because of the common occurrence of multifocal dermal lesions in animals with dermal mast cell neoplasia, thorough examination and regular reexamination of the entire dermis is recommended.

CANCER THERAPY

Once the diagnosis of cancer has been made and staging is completed, definitive therapy can be conducted. Factors to be considered in establishing a treatment protocol include the presence of other life-limiting illnesses, the animal's performance status, the owner's attitudes and expectations, and cost of treatment. Additionally, aged animals have decreased physiologic reserve and thus increased potential for toxicity during therapy with cancer drugs. Because of these considerations, veterinarians and owners often opt for conservative treatment regimens for elderly animals.

Surgery

The basic principles of cancer treatment apply equally to all animals with cancer regardless of age at diagnosis. The best cure rates for locally confined tumors are achieved when appropriate oncologic surgical principles are applied to their removal. The first surgery represents the best chance to achieve a complete cure, and for this reason, careful surgical planning is paramount. Furthermore, geriatric animals are less likely to tolerate repeated subcurative surgeries, so this principle certainly applies to them. En bloc resection techniques should be carried out, followed by careful evaluation of the submitted surgical margins by the pathologist. Veterinarians should contact surgical specialists for guidance before undertaking a procedure, and for animals that would benefit from referral, owners should be offered that option regardless of the animal's age.[3] Careful pretreatment planning and anesthetic management are essential for a successful outcome, as is aggressive supportive care in the preoperative and postoperative periods.

Radiotherapy

Radiation therapy is equally effective in killing cancer cells in elderly and young animals. Individualization of treatment programs by changes in fractionation, duration of therapy, total dose delivered, or total tissue volume treated is recommended for geriatric cancer animals. Most animals need brief anesthesia with each fraction of radiotherapy. This may be deleterious to elderly dogs and cats. With appropriate management and precautions, potentially curative or palliative radiation therapy may be administered.[3]

Chemotherapy

Cancer chemotherapy agents have a low therapeutic index. That is, the dose that produces a desired treatment response is very close to the dose that produces an undesired toxic response. With careful management and clear treatment goals, it is possible to use these drugs safely and effectively.[3] Myelotoxicity is the most universal adverse effect of chemotherapy and is due to the constant and relatively rapid replication of hematopoietic precursor cells. In theory, replacement of chemotherapy-destroyed hematopoietic elements may be delayed in the elderly because of exhaustion of pluripotent hematopoietic stem cells, impaired production of hematopoietic growth factors, and a dysfunctional hematopoietic microenvironment.[6] The administration of other myelodepressive drugs such as sulfamethoxazole-trimethoprim might contribute to delayed regeneration.[6] Recombinant hematopoietic growth factors may further aid in preventing myelotoxicity in the elderly.[7] Mucositis is caused by the destruction of rapidly proliferating cells of the gastrointestinal tract. Elderly animals should be treated aggressively if signs of vomiting or diarrhea develop after treatment with anticancer drugs. Fluid and electrolyte support, glucocorticoids, and sucralfate may be indicated in these animals.[6]

Nausea and vomiting may occur as a result of several mechanisms. Drugs may have direct action on the chemoreceptor trigger zone of the medulla, or mucositis may occur as described previously. Delayed nausea and vomiting may occur 2 days after treatment and may persist for days. Dexamethasone and metoclopramide have been used successfully as antiemetics in cancer therapy.[8] Butorphanol has been used specifically to block nausea and vomiting associated with the administration of cisplatin in dogs.[9]

Cardiotoxicity can be a complication of anthracyclines, mitoxantrone, mitomycin C, and high doses of cyclophosphamide.[6] Because anthracycline cardiotoxicity may be associated with increased free radical formation in the sarcoplasm, geriatric heart muscle may be at greater risk as a result of decreased content of free radical scavengers.[6] Certainly the presence of preexisting cardiac disease is a major factor in induction of doxorubicin cardiotoxicity, and careful cardiac evaluation should precede use of this drug.[10] Mitoxantrone, an anthracenedione derivative of the anthracyclines, is approximately 10 times less cardiotoxic and thus may be useful in geriatric animals.[6] Mitoxantrone appears to have a similar spectrum of anticancer activity as doxorubicin in dogs and cats.[11,12]

Cats are affected by pulmonary edema from systemic administration of cisplatin, and the use of the drug in cats is not appropriate.[13]

Neurotoxicity from vinca alkaloids (vincristine and vinblastine), and epipodophyllotoxins (etoposide and teniposide) may be more significant in the elderly because of an effect of unmasking subclinical neuropathies. Manifestations include paresthesias, weakness, and loss of deep tendon reflexes.[6] Vincristine neurotoxicity is reversible over time. Cisplatin neurotoxicity is an idiosyncratic effect that is not dose related and is often irreversible. Veterinarians should be aware that vincristine and cisplatin may induce acoustic neuropathy with associated hearing loss.[6] Geriatric dogs, in particular, may manifest deafness when treated with these agents, perhaps through unmasking of underlying hearing loss. Central neurotoxicity may be seen in animals receiving high-dose cytarabine, 5-fluorouracil, nitrosureas, and dacarbazine. The central nervous system of older animals may be more sensitive because of age-related neuron loss.[6] Again, cats are exquisitely sensitive to the neurotoxic effects of 5-fluorouracil, and its use is contraindicated in cats.[14]

Nephrotoxicity may be induced by cisplatin, mitomycin C, nitrosureas, and ifosfamide. Carboplatin, a nonnephrotoxic analog of cisplatin, may be substituted in animals with abnormal renal function. As carboplatin is excreted by the kidneys, the dose must be reduced in animals with reduced creatinine clearance to avoid myelosuppression from prolonged exposure.[6] Cats also have a tendency to develop renal insufficiency on high-dose doxorubicin therapy.[15]

Various chemotherapy protocols are listed in the appendix to this chapter.

Supportive Care

Adequate supportive care is paramount to successful management of all animals diagnosed with cancer, but this principle is particularly applicable to the care of the elderly. All methods of care that optimize quality of life should be used. Monitoring food intake, water consumption, and elimination are important in managing geriatric animals. Cats especially will benefit from grooming when they are debilitated.[4]

Pain may be managed with various approaches, including aspirin, corticosteroids, nonsteroidal antiinflammatory drugs, and even acupuncture in select cases. Corticosteroids may have direct anticancerous activity against lymphomas, myeloma, lymphocytic leukemia, and mast cell disease. Corticosteroids are useful for appetite stimulation and promoting a general sense of well-being in animals diagnosed with cancer. However, corticosteroid administration may compound immunosuppression, may cause liver toxicity, and has been implicated in the development of pleiotropic drug resistance. The potential benefits of corticosteroid administration should be weighed against these detrimental aspects. Nonsteroidal antiinflammatory drugs such as piroxicam have been used as palliative agents in the treatment of a variety of canine malignancies.[16] Most dogs that receive piroxicam at a dose of 0.3 to 0.5 mg/kg body weight once daily for 1 week, then on alternate days, experience enhanced quality of life as a result of decreased pain from arthritis and inflammation. This drug should be used very cautiously because it can cause severe gastrointestinal ulceration. Piroxicam should not be used in conjunction with agents such as corticosteroids and aspirin, to avoid compounding the ulcerogenic effects.[16]

Cancer-induced malnutrition may be a more severe problem for geriatric animals. Nausea and vomiting can exacerbate preexisting nutritional deficits. Food aversions may form as a result of receiving chemotherapy after a meal, in which case the animal associates the sensation of nausea with the food rather than with the treatment.[3,4] A change in diet, hand feeding, and the use of appetite stimulating agents such as diazepam (0.05 to 0.4 mg/kg intravenously [IV] or orally [PO]) may prove helpful. Metoclopramide (0.1 to 0.3 mg/kg IV, subcutaneously [SC], or PO three times daily) may help with appetite support by suppressing subclinical nausea and overt vomiting.[3,4,8] The potential negative consequences of aggressive nutritional support (sepsis from feeding tubes or hyperalimentation) should be weighed against the benefits.[17]

Assessing Response to Therapy

Analysis of survival from cancer becomes especially difficult in the geriatric animal. Competing causes of death and the availability of euthanasia as an end point in veterinary medicine make it especially difficult to determine the efficacy of cancer treatment for geriatric animals. Perhaps owner evaluation of improved quality of life should be weighed as heavily as remission and survival times in assessing the response to geriatric animals to cancer therapy.

References

1. Lyman GH: Decision analysis: a way of thinking about health care in the elderly. In Balducci L, Lyman GH, Ershler WB, eds: *Geriatric oncology,* Philadelphia, 1992, JB Lippincott.
2. Balducci L, Wallace C, Khansur T et al: Nutrition, cancer and aging: an annotated review. I. Diet, carcinogenesis, and aging, *J Am Geriatr Soc* 34:127, 1986.
3. Kitchell BE: Cancer therapy for geriatric dogs and cats, *J Am Anim Hosp Assoc* 29:41, 1993.
4. Kitchell BE: Feline geriatric oncology, *Compend Contin Educ Pract Vet* 11:1079, 1989.
5. Holmes FF: Clinical evidence for change in tumor aggressiveness with age. In Balducci L, Lyman GH, Ershler WB, eds: *Geriatric oncology,* Philadelphia, 1992, JB Lippincott.
6. Balducci L, Mowrey K, Parker M: Pharmacology of antineoplastic agents in older patients. In Balducci L, Lyman GH, Ershler WB, eds: *Geriatric oncology,* Philadelphia, 1992, JB Lippincott.
7. Shank W: Clinical use of hematopoietic growth factors in older patients with cancer. In Balducci L, Lyman GH, Ershler WB, eds: *Geriatric oncology,* Philadelphia, 1992, JB Lippincott.
8. Couto CG: Management of complications of cancer chemotherapy, *Vet Clin North Am Small Anim Pract* 20:1037, 1990.
9. Moore AS, Cardona A, Shapiro W et al: Cisplatin (cis-diaminedichloroplatinum) for treatment of transitional cell carcinoma of the urinary bladder or urethra, *J Vet Intern Med* 4:148, 1990.
10. Susaneck SJ: Topics in drug therapy: doxorubicin therapy in the dog, *J Am Vet Med Assoc* 182:70, 1983.
11. Helfand SC: Principles and applications of chemotherapy, *Vet Clin North Am Small Anim Pract* 20:986, 1990.
12. Ogilvie GK, Obradovich JE, Elmslie RE et al: Efficacy of mitoxantrone against various canine neoplasms, *J Am Vet Med Assoc* 198:1618, 1991.
13. Knapp DW, Richardson RC, DeNicola DB et al: Cisplatin toxicity in cats, *J Vet Intern Med* 1:29, 1987.
14. Theilen GH, Madewell BR: Clinical application of cancer chemotherapy. In Theilen GH, Madewell BR, eds: *Veterinary cancer medicine,* ed 2, Philadelphia, 1987, JB Lippincott.
15. Cotter SM, Kanki PJ, Simon M: Renal disease in five tumor-bearing cats treated with Adriamycin, *J Am Anim Hosp Assoc* 21:405, 1985.
16. Knapp DW, Richardson RC, Bottoms GD et al: Phase I trial of piroxicam in 62 dogs bearing naturally occurring tumors, *Cancer Chemother Pharmacol* 29:214, 1992.
17. Ogilvie GK, Vail DM: Nutrition and cancer: recent developments, *Vet Clin North Am Small Anim Pract* 20:969, 1990.

Supplemental Reading

Phillips B: Staging the veterinary oncology patient. Proceedings of the Twentieth Annual Forum, *Am Coll Vet Intern Med* 20:445, 2002.

Appendix: CHEMOTHERAPY PROTOCOLS

Canine Lymphoma—Single Agent Doxorubicin Protocol

- Thirty minutes prior to drug administration, inject diphenhydramine at 2 mg/kg SC in dogs. Anaphylaxis is rare in properly premedicated dogs.
- Doxorubicin: 30 mg/m^2 IV at weeks 1, 3, 6, 9, and 12. In animals that have had relatively few doses of doxorubicin, reinduction with doxorubicin may be possible. Cardiotoxicity becomes a threat, however, when cumulative doses of doxorubicin approach or exceed 240 mg/m^2.
- Draw up doxorubicin into a syringe and dilute it with preservative-free 0.9% sodium chloride solution to a volume of 10 ml for small dogs (20-ml syringe) and 20 ml for large dogs (35-ml syringe). Personnel responsible for the handling and infusion of the doxorubicin should be gloved and protected from any direct contact with the doxorubicin.
- Immediately prior to administration, place an indwelling IV catheter (20 or 22 gauge) in a peripheral vein with an intermittent infusion plug. The catheter should be secured with tape, but the insertion site of the catheter and the limb area proximal to the catheter site should be visible at all times so that catheter patency can be monitored. Perivascular necrosis occurs if doxorubicin is extravasated; extravasation can be prevented with careful catheter placement.
- Start a rapid drip of 0.9% sodium chloride solution into the catheter through an IV administration set.
- Confirm catheter patency by aspiration and by unimpeded flow of the 0.9% sodium chloride solution.
- Connect the doxorubicin syringe to the IV set and slowly infuse the doxorubicin over 5 to 10 minutes.
- Observe the dog for signs of distress, including erythema of the pinna, pruritus, and urticaria. If these signs develop, stop the doxorubicin infusion. When the signs cease, resume the infusion at a slower rate. If the signs continue, administer diphenhydramine, 1 mg/kg IV slowly, followed by dexamethasone sodium phosphate at 2 mg/kg IV. Resume infusion if rapid and complete resolution of the signs occurs. If signs do no resolve quickly or if signs progression is noted, do not resume doxorubicin infusion and treat for shock as needed. Some generic doxorubicin products have been related to an increased incidence of anaphylaxis episodes; switching brands can prevent this outcome.
- When doxorubicin infusion is complete, carefully withdraw the doxorubicin syringe and carefully catch small drops of the doxorubicin that may be leaking. After disconnecting the syringe, start the IV of 0.9% sodium chloride solution again and continue its administration until the IV line is absolutely clear.
- Disconnect the IV administration set from the intermittent infusion plug, inject 6 ml of 0.9% sodium chloride solution into the catheter, and then remove the catheter and apply a pressure wrap to the catheter site.

Combination Chemotherapy—Madison-Wisconsin Protocol

- Vincristine: 0.5 to 0.7 mg/m^2 IV on weeks 1, 3, 6, 8, 11, and 15
- L-Asparaginase: 400 IU/kg intramuscularly [IM] on week 1
- Cyclophosphamide: 200 mg/m^2 IV on weeks 2, 7, and 13
- Doxorubicin: 30 mg/m^2 IV on weeks 4 and 9
- Methotrexate: 0.5 to 0.8 mg/kg IV on week 17
- Prednisone: 2 mg/kg PO daily for week 1; then 1.5 mg/kg PO daily for week 2; then 1 mg/kg PO daily for week 3; and then 0.5 mg/kg PO daily for week 4

After completion of week 17, weeks 11 to 17 are repeated every 2 weeks until week 25, then every 3 weeks until week 49, and then every 5 weeks. Chlorambucil at 1.4 mg/kg PO replaces cyclophosphamide after week 11 for dogs in complete remission.

Combination Chemotherapy—ACOPA I Protocol

- Vincristine: 0.75 mg/m^2 IV weekly for weeks 1 to 4 and then weeks 7, 10, 13 and 16
- L-Asparaginase: 10,000 IU/m^2 IM weekly for weeks 1 to 4 and then weeks 7, 10, 13, and 16
- Cyclophosphamide: 250 mg/m^2 PO on weeks 7, 13, and 16
- Doxorubicin: 30 mg/m^2 IV on week 10
- Prednisone: 40 mg/m^2 PO daily for 7 days and then every other day

ACOPA I is maintained by repeating weeks 10 to 16 every 9 weeks until week 75. Melphalan is substituted for cyclophosphamide in the case of sterile hemorrhagic cystitis.

Combination Chemotherapy—ACOPA II Protocol

- Vincristine: 0.75 mg/m^2 IV on weeks 4, 10, 13 16, 19, and 22
- L-Asparaginase: 10,000 IU/m^2 IM on weeks 7, 8, 25, and 26
- Cyclophosphamide: 250 mg/m^2 PO on weeks 4, 7, 13, 16, and 22
- Doxorubicin: 30 mg/m^2 IV on weeks 1, 10, and 19
- Prednisone: 40 mg/m^2 PO daily for 7 days and then every other day

This protocol is maintained after week 29 by repeating weeks 10 to 16 every 9 weeks until week 75. Melphalan is substituted for cyclophosphamide in the case of sterile hemorrhagic cystitis.

Combination Chemotherapy—COPLA Protocol

- Cyclophosphamide: 50 mg/m^2 PO every other day for 8 weeks, then substitute chlorambucil 4 mg/m^2 PO every other day until relapse or 2 years of therapy
- Vincristine: 0.5 to 0.7 mg/m^2 IV once a week for 8 weeks and then step down to every other week for two cycles, every third week for three cycles, and then every 4 weeks thereafter until relapse or 2 years of therapy
- Prednisone: 20 mg/m^2 PO once a day for 1 week and then every other day until relapse or adverse corticosteroid effect, in which case taper and discontinue
- L-Asparaginase: 10,000 IU/m^2 IM or SC on days 1 and 8 and again at relapse
- Doxorubicin: 30 mg/m^2 IV on weeks 6, 9, and 12 and again at relapse

Rescue Protocol for Lymphoma

- Doxorubicin: 30 mg/m^2 IV every 3 weeks
- Dacarbazine: 200 mg/m^2 IV daily for 5 days or 800 mg/m^2 administered as an 8-hour IV infusion

Care should be taken to screen for cardiac toxicity if high cumulative doses of doxorubicin have been administered in the initial induction protocol (more than 200 to 240 mg/m^2 total).

Feline Lymphoma

- Induction for combination chemotherapy—vincristine (0.5 mg/m^2 IV once weekly), cyclophosphamide (50 mg/m^2 PO q48h), and prednisone (40 mg/m^2 q24h for 1 week; then 20 mg/m^2 PO q48h); use for 6 weeks
- Maintenance for combination chemotherapy—use one of the following maintenance approaches:
  - Doxorubicin at 1 mg/kg IV every 3 weeks for at least five times, or
  - Methotrexate (2.5 mg/m^2 PO three times a week), chlorambucil (20 mg/m^2 PO every 2 weeks), prednisone (20 mg/m^2 PO q48h), and vincristine (0.5 mg/m^2 IV every 4 weeks)

Urinary Bladder Neoplasia

- Chemotherapy with mitoxantrone (dosage of 5.5 mg/m^2 and given IV at 3-week intervals) and piroxicam is the preferred way to treat urinary bladder neoplasia. This therapy should be continued as long as no adverse side effects are noted. The hemogram should be monitored before each mitoxantrone treatment and 1 week after its administration for myelosuppression. Administration of piroxicam (0.3 mg/kg PO once a day with food for affected dogs; those dogs with compromised liver or kidney function and cats use the initial dose of 0.15 mg/kg PO once a day with food) will minimize animal discomfort and somewhat decrease the size of the urinary bladder mass(es). Owners should watch for signs of gastrointestinal upset such as inappetence, vomiting, diarrhea, and change in color of stools passed when the animal is receiving piroxicam. In addition, the hemogram and renal function should be monitored.
- Symptomatic therapy usually includes treatment of secondary urinary tract infection and urolithiasis. In those animals with profuse bleeding to the point of declining packed cell volume (PCV) values, surgical resection or chemical cauterization of the urinary bladder lining may be needed. Intravesicular instillation of 10 to 20 ml of 1% formalin solution for 20 minutes followed by thorough rinsing with sterile saline solution may be used to cauterize the urinary bladder lining.

Mast Cell Tumors in Dogs

- When a mast cell tumor appears in the axilla, mammary tissue, groin, perineum, or genitals, or in any of the mucocutaneous tissue, the tumor usually acts as a grade 3 mast cell tumor with metastatic intentions. Intraoperative radiation therapy and intralesional methylprednisolone acetate or triamcinolone are adjunctive therapies that may also enhance the possibility of successful excisional surgery.
- All dogs receiving chemotherapy for cancer require regularly scheduled complete blood cell counts to monitor for drug-induced myelosuppression. Chemotherapy protocols for mast cell tumors in dogs vary with the severity of disease. Prednisone at 40 mg/m^2 PO q48h for 10 to 14 days then 20 mg/m^2 q48h along with chlorambucil at 4 to 6 mg/m^2 PO q48h should be administered for maintenance of dogs with mild clinical disease. Vinblastine at 2 mg/m^2 or vincristine at 0.7 mg/m^2 IV weekly for six times and then every other week for six times, and every 3 weeks as maintenance may be added to the previous protocol for high-grade or metastatic disease. If chlorambucil is not effective, cyclophosphamide at 200 to 300 mg/m^2 given PO during a 4-day period may be used on the alternate weeks when vinblastine or vincristine is not being used. For severe disease, lomustine at 50 to 85 mg/m^2 PO divided over 4 days every 3 weeks is an additional approach. Lomustine causes significant myelosuppression after three or four treatment cycles; therefore, increasing the interval between treatments to 5 weeks to 8 weeks seems to help the myelosuppressed dog.

Tumor-Bearing Cats

Lomustine at 50 to 60 mg/m^2 given as a single oral dose every 6 weeks for six times appears to be an appropriate therapy for tumor-bearing cats. Because the time of the nadir is variable, complete blood cell and platelet counts should be done weekly after treatment to determine an individual cat's nadir. Some cats may develop myelosuppression early and recover by 21 days after treatment. A shorter dosage interval may be feasible in these cats. Serum chemistry profiles are recommended after every other lomustine treatment to monitor for potential organ toxicity. Myelosuppression, specifically neutropenia, is the acute dose-limiting toxicity of lomustine in cats. The neutrophil nadir is variable, occurring 7 to 28 days after treatment. The median neutrophil count at the nadir is approximately 1000 cells/μL (range, 0 to 9694 cells/μL). Neutrophil counts may not return to normal for up to 14 days after the nadir. The nadir of the platelet count may occur 14 to 21 days after treatment (median, 43,500 cells/μL). No gastrointestinal, renal, or hepatic toxicity has been observed after a single dose of lomustine.

Angiogenesis Inhibitory Protocol for Dogs

Celecoxib, tamoxifen citrate, and doxycycline are three angiogenesis inhibitory drugs that can be used for management of cancer with growing blood supply. Reducing the blood supply assists in control or eradication of the cancerous process.

Each drug is available in a capsule that can be opened, or the combination can be prepared by a pharmacy compounder into a suspension or a single capsule. The schedule for each drug is twice daily.

SIZE OF DOG	WEIGHT (LB)	CELECOXIB	TAMOXIFEN CITRATE	DOXYCYCLINE
Largest	≥85	100 mg	5 mg	300 mg
Large	Approximately 50	75 mg	3 mg	200 mg
Medium	Approximately 25	50 mg	2 mg	100 mg
Small	Approximately 10	25 mg	1 mg	50 mg

Nonresectable or Metastatic Feline Squamous Cell Carcinoma

- Bleomycin: 10 mg/m^2 IV or SC, every day for 3 to 4 days; then every 7 days to a maximum dose of 200 mg/m^2. (Pretreat with diphenhydramine 0.5 mg/lb 15 minutes before drug injection.)

Chronic Granulocytic Leukemia

- Busulfan: 3 to 4 mg/m^2 PO, daily

Chronic Lymphocytic Leukemia

- Chlorambucil: 2 to 4 mg/m^2 PO, every other day
- Prednisone: 20 to 40 mg/m^2 PO, every other day, given on nonchlorambucil days

Multiple Myeloma

- Melphalan: 2 to 4 mg/m^2 PO, every other day
- Prednisone: 20 to 40 mg/m^2 PO, every other day, given on nonmelphalan days

Transmissible Venereal Tumor

- Vincristine: 0.025 mg/kg IV, every 7 days until tumor not grossly visible

Canine Osteosarcoma, Squamous Cell Carcinoma, Transitional Cell Carcinoma, Pulmonary Carcinoma

- Cisplatin: 60 to 70 mg/m^2 IV, every 30 days

Administrative Procedure

- Secure IV catheter and administer 0.9% saline solution at 8 ml/lb/h for 4 hours
- Administer butorphanol at 0.4 mg/kg IM, 30 minutes before cisplatin injection
- Administer cisplatin (1 mg/ml saline solution) IV over 20 minutes
- Administer 0.9% saline solution at 8 ml/lb/h for additional 2 hours

Give two treatments after suture removal in osteosarcoma amputees with no pulmonary metastasis and in cases of pulmonary carcinoma, squamous cell carcinoma, and transitional cell carcinoma with lymphatic or blood vessel invasion. If contaminated surgical margins exist, attempt a second surgical procedure; if this is not possible, treat twice with cisplatin.

CHAPTER 7

Anesthesia

ROBERT R. PADDLEFORD

The anesthetic management of the geriatric dog or cat can be challenging for the veterinarian. These animals are often suffering from multiple pathophysiologic conditions as well as decreased organ reserve capacity. Thus, the anesthetic episode may exacerbate a preexisting subclinical organ dysfunction and produce overt organ failure. The primary goals in the anesthetic management of the geriatric dog or cat are to keep anesthesia time to a minimum; to use anesthetic drugs that produce minimal cardiopulmonary depression; to use anesthetic drugs that can be antagonized, are readily metabolized, or require no metabolism; to maintain adequate renal function; and to monitor physiologic parameters closely.[1-5]

PHYSIOLOGIC CHANGES ASSOCIATED WITH AGING

It is often difficult to define a geriatric dog or cat simply on the basis of chronologic age. Young dogs and cats may have organ system dysfunction more typical of a geriatric animal, whereas some older dogs and cats have organ systems more typical of younger animals. Some authors have suggested that animals be considered as aged or geriatric when they have reached 75% to 80% of their life expectancy; however, each animal must ultimately be evaluated as an individual and not simply as a "geriatric" animal.

Some general considerations apply to the physiologic changes associated with aging. The aged animal is likely to have more diseases and organ dysfunction than a young animal. In addition, the geriatric animal is more likely to have less functional organ reserve capacity than a young animal. This decreased organ reserve, termed *elderly normal,* may not become apparent until the animal is stressed by disease, hospitalization, anesthesia, or surgery; then overt organ failure may occur.

Much of the knowledge regarding physiologic changes associated with aging has been derived from human studies. However, this information may be very applicable to the geriatric dog and cat.

Pulmonary System

Respiratory function progressively diminishes as an animal ages, resulting in a decreased functional reserve. A loss of strength occurs in the muscles of respiration, the chest wall compliance decreases, and elastic recoil is reduced.[1] The net effect of these changes is an increase in small airway closure, which produces a decrease in the vital capacity and an increase in the residual volume.[2] In addition, decreases occur in lung elasticity, respiratory rate, tidal volume, minute volume, oxygen consumption, carbon dioxide production, maximal diffusion capacity for oxygen, capillary blood volume, and protective airway reflexes in the aged animal.[2] The decrease in protective airway reflexes (pharyngeal and laryngeal reflexes) puts the geriatric animal at a greater risk of aspiration in the perioperative period.[3] Finally, anatomic dead space and functional residual capacity increase.[2]

Aging produces histologic changes in the lungs that include dilatation of alveolar ducts, loss of intraalveolar septa, decreased numbers of alveoli, and a reduction in total lung surface area.[4] Geriatric humans have a marked reduction in their ability to respond to induced hypercarbia and hypoxia.[5]

These changes in the respiratory system are significant in that even mild to moderate respiratory depression due to anesthesia may produce marked hypoxia and hypercarbia, and any pathologic disease of the respiratory system (such as pneumonia, edema, pulmonary fibrosis) will be greatly exacerbated in the geriatric animal. What may be mild anesthetic depression in the young animal may be disastrous in the aged animal.

Cardiovascular System

Geriatric animals have a decreased cardiac reserve compared with younger animals and may have difficulty compensating for cardiovascular changes that occur during anesthesia. Geriatric animals have decreased baroreceptor activity, blood volume, cardiac output, blood pressure, circulation time, and vagotonia.[6] The conduction system of the heart is also affected by aging. In human patients it is not uncommon to see left bundle branch block, intraventricular conduction delay, ST segment and T wave changes, and atrial fibrillation.[7] This may make the geriatric animal more prone to anesthetic-induced dysrhythmias.

In addition, the geriatric animal may suffer from progressive and degenerative myocardial disease. This usually is associated with chronic valvular disease, which can lead to an increased myocardial workload and oxygen consumption and demand and make the myocardium extremely sensitive to hypoxia. Geriatric animals often develop thickened elastic fibers and an increase in collagen and calcium in the walls of large arteries, which results in an increased peripheral vascular resistance. The ability of the geriatric animal's cardiovascular system to adapt to hypotension is limited, and autoregulation is decreased.[8]

The decreased cardiovascular capabilities of geriatric animals make them very susceptible to anesthetic-induced cardiovascular depression, hypotension, and dysrhythmias.

Hepatic System

The aging process results in a reduction in the functional state of the microsomal enzyme systems in the liver. This reduction is present even when the results of standard biochemical function tests are normal.[9] Geriatric animals often have a decreased hepatic blood flow, most likely as a result of decreased cardiac output. The plasma half-life of drugs dependent on hepatic excretion, metabolism, or conjugation is, therefore, often increased in the geriatric animal. Altered hepatic function in the aged animal may lead to hypoproteinemia, delayed clotting function, and a greater susceptibility to hypoglycemia.

Renal System

The kidney is the major effective organ in fluid and electrolyte balance. Normal aging affects the kidneys in several ways.[10] Renal blood flow is decreased, most likely as a result of the decreased cardiac output. Total number of glomeruli decreases to one half to two thirds of that of a young animal, and the nephron mass is reduced. Tubular changes, which include atrophy, decreased tubular diameter, tubular disruption, and tubular hypertrophy, occur. Glomerular filtration rate may be decreased by as much as 45% to 50% in the aged animal. There is also a decreased ability to concentrate urine and excrete hydrogen ion because of decreased distal tubular function. The urine volume necessary for excretion of the obligatory solute load increases.

The result of these alterations is a diminished functional renal reserve, which makes the geriatric animal much less tolerant of body water deficits and the excessive administration of fluids. Aged animals have a decreased capacity to excrete certain drugs. They are more prone to acidosis, thus prolonging the plasma half-life of drugs dependent on renal excretion.

The effects of anesthesia and surgery on the kidney can be greatly exacerbated in the geriatric animal. Anesthesia and surgery generally cause an increased activity of the sympathetic nervous system and of the renin-angiotensin system, resulting in a decreased total renal blood flow and a redistribution of intrarenal blood flow away from the renal cortex. General anesthesia may decrease renal blood flow and the glomerular filtration rate by up to 40%. However, when the effects of the anesthetic agents terminate, renal function will usually return to normal. In addition, anesthesia and surgery may cause hypovolemia, hypotension, hypoxia, and hypercarbia, all of which will worsen preexisting decreased renal function. All the foregoing factors make the geriatric animal much more susceptible to renal failure following anesthesia and surgery.

Central Nervous System

Aging produces changes in the central nervous system (CNS) in human patients. Alterations occur in cognitive, sensory, motor, and autonomic functions. Cerebral perfusion and cerebral oxygen consumption decline. Aging is also associated with a reduction in brain weight, which is most likely a result of individual neuron degeneration.[11] The loss of brain weight is most evident in the cerebral cortex and the cerebellar cortex.[12] Myelin sheaths also degenerate in the aged animal.

Strong evidence suggests that neurotransmitters change with age. In the geriatric animal, destruction of neurotransmitters increases and production of neurotransmitters decreases. The reduction in neurotransmitter function may be a result of the decreased quantity of neurotransmitters or perhaps a change in the receptors themselves.

The overall effects of these alternations in the CNS on the anesthetic management of the geriatric animal are not fully understood. The effects of local anesthetic agents seem to be enhanced in the aged animal, and the effects of the neuromuscular blocking agents are prolonged. In addition, thermoregulatory center function is decreased, making the geriatric animal more susceptible to anesthesia-induced hypothermia.

Autonomic Nervous System

The autonomic nervous system loses some of its ability to respond to stress in the human geriatric patient. This appears to be most marked in the sympathetic nervous system. The aged animal has decreased vasoconstrictor responses and a decreased response to decreased cardiac preload.[13] Despite this reduced response, there appears to be an enhanced response to iatrogenic epinephrine and norepinephrine, leading to the conclusion that perhaps the autonomic nervous system output is decreased but the receptors are more sensitive.

Endocrine System

Although aging does not appear to alter adrenocorticotropic hormone (ACTH)—stimulated plasma cortisol levels,[14] there are reports that human geriatric patients may not have the adrenal gland reserves necessary to protect themselves adequately during stress from anesthesia and surgery.[11] Renin and aldosterone—hormones that are necessary for water, sodium, and potassium balance as well as blood pressure control—are attenuated when the human geriatric patient is stressed.[15]

Hyperadrenocorticism can be seen in middle-aged and older dogs.[16] Clinical findings in animals with hyperadrenocorticism include muscle weakness, reduced expiratory reserve volume, decreased chest wall compliance, expanded vascular volume leading to increased systolic and diastolic pressure, and pyelonephritis. The ability of these animals to ventilate adequately under anesthesia may be greatly attenuated.

Hypothyroidism is the most common endocrine disease in the dog.[17] Hypothyroid animals may have several clinical abnormalities that can be significant with regard to anesthetic management. These animals are more prone to hypothermia because of thermoregulation abnormalities.[17] Cardiovascular problems may include sinus bradycardia, decreased myocardial contractility, cardiomyopathy, ischemic heart disease, and anemia.[17] These cardiovascular abnormalities make the animal with hypothyroidism more sensitive to the cardiovascular depressant effects of anesthetic agents. Animals with hypothyroidism also have a decreased ability to metabolize drugs.[17] This will prolong the effects of any preanesthetic and anesthetic agents that require metabolism and biodegradation to terminate their effects. Finally, many hypothyroid animals are obese. This obesity can lead to a decrease in tidal volume and minute volume, which can be greatly exacerbated by hypoventilation during anesthesia.

Antidiuretic hormone level increases with age owing to an increased resistance of the distal renal tubules to its effects.[6] This can lead to impaired renal concentrating ability.

Pancreatic function may be altered in the geriatric animal. Glucose tolerance decreases with age. This may result from a decline in the ability of the insulin receptors to respond, or there may be an actual decrease in the number of receptors.[18] Diabetes mellitus is an endocrine disease often encountered in the older animal. It can be associated with osmotic diuresis, ketoacidosis, liver dysfunction caused by fat deposition and cirrhosis, and concurrent infectious diseases. Hypoglycemia during and after anesthesia can be a problem in the aged animal owing to altered pancreatic and liver function. The administration of fluids containing glucose may be warranted in the geriatric animal during and after anesthesia.

PHARMACOKINETICS AND PHARMACODYNAMICS

Pharmacokinetics

Pharmacokinetics is the study of drug disposition in an animal. The most important age-related changes in the handling of anesthetic and preanesthetic drugs in the geriatric animal are in disposition (partitioning within the various distribution volumes) and in clearance (excretion, metabolism, or conjugation of drugs). The slight reduction of plasma albumin concentrations in the aged animal is most likely not sufficient to produce clinically important changes in the amount of active or unbound drug in plasma after intravenous (IV) drug administration. Data also do not suggest that the aging process plays any significant role in altering the parenteral uptake of drugs.[19]

The physical characteristics of drug molecules make them either lipophilic or hydrophilic and thus determine their ultimate partitioning between lipid tissues (brain, adipose, and viscera) and aqueous body compartments (blood, extracellular fluid, and skeletal muscle). As an animal ages, it experiences a progressive decrease in the absolute volume of the aqueous fraction and an increase in the lipid compartments.[20] Therefore, for hydrophilic drugs, the decrease in the aqueous fraction of the body of an aged animal could produce higher than expected initial plasma levels following IV administration of recommended dosages of drugs, even when the dose has been adjusted for total body weight. The net pharmacokinetic effect would be an enhancement of drug potency.

Because lipophilic drugs undergo some initial distribution to highly perfused nonadipose lipid tissues, the effects of the decreased aqueous fraction on the body are offset. However, because of the significant increase in total body lipid into which lipophilic drug molecules are ultimately distributed, the elimination process is markedly delayed because the volume of the drug that must be cleared is increased in the geriatric animal.[21]

Age also alters drug disposition or pharmacokinetics by significantly reducing both renal and hepatic function and thereby decreasing the clearance of drugs eliminated through these pathways. This occurs regardless of whether a drug is lipophilic or hydrophilic.

Pharmacodynamics

Pharmacodynamics is the relationship between drug quantity and drug effect and is frequently altered in the geriatric animal. The geriatric animal has a decrease in the circulating blood volume, which can produce high initial plasma concentrations of anesthetic drugs. However, this cannot solely explain the many observed cases of a need for reduced doses of anesthetic agents in geriatric animals.[22] Studies involving tranquilizer and sedative drugs in humans confirm that geriatric animals achieve a given drug effect at plasma concentrations that are significantly lower than those required for young adults.[23] In addition, the minimum alveolar concentration (MAC) of volatile anesthetic agents is less in aged animals than in young adult animals.[24] The mechanism by which age reduces the need for anesthetic agents is unclear, but anesthetic and analgesic requirements in the aged animal are decreased [25,26]; the decrease seems to correlate with the reduction in brain mass, the decrease in brain blood flow, and the decrease in the number and density of neurons and axons in both the central and peripheral nervous systems. These decreases and reductions occur in geriatric animals even in the absence of disease.

Other factors may play a significant role in reducing anesthetic requirements in the geriatric animal. The alterations in neurotransmitter activity have already been discussed. Other unknown factors may also play a role. It may be that the decreased anesthetic requirement is more the result of a decreased functional reserve of the nervous system as opposed to the actual level of nervous system function.

Regardless of the reasons for the pharmacokinetic and pharmacodynamic alterations of the anesthetic agents observed in the geriatric animal, each animal must be examined on an individual basis because no reliable universal guidelines are available. Some of the clinical consequences of these alterations are predictable, but they do not apply consistently to all the preanesthetic and anesthetic agents used.

ANESTHETIC CONSIDERATIONS

Any geriatric dog or cat requiring anesthesia should be considered on an individual basis. Each geriatric animal will have specific and unique physiologic alterations or diseases. Thus, the anesthetic protocol that suits one aged animal may of necessity be different for the next animal.

As with any animal, a thorough and complete preanesthetic examination should be done. A complete history should be taken, with a special emphasis on present medical or surgical problems, current medications the animal is receiving, and previous medical or surgical problems. Any previous anesthetic experience the animal has had should be noted, and close attention should be paid to any anesthetic complications or abnormal responses that occurred. A thorough preanesthetic physical examination should be performed to determine physiologic baseline values for future monitoring, as well as to ascertain any existing pathologic conditions. A complete blood count and serum biochemical profile with special emphasis on renal and hepatic function and electrolyte balance should be obtained. Thoracic radiographs and a baseline electrocardiogram should be considered. If any abnormal preanesthetic findings are found, they should be thoroughly evaluated, and delay of the anesthesia and surgery should be considered.

Preanesthetic Drugs

The preanesthetic medications used in a particular geriatric animal depends on that animal's physical condition, the amount of sedation or analgesia required, and the experience and preference of the veterinarian. Preanesthetic medications that are commonly used are the anticholinergic agents, tranquilizers or sedatives, opioids, and neuroleptanalgesic agents (Table 7-1).

Anticholinergic Agents. The anticholinergic agents are used to decrease respiratory secretions and to counteract sinus bradycardia. The two drugs available are atropine and glycopyrrolate. The drugs have similar actions except that glycopyrrolate does not cross the blood-brain barrier. Glycopyrrolate takes longer to exert its effects, but it lasts longer than atropine and is less likely to produce sinus tachycardia. Glycopyrrolate does not seem to counteract severe sinus bradycardia as well as does atropine.

The indiscriminate use of atropine or glycopyrrolate should be avoided in the geriatric animal, to prevent an unwanted and potentially dangerous sinus tachycardia from occurring. The geriatric animal's heart may not be able to withstand the increased oxygen consumption and demand needed when sinus tachycardia occurs, and the sinus tachycardia may precipitate acute myocardial failure.

If sinus bradycardia does occur, atropine may be given intravenously to effect. If potent vagotonic drugs, such as the opioids, α_2 agonists (xylazine, medetomidine), or fentanyl-droperidol, are to be used, administration of an anti-

TABLE 7-1. SUGGESTED DOSAGES FOR PREANESTHETIC MEDICATIONS IN THE GERIATRIC DOG AND CAT

DRUG	DOSE: DOG	DOSE: CAT	DURATION OF ACTION
Anticholinergic Agents			
Atropine sulfate	0.22 mg/kg IM, SC	Same	1-1½ h
Glycopyrrolate (Robinul-V)	0.01 mg/kg IM, SC	Same	2-3 h
Tranquilizers or Sedatives			
Acetylpromazine (Acepromazine)	0.1-0.2 mg/kg IM, IV to a maximum total dose of 2 mg	Same	3-6 h
Diazepam (Valium)	0.4 mg/kg IM, IV to a total dose of 10 mg	0.4 mg/kg IM, IV	½-3 h IV
Midazolam (Versed)	0.2-0.4 mg/kg IM, IV	Same	<2 h
Xylazine (Rompun)	0.1-0.2 mg/kg IM, IV	Same	1-2 h
Medetomidine	0.01-0.04 mg/kg IM	0.08-0.1 mg/kg IM	1 h
Narcotic Analgesics (Agonists-Antagonists)			
Pentazocine (Talwin)	1-3 mg/kg IM, IV	Same	1-2 h
Butorphanol (Torbugesic)	0.1-0.5 mg/kg IM, IV	Same	Up to 4 h
Buprenorphine	0.1-0.5 mg/kg IM, IV	Same	Up to 12 h
Narcotic Analgesics (Agonists)			
Morphine	0.05-1 mg/kg SC	0.002-0.1 mg/kg SC	3-6 h
Meperidine	0.5-3 mg/kg IM, IV	1-5 mg/kg IM, IV	2-4 h
Oxymorphone	0.1-0.2 mg/kg IM, IV to a maximum total dose of 4 mg	0.2 mg/kg IM, IV	2-4 h

IM, Intramuscular; *IV*, intravenous; *SC*, subcutaneous.

cholinergic agent may be warranted. Half the normal dose of anticholinergic may be given intramuscularly as a premedicant, with additional anticholinergic given intravenously to effect if needed.

Tranquilizer-Sedatives. The primary tranquilizer-sedative preanesthetic agents available are the phenothiazine derivatives, butyrophenone derivatives, benzodiazepine derivatives, and thiazine derivatives.

Acetylpromazine is the most common phenothiazine-derivative tranquilizer in use. For the healthy geriatric animal, the use of low-dose acetylpromazine is a reasonable choice for preanesthesia. Acetylpromazine causes general CNS depression without producing analgesia. It lowers the seizure threshold, so it should not be used in animals with epilepsy. Acetylpromazine can produce hypotension because of a peripheral vasodilating effect as opposed to direct myocardial depression. It does possess antidysrhythmic activity because of either a quinidine-like effect or a local anesthetic effect on the myocardium, and it does inhibit myocardial sensitization to catecholamines. At low doses, the effect of acetylpromazine on the respiratory system is usually negligible. A slight decrease in respiratory rate may occur, but this is usually compensated for by an increase in tidal volume resulting in normal minute ventilation. Acetylpromazine does not delay the respiratory center response (threshold) to increases in partial arterial carbon dioxide pressure ($PaCO_2$), although the maximum ventilatory response (sensitivity) may be decreased. Acetylpromazine undergoes extensive biodegradation in the liver; therefore, animals with hepatic dysfunction may have extremely long recovery times. This may explain why aged animals may have prolonged recovery times after receiving acetylpromazine.

The three butyrophenone derivatives used in veterinary anesthesia are droperidol (Inapsine), azaperone (Stresnil), and lenperone (Elanone-V). These drugs have similar physiologic effects. They have little or no direct effect on cardiac output, but they do decrease arterial blood pressure, total peripheral resistance, and heart rate. Respiratory depression can occur. The butyrophenones are biodegraded by the liver. Lenperone has been approved for dogs and cats; azaperone is primarily used in swine, and droperidol is mainly used in combination with the narcotic fentanyl.

The main benzodiazepine derivative tranquilizer used in small animal anesthesia is diazepam. Diazepam is dissolved in propylene glycol; therefore, its absorption from intramuscular (IM) injection sites may be unpredictable and erratic. In addition, propylene glycol is a cardiopulmonary depressant, and rapid IV administration may cause hypotension, bradycardia, and apnea. Benzodiazepine tranquilizers are considered "minor" tranquilizers, meaning they have minimal CNS-depressant activity. They produce a calming or taming effect and reduce fear and anxiety without marked sedation. They are good muscle relaxants. The benzodiazepines have broad-spectrum anticonvulsant activity and usually produce minimal cardiopulmonary depression. Because of the minimal cardiopulmonary depression, they are often used as a preanesthetic agent in aged animals. When combined with an opioid, they can be very effective. These drugs are highly protein bound and are metabolized in the liver.

Midazolam (Versed) is a water-soluble benzodiazepine. It is highly lipid soluble and has a short duration of action with a rapid elimination half-life and total body clearance. Midazolam has been used at a dose of 0.1 to 0.2 mg/kg intravenously or intramuscularly as a preanesthetic tranquilizer. It has been used in combination with opioids, barbiturates, dissociative agents, and inhalant agents. The cardiopulmonary effects of midazolam are similar to those of the other benzodiazepines. Higher doses of midazolam have produced dysphoria in dogs. Behavioral effects, including restlessness, pacing, vocalization, and difficulty in handling have been reported in cats following midazolam administration. If midazolam is used in combination with an opioid, the behavioral effects can be attenuated.

A specific antagonist has been developed for the benzodiazepine tranquilizers. Flumazenil (Mazicon) is a benzodiazepine antagonist that competitively and reversibly binds with the benzodiazepine CNS receptor sites. It reverses the sedative, muscle relaxant, amnesic, and anxiolytic effects of the benzodiazepine tranquilizers but has minimal intrinsic pharmacologic activity itself. Flumazenil does have weak agonistic effects with high doses. A dose of 0.1 mg/kg intravenously of flumazenil will antagonize the effects of diazepam or midazolam in dogs and cats.

There are two α_2 agonists that are being used in small animal practice: xylazine and medetomidine. Xylazine (Rompun) is a thiazine derivative that has sedative, analgesic, and muscle-relaxant properties. Its marked cardiovascular effects and its unpredictable respiratory effects may limit its use in geriatric animals. Xylazine can produce significant bradycardia as well as second-degree atrioventricular heart block. It also appears to sensitize the myocardium to catecholamines, thereby making dysrhythmias more likely. The bradycardia and heart block are vagally induced; atropine can counteract these effects. Xylazine's effect on respiration is extremely variable and may range from minimal to marked depression of the rate and tidal volume, leading to hypoxemia and hypercarbia. Xylazine should be used with extreme caution in geriatric animals or debilitated animals with cardiovascular or pulmonary dysfunction.

Medetomidine differs from xylazine in that it has more potency and efficacy at α_2 receptors, is more lipophilic and is eliminated more quickly.[27] The physiologic effects of medetomidine are very similar to those of xylazine, and the precautions for its use in geriatric animals should be the same as for xylazine.

One advantage to the use of xylazine and medetomidine is that specific antagonists are available to counteract their effects (Table 7-2). Yohimbine, tolazoline, idazoxan, and atipamezole are α_2 antagonists. Yohimbine and tolazoline are commercially available and will completely and rapidly antagonize the CNS and cardiopulmonary depressant effects of xylazine and medetomidine.

Opioids. Opioids and narcotic analgesics are often used alone or in combination with tranquilizers in geriatric animals as preanesthetic medications. Various opioid agonists have been used, including morphine, meperidine, oxymorphone, and fentanyl. In addition, the opioid agonist-antagonists such as butorphanol, buprenorphine, pentazocine, and nalbuphine have also been used.

There are at least four major opioid receptor sites. The mu receptors are associated with respiratory depression, supraspinal analgesia, euphoria, and physical dependence; the kappa receptors are associated with spinal analgesia, sedation, and miosis; the sigma receptors are associated with dysphoria, hallucinations, and respiratory and vasomotor stimulation; and the delta receptors are associated with dependency and behavioral alterations. Opioids such as morphine, meperidine, oxymorphone, and fentanyl act as agonists at all four receptors. Butorphanol, buprenorphine, pentazocine, and nalbuphine are agonists at the kappa and sigma receptors but are antagonists or partial antagonists at the mu and delta receptors. Thus, they are less likely to produce the degree of respiratory depression and addiction that pure opioid agonists do.

The advantages of the opioids are that they produce analgesia and sedation, they produce minimal direct myocardial depression, and their effects can be readily antagonized (see Table 7-2). One must be aware, however, that they can produce mild to significant depression of minute ventilation; therefore, respiratory rate and depth should be closely monitored. Opioids often slow the heart rate; however, this may be advantageous in the geriatric animal in that the slow heart rate may lead to a decreased myocardial oxygen consumption and demand and more forceful contractions. Because the bradycardia is vagal induced, an anticholinergic may be used to counteract it if deemed necessary.

Butorphanol (Torbugesic, Torbutrol, Stadol) has been used as an effective preanesthetic and postanesthetic analgesic in the dog and cat. However, at the present it has been approved only for use as a cough suppressant in small animals. Butorphanol is an uncontrolled synthetic opioid agonist-antagonist of the nalophane-cyclazocine class, with a chemical structure similar to morphine but with pharmacologic activity similar to pentazocine. Its analgesic potency is five times that of morphine, 15 to 30 times that of pentazocine, and one third to one half that of oxymorphone. Butorphanol can produce a dose-related

TABLE 7-2. VARIOUS ANTAGONISTS, THEIR DOSAGES, AND DURATION OF ACTION

ANTAGONIST	DOSE	ANTAGONIZES THE EFFECTS OF	DURATION OF ACTION
Levallorphan (Lorfan)	0.02 to 0.2 mg/kg IV	Narcotic agonist-antagonist	1½-3 h
Nalorphine (Nalline)	1 mg/kg IV, IM, SC	Narcotic agonist-antagonist	1½-3 h
Naloxone (Narcan)	20-100 μg/kg IV, IM, SC	Pure narcotic antagonist (only antagonist for pentazocine)	15-45 min
4-Aminopyridine	0.3 mg/kg IV	Partial antagonist, for xylazine, ketamine, and barbiturates	
Yohimbine (Yobine)	0.15 mg/kg IV	α_2 agonists (xylazine, medetomidine)	
Tolazoline (Priscoline)	0.4-2 mg/kg IV	α_2 agonists (xylazine, medetomidine)	
Flumazenil (Mazicon)	0.1 mg/kg IV	Benzodiazepine derivatives	1 h

IM, Intramuscular; *IV*, intravenous; *SC*, subcutaneous.

respiratory depression similar to that caused by morphine; however, butorphanol seems to reach a "ceiling" beyond which higher doses do not cause significantly more depression. Butorphanol can produce decreases in heart rate, cardiac output, and blood pressure, but the depression is less than with morphine and oxymorphone. It is rapidly absorbed following IM injection, with peak blood levels occurring in 15 to 30 minutes. Butorphanol is extensively metabolized in the liver, with its analgesic activity lasting 2 to 4 hours. It is rapidly and completely absorbed from the gastrointestinal tract; however, because of significant first-pass hepatic metabolism, only about 17% of the administered dose is available systemically. Its effects are readily antagonized with naloxone.

Butorphanol has good analgesic properties and fair sedative properties. When it is combined with a tranquilizer such as diazepam or acetylpromazine a very acceptable neuroleptanalgesic agent is produced. Butorphanol's main advantages in the geriatric animal are that it produces minimal respiratory depression, it produces minimal-to-moderate cardiovascular depression, it provides good analgesia, and it is an uncontrolled opioid.

Neuroleptanalgesics. A neuroleptanalgesic is a combination of a tranquilizer (neuroleptic) and an opioid (analgesic). The use of neuroleptanalgesics may be very beneficial in the geriatric animal. Various neuroleptanalgesic combinations are available (Table 7-3). The pharmacologic effects of a neuroleptanalgesic depend on the tranquilizer and opioid used.

Neuroleptanalgesics used alone or in combination with local anesthetic agents may be all that is needed for minor diagnostic or surgical procedures in the geriatric animal. As with any animal, cardiopulmonary function should be closely monitored when neuroleptanalgesics are used, as these drugs may produce respiratory depression ranging from slight to significant.

Injectable General Anesthetic Agents

Injectable general anesthetic agents can be used in the geriatric animal, but they should be used with care because of the often altered hemodynamics, the decreased plasma protein binding, and the decreased ability of the liver in the aged animal to biodegrade drugs. The two major types of injectable agents in use in the dog and cat are the ultra–short-acting thiobarbiturates and the dissociative agents. In addition, two newer injectable agents—propofol and etomidate—are also being used in the small animals.

Ultra–short-acting Barbiturates. Ultra–short-acting thiobarbiturates (thiamylal, thiopental) can be used to induce anesthesia and for short surgical procedures; however, the lowest possible dose necessary for the procedure should be used. These drugs are highly protein bound, and their effects will be greatly exacerbated in any animal that is hypoproteinemic. Acidosis will also greatly enhance their effects in an animal by causing more nonionized barbiturate to be available and by decreasing the amount of protein-bound barbiturate. Both factors increase the amount of active barbiturate available.

The effects of the ultra–short-acting barbiturates on the cardiovascular system are variable, depending on species, specific barbiturate, and dose given. In general, there is usually an increase in the heart rate because of depression of the vagal center and/or arterial pressoreceptor reflexes, a decrease in stroke volume and myocardial contractility related to calcium-dependent mechanisms, an initial increase in cardiac output followed by a decrease, and an initial decrease in total peripheral resistance followed by a return to nor-

TABLE 7-3. NEUROLEPTANALGESIC COMBINATIONS FOR THE GERIATRIC DOG AND CAT

NEUROLEPTIC (TRANQUILIZER)	ANALGESIC (NARCOTIC)
Acetylpromazine 0.1 mg/kg IM or IV not to exceed a maximum total dose of 1.5 mg	Oxymorphone 0.2 mg/kg IM or IV not to exceed a maximum total dose of 3 mg
Diazepam 0.25 to 0.45 mg/kg IM or IV to a maximum total dose of 10 mg	Oxymorphone—same as above
Acetylpromazine—same as above	Meperidine 1 to 4.5 mg/kg IM or IV
Acetylpromazine—same as above	Butorphanol—0.2 to 0.45 mg/kg IM or IV
Diazepam—same as above	Butorphanol—same as above

IM, Intramuscular; *IV*, intravenous.

mal. The ultra–short-acting thiobarbiturates may produce transitory cardiac dysrhythmias, which are usually premature ventricular contractions and of a bigeminal nature.

The ultra–short-acting barbiturates are potent respiratory depressants, depressing both rate and tidal volume and therefore minute ventilation. The respiratory center response to increases in $PaCO_2$ is delayed, and the maximum ventilatory response is decreased. The carotid-aortic chemoreceptors are also depressed. Although initial arousal from an ultra–short-acting thiobarbiturate is dependent on redistribution of the drug into the various body tissue compartments, ultimately they must be metabolized in the liver to be excreted. If an animal receives an overdose of a thiobarbiturate or redistribution is hindered because of a lack of body fat, hepatic biodegradation then becomes the main factor for arousal and awakening. Because the dog and cat do not readily metabolize the thiobarbiturates, very prolonged recovery times (6 to 24 hours) may be observed. If, in addition, hepatic dysfunction is also evident in the animal, the recovery from a thiobarbiturate may take even longer if tissue redistribution is altered.

Because of the ability of the ultra–short-acting thiobarbiturates to depress the cardiovascular system and especially the respiratory system, they should be used with extreme care in the geriatric animal that may already have cardiopulmonary compromise. In addition, the geriatric animal may have decreased plasma protein-binding capabilities, hepatic dysfunction, and an increase in the total body lipid into which the thiobarbiturates are ultimately distributed. These three factors may cause a marked increase in the physiologic effect and the duration of action of a given dose of ultra–short-acting thiobarbiturate.

Dissociative Anesthetic Agents. Dissociative anesthetic agents are cyclohexanone derivatives that produce a cataleptic state characterized by CNS excitement rather than depression, analgesia, immobility, dissociation from one's environment, and amnesia. The two drugs in this group available for veterinary anesthesia are ketamine and tiletamine.

The drugs have the same basic pharmacologic effects. They appear to depress the thalamocortical system (the association region of the cerebral cortex) selectively while stimulating the reticular-activating and limbic systems. Ketamine and tiletamine appear to potently inhibit gamma-aminobutyric acid (GABA)-binding in the CNS, enhance inhibitory mechanisms through the action of the GABA systems, and block neuronal transport processes for the monoamine transmitters such as 5-hydroxytryptamine (serotonin), dopamine, and norepinephrine.

These drugs tend to stimulate the cardiovascular system. The mechanism(s) by which this occurs is not completely understood. Ketamine and tiletamine exert a selective positive inotropic effect on heart muscle that is independent of heart rate and/or the autonomic nervous system. They tend to cause an increase in heart rate, cardiac output, mean arterial blood pressure, pulmonary arterial blood pressure, and central venous pressure either by directly stimulating the central adrenergic centers or by indirectly preventing the uptake of the catecholamines. Both dissociative agents seem to have antidysrhythmic activity. As a result of the increase in the heart rate, there can be a marked increase in myocardial oxygen consumption and demands. Large doses of ketamine and tiletamine, especially when administered intravenously, can have a marked depressant effect on the cardiovascular system.

Both drugs can produce apneustic ventilation, that is, a ventilatory pattern characterized by a prolonged pause after inspiration. Although the respiratory rate may decrease, the tidal volume usually remains normal. In general, the respiratory alterations do not affect the blood gases; however, in some animals the dissociative agents can produce marked hypoxia and hypercarbia, especially when additional CNS-depressant drugs, such as tranquilizers, sedatives, or opioids, are used in combination with them. Dissociative agents do not depress the pharyngeal or laryngeal reflexes, although they may only be activated with stimulation; therefore, an animal may be more prone to laryngospasm, bronchospasm, and coughing because of these agents' activity. The dissociative agents increase salivation and respiratory secretions, sometimes to the point of aspiration and respiratory obstruction. For this reason, the use of an anticholinergic in combination with these drugs may be indicated.

The dissociative agents produce muscle tonus and increased limb rigidity, often necessitating the additional use of a tranquilizer-sedative to produce better muscle relaxation. Animals under the effects of these drugs may have spontaneous, random limb movements not associated with pain. Eyelid and corneal reflexes remain intact, and the eyes remain open; therefore, eye ointment should be used to prevent corneal drying. Because coughing, swallowing, corneal, and pedal reflexes are maintained, these reflexes cannot be used to adequately judge the depth of anesthesia.

In the dog, ketamine and tiletamine undergo extensive hepatic biodegradation, with the water-soluble metabolites being excreted in the urine. Because both drugs are rapidly metabolized in the dog, the duration of anesthesia from an IM dose is approximately 20 to 30 minutes, with full recovery in 2 to 4 hours. In the cat, the majority of the injected dissociative agent is eliminated intact by the kidneys, with only 25% to 35% of the dose metabolized by the liver. Therefore, even though anesthesia time from a single IM dose of one of these drugs may last 20 to 40 minutes in the cat, full recovery may take 5 hours or more. Both drugs are highly lipid soluble. This accounts for the rapid induction of anesthesia following IM administration.

Ketamine has been used intravenously in the dog and cat at a dose of 2 to 4 mg/kg to induce general anesthesia and for short surgical procedures (lasting less than 10 minutes). Ketamine may produce seizures, especially in the dog, and for this reason diazepam, at a dose of 0.4 mg/kg IV is often administered with it. Acetylpromazine may also be used with ketamine at a dose of 0.1 mg/kg IV or IM (to a maximum total dose of 2 mg). Acetylpromazine aids in providing better muscle relaxation and will help prevent ketamine-induced seizures because of its dopamine-blocking capabilities.

Telazol is a combination of equal parts by weight of tiletamine and zolazepam (a nonphenothiazine diazepinone tranquilizer). It is supplied in sterile vials containing 500 mg of active drug (250 mg of tiletamine and 250 mg of zolazepam). Sterile diluent (5 ml) is added to produce 100 mg/ml of active drug. Telazol is a class III controlled substance approved only for IM use in the dog and cat.

In the dog, Telazol is recommended as an anesthetic for diagnostic examinations, restraint, treatment of lacerations and wounds, castrations, and any procedure requiring mild-to-moderate analgesia. The dose range is 6 to 12 mg/kg IM. Supplemental doses may be given, but any supplemental dose should be less than the initial dose, and the total dose given (initial dose plus supplemental dose or doses) should not exceed 20 mg/kg in the dog. Telazol is not recommended as the sole agent for use in the dog for procedures requiring major analgesia such as abdominal or thoracic procedures.

In the cat, Telazol is recommended as an anesthetic for procedures ranging from diagnostic examinations and restraint to declawing and ovariohysterectomies. The dose range is 9 to 15 mg/kg IM. As with the dog, supplemental doses may be given, but any supplemental dose should be less than the initial dose, and the total dose given (initial dose plus supplemental dose or doses) should not exceed 50 mg/kg. Telazol has a wider margin of safety in cats than in dogs.

Repeated doses of Telazol increase the duration of effect of the drug but may not further diminish muscle tone, and the recovery is extended with multiple doses. The quality of anesthesia varies with repeated doses, because the ratio between tiletamine and zolazepam within the animal changes with each injection. Therefore, giving repeated doses of Telazol to prolong anesthesia time should be avoided if possible.

In the dog, both tiletamine and zolazepam undergo extensive biodegradation in the liver, with less than 4% of the injected dose excreted unchanged. In the cat, both drugs are excreted virtually intact by the kidneys. Following IM injection, animals lose the righting reflex in 3 to 4 minutes, with the onset of surgical anesthesia in 6 to 7 minutes. The duration of surgical anesthesia ranges from 20 to 30 minutes. Righting reflexes return in 2 to 3 hours, with full recovery in 4 to 6 hours. Supplemental doses will prolong the recovery period.

Ketamine and Telazol should be used with caution in geriatric animals with preexisting cardiovascular or pulmonary dysfunction. The sinus tachycardia produced by both these drugs may be disadvantageous in the geriatric animal because of the marked increase in oxygen consumption and demands. The geriatric animal may not have the cardiac reserve to withstand this increased heart rate. The dissociative agents may also exacerbate any preexisting pulmonary dysfunction and further compromise the animal. Animals with renal or hepatic dysfunction may be expected to have prolonged recovery times.

Propofol (Diprivan). Propofol is a highly lipid-soluble alkylphenol that is a rapid-acting IV anesthetic agent. It is insoluble in water and must be solubilized in a lecithin-containing emulsion. Propofol is formulated as 1% emulsion containing 10% soybean oil, 1.2% egg lecithin, and 2.25% glycerol. Propofol can be used for short periods of anesthesia (5 to 10 minutes) following a single bolus. More prolonged anesthesia can be maintained using repeated bolus injections or continuous infusion.

Propofol's rapid onset time is similar to that of thiamylal and thiopental. A single bolus injection of propofol produces a rapid onset of anesthesia (less than 60 seconds), lasting 5 to 10 minutes

TABLE 7-4. PHARMACOKINETICS OF INTRAVENOUS GENERAL ANESTHETIC AGENTS

DRUG GROUP	DRUG NAME	DISTRIBUTION HALF-LIFE (MINUTES)	ELIMINATION HALF-LIFE (HOURS)
Barbiturates	Thiopental	2-4	10-12
	Methohexital	5-6	3-5
Imidazoles	Etomidate	2-4	2-5
Arylcyclohexylamines	Telazol	11-17	2-3
Alkylphenols	Propofol	2-4	1-3

(Table 7-4). The induction is smooth and excitement free; however, transient local pain due to venoirritation may occur during induction. Propofol-induced excitatory activity, such as movements, myoclonic twitching, and muscle tremors, has been reported in some animals.

Recovery is very rapid following even repeated doses of propofol. It is rapidly redistributed and rapidly metabolized by glucuronidation and sulfonation. After 30 minutes, less than 20% of the dose can be recovered as unchanged compound. Total body clearance exceeds hepatic blood flow, and, although hepatic metabolism plays a major role in clearance, other tissues (lung) are also involved. Excretion of 90% of propofol is via the urine in the form of water-soluble glucuronide and sulfate conjugates, and there are no known active metabolites. Cats have a deficiency in their ability to conjugate phenols and, although the reported recovery times following single or repeated doses of propofol are similar in dogs and cats, continuous infusion may produce more prolonged recoveries in cats.

The total calculated dose used for anesthetic induction in the dog and cat is 6 mg/kg IV. The drug is administered to effect much the same way thiamylal and thiopental are. Approximately one quarter to one third of the dose is administered every 30 to 45 seconds until the desired level of anesthesia is produced. The total dose given will depend on the preanesthetic sedatives used, the degree of animal sedation, and the physical status of the animal. Following propofol induction, anesthesia can be maintained with inhalation agents or by repeated bolus injections or continuous infusions of propofol. Propofol can be used at a maintenance infusion of 0.2 to 0.4 mg/kg/min. The maintenance infusion is increased or decreased depending on the desired anesthetic level of the animal.

The cardiopulmonary effects of propofol are similar to those of the barbiturates (Table 7-5). Propofol causes a decrease in cerebral blood flow and oxygen consumption. It causes direct myocardial depression, peripheral vasodilation, venodilation, and hypotension. Propofol can produce respiratory depression. The incidence of apnea with propofol is comparable to the barbiturates, but the duration of apneic episodes may be slightly longer. The cardiopulmonary effects of propofol are dose dependent.

The pharmacokinetic action of propofol in animals with renal and hepatic dysfunction is similar to that in nondiseased animals, suggesting it would be suitable for animals with renal and/or hepatic impairment. Propofol has been safely used in sighthound dog breeds.

Propofol is a drug that seems ideally suited for use as a continuous infusion for the maintenance of anesthesia. Recovery is rapid with minimal "drug hangover." Drug buildup does not appear to be a problem with propofol when compared with the barbiturates or the dissociative agents. Myoclonic twitching, muscle tremors, and muscle movements have been reported in humans and dogs during maintenance of anesthesia with propofol. During these episodes, anesthetic depth appears adequate, and arterial blood gases and pH are normal. Diazepam, 2.5 to 5 mg IV given slowly, has been used to control the myoclonus when necessary.

Propofol may be suited for use in the geriatric animal, because recovery times do not seem to be prolonged in animals with renal or hepatic dysfunction. However, because its cardiopulmonary depressant effects are very similar to those of the thiobarbiturates, it should be used with caution in any animal with preexisting cardiopulmonary disease or dysfunction.

Etomidate (Amidate). Etomidate is a carboxylated imidazole-containing compound that is structurally unrelated to any other IV anesthetic. It is a sedative-hypnotic with a rapid onset of action and a rapid recovery. It is a weak base dissolved in propylene glycol; therefore, IV infusion can be associated with pain and venoirritation.

Etomidate has been used in veterinary anesthesia although it has not been approved for use at this time. The induction dose of etomidate in

TABLE 7-5. SUMMARY OF COMPARATIVE PHARMACOLOGIC PROPERTIES OF INTRAVENOUS INDUCTION AGENTS

PROPERTIES	THIOPENTAL	ETOMIDATE	TELAZOL	PROPOFOL
Solubility	Water	Propylene glycol	Water	Egg lecithin
Dose (mg/kg)	8-12 (IV)	1.5-3 (IV)	4-16 (IM) 1-2 (IV)	2-6 (IV)
Onset	Rapid	Rapid	Rapid	Rapid
Induction	Smooth	Pain/myoclonus	Excitatory/smooth	Smooth/pain
Cardiovascular effects	Depression	Minimal	Stimulation	Depression
Respiratory effect	Depression	Minimal	Minimal/Moderate depression	Depression
Analgesia	None	None	Superficial—yes Deep visceral—?	None
Amnesia	Minimal	Minimal	Minimal	Minimal
Recovery	Rapid	Rapid	Intermediate	Rapid

IM, Intramuscular; *IV,* intravenous.

the dog and cat is 1.5 to 3 mg/kg IV. The dose is given to effect and will depend on the preanesthetic sedatives given to the animal and the physical status of the animal. A single bolus injection produces a rapid loss of consciousness with duration of action of 5 to 10 minutes. Etomidate undergoes rapid hepatic hydrolysis to inactive metabolites. This results in a rapid recovery and a lack of accumulation when used in repeated boluses or as an infusion.

At doses used to produce general anesthesia (3 mg/kg IV), etomidate produces no change in heart rate, cardiac output, or mean arterial blood pressure. Cardiovascular stability may be better with etomidate because it better maintains baroreceptor-mediated responses. Etomidate can produce a mild-to-moderate dose-dependent respiratory depression (see Table 7-5).

Several adverse side effects have been reported with etomidate. Pain and phlebitis have been associated with the IV injections of etomidate. These effects may be due to the carrier agent propylene glycol. Excitement during induction and recovery has been reported. This can be partially or completely eliminated by using preanesthetic sedatives. Retching, myoclonus, and apnea have been reported in humans and dogs during induction. Etomidate has been demonstrated to temporarily inhibit adrenal steroidogenesis in humans and dogs. Whether or not this inhibition is significant to the animal is controversial.

Etomidate's minimal cardiopulmonary depressant effects and its rapid metabolism and recovery would make it seem ideally suited for the geriatric animal. However, the adverse side effects during induction may limit its use, at least at the present time.

Inhalant General Anesthetic Agents

Inhalant general anesthetic agents are probably the anesthetic agents of choice in the geriatric animal, especially for procedures lasting longer than 10 to 15 minutes and in the very debilitated animal. Methoxyflurane, halothane, or isoflurane can all be used either with or without nitrous oxide.

Methoxyflurane. Methoxyflurane is a methyl-ethyl-ether that is the most potent (lowest MAC requirement) of the volatile inhalant anesthetic agents. Because of its high blood and rubber solubility, induction and recovery from methoxyflurane when compared with the other inhalant agents is slow. Methoxyflurane depresses the cardiovascular system in a dose-dependent fashion. It depresses heart rate, stroke volume, and cardiac output. Spontaneous cardiac dysrhythmias are not common during methoxyflurane anesthesia.

Methoxyflurane can produce hypotension primarily because of the decreased cardiac output. At normal anesthetic concentrations, peripheral resistance is usually maintained; therefore, large falls in arterial blood pressure may not be observed. However, with high doses of methoxyflurane, peripheral resistance decreases, and significant falls in arterial blood pressure may occur. Methoxyflurane produces a dose-dependent respiratory depression by decreasing the respiratory rate and tidal volume. Methoxyflurane can produce a transitory hepatic depression, but it does not appear to be directly hepatotoxic. Methoxyflurane may alter renal function by decreasing renal blood flow. It has also been shown to produce direct renal toxicity in humans through its metabolic by-products, primarily oxalic acid and inorganic fluoride ion. The renal toxicity produced by methoxyflurane is characterized by proximal renal tubular necrosis with a high-output renal failure, hypernatremia, elevated blood urea nitrogen, and dehydration. As much as 80% of the inspired methoxyflurane is metabolized by the liver. Although there are no specific contraindications to the use of methoxyflurane, it should be used with caution in the presence of renal or hepatic dysfunction.

Halothane. Halothane is a halogenated hydrocarbon that produces a fairly rapid induction and recovery from anesthesia. Halothane can produce significant cardiovascular depression that is directly related to the administered concentration. Myocardial contractility, heart rate, and cardiac output are decreased in a dose-dependent manner. Halothane can produce marked arterial hypotension owing to direct myocardial depression, decreased peripheral resistance, and direct depression of the vasomotor center. Spontaneous cardiac dysrhythmias are more common with halothane than with methoxyflurane because halothane sensitizes the myocardium to catecholamines and also slows the conduction impulses through the His-Purkinje system, allowing for reentry of impulses. Halothane, like most inhalant and injectable anesthetic agents, has an additive effect on sinoarterial or atrioventricular conduction disturbances. Halothane has the lowest cardiac index (a low cardiac index equates to more myocardial depression) of the volatile anesthetic agents. Halothane produces the same amount of respiratory depression as does methoxyflurane at equipotent doses. Halothane does not have direct nephrotoxic effects, although it can produce a transitory decrease in renal function by decreasing blood flow. Up to 50% of the inspired halothane can be metabolized by the liver.

Halothane has been implicated as a possible cause of postanesthetic hepatitis in human patients. The phenomenon is extremely rare and is most likely related to the metabolites of halothane biodegradation. Halothane can be metabolized via an oxidative hepatic microsomal enzyme pathway (major pathway), which produces relatively harmless metabolites, or it can occur via a reductive pathway (non–oxygen-dependent and minor pathway), which produces potentially harmful metabolites. The reactive intermediate metabolites produced by the reductive pathway can covalently bind to hepatic proteins, lipoproteins, and lipids, altering their function and resulting in hepatic necrosis. Certain factors seem to increase the risk of "halothane hepatitis" in human patients, including intraoperative hepatic hypoxia, reductive metabolism of halothane by the liver, and genetics of the animal. Repeated halothane exposure seems to be less important.

Halothane should be used with extreme caution in animals with cardiac conduction problems or other dysrhythmias and in animals with myocardial disease. Halothane is contraindicated in animals that have developed an unexplained postanesthetic hepatitis following its use or in animals with active hepatitis. Chronic liver dysfunction should also preclude the use of halothane.

Isoflurane (AErrane). Isoflurane is halogenated ether that is the newest of the volatile inhalant agents. It is the least soluble of the volatile inhalation anesthetic agents in blood, body tissues, and conductive rubber components of the anesthetic circuit. This accounts for its very rapid induction time (3 to 5 minutes) and its very rapid recovery time (often less than 5 minutes). The MAC for isoflurane is 1.3 and 1.6 in the dog and cat, respectively; therefore it is less potent than methoxyflurane or halothane. In normal animals, the isoflurane concentrations needed to provide clinical surgical anesthesia will have minimal depressant effects on the cardiovascular system. Its cardiovascular margin of safety seems to be greater than that for halothane or methoxyflurane; in fact, it has the highest cardiac index of the volatile inhalant anesthetic agents. Although isoflurane does decrease the stroke volume, the heart rate remains the same or increases slightly and compensates for the decreased stroke volume; therefore, cardiac output does not fall significantly. Isoflurane does decrease arterial blood pressure in a dose-related fashion primarily because of a decreased vascular resistance (vasodilation) and not to a decreased cardiac output. Peripheral perfusion is adequately maintained at the normal anesthetic concentrations clinically used. Isoflurane decreases myocardial oxygen consumption and coronary vascular resistance without decreasing coronary blood flow. It produces an extremely stable heart rhythm, because isoflurane does not seem to sensitize the myocardium to catecholamines, and it does not slow the conduction of impulses through the His-Purkinje system. Isoflurane depresses respiration in a dose-related fashion and is slightly more depressant than methoxyflurane and halothane. It does not appear to produce any liver damage even when used for long procedures or during hypoxia. Isoflurane, like the other inhalant anesthetic agents, produces a transitory decrease in renal blood flow, glomerular filtration rate, and urine flow. No direct renal toxicity has been reported. Only about 0.2% of the inhaled isoflurane undergoes hepatic biodegradation. There are no major precautions or contraindications to the use of isoflurane, and, in fact, it is probably the volatile inhalant anesthetic of choice in the geriatric animal.

Nitrous Oxide. Nitrous oxide is an inorganic gas that can be used in combination with any of the volatile anesthetic agents. The minimum alveolar concentration in the dog and cat is 200% and 250%, respectively. This means it is a very weak CNS depressant and is not capable of producing general anesthesia by itself; therefore, to obtain surgical anesthesia, one must use hypnotics, narcotics, or other inhalation anesthetic agents in combination with it. Nitrous oxide has minimal effects on cardiopulmonary function unless hypoxia occurs, and it has no appreciable effects on other organ systems. Nitrous oxide can be used with the more potent inhalant anesthetic agents during mask induction to induce anesthesia more rapidly in the animal owing to a concentrating or "second gas effect" of the nitrous oxide.

Nitrous oxide must be combined with other CNS depressant drugs or anesthetic agents for maintenance of anesthesia. For maintenance, it is recommended that 50% to 66% nitrous oxide be used in combination with 50% to 33% oxygen. At least 30% oxygen should always be administered with the nitrous oxide. The concentration of the other, more potent inhalation anesthetic agents can be decreased by one third to one half when nitrous oxide is used in combination with them. Nitrous oxide and oxygen can be used in combination with hypnotics, narcotics, or local anesthetic agents for minor procedures in the geriatric animal.

There are several precautions to be aware of with nitrous oxide. General anesthesia cannot be produced with nitrous oxide alone. Nitrous oxide may cause increased tension in the gas pockets of the body; therefore, it may compound problems when used in the presence of a pneumothorax or intestinal obstruction. Diffusion hypoxia may occur when nitrous oxide is discontinued and the animal is allowed to breathe room air immediately. Therefore, the animal should be allowed to breathe 100% oxygen for a minimum of 5 minutes following its discontinuation. Hypoxia is always a danger with nitrous oxide unless at least 30% oxygen is administered with it. If the animal develops cyanosis while receiving nitrous oxide, it should be discontinued immediately and 100% oxygen should be administered.

MISCELLANEOUS CONSIDERATIONS

Regardless of the anesthetic techniques used in a particular geriatric animal, certain protocols should be incorporated. Geriatric animals should be preoxygenated for 2 to 5 minutes before anesthetic induction to help prevent hypoxia from developing during induction. The animal should be intubated when a general anesthetic is used to provide a patent airway. Close monitoring of cardiovascular and respiratory parameters are essential and, if necessary, the geriatric animal's ventilation should be assisted or controlled.

Adequate fluid replacement should be given to prevent a renal crisis and to help maintain a proper hemodynamic state in the geriatric animal. The specific fluid used will be dictated by the particular animal's needs; however, in most situations, a balanced electrolyte solution, such as lactated Ringer's or Normosol-R solution, is a reasonable choice. Because hypoglycemia during and after anesthesia can be a problem in the geriatric animal, administering fluids containing glucose may be warranted. The rate of IV fluid administration again depends on the particular animal's needs but will most likely be in the range of 10 to 20 ml/kg/h. Obviously, the rate will be decreased in a geriatric animal where the risk of cardiovascular overload, with the subsequent development of pulmonary edema, is a concern. Fluid therapy may need to be continued for several hours to several days following anesthesia and surgery.

Methods should be used to prevent or decrease hypothermia during and after the surgical procedure. The intraoperative monitoring techniques should be continued into the postoperative period or until the geriatric animal has returned to the preanesthetized state.

References

1. Knudson RJ, Clark DF, Kennedy TC et al: Effect of aging alone on mechanical properties of the normal adult lung, *J Appl Physiol* 43:1054, 1977.
2. Muiesan G, Sorbini CA, Grassi V: Respiratory function in the aged, *Bull Physiopathol Respir* 7:973, 1971.
3. Pontoppidan H, Beecher HK: Progressive loss of protective reflexes in the airway with the advance of age, *JAMA* 174:2209, 1960.
4. Ryan SF, Vericent TN, Mitchell RS et al: Ductasia—an asymptomatic pulmonary change related to age, *Med Thorac* 22:181, 1965.

5. Kronenberg RS, Drage CW: Attenuation of the ventilatory and heart rate responses to hypoxia and hypercapnia with aging in normal men, *J Clin Invest* 52:1812, 1973.
6. Dodman NH, Seeler DC, Court MH: Aging changes in the geriatric dog and their impact on anesthesia, *Compend Contin Educ Pract Vet* 6:1106, 1984.
7. Fisch C: Electrocardiogram in the aged—an independent marker of heart disease? *Am J Med* 70:4, 1981.
8. Owens W: The geriatric animal—physiology of aging, *Proc Am Soc Anesthesiologists* 275A:1, 1985.
9. Greenblatt DJ, Sellers EM, Shader RI: Drug disposition in old age, *N Engl J Med* 306:1081, 1982.
10. McLachlan MSF: The aging kidney, *Lancet* 2:143, 1978.
11. Lorhan PH: Physiological considerations. In Lorhan PH, ed: *Anesthesia for the aged,* Springfield, Ill, 1971, Charles C Thomas.
12. Devaney KO, Johnson HA: Neuron loss in the aging visual cortex of man, *J Gerontol* 35:836, 1980.
13. Collins KJ, Exton-Smith AN, James MH et al: Functional changes in autonomic nervous responses with aging, *Age Ageing* 9:17, 1980.
14. Cherondache CN, Romanoff LP: Hormones in aging men. In Gitman L, ed: *Endocrines and aging,* Springfield, Ill, 1967, Charles C Thomas.
15. Weidman P, DeMyttenoere-Buraztein S: Effect of aging on plasma renin and aldosterone in normal man, *Kidney Int* 8:325, 1975.
16. Feldman EC: The adrenal cortex. In Ettinger SJ, ed: *Textbook of veterinary internal medicine: diseases of the dog and cat,* Philadelphia, 1983, WB Saunders.
17. Rosychuk R: Management of hypothyroidism. In Kirk RW, ed: *Current veterinary therapy VIII,* Philadelphia, 1983, WB Saunders.
18. Davis PJ, Davis FB: Endocrinology and aging. In Reichel W, ed: *Clinical aspects of aging,* Baltimore, 1983, Williams & Wilkins.
19. Ouslander JG: Drug therapy in the elderly, *Ann Intern Med* 95:711, 1981.
20. Ritchel WA: Pharmacokinetics in the aged. In Pagliaro LA, Pagliaro AM, eds: *Pharmacologic aspects of aging,* St Louis, 1983, Mosby.
21. Richey DP, Bender AD: Pharmacokinetic consequences of aging, *Ann Rev Pharmacol Toxicol* 17:49, 1977.
22. Berkowitz BA, Ngai SH, Yang JC et al: The disposition of morphine in surgical animals, *Clin Pharmacol Ther* 17:629, 1975.
23. Giles HG, MacLoed SM, Wright JR et al: Influence of age and previous use on diazepam dosage required for endoscopy, *CMAJ* 118:513, 1978.
24. Quasha AL, Eger EI III, Tinker JH: Determination and application of MAC, *Anesthesiology* 53:315, 1980.
25. Bellville JW, Forrest WH, Miller E: Influence of age on pain and relief from analgesics: a study of postoperative animal, *JAMA* 217:1835, 1971.
26. Muravchick S: Effect of age and premedication on thiopental sleep dose, *Anesthesiology* 61:333, 1984.
27. Tranquilli WJ, Benson GJ: Advantages and guidelines for using alpha-2 agonists as anesthetic adjuvants, *Vet Clin North Am* 22:289, 1992.

Supplemental Reading

Lytle LD, Altar A: Diet, central nervous system and aging, *Fed Proc* 38:2017, 1979.

CHAPTER 8

Surgery and Its Application

DON R. WALDRON

The increased numbers of animals under veterinary care has seemingly increased the number of geriatric animals presented for medical and surgical care.[1] Improvement in veterinary nutrition, the quality of veterinary care, and the numbers of owners seeking improved veterinary care are likely causes of this increase in geriatric patients. It has been stated repeatedly that aging is not a specific disease but rather a complex process influenced by genetics, environment, and nutrition.[2] The veterinary profession has advanced over the past dozen years, allowing a distinction to be made between processes of aging as opposed to age-related disease. Nevertheless, increasing age does negatively affect an animal's ability to respond to stress. Furthermore, the geriatric animal is more likely to have multiple organ system disease and less functional organ reserve capacity than the young patient.[3,4] Surgery should not be viewed as impractical or prohibitive in the aged patient; however, complete and thorough evaluation of the animal is necessary to identify subclinical organ dysfunction that may become significant after hospitalization, anesthesia, and surgery. Similarly, there are known physiologic changes that occur in the aging animal that may affect the morbidity or mortality associated with surgical procedures.

Identification of specific problems that may affect an animal requires a complete and thorough history and physical examination, and collection of data regarding both the animal's surgical problem and any other clinical disease (Table 8-1). Focusing on the surgical problem is to be avoided initially; rather, the emphasis should be placed on identification of covert clinical disease by means of appropriate laboratory testing and imaging techniques.[5] Complete evaluation of the animal as a whole and specific evaluation of the surgical problem will allow the veterinarian to develop a rational plan of therapy that may or may not include surgery. If surgery is deemed necessary or appropriate, proper surgical planning should include consideration of the preoperative, intraoperative, and postoperative needs of the animal.

PHYSIOLOGY OF THE GERIATRIC ANIMAL AND ITS CLINICAL SIGNIFICANCE

Many organ systems undergo change with aging. Organ changes have been described in geriatric humans, and it is thought these same changes occur in animals.[3] In addition to physiologic changes in organ systems, aging may increase the role of other extrinsic factors that may affect the morbidity related to surgery in the aged animal. The risk of any surgical procedure is the sum of risks inherent in the animal's physical condition and the direct risk factors associated with the specific surgical procedure. In many cases, increased risk in the geriatric patient is due to the previously described impaired ability to maintain normal homeostasis. The stress of disease, hospitalization, anesthesia, and surgery may cause a compensated geriatric animal to decompensate, thus causing overt clinical disease in addition to the primary surgical problem.

TABLE 8-1. GERIATRIC SURGICAL DISEASE

SYSTEM OR ORGAN	PATHOLOGY	THERAPEUTIC OPTIONS
Digestive System		
Oral cavity	Neoplasia	Maxillectomy or mandibulectomy
	Inflammation or abscess	Dentistry
	Gingival hyperplasia	Gingivectomy
	Oronasal fistula	Mucoperiosteal flap
Tongue	Neoplasia	Partial glossectomy
Salivary gland	Mucocele	Mandibular or sublingual salivary gland, excision, drain mucocele
	Neoplasia	Excision of affected gland
Esophagus	Neoplasia	Resection and anastomosis, local excision for benign lesions (leiomyomas)
Stomach	Neoplasia	Partial gastrectomy or gastroduodenostomy
	Gastric dilation-volvulus	Decompression, permanent gastropexy
	Ulceration	Local excision or partial gastrectomy, consider underlying cause (nonsteroidal antiinflammatory drugs, mast cell tumor, gastrinoma, hepatic disease)
	Outlet obstruction	Gastroduodenostomy, Y-U pyloroplasty if benign
Small intestine	Neoplasia	Resection and anastomosis if localized, chemotherapy for lymphosarcoma
Cecum	Neoplasia	Typhlectomy
Colon	Neoplasia	Resection and anastomosis for malignancy, colonoscopic polyp excision
	Idiopathic megacolon	Subtotal colectomy
Rectum	Neoplasia	Submucosal resection, partial pull-through, Swenson's pull-through, dorsal approach for resection and anastomosis or extramural tumor excision
Perineum	Perineal hernia	Herniorrhaphy with internal obturator muscle flap and castration
	Perianal neoplasia	Surgical excision and castration for adenomas, castration and delayed local aggressive resection for sebaceous adenocarcinoma, excision for large adenomas
Anal sac	Neoplasia	Anal sacculectomy and abdominal lymphadenectomy, chemotherapy
	Abscess or inflammation	Anal sacculectomy
Liver	Neoplasia	Partial or total lobectomy if disease is localized to one lobe
Gall bladder	Cholelithiasis	Cholecystectomy
	Cholecystitis	Cholecystectomy
Pancreas	Beta-cell neoplasia	Tumor excision, metastases are functional; corticosteroids, diazoxide, or streptozotocin
	Adenocarcinoma	Partial pancreatectomy if localized
	Gastrinoma	Partial pancreatectomy, H_2 blockers, octreotide, proton pump inhibitors
	Abscess	Drainage, lavage
Respiratory System		
Nasal planum	Neoplasia	Nosectomy
Nasal cavity	Neoplasia	Radiation therapy (megavoltage or cobalt), rhinotomy plus orthovoltage radiation
Larynx	Paralysis	Unilateral arytenoid lateralization
	Collapse	Permanent tracheostomy, unilateral arytenoid lateralization, partial laryngectomy
Trachea	Collapse	Prosthetic rings for extrathoracic collapse, intraluminal stent for intrathoracic collapse
Lung	Neoplasia	Lobectomy, lymph node biopsy
Pleural space	Chylothorax	Thoracic duct ligation or embolization, pleuroperitoneal shunt
Cardiovascular System		
Cardiac	Right atrial neoplasia	Excision of right atrial appendage and tumor and pericardiectomy
	Atrioventricular block	Pacemaker implantation if second or third degree
	Pericardial effusion	Pericardiectomy if caused by neoplasia or idiopathic
Urologic System		
Renal	Lithiasis	Lithotripsy or nephrotomy and calculus removal if obstructive disease is present, "watchful waiting" if no infection or obstruction, nephrectomy if kidney is nonfunctional
	Neoplasia	Nephrectomy if unilateral
	Chronic renal failure or acute renal failure	Medical management, renal transplantation

TABLE 8-1. GERIATRIC SURGICAL DISEASE—cont'd

SYSTEM OR ORGAN	PATHOLOGY	THERAPEUTIC OPTIONS
Urologic System—cont'd		
Ureter	Lithiasis	Ureterotomy, lithotripsy
Urinary bladder	Lithiasis	Cystectomy, lithotripsy, or medical management if calculi are magnesium ammonium phosphate
	Neoplasia	Partial cystectomy if possible and/or chemotherapy, tube cystostomy for palliation
	Incontinence	Colposuspension if unresponsive to medical management
Urethra	Lithiasis	Urohydropulsion, scrotal, perineal, or antepubic urethrostomy
	Neoplasia	Vaginourethroplasty
	Stricture	Tube cystostomy for palliation
Endocrine System		
Thyroid	Neoplasia, canine	Thyroidectomy if freely movable and noninvasive, radiation
	Neoplasia, feline	I-131 therapy, thyroidectomy or medical management with methimazole
Parathyroid	Neoplasia	Parathyroidectomy
Adrenal	Neoplasia	Adrenalectomy
Pituitary	Neoplasia	Hypophysectomy
Reproductive System		
Testes	Neoplasia	Neutering
Prostate	Hyperplasia	Neutering
	Cyst	Drainage procedure, excision of cyst
	Inflammation	Omentalization of abscess
	Abscess	
	Neoplasia	
Mammary	Neoplasia, canine	Lumpectomy, regional or unilateral mastectomy, ovariohysterectomy
	Neoplasia, feline	Regional or unilateral mastectomy
Uterus or ovary	Pyometra	Ovariohysterectomy
	Neoplasia	Ovariohysterectomy
Vagina	Neoplasia	Excision of tumor, with or without episiotomy
Hematopoietic System		
Spleen	Neoplasia	Splenectomy
	Hematoma	Splenectomy, partial splenectomy
Nervous System		
Brain	Neoplasia	Excision, radiation therapy
Spinal Cord	Disk	Medical treatment or laminectomy if motor impairment or chronic pain
	Neoplasia	Excision by laminectomy if extradural or intradural or extramedullary
Nerve	Neoplasia	Excision with or without amputation
	Cauda equina	Laminectomy with or without foraminotomy
Skeletal System		
Joints	Degenerative joint disease	Treatment of underlying cause, weight control, exercise modification, analgesics, arthrodesis, excision arthroplasty, joint replacement
Coxofemoral	Hip dysplasia	Weight control, exercise modification, medical management, total hip arthroplasty, femoral head ostectomy
Stifle	Cranial cruciate rupture	Arthrotomy, joint stabilization, tibial plateau leveling osteotomy, fibular head transposition, conservative in small dogs and cats
Bone	Neoplasia	Amputation plus chemotherapy, limb-sparing treatment plus chemotherapy
Special Senses		
Skin	Neoplasia	Excision, laser ablation, cryosurgery
Ear	Neoplasia	Excision of tumor, vertical or total ear canal ablation
	Inflammation	Lateral ear canal resection, vertical or total ear canal ablation
	Hypertrophy	Lateral ear canal resection, vertical or total ear canal ablation
Eye	Neoplasia	Observation or enucleation
	Cataracts	Observation, phacoemulsification, intraocular lens implantation

Hepatic System

Altered hepatic microsomal enzyme systems may cause a decreased ability to metabolize drugs in the geriatric animal.[4] Elimination of some drugs is dependent on hepatic blood flow, which decreases with aging.[6] This decreased metabolic function may be present in spite of normal laboratory values. A decreased ability to metabolize or eliminate drugs has obvious implications from an anesthetic point of view but also affects administration of other drugs in the perioperative period such as antimicrobial and nonsteroidal antiinflammatory agents (NSAIDs). Severe liver disease may be responsible for hypoproteinemia, which delays wound healing. Similarly, severe disease may result in a decrease in blood clotting factors, thereby prolonging normal clotting times. Serum liver enzymes, albumin, and total protein levels and prothrombin and partial thromboplastin times may assist in assessing liver function. Fasted and postprandial serum bile acids more accurately reflect true liver function.

Renal System

Decreased renal function and decreased renal reserve are of utmost concern in the geriatric animal in the perioperative period (Table 8-2). The kidneys of the geriatric animal have decreases in glomerular numbers, tubular size and weight, and increased fibrosis.[7] It should be recalled that decreases in renal function as indicated by abnormal elevations in laboratory values (blood urea nitrogen and serum creatinine) are not linearly related. At least 65% to 75% of renal function is lost before there are increases in the commonly obtained laboratory values; therefore small increases in blood urea nitrogen may indicate large decreases in glomerular filtration rate. As always, blood urea nitrogen and serum creatinine values are interpreted in conjunction with urinalysis. Chronic renal failure produces mild to moderate elevations in blood urea nitrogen and serum creatinine, an isosthenuric urine, and mild anemia in some cases. More specific testing for renal function involves the use of creatinine clearance or glomerular filtration rates as determined by nuclear scintigraphy.

Even in the face of normal renal laboratory values, decreased renal blood flow as a result of less than normal cardiac output causes glomerular filtration rates of the kidneys to decrease. Glomerular filtration rates as determined by nuclear scintigraphy are not widely available in practice; however, they represent an excellent noninvasive means of evaluating the contribution of each kidney to overall renal function. This information is especially valuable when one is

TABLE 8-2. PRACTICAL GUIDE TO THE PREVENTION OF PERIOPERATIVE RENAL FAILURE IN GERIATRIC ANIMALS

PRINCIPLE	METHOD OR MEASUREMENT
Assess renal function accurately	Blood urea nitrogen Serum creatinine Urine output Glomerular filtration rate measured via scintigraphy
Assess and monitor volume status	Physical examination Serial body weights Packed cell volume and total solids Central venous pressure
Control and maintain blood pressure	Avoid hypotension by assuring normal volume status and surgical hemostasis Reverse severe hypotension with crystalloid fluids, blood products, and vasopressors
Relieve urinary tract obstruction	Prompt radiographic diagnosis Catheter drainage Surgical correction
Avoid known nephrotoxins	Limit use of aminoglycosides or nonsteroidal antiinflammatory drugs Limit use of intravenous contrast agents Adjust drug doses
Prevent sepsis	Abscess drainage (local, pancreatic, prostate) Catheter care Appropriate antibiotics
Consider diuresis	Crystalloid fluids in correct volume Mannitol, furosemide, dopamine Monitor urine output

Modified from Monroe WE, Waldron DR: Renal failure: surgical considerations. In Bojrab MJ, ed: *Disease mechanisms in small animal surgery*, ed 2, Philadelphia, 1993, Lea & Febiger.

considering surgery on the kidney itself, for example, nephrotomy or nephrectomy.

Animals with compensated renal disease may be anesthetized and operated on successfully; however, attention to perioperative fluid needs and urine production is critical in ensuring that the animal is not pushed into decompensated renal failure or that, conversely, overly zealous fluid administration does not cause pulmonary edema. Drugs that are potentially nephrotoxic such as NSAIDs and aminoglycoside antibiotics are used cautiously in the geriatric animal.

Cardiopulmonary Function

As with other organ systems, there is a decrease in cardiac reserve in geriatric patients compared with healthy young animals.[3] Although animals are not routinely diagnosed with primary vascular disease and hypertension as geriatric humans are, there is a decrease in cardiac output, baroreceptor activity, and circulation time in the geriatric animal.[8,9] Although the geriatric heart has normal contractile elements, its ability to respond to catecholamines is reduced.[5] The changes that occur negatively affect the animal's ability to maintain blood pressure during stress and anesthesia.[3,10] Valvular disease is extremely common in the geriatric canine, and myocardial disease may be seen in both the aging canine and feline. Valvular disease by itself, as evidenced by cardiac murmurs detected on physical examination, does not prohibit anesthesia or surgery; however, judicious use of crystalloid fluids is indicated, especially if renal function is also compromised.

In addition to careful auscultation and pulse examination, thoracic radiography, electrocardiography, and ultrasonography of the heart may aid in identifying specific disease, which may affect anesthesia and surgical planning.

Respiratory function decreases as the animal ages. Respiratory rate, tidal volume, lung elasticity, and partial pressure of arterial oxygen all decrease in the geriatric animal.[11,12] Gas exchange is less efficient, and ventilation-perfusion mismatch is potentially more prevalent and severe than in the young animal.[13] Clinically, the decreased function may result in hypoxia and hypercarbia, which may in turn negatively affect cardiac function by predisposing the animal to arrhythmias. Mild anesthetic depression of respiration in the normal young animal may be critical to the geriatric animal.[3]

Pulmonary function testing is not routinely performed in animals. Auscultation, thoracic radiography, and blood-gas analysis are available to aid in assessment of pulmonary function. Aspiration pneumonia may occur more commonly in geriatric humans and is especially common in the perioperative period in animals with laryngeal paralysis or esophageal disease.

Endocrine Disease

Endocrine diseases are diagnosed more commonly in the geriatric dog and cat. Diseases of the endocrine system often have a primary affect and also may affect other organ systems important in anesthesia and surgery. For example, parathyroid adenomas cause hypercalcemia, which may cause peripheral weakness and renal disease. Hyperthyroidism in cats causes primary gastrointestinal disturbances but has profound secondary effects on cardiac function. Hyperadrenocorticism, either naturally occurring or iatrogenic, may affect wound healing or wound infection rates in surgery of any type performed in the geriatric animal.

Some of the endocrine diseases diagnosed in geriatric animals are potentially surgical in nature, such as beta-cell tumors of the pancreas, hyperthyroidism in the cat, parathyroid adenomas, and functional adrenal tumors. Careful assessment of multiorgan systems before surgery is indicated in these animals. In some cases, the animal can be treated medically in the short term before surgery, and the risks associated with anesthesia and surgery are reduced. A hyperthyroid feline made euthyroid with methimazole and an animal with hyperadrenocorticism that is treated medically are examples of geriatric disease states in which the animal may be improved with medical therapy prior to definitive surgical therapy.

INFECTION AND WOUND HEALING

Wound infection rates in geriatric humans with clean or clean-contaminated wounds have been reported to be higher than in the younger population. Other authors, however, have not found age to be an independent predictor of wound infection.[14] Similarly, wound infection rates in animals, when assessed by univariate analysis, appear increased in the geriatric animal. However, when the same data are assessed by multivariate analysis, infection rates in the geriatric population appear the same as in younger populations; therefore, it appears that other factors including concurrent infections at distant sites or the presence of endocrinopathies likely influence wound infection rates.[15]

Wound healing is reported as delayed in geriatric humans[16] and in rats.[17,18] The effect of increasing age on wound healing in dogs and cats is questionable and probably not clinically significant; however, concurrent pathologic problems such as hyperadrenocorticism, diabetes mellitus, or hypoproteinemia negatively affects wound healing.[5]

Supplementation with vitamin A and anabolic steroids may correct the adverse effects of diabetes mellitus, corticosteroids, or radiation on healing and is commonly used in human surgical patients.[19]

PREOPERATIVE ASSESSMENT

History and Physical Examination

A thorough history and detailed physical examination are essential in assessing the geriatric animal's surgical needs. Information acquired may affect both the anesthesia and surgical protocols. Attention to possible drug interactions or their specific effects is especially important. Prolonged administration of corticosteroids or certain antibiotics for dermatologic disease or NSAIDs for degenerative joint disease is common in geriatric animals. These agents may affect wound healing, wound infection, renal function, microbial susceptibility, and blood clotting.[5,20]

History or physical findings of polydipsia, polyuria, lack of exercise tolerance, persistent cough, lameness, or undiagnosed mass may indicate a serious problem that requires further attention prior to surgery. History regarding the primary clinical problem is also important. A spontaneously occurring long bone or facial fracture in a geriatric animal with minor trauma may be secondary to neoplasia, infection, dental disease, or metabolic bone disease. Acute clinical signs seemingly associated with chronic problems may, in fact, be due to secondary disease. An acute rear limb lameness in a canine with a chronically luxating patella may indicate a cranial cruciate ligament injury. Similarly, a dyspneic geriatric animal of a brachycephalic breed may have an obstructed airway from laryngeal collapse or neoplasia rather than an elongated soft palate.

Physical examination includes careful thoracic auscultation and abdominal palpation. Superficial palpation of the entire body is advised to diagnose skin and mammary tumors, both of which have an increased prevalence in the geriatric animal.[21,22]

Preoperative Evaluation

The extent of preoperative evaluation is dictated by the primary surgical problem and any problems identified historically or on physical examination. A problem list should be made to guide the veterinarian in formulating differential diagnoses and a diagnostic plan. For elective surgery, a minimum database for geriatric animals should include a complete blood count, serum chemistry panel, urinalysis, and a lead II electrocardiogram. Thoracic radiographs are taken in many animals to identify cardiac or lung pathology that may affect anesthetic administration, although the value of such screening has been questioned in asymptomatic animals.[13] Three-view thoracic radiographs are considered mandatory in the animal with suspected or known cancer to identify possible metastatic disease prior to surgery. Thoracic metastatic lesions must be 3 to 5 mm in diameter before they are visible radiographically. A lead II electrocardiogram tracing is valuable as a screening tool for cardiac arrhythmias.

Undiagnosed lesions or masses identified on or within an animal can be initially assessed by fine needle aspiration and cytologic examination. Aspiration of superficial masses is routine; aspiration of abdominal or thoracic masses may require ultrasound guidance. In many animals, these procedures may be performed without anesthesia; however, sedation may be required for aspiration of masses within body cavities. Similarly, tissue biopsies from a sedated animal may be obtained using ultrasound guidance, local anesthesia, and a biopsy punch or Tru-Cut needle (Travenol Laboratories, Deerfield, Ill) technique. Biopsies of the liver, spleen, prostate, and kidneys are commonly performed by this method. A diagnosis obtained from biopsy specimens can be vital to constructing a rational therapeutic plan that may or may not include surgery.

Ultrasonography, magnetic resonance imaging, and computed tomography are valuable noninvasive tools for more complete evaluation of the geriatric animal. Sonographic evaluation of the abdomen by a skilled examiner is a sensitive means of screening for either primary or metastatic masses in the animal with suspected or known cancer. Advanced imaging techniques, such as magnetic resonance imaging or computed tomography, require general anesthesia but allow for more accurate assessment of normal and diseased tissue than conventional radiography and may further assist the surgeon in developing a therapeutic plan. The increased ability to image diseased tissue accurately may allow the surgeon to avoid unnecessary surgery when successful resection of diseased tissue is not possible. Endoscopic examination of the upper and/or lower gastrointestinal tract may provide tissue for diagnosis of enteric disease. Endoscopic examination may also characterize disease as focal or more diffuse in nature, thereby contributing to accurate therapeutic planning.

Preoperative Care

In the case of elective geriatric surgery, it is desirable that the animal be as "normal" as possible for anesthesia and surgery. This implies that any current therapy for preexisting defined disease be optimal. In addition to treatment of defined disease, provision of preoperative nutrition may be indicated to improve the overall health of the animal, especially if the animal has had chronic disease.[5] The stress of anesthesia and surgery can increase the basal metabolic rate significantly; therefore, attention to nutritional needs preoperatively and postoperatively is important. A high-energy, high-protein diet can meet these needs. Alternatively, a nasogastric, esophagostomy, or gastrostomy tube may be placed to assure that caloric and energy needs are met in the perioperative period. The importance of maintaining adequate nutrition in the feline to prevent hepatic lipidosis is well known.

Attention to fluid and electrolyte needs is important in the perioperative period. Electrolyte abnormalities should be corrected by oral or parenteral means prior to general anesthesia. During the preoperative fasting period, the well-hydrated animal is allowed free access to water until anesthesia is induced. If the animal's hydration status is questionable or there is evidence of renal disease, preoperative fluid therapy is advisable prior to anesthesia. Effects of fluid therapy may be monitored by packed cell volume and total solids measurement, body weight, serum chemistries, and quantitative urine production. The latter requires placement of an indwelling urinary catheter that is connected to a closed collection system.

The need for blood transfusion is a clinical judgment; however, existing anemia in which the packed cell volume is less than 25% is an indication for cross-matched packed cells or whole blood transfusion prior to general anesthesia and surgery.

Surgical Planning

The critical periods for the geriatric animal undergoing surgery are at anesthesia induction, intraoperatively, and in the immediate postoperative period.[5] Every effort is made to minimize stress on the animal preoperatively. For elective surgery, geriatric animals may be evaluated as outpatients and then presented fasted (free-choice water) on the morning of surgery. Proper planning and preparation for both general and specific needs during surgery will allow the surgeon to minimize the animal's time under general anesthesia. Consideration of the following guidelines may decrease anesthesia time and improve operative efficiency in the geriatric animal.[5,20]

- Consider the need for equipment appropriate to the specific surgery.
- Have a specific operative goal or goals prior to surgery; have contingency or alternative plans should problems arise. Plan on biopsy of diseased tissue if resection is not possible.
- Be familiar with the surgical procedure and know the appropriate anatomy.
- Consider the need for cross-matching and possible intraoperative or postoperative blood transfusion if blood loss is likely. Consider the possibility of using colloids such as plasma or hetastarch.
- If the animal is cooperative clip the surgical site immediately prior to induction of anesthesia; alternatively the clip may be performed in the premedicated animal.
- Once anesthesia is induced and the animal is stabilized, complete the preoperative surgical site preparation as expeditiously as possible and move the animal to the operating room.
- Consider the need for appropriate antibiotics in the intraoperative and postoperative periods.

Surgical procedures that are expected to last longer than 90 minutes have a higher rate of bacterial wound contamination, and prophylactic antibiotic therapy is indicated. In addition, procedures that are clean-contaminated (entry into the gastrointestinal, respiratory, or infected urinary tract) or contaminated (entry into the colon) require the administration of antibiotics effective against suspected pathogens. Perioperative antimicrobial agents should be given in these cases in the immediate preoperative period after anesthetic induction and intraoperatively if the procedure exceeds 90 minutes; one or two doses should be given postoperatively.

Intraoperative Monitoring and Support

Close monitoring of the animal is indicated during surgery. Routine intraoperative monitoring should include electrocardiogram and pulse oximetry in addition to physical monitoring of pulse quality (Figure 8-1). End-tidal CO_2 monitoring is a sensitive means of measuring the adequacy of ventilation, but the equipment is expensive. Blood pressure may be monitored noninvasively with Doppler equipment or oscillometric monitoring using a pneumatic cuff. Urine production as measured by use of an indwelling urinary catheter and closed collection system is an indirect measure of the adequacy of blood pressure and a direct measure of renal function, which is important in any animal with renal compromise or in an animal that undergoes renal surgery. Normal urine output should be at least 1 to 2 ml/kg/h.

Intraoperative administration of crystalloid intravenous fluids is routinely provided at 10 to 20 ml/kg/h to provide cardiovascular and renal support. In general, a balanced electrolyte solution such as lactated Ringer's is used, although specific disease processes may dictate the selection of other fluids. Pharmacologic management of oliguria during surgery is indicated in some cases. If the animal has been adequately volume expanded, the use of a dopamine drip (2 to 5 μg/kg/min), furosemide (2 to 4 mg/kg bolus), or mannitol 0.5 g/kg given over 15 minutes) may be considered to increase urine production.

The older animal has less efficient thermoregulatory control, so attempts should be made during surgery to keep the animal warm.[5] Core body temperature is usually monitored with rectal or esophageal thermometers or by other intermittent manual methods. Maintenance of body temperature is especially difficult in animals weighing <5 kg when body cavities are opened. Warm water–circulating blankets (Gaymar Industries, Orchard Park, N.Y.) (Figure 8-2), circulating hot air blankets (Bair Hugger, Augustine Medical, Eden Prairie, Minn.) (Figure 8-3), and warm lavage solutions are useful in prevention and treatment of hypothermia.

SURGICAL PRINCIPLES

Appropriate surgical planning, as suggested previously, will expedite the surgical procedure and reduce the need for crisis-based decisions. In addition to a surgical plan, specific techniques and equipment are available to maximize the surgeon's efficiency. Maximizing the efficiency of

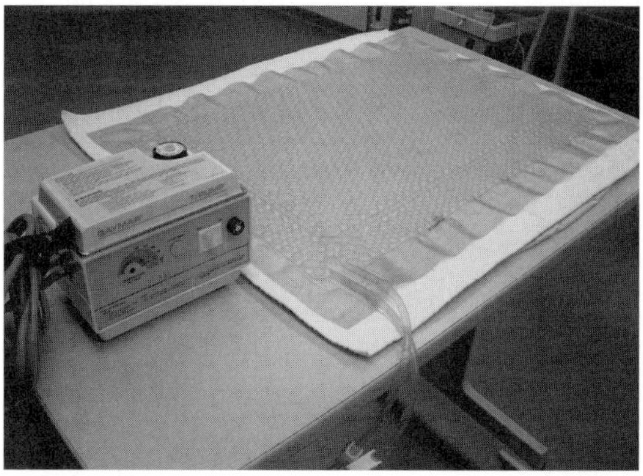

Figure 8-2. Circulating warm water blanket that is useful in preventing hypothermia.

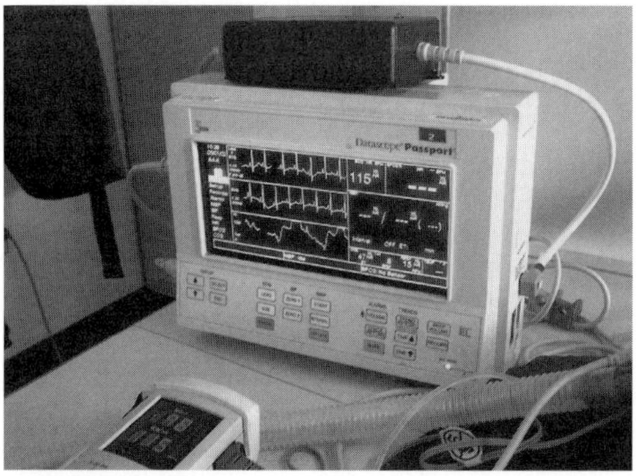

Figure 8-1. Intraoperative monitoring of electrocardiographic tracing, heart rate, and pulse oximetry with one monitor.

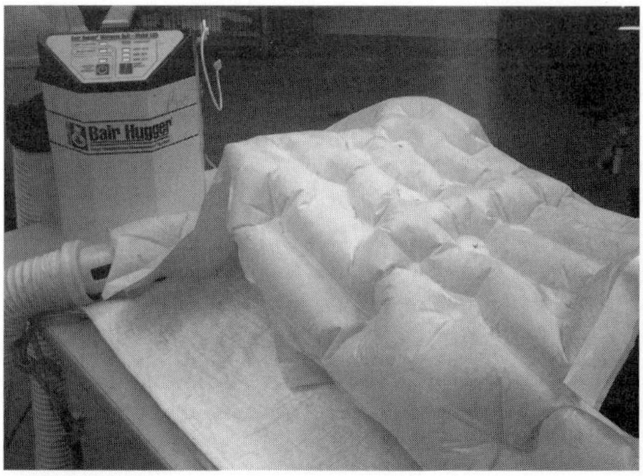

Figure 8-3. Circulating hot air blankets also assist in preventing hypothermia and provide more uniform body coverage than water blankets.

the surgical procedure will reduce anesthesia time and stress on the geriatric animal.[5]

Adequate surgical exposure is extremely important for any surgical procedure. A generous incision that is appropriate for the specific procedure is made. Small incisions made in an effort to decrease operative time compromise surgical exposure and tend to increase operative time. Another technique to assist in exposure involves the use of self-retaining retractors. Balfour retractors are especially valuable to maintain exposure during abdominal procedures; Gelpi or Weitlander retractors are useful for orthopedic or neurologic cases. Direct surgical assistance from and tissue retraction by a technician are invaluable during many surgical procedures.

Appropriate tissues should be excised or biopsies obtained. If neoplastic masses or organs are excised, regional lymph nodes should be excised or biopsied to stage the disease. Liver biopsies are easily obtained by the "guillotine" method using a loop of absorbable suture to attain hemostasis and cut through the edge of a liver lobe. Simple incisional biopsies are appropriate for obtaining renal, intestinal, bladder, or prostatic biopsies. Simple interrupted or mattress sutures of 3-0 or 4-0 polydioxanone (PDS II, Ethicon, N.J.) are used postbiopsy for hemostasis and to provide a leak-proof closure of hollow viscus.

The use of mechanical surgical stapling equipment saves considerable time for the surgeon and results in decreased anesthesia time. Thoracoabdominal surgical instruments (TA, United States Surgical Corporation, Norwalk, Conn.) are easy to use and place two or three staggered rows of staples that provide good hemostasis and leak-proof closure of soft tissues. These instruments place staple lines measuring 90, 55, or 30 mm in length and have been used for complete lung lobectomy, partial lung lobectomy, partial hepatectomy and splenectomy, closure of the stomach following partial gastrectomy, cecal removal, and prostatic and paraprostatic cyst removal.[23] Ligate-and-divide staplers (LDS, United States Surgical Corporation, Norwalk, Conn.) place two staples while a cutting blade cuts between them. This instrument is extremely useful for procedures such as splenectomy or in which the well-vascularized omentum must be dissected from abdominal masses. Vascular staples (Surgiclips, United States Surgical Corporation, Norwalk, Conn.) place a single vascular clip on vessels and are very convenient for use in deep cavities. The LDS stapler and Surgiclips are "user friendly" with essentially little or no learning curve for the surgeon.

Other stapling devices such as the gastrointestinal anastomosis (GIA, United States Surgical Corporation, Norwalk, Conn.) and end-to-end anastomosis (EEA, United States Surgical Corporation, Norwalk, Conn.) can save time when one performs gastrointestinal anastomoses, but efficient and safe use of these instruments requires considerable training and experience.

Simple continuous suture closure of the linea alba is a safe and quick alternative to simple interrupted patterns. Monofilament absorbable suture with prolonged tensile strength such as polydioxanone or polyglyconate (Maxon, United States Surgical Corporation, Norwalk, Conn.) or nonabsorbable material such as polypropylene (Prolene, Ethicon, NJ) or nylon (Dermalon, Ethicon, N.J.) is recommended for continuous closure. General suture size guidelines for continuous closure are as follows: for animals weighing <5 kg, use 3-0 suture; for those weighing 5 to 25 kg, use 2-0 suture; for those weighing 25 to 50 kg, use 0 suture; and for animals weighing >50 kg, use size 1 suture.

Skin staples are a time-saving adjunct to efficient surgery, especially when long linear incisions such as celiotomy or thoracotomy incisions are closed. Skin stapling is reported to be three to five times faster than suturing for wound closure.[24] Staplers are available from several manufacturers and generally come in two widths. Wide staples are preferred for use in animals and are most easily placed after an intradermal closure of the incision, which enhances skin alignment.

In recent years, minimally invasive surgical techniques have become more widely used in veterinary surgery. Arthroscopy, laparoscopy, thoracoscopy, and urethrocystoscopy have been used for diagnosis and therapy of some disease processes. Advantages include less morbidity and mortality than with open surgical techniques, and definitive tissue biopsy is possible under direct visualization. Disadvantages include the expense of the equipment, the need for training in specialized techniques, and in some cases limited visualization of complete body cavities. Considerable time may be saved depending on the specific procedure and the experience of the surgeon.

POSTOPERATIVE CONSIDERATIONS

Monitoring and Support

During the postoperative period, respiratory, cardiovascular, and renal compensatory mechanisms may be diminished and susceptible to dysfunction. Repetitive monitoring and evaluation of circulatory and metabolic parameters can clearly show the progression of a normal recovery or allow early detection of abnormalities that threaten normal recovery. Immediately following surgery, the animal should be placed on a preheated circulating water blanket and monitored constantly until extubation. Continuous monitoring of body temperature is advised until core body temperature reaches 37.8° C (100° F). Pulse and capillary refill time, respiration rate, and anesthetic depth are monitored closely until the animal is sternal, alert, and responsive. Thoracic auscultation is indicated, especially if aggressive fluid therapy is being administered. Blood pressure, central venous pressure, urine output, and electrocardiography monitoring may be indicated in animals whose condition is critical.

Fluid therapy is continued for at least 12 hours following any major surgical procedure; however, duration and volume ultimately depends on the animal's needs. After surgery, a packed cell volume and total solids should be recorded to establish a baseline for monitoring hydration status. Fluids at maintenance rates (40 to 60 ml/kg/day) are administered routinely; however, significant blood loss or concerns about renal function may dictate that higher rates be used.

Supplemental oxygen should be available for animal support as needed. Placement of a nasopharyngeal oxygen tube may be indicated in brachycephalic animals or geriatric animals with preexisting respiratory disease. Supplemental oxygen may also be administered by oxygen cage or face mask, although the latter is labor intensive. The need for mechanically assisted ventilation or placement of a tracheostomy tube is rare but should be anticipated and prepared for in some critical care cases.

Analgesia

Appropriate administration of analgesics to the geriatric animal can eliminate or reduce the stress and distress of postoperative pain. Opioids are the most reliable and predictable drugs for the relief of major postoperative pain. They may be administered parenterally or orally in some cases, and opioid cutaneous patches are available for longer duration analgesia.

NSAIDs are useful for minor postoperative pain but should not be used concurrently with corticosteroids because of the risks of gastrointestinal ulceration. Caution is advised if NSAIDs are used in animals with chronic renal failure.

Other methods of postoperative analgesia include the use of epidurally administered drugs and blocking of the pain response by local injection of lidocaine or marcaine.

Nutrition

Anticipation of the geriatric animal's nutritional needs in the perioperative period is important. Animals that have questionable nitrogen balance or those animals undergoing a surgical procedure that may impair eating should have a feeding tube placed while the animal is under anesthesia. Esophagostomy, percutaneous gastrostomy, or endoscopically assisted gastrostomy tubes have all been placed and used successfully to support animals nutritionally. It is important that nutritional therapy be administered early in the course of the animal's anorexia rather than after it has not eaten for several days.[5]

References

1. Kraft W: Geriatrics in canine and feline internal medicine, *Eur J Med Res* 3:31, 1998.
2. Goldston RT: Introduction and overview of geriatrics. In Goldston RT, Hoskins JD, eds: *Geriatrics and gerontology of the dog and cat,* Philadelphia, 1995, WB Saunders.
3. Harvey RC, Paddleford RR: Management of geriatric patients: a common occurrence, *Vet Clin North Am Small Anim Pract* 29:683, 1999.
4. Paddleford RR: Anesthetic considerations for the geriatric patient, *Vet Clin North Am Small Anim Pract* 19:13, 1989.
5. Hosgood G: Surgical protocol. In Goldston RT, Hoskins JD, eds: *Geriatrics and gerontology of the dog and cat,* Philadelphia, 1995, WB Saunders.
6. Aucoin DP: Drug therapy in the geriatric animal: the effect of aging on drug disposition, *Vet Clin North Am Small Anim Pract* 19:41, 1989.
7. Krawiec DR: Urologic disorders of the geriatric dog, *Vet Clin North Am Small Anim Pract* 19:75, 1989.
8. Dodman NH, Deeler DC, Court MH: Aging changes in the geriatric dog and their impact on anesthesia, *Compend Contin Educ Pract Vet* 6:1106, 1984.
9. Meurs KM, Miller MW, Slater MR: Arterial blood pressure measurement in a population of healthy geriatric dogs, *J Am Anim Hosp Assoc* 36:497, 2000.
10. Hamlin RL: Identifying the cardiovascular and pulmonary diseases that affect old dogs, *Vet Med* 85:483, 1990.
11. Robinson NE, Gillespie JR: Lung volumes in aging beagle dogs, *J Appl Physiol* 35:317, 1973.
12. Meyer RE: Anesthesia for neonatal and geriatric patients. In Short CE, ed: *Principles and practice of veterinary anesthesia,* Baltimore, 1987, Williams & Wilkins.
13. Muravchick S: Preoperative assessment of the elderly patient, *Anesthesiol Clin North Am* 18:71, 2000.
14. Sawyer RG, Pruett TL: Wound infections, *Surg Clin North Am* 74:519, 1994.

15. Brown DC: Personal communication, February, 2002.
16. Holt DR, Kirk SJ, Regan MC et al: Effect of age on wound healing in healthy human beings, *Surgery* 112:293, 1992.
17. Quirinia A, Viidik A: The influence of age on the healing of normal and ischemic skin wounds, *Mech Ageing Dev* 5:221, 1991.
18. Petersen TI, Kissmeyer-Nielsen P, Laurberg S et al: Impaired wound healing but unaltered colonic healing with increasing age: an experimental study in rats, *Eur Surg Res* 27:250, 1995.
19. Hunt TK, Hopf HW: Wound healing and wound infection: what surgeons and anesthesiologists can do, *Surg Clin North Am* 77:587, 1997.
20. Waldron DR, Budsberg SC: Surgery of the geriatric patient, *Vet Clin North Am Small Anim Pract* 19:33, 1989.
21. MacDonald J: Neoplastic diseases of the integument, *Proc Am Anim Hosp Assoc*, 1987.
22. Rutteman GR, Withrow SJ, MacEwen GE: Tumors of the mammary gland. In Withrow SJ, MacEwen GE, eds: *Small animal clinical oncology*, Philadelphia, 2001, WB Saunders.
23. Pavletic MM, Schwartz A: Stapling instrumentation, *Vet Clin North Am Small Anim Pract* 24:247, 1994.
24. Brickman KR, Lambert RW: Evaluation of skin stapling for wound closure in the emergency department, *Ann Emerg Med* 18:122, 1989.

Supplemental Readings

Willard MD: Endoscopy of body cavities. In Fossum TW, ed: *Small animal surgery*, St Louis, 2002, Mosby.

CHAPTER 9

The Respiratory System

JOSEPH TABOADA

Few diseases of the respiratory system, other than neoplasia, are exclusive diseases of geriatric dogs and cats. This chapter will discuss the effects of senescence on respiratory function and the diseases of the respiratory system that may occur in the geriatric dog and cat.

EFFECTS OF AGING ON THE RESPIRATORY SYSTEM

The determinants of static lung volumes are the elastic properties of the lungs and chest wall and the forces that can be generated by the muscles of respiration. With advancing age, there is progressive loss of pulmonary elasticity that results in changes in lung volumes, expiratory flow rates, and arterial blood gas values.[1] Chest wall compliance gradually decreases with age.[2] Age-related decreases in chest wall compliance, pulmonary compliance, and pulmonary elastic fiber properties are well tolerated. In one study of lung recoil pressure in elderly people, decreased recoil was evident only at lung volumes greater than 40% of total lung capacity (TLC).[3] TLC remains virtually constant as aging occurs, but vital capacity decreases by about 25%, whereas residual volume increases by about 50%.

Dynamic properties of airway resistance and respiratory muscle function are also affected by aging. As an animal reaches middle age, forced vital capacity and maximal expiratory flow rates decline.[4] Smaller airway caliper plays an important role in increased airway resistance. Lower levels of cyclic adenosine monophosphate (cAMP) may contribute to bronchial constriction, and decreased mucociliary transport function results in increased quantities of small airway mucus. The amount of smooth muscle in the walls of dog bronchi also decreases with age.

Distribution of ventilation changes with age. Closing capacity (closing volume [the lung volume at which dependent lung zones cease to ventilate] plus residual volume, expressed as percentage of TLC) increases until dependent airways are not routinely ventilated. This change is more important in bipedal animals such as humans but probably occurs in large deep-chested quadrupeds as well. Uniformity of ventilation is improved by increasing the depth of respiration and may account for observations of increased respiratory depth in aging patients. Membrane diffusing capacity has also been shown to decrease with advancing age.[5] These changes in closing capacity, ventilation, and diffusing capacity are important determinants of age-related changes in arterial PO_2.

Senescence results in a gradual reduction in arterial PO_2 by 15% to 20%.[1] The most important cause would appear to be ventilation-perfusion inequities associated with the age-related changes discussed above. Despite changes in arterial PO_2, arterial PCO_2 and arterial pH remain constant. Ventilatory response to hypoxia and hypercapnia is diminished with age.[6] Attenuation of response of both peripheral and central chemoreceptors and decreased central nervous system integrative functions are probably involved. This aging change results in diminution of an important protective mechanism in the patient that is most likely to be afflicted with chronic pulmonary diseases.

Respiratory muscle mass decreases with age, as does total muscle mass, resulting in decreased respiratory efforts during exercise or hypoxia from respiratory disease. Pulmonary intravascular pressure also progressively increases during exercise in the aged.[7] This can increase the potential risks of pulmonary hypertension or pulmonary thromboemboli as seen in hyperadrenocorticism, renal amyloidosis, or immune-mediated hemolytic anemia. The consequences of aging on the normal respiratory system are summarized in Table 9-1.

DISEASES OF THE NASAL CAVITY

History and Clinical Findings

Sneezing and nasal discharge are the most common clinical signs associated with nasal cavity disease. Nasal disease can occur in any aged dog and is of concern because of the high incidence of nasal or paranasal sinus neoplasia and chronic rhinitis secondary to dental disease.[8,9] When nasal discharge is reported, the veterinarian should question the owner about its color and consistency. Any changes in the discharge following treatment should also be noted. The initial

TABLE 9-1. EFFECTS OF AGING ON THE NORMAL RESPIRATORY SYSTEM

FUNCTION	AGE-RELATED EFFECT	CAUSE
Static Lung Volumes		
Total lung capacity	Unchanged	Changes in chest wall compliance, pulmonary compliance, pulmonary elasticity, and pulmonary fibrosis
Vital capacity	Decreased	
Compliance		
Chest wall compliance	Decreased	Decreased muscle strength, costal and costochondral ossification, and changes in rib conformation
Pulmonary compliance	Decreased	Remodeling of pulmonary elastic fibers and pulmonary fibrosis
Airway resistance	Increased	Decreased airway caliper resulting from bronchoconstriction and increased small airway mucus
Respiratory Muscle Function	Decreased	Decreases in muscle mass and strength, as well as increases in body fat content
Forced vital capacity	Decreased	
Maximal expiratory flow rate	Decreased	
Distribution of Ventilation		
Closing capacity	Increased	Dependent areas of lung are aerated less efficiently, resulting in ventilation-perfusion mismatch
Membrane diffusing capacity	Decreased	Morphologic changes in the alveolar-capillary membrane and inhomogeneities in ventilation and/or blood flow
Arterial Blood Gases		
PaO_2	Decreased	Ventilation-perfusion inequities
$PaCO_2$	Unchanged	
pH	Unchanged	
Ventilatory responses to hypoxia and hypercapnia	Decreased	Diminution of both peripheral and central chemoreception and decreased central nervous system integration appear to be involved
Pulmonary Defense Mechanisms		
Alveolar macrophage function	Decreased	
Circulating phagocyte function	Unchanged	
Humoral immunity	Decreased	Decreased concentrations of both immunoglobulin G and immunoglobulin M, but mucosal immunity appears to be unaffected by age
Cell-mediated immunity	Decreased	Helper T-cell function is decreased, and suppressor T-cell function is enhanced

character of the discharge or the character following antibiotic therapy is important to determine, as it probably more accurately reflects the primary underlying disease process than the discharge that will be present in chronic diseases with secondary bacterial infection. Secondary bacterial infection results in purulent or mucopurulent discharge regardless of the primary underlying cause.

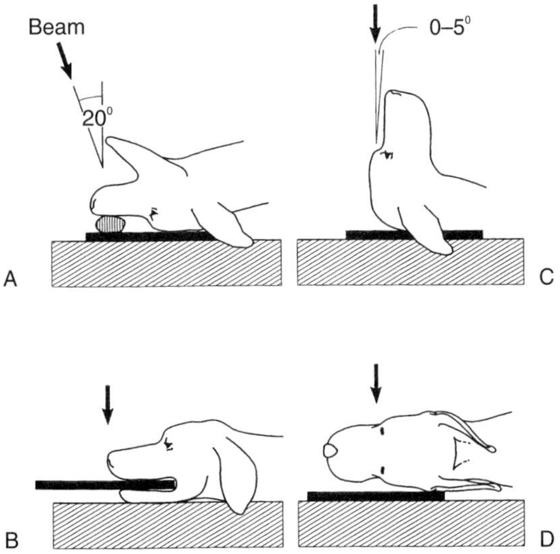

Figure 9-1. Positions for radiographic views of the nasal cavity. **A,** Open-mouth ventrodorsal position. **B,** Occlusal dorsoventral position. **C,** Rostrocaudal skyline position for frontal sinus projection. **D,** Lateral position.

Diagnostic Evaluation of the Nasal Cavity

A complete physical examination should be part of the evaluation of every animal with nasal disease. Complete evaluation of the nasal cavity requires general anesthesia and should include a complete dental examination, radiographs of the nasal cavity, rhinoscopy, and visual examination of the nasopharynx and internal nares. Radiography is an important diagnostic tool in the evaluation of the nasal cavity; however, radiographs are virtually useless if appropriate views are not taken with the dog or cat under general anesthesia. Lateral, open-mouth ventrodorsal, rostrocaudal projection through the frontal sinuses, and dorsoventral (occlusal) projections should be taken (Figure 9-1). If dental disease is suspected, lateral oblique projections will help rule in periapical abscess or destruction of periodontium. Advanced diagnostic imaging techniques, such as computed tomography (CT) and magnetic resonance imaging (MRI), are also ways to evaluate the nasal cavity and are often available on a referral basis.[10,11] Rhinoscopy can be performed using an otoscope, a rigid arthroscope, or a flexible endoscope (Table 9-2).[12] An otoscope will allow visualization only of the rostral 20% of the nasal cavity, whereas an arthroscope or flexible endoscope will allow more complete visualization of the rostral nasal cavity (50% or more) and occasionally the caudal nasal cavity and nasopharynx. Rhinoscopy is most useful when it affords both visual recognition of lesions and the ability to obtain sample material directly from sites of disease. It is especially useful in differentiating fungal from neoplastic nasal disease. The caudal portion of the nasopharynx

TABLE 9-2. RHINOSCOPIC INSTRUMENTATION ALTERNATIVES

INSTRUMENT	GENERAL ADVANTAGES	LIMITATIONS
Otoscope	Inexpensive tool that can be used for many routine procedures. Multiple tip sizes (2 to 9 mm) allow for flexibility of use in different sizes of dogs and cats. Biopsy and foreign body retrieval are possible through larger sized tips but are cumbersome.	Visualization is only fair and is limited to the rostral 20% of the nasal cavity, which does not allow visualization of the nasopharynx. The viewing angle is limited by the tip diameter.
Rigid endoscopy (arthroscope)	Good visualization of the rostral 50% or more of the nasal cavity is allowed. The angle of view varies from 5 to 70 degrees with equipment. This may be the easiest system for visualization of the nasal cavity.	Relatively expensive and requires a separate light source and visualization equipment. Through-the-scope biopsy and foreign body retrieval are not possible. Does not allow visualization of the nasopharynx.
Flexible endoscopy (bronchoscope or pediatric gastroscope)	Good visualization of the rostral 50% or more of the nasal cavity and the nasopharynx. The angle of view is generally greater than with other instrumentation alternatives (up to 100 degrees). Through-the-scope biopsy and suction, as well as saline flush, are usually available.	Expensive and requires a separate light source and visualization equipment. Generally, the larger diameter tube limits usefulness in small dogs and cats. Technique is more difficult to learn.

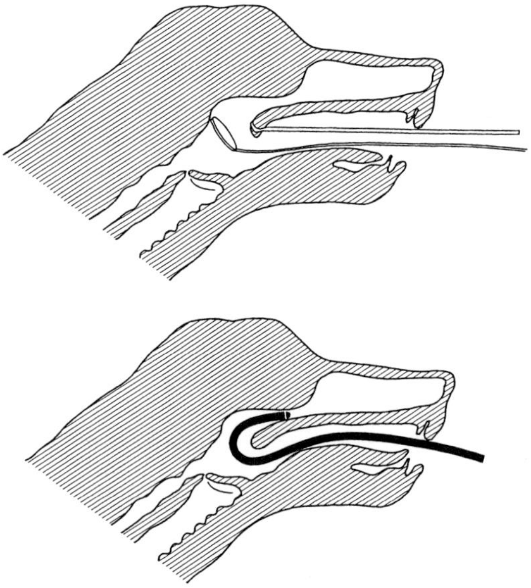

Figure 9-2. A dental mirror *(top)* or a flexible endoscope with a 180-degree tip deflection *(bottom)* can be used to visualize nasal disease in the caudal portion of the nasal cavity.

should be examined with a dental mirror placed in the pharynx or with an endoscope equipped with tip deflection of greater than or equal to 180 degrees in at least one direction (Figure 9-2). Tissue samples from the nasal cavity should be collected for fungal culture, cytology, and histopathologic evaluation. Material for culture should be obtained from within the nasal cavity; swabs of the discharge are rarely useful. Bacterial culture of the nasal cavity is rarely of benefit; the nasal environment is normally a rich source of bacteria. In most cases, histopathologic evaluation is going to be critical in the definitive diagnosis of nasal disease.[13] Methods of obtaining nasal samples for fungal culture, cytology, and histopathology include deep nasal swab, nasal flush, nasal suction biopsy, pinch biopsy, curettage biopsy, and rhinotomy (Figures 9-3 and 9-4).

Nasal flushing procedures are done with the animal under general anesthesia with the cuff on the endotracheal tube inflated. The animal should be in lateral recumbency and tilted toward the floor or a sink so that excess fluid or blood flows out the mouth and nose. Like nasal swabs, nasal flushing procedures are generally noninvasive and tend to be less diagnostic than more aggressive biopsy techniques. Aspiration biopsy (Figure 9-5) is the best technique for diagnosis of nasal tumors and diseases resulting in a large amount of thick exudate.[14] The outer casing of a stiff intravenous catheter is connected to a 10- to 12-ml syringe and aggressively inserted into the nasal cavity to the level of the medial canthus of the eye or to the level of radiographic apparent disease. Care must

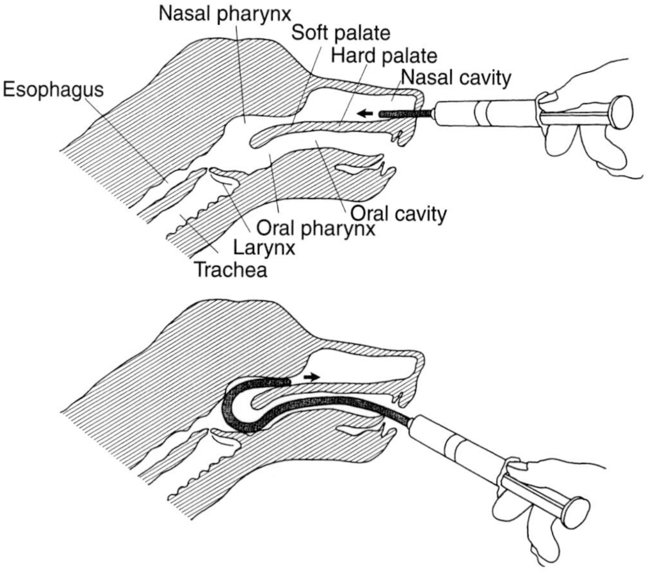

Figure 9-3. Two techniques for nasal flush. Sterile saline is flushed through a catheter into the nasal cavity either from the nares *(top)* or from the nasopharynx *(bottom)*. Diagnostic samples can be collected in gauze at the back of the nasopharynx *(top)*, or the nose can be lowered and samples collected as saline falls from the nares. Samples of mucus, tissue, and other debris can be used for cytologic and histopathologic analysis and fungal culture. Nasal flushing techniques are generally not as diagnostically effective as biopsy techniques. Note that this procedure should not be performed unless a cuffed endotracheal tube is in place.

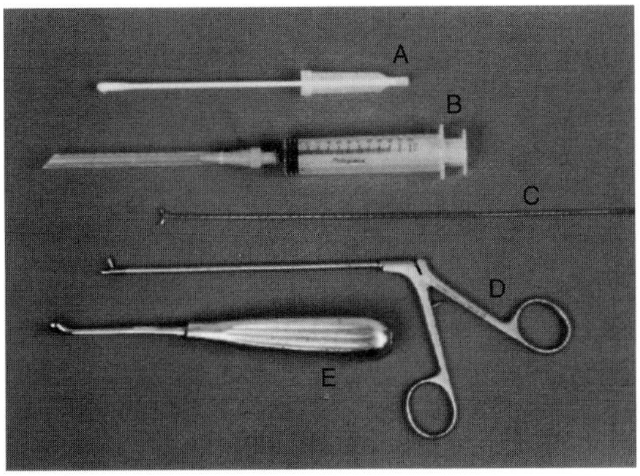

Figure 9-4. Tools for obtaining biopsy and cytology samples from the nasal cavity. **A,** Swab for collecting material for cytologic analysis and culture. **B,** Material for suction biopsy. **C,** Endoscopic biopsy forceps for pinch biopsy. **D,** Pituitary forceps for larger biopsy samples. **E,** Bone curette for largest biopsy samples.

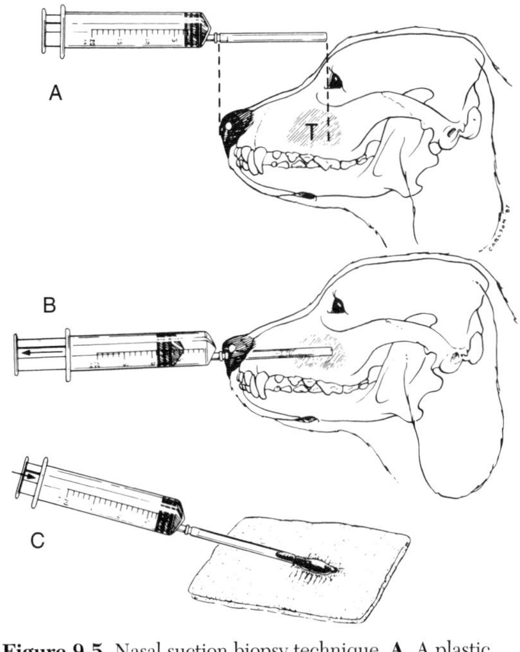

Figure 9-5. Nasal suction biopsy technique. **A,** A plastic cannula is connected to a syringe and measured to the medial canthus of the eye. **B,** The cannula is inserted into the nasal cavity through the nares and advanced to the level of the radiographically defined mass while suction is applied to the syringe. The suction is then released, and the cannula is withdrawn. The sample will be in the cannula and can be expressed onto gauze **(C)** or into a formalin container. (From Withrow SJ: Tumors of the respiratory system. In Withrow SJ, MacEwen EG, eds: *Small animal clinical oncology*, ed 3, Philadelphia, 2001, WB Sanders.)

be taken not to extend the casing beyond the medial canthus of the eye. As the plastic casing is inserted, negative pressure is applied to the syringe to aspirate a core of tissue. The tissue is then submitted for culture and histopathologic evaluation. Bleeding is common with this technique but rarely continues for more than a few minutes. If bleeding persists, diluted epinephrine (1:100,000) can be flushed over the bleeding area or umbilical ties can be inserted into the nasal cavity. In severe cases a Foley catheter can be inserted into the nasal cavity until the cuff is at the level of the biopsy site; the cuff is then inflated to apply pressure to the bleeding area. I have also had success using the pituitary cup forceps technique.

Nasal cavity exploratory surgery is still occasionally needed for a definitive diagnosis. Indications include diagnosis of intranasal disease not diagnosed by other means and resection of lesions.[15] Samples should always be obtained from the nasal cavity for both histopathology and fungal culture.

Nasal Diseases

Chronic Rhinitis. Dental disease–induced chronic rhinitis is common in older dogs and cats. It can be caused by periodontal or endodontal disease and sequelae such as osteomyelitis, bony sequestra, and intranasal tooth migration. Communication between the oral and nasal cavity is referred to as *oronasal fistula*, and communication between the oral cavity and the maxillary sinus is referred to as *oroantral fistula.* Oronasal and oroantral fistulas often occur after dental extractions. The extension of periodontal pockets into the nasal cavity or maxillary sinus also may result in oronasal or oroantral fistulas. Therapy for oronasal and oroantral fistulas involves recreating the barrier between the oral and nasal cavities (see Chapter 11). If periapical tissue is involved or if the veterinarian is not skilled in endodontal management, the tooth can be extracted and the oronasal barrier can be recreated using a mucoperiosteal flap.[16,17] Tetracycline therapy has been recommended (22 mg/kg PO tid) for 3 weeks after repair to treat infection.[18] Alternatively, metronidazole (30 to 60 mg/kg PO sid) or clindamycin (11 mg/kg PO bid) can be used.

Lymphoplasmacytic rhinitis, a steroid-responsive chronic nasal disease, should be considered in the evaluation of a dog with clinical signs of chronic nasal disease. Although not limited to geriatric dogs, the disease should be considered in any middle-aged to older dog that presents with signs of sneezing, upper airway stertor, or nasal discharge. The clinical signs are similar to those of other nasal diseases; sneezing and stertor predominate. Nasal discharge may be serous to mucopurulent. The diagnosis is based on histologic changes characterized by mixed inflammatory cell infiltration of nasal mucosa and submucosa composed predominantly of mature lymphocytes and plasma cells. Because the underlying pathogenesis and cause is unknown, treatment recommendations are usually based on trial and error experience. Antimicrobial therapy using ampicillin, chloramphenicol, trimethoprim-sulfonamide combination, or cephalexin is unsuccessful.[19] I have had some success using metronidazole (30 to 60 mg/kg PO sid). If the condition does not respond to treatment with antibacterial agents, immunosuppressive therapy should be considered. Immunosuppressive doses of prednisone (2 to 4 mg/kg prednisone) should initially be given, followed by a tapering course to the lowest dose that successfully controls the clinical signs. Most dogs will improve, although they may not become completely normal. Other immunosuppressive drugs should be used to treat dogs that cannot tolerate prednisone or can only be controlled with high daily doses. Azathioprine (2 mg/kg q24h for a week then 1 to 2 mg/kg q48h), chlorambucil (2 mg/m^2 q48h), or 6-mercaptopurine (50 mg/m^2 q24h for a week then q48h) can be used.

Fungal Diseases. Fungal diseases of the nasal cavity should also be considered in aged dogs and cats that have signs referable to the nasal cavity.[20] Although most pathogenic or opportunistic fungi can infect the nasal cavity, *Aspergillus* species, *Penicillium* species, and *Cryptococcus neoformans* are the most common. Canine aspergillosis and penicilliosis occur most commonly in young to middle-aged dogs with dolichocephalic conformation; brachycephalic breeds are rarely affected. Radiographs of the nasal cavity reveal a mixed pattern of osteolysis and increased radiodensity, and rhinoscopic examination may reveal hyperemic nasal mucosa with plaque-like yellow-green to gray-black *Aspergillus* colonies on the mucosal surface.[21] Positive fungal cultures should be interpreted together with the results of cytology and histopathology, because *Aspergillus* and *Penicillium* are both common contaminants of cultures collected from the nasal cavity. Serologic techniques to detect serum antibodies against *Aspergillus* are widely available. Positive results support active infection, but a rate of up to 15% false-positive results has been reported.[22] Antibody titers are often negative early in the disease course. Treatment of nasal aspergillosis or penicilliosis may entail systemic or topical therapy. Topical therapy using either enilconazole (10 mg/kg bid for 7 to 10 days) or clotrimazole (1 g in 100 ml polyethylene glycol applied over 1 hour) appears to be most effective.[23,24] Systemic therapy using ketoconazole (5 to 10 mg/kg PO bid), itraconazole (5 mg/kg PO sid), fluconazole (5 mg/kg PO sid), or thiabendazole (10 mg/kg PO bid) for 6 to 8 weeks appears to be less efficacious.[24-26]

Cryptococcosis is rhinotropic to the nasal cavity in geriatric cats. Feline leukemia virus (FeLV) antigen and feline immunodeficiency virus antibody tests are usually negative in cats with cryptococcosis restricted to the nasal cavity, but cats with disseminated disease may be infected with feline immunodeficiency virus. Radiographs of the nasal cavity will likely reveal an increased soft-tissue density early in the course of disease, with nasal turbinate and nasal bone destruction occurring later. Definitive diagnosis of cryptococcosis can be made based on cytologic identification of cryptococcal organisms from aspirates or swabs of the nasal cavity. The organisms are 1 to 7 μm with a nonstaining 1 to 30 μm capsule.[22] Detection of cryptococcal capsular polysaccharide antigen in serum and cerebrospinal fluid via a latex cryptococcal antigen test (LCAT) has been shown to be highly sensitive and specific in the diagnosis of cryptococcosis. Additionally, antigen titers increase with the severity of the disease, and their decline can be used to monitor response to therapy.[27] Treatment with ketoconazole (10 mg/kg sid to bid) or itraconazole (10 mg/kg PO sid) appears to be effective.[28] Treatment should be continued for 1 month after the remission of clinical signs. Alternatively, the LCAT can be used to monitor response to therapy, and the treatment can be discontinued when the test becomes negative.

Neoplasia. Nasal and paranasal neoplasia in the dog are uncommon, yet they are the most common cause of unilateral epistaxis and facial deformity in geriatric dogs (average age being 10 years). Clinical signs of nasal and paranasal tumors are similar to those seen with other chronic nasal diseases.[29,30] Neurologic signs (seizures, postural reaction deficits, blindness, circling, behavior changes, alterations of consciousness, and contralateral facial hypalgesia) may be the predominant or only sign noted in some dogs.[11,31]

Adenocarcinoma and squamous cell carcinoma are most common, but other carcinomas are occasionally encountered.[8,30] A wide variety of sarcomas are diagnosed, with tumors of skeletal origin (chondrosarcoma, osteosarcoma) making up about 18% and soft-tissue sarcomas (lymphosarcoma, fibrosarcoma, hemangiosarcoma, fibrous histiocytoma, myosarcoma, nerve sheath tumor, undifferentiated sarcoma) making up about 16%.[30] Transmissible venereal cell tumor, neuroendocrine tumors, melanoma, esthesioneuroblastoma, and extramedullary plasmacytoma are seen rarely.[30] Despite the fact that most nasal tumors are malignant, it is rare for clinical evidence of metastasis to have occurred. In one study, 41% of 120 dogs with sinonasal neoplasia diagnosed at necropsy had evidence of distant metastasis,[30] whereas only 17.6% of soft-tissue sinonasal neoplasia in a follow-up study had metastasized (lymphosarcoma, hemangiosarcoma). Metastasis may occur late in the disease course to local lymph nodes, lung, bone, and brain.[30,32] Although nasal tumors are slow to metastasize, they are locally very aggressive, making surgical resection largely unrewarding.

Radiographic abnormalities that may be seen in an animal with nasal neoplasia include loss of nasal and fine trabecular turbinate pattern, increased soft-tissue density in the nasal cavity and frontal sinus, deviation or destruction of the vomer bone or surrounding nasal and maxillary bones, periosteal new bone formation, and the presence of an external soft tissue mass[33] (Figure 9-6). It is difficult or impossible to consistently differentiate neoplasia from an inflammatory process solely by radiographic criteria, however. CT imaging is becoming a widely used tool in the evaluation of nasal cavity disease in many referral institutions. In one study of dogs with malignant tumors and advanced clinical signs of nasal disease, CT imaging was not shown to be more sensitive than conventional radiography for detection of nasal cavity abnormalities. Increased nasal cavity opacity was observed radiographically in all of the dogs in the study.[34] However, CT images were more sensitive than radiographs at demonstrating bony lysis and predicting the extent of nasal cavity involvement in early disease.[34] MRI is optimal for demonstration of detailed anatomic features of nasal neoplasia and involvement of the nasal cavity and central nervous system.[11] Availability of MRI is presently limited to referral practices, and the procedure generally costs more than CT.

Reported life expectancies are generally 2 to 5 months without treatment.[35] Chemotherapy, immunotherapy, cryosurgery, or conventional nasal surgery alone does not appear to increase survival times.[8,29,35] A recent study evaluated

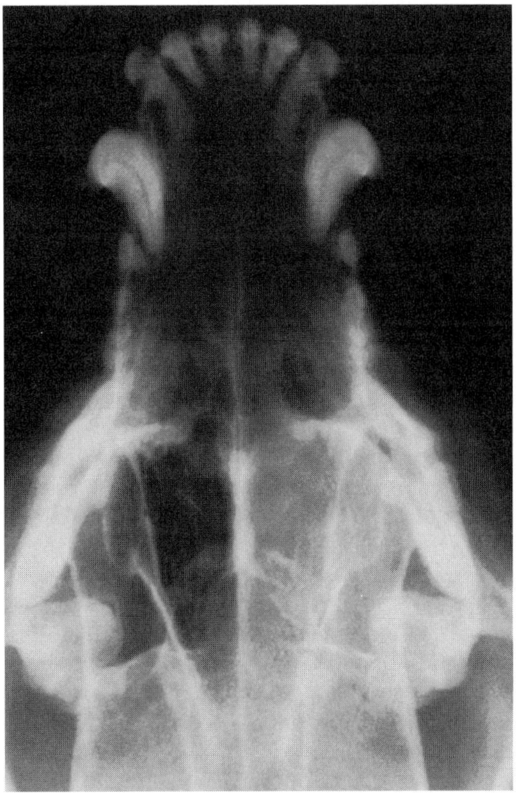

Figure 9-6. Open-mouth ventrodorsal radiograph of the nasal cavity of a dog with a nasal adenocarcinoma.

response of nasal adenocarcinoma to cisplatin (60 mg/m^2 of body surface, IV, given at 3-week intervals for two to eight doses) in 11 dogs.[36] Median survival was only approximately 4 months.

Radiation therapy is the only treatment modality effectively increasing survival time of dogs with nasal tumors.[37-39] Orthovoltage x-rays, megavoltage gamma-rays produced by a cobalt 60 source, or high energy x-rays produced by a linear accelerator are types of external beam radiation that have been used to treat nasal tumors. Protocols call for animals to be treated multiple times a week (often on a Monday, Wednesday, and Friday schedule) for 3 to 4 weeks.

Orthovoltage radiation is delivered from a therapeutic x-ray machine that delivers low milliampere values (5 to 20 mA) and high kilovolt peak values (150 to 300 kVp). Orthovoltage radiation is absorbed by the bone of the nasal cavity and delivers a high dose of radiation at the level of the overlying skin resulting in epilation, mucositis, and desquamating dermatitis. Median survival times of 16 to 23 months have been reported when orthovoltage radiation is used in conjunction with aggressive cytoreduction.[38] The

1- and 2-year survival rates were 54% to 57% and 43% to 48%, respectively. Orthovoltage radiation without surgical cytoreduction resulted in shorter survival.

Megavoltage radiation is higher energy gamma-rays and high energy x-rays produced by a cobalt 60 source or a linear accelerator. The maximum delivered dose is 5 mm below the skin surface, which limits the mucocutaneous side effects that are prevalent when orthovoltage radiation is used. Ocular complications are the most often reported side effects seen when megavoltage radiation is used in treatment of nasal tumors. Complications include keratitis, corneal ulceration, keratoconjunctivitis sicca, conjunctivitis, and cataracts.[40] Median survival times for dogs treated with megavoltage radiation and no surgical cytoreduction are generally shorter than with orthovoltage radiation following surgical cytoreduction, ranging from 8 to 12.8 months.[37,39] Longer survival in McEntee's study (1- and 2-year survival of 59% and 22%, respectively) was attributed to the use of CT for tumor localization and computer-generated treatment plans.

A third form of radiation therapy that is being used is brachytherapy. Brachytherapy is the local delivery of radiation at the tumor site. It is usually accomplished by implanting radioactive material directly into the tumor bed. When treating nasal tumors in this manner the tumor is aggressively removed, and iridium 192 is implanted into the nasal cavity. The iridium 192 implants are left in the nasal cavity for an average time of 4 to 9 days and then removed.[41] In the single study reporting the results of iridium 192 nasal implants in dogs with nasal neoplasia, eight dogs were treated. Median survival of only 3.1 months was reported, but one of the dogs was alive at 587 days.[41]

Nasal and paranasal tumors are uncommon in cats compared with dogs.[29,42] Nasal tumors occur more commonly in older, male cats (mean age approximately 9 years).[42,43] The clinical signs seen in cats with nasal and paranasal tumors are similar to those seen in dogs. Sneezing and nasal discharge are common. Nasal tumors in cats are more likely to cause facial and oral deformity and epiphora.[43] Systemic evidence of disease (depression, anorexia) is more common in cats than in dogs.[43] Diagnosis is based on biopsy and histopathologic demonstration of tumor type.

Of feline nasal tumors, adenocarcinomas (or undifferentiated carcinomas) and lymphosarcomas are the most common (Table 9-3). Although benign tumors such as chondroma and hemangioma have been reported,[42,44] most nasal tumors of cats are malignant, with distant metastasis rare. Regional lymph nodes are the primary site of metastasis when it occurs.[42] Feline nasal tumors are locally very aggressive, commonly resulting in facial deformity and bony lysis. Type C retroviral expression has been demonstrated in three olfactory neuroblastomas from cats with FeLV infection.[45] The diagnostic evaluation of cats suspected of having a nasal tumor is the same as that of dogs; the smaller nasal cavity makes rhinoscopic evaluation less rewarding. Increased nasal cavity opacity is seen radiographically most commonly, with frontal bone, vomer bone, or palatine lysis occurring less commonly.[42,43] The veterinarian is more dependent on blind nasal biopsy procedures because of the difficulty encountered with rhinoscopy, although cats have a higher incidence of facial and oral lesions, which may make extranasal biopsy sites easy to identify. Care must be taken in the interpretation of nasal biopsies. Inflammation is common, and biopsies may not include representative areas of neoplasia. Nasal lymphosarcoma may be especially difficult to confirm on nasal biopsy.[43]

In general, cats respond well to radiotherapy.[46] In one study, orthovoltage radiation therapy following rhinotomy resulted in median survival of 20.8 months.[43] A mean survival of 19 months was achieved without rhinotomy using high energy x-ray radiation generated by a linear accelerator.[46] Localized nasal lymphoma is ideally suited for radiation therapy.[47] With the exception of lymphosarcoma, chemotherapy has not been reported for nasal tumors in cats. An algorithm for approaching the geriatric animal with nasal disease is presented in Figure 9-7.

DISEASES OF THE LARYNX

Disease of the larynx is uncommon in the aged animal. When present, it is usually obstructive in nature and most frequently due to degenerative (idiopathic laryngeal paralysis) or neoplastic causes.[48]

History and Clinical Findings

Laryngeal disease is suggested by failure of laryngeal function resulting in stridor, inspiratory dyspnea, loss or change of voice, exercise intolerance, or coughing. Stridor is a wheeze or noise that occurs typically during inspiration. In mild disease it may occur only when the animal is exerted or excited, being noticeable only during inspiration. In severe disease it may be heard at

TABLE 9-3. FELINE NASAL NEOPLASIA

TUMOR TYPE	SIGNALMENT	DURATION OF SIGNS	THERAPY	REFERENCE	OUTCOME
Adenocarcinoma	8 yr FS	3 months	Surgery	Cox et al., 1991	Died 5 days after surgery
	11 yr M	6 months	Surgery	Cox et al., 1991	Euthanized 4-6 weeks after diagnosis
	4 yr MC	1 month	None	Cox et al., 1991	Euthanized
	14 yr MC	1 year	Surgery, cobalt irradiation	Cox et al., 1991	Tumor recurred at 10 months
	12 yr MC	Unknown	Surgery, cobalt irradiation	Cox et al., 1991	Recurred at 8 months; reirradiation, followed by recurrence at 24 months
	12 yr MC	Not reported	Linear accelerator irradiation	Straw et al., 1986	Died 2 months after treatment; unrelated cause of death, but tumor noted in nasal cavity at necropsy
	4 yr M	Not reported	Chemotherapy, orthovoltage irradiation	Evans et al., 1989	Died 5 months after treatment; unrelated cause of death
	12 yr FS	Not reported	Orthovoltage irradiation	Evans et al., 1989	Died 62.3 months after treatment; unrelated cause of death, but recurrence noted at necropsy
	14 yr MC	3 months	None	Unreported	
	12 yr MC	1 month	None	Unreported	
Undifferentiated carcinoma	6 yr MC	1 year 5 months	None	Cox et al., 1991	Euthanized
	11 yr MC	1.5 weeks	Surgery	Cox et al., 1991	Died 3 weeks after diagnosis
	10 yr FS	7 months	Surgery	Cox et al., 1991	Died postoperatively
	6 yr M	4.5 months	None	Cox et al., 1991	Euthanized 4 months after diagnosis
	13 yr MC	Not reported	Linear accelerator irradiation	Straw et al., 1986	Died 41 months after treatment; unrelated cause of death
	4 yr MC	Not reported	Orthovoltage irradiation	Evans et al., 1989	Died 5.3 months after treatment, unrelated cause
	8 yr MC	Not reported	Orthovoltage irradiation	Evans et al., 1989	Alive 26.3 months after treatment
Carcinoma	11 yr F	2 months	Cobalt irradiation	Cox et al., 1991	Died 3 weeks after therapy
	12 yr FS	Not reported	Orthovoltage irradiation	Evans et al., 1989	Died 39.8 months after treatment; unrelated cause of death
	11 yr MC	Not reported	Orthovoltage irradiation	Evans et al., 1989	Died 20.8 months after treatment, recurrence noted
Mucinous carcinoma	13 yr FS	5 months	None	Unreported	
Fibrosarcoma	9 yr MC	6 months	None	Cox et al., 1991	Died 10 days after diagnosis
	7 yr M(?)	Not reported	Surgery	Neumann et al., 1990	Alive without recurrence 10 months after surgery
Undifferentiated sarcoma	8 yr MC	3 months	None	Unreported	
Sarcoma	11 yr MC	2 months	None	Unreported	
Chondrosarcoma	9 yr FS	4 months	Surgery	Cox et al., 1991	Euthanized 24 months after therapy for unrelated reason
	13 yr FS	Not reported	Linear accelerator irradiation	Straw et al., 1986	Died 6 months after treatment, recurrence noted
Chondroma	3 yr M	1 year	Surgery	Cox et al., 1991	Lost to follow-up
Olfactory neuroblastoma	10 yr FS	3 months	None	Cox et al., 1991	Died day of presentation
	15 yr FS	1 week	None	Cox et al., 1991	Euthanized
	5 yr M	Weeks	None	Smith et al., 1989	Dead at presentation
	8 yr F	Weeks	None	Smith et al., 1989	Dead at presentation
	Adult F	Unknown	None	Schrenzel et al., 1990	FeLV positive, euthanized
	8 yr FS	Not reported	None	Schrenzel et al., 1990	Euthanized

Continued

TABLE 9-3. FELINE NASAL NEOPLASIA—cont'd.

TUMOR TYPE	SIGNALMENT	DURATION OF SIGNS	THERAPY	REFERENCE	OUTCOME
	5 yr MC	Not reported	None	Schrenzel et al., 1990	Euthanized, FeLV identified in tumor
Histiocytic lymphosarcoma	10 yr MC	Not reported	Chemotherapy, linear accelerator irradiation	Straw et al., 1986 Elmslie et al., 1991	Alive 277 weeks after treatment
	10 yr FS	Not reported	Linear accelerator irradiation	Straw et al., 1986 Elmslie et al., 1991	Lost to follow-up 180 weeks after treatment
	9 yr MC	Not reported	Chemotherapy, orthovoltage irradiation	Evans et al., 1989	Died 67 months after treatment, unknown cause
Lymphosarcoma	3 yr M	2 months	None	Cox et al., 1991	Euthanized
	8 yr MC	Not reported	Linear accelerator irradiation	Straw et al., 1986	Lost to follow-up 41 months after treatment
	Not reported	Not reported	Chemotherapy	Cotter, 1983	5 month remission
	Not reported	Not reported	Chemotherapy	Cotter, 1983	10 month remission
	Not reported	Not reported	Chemotherapy	Cotter, 1983	Remission not achieved
	9 yr FS	Not reported	Orthovoltage irradiation	Evans et al., 1989	Died 18.8 months after treatment, unknown cause
	8 yr MC	Not reported	Orthovoltage irradiation	Evans et al., 1989	Died 6.3 months after treatment, recurrence noted
	Not reported	Not reported	Linear accelerator irradiation	Elmslie et al., 1991	Died 97 weeks after treatment, unrelated cause
	7 yr MC	6 weeks	None	Legendre et al., 1975	Euthanized 1 month after diagnosis
Cavernous hemangioma	11 yr MC	1 month	Surgery	Anderson et al., 1989	Recurrence 5 months after surgery; alive 4 months after second surgery
Mast cell tumor	6 yr MC	1 month	Chemotherapy	Unreported	

F, Female; *FeLV,* feline leukemia virus; *FS,* spayed female; *M,* male; *MC,* castrated male.

rest and during both inspiration and expiration. The wheeze is soft and rasping with mild obstructive disease and becomes loud and high pitched when severe, life-threatening disease is present. Severe, high pitched stridor is usually accompanied by relentless inspiratory and expiratory dyspnea and cyanosis. In most cases the lungs function normally and transtracheal or endotracheal intubation will rapidly result in relief of the dyspnea, stridor, and cyanosis. Hyperthermia is occasionally noted in animals with significantly increased respiratory efforts or pneumonia. Pneumonia is seen in animals in which poor laryngeal and pharyngeal function has led to tracheal aspiration of foreign material.

Diagnostic Evaluation

The combined signs of inspiratory dyspnea and stridor should lead the veterinarian to suspect laryngeal disease. Diagnostic evaluation includes a thorough physical examination followed by sedation and laryngoscopy. If the animal has severe dyspnea or if its condition is rapidly deteriorating, emergency tracheal or transtracheal intubation should precede diagnostic evaluation. If dyspnea is severe but not considered life threatening, sedation may alleviate anxiety and frantic behaviors that tend to traumatize the larynx, contribute to laryngeal swelling, and result in a vicious spiral of dyspnea and stridor. Neuroleptanalgesic combinations are recommended for this purpose.[49] Oxygen therapy may be useful early, but once dyspnea and stridor have become life threatening, oxygen therapy alone is rarely of much benefit.

Lateral radiographs of the cervical region may confirm the presence of ossified laryngeal cartilages or laryngeal neoplasia but are rarely otherwise helpful in the diagnosis of laryngeal disease.[50] Radiography may, however, be useful in ruling out proximal tracheal collapse or intraluminal obstructive disease. Care must be taken in the interpretation of mild laryngeal distortion or air pockets in and around the laryngeal structures, as even moderate respiratory distress can influence these findings. Thoracic radiographs

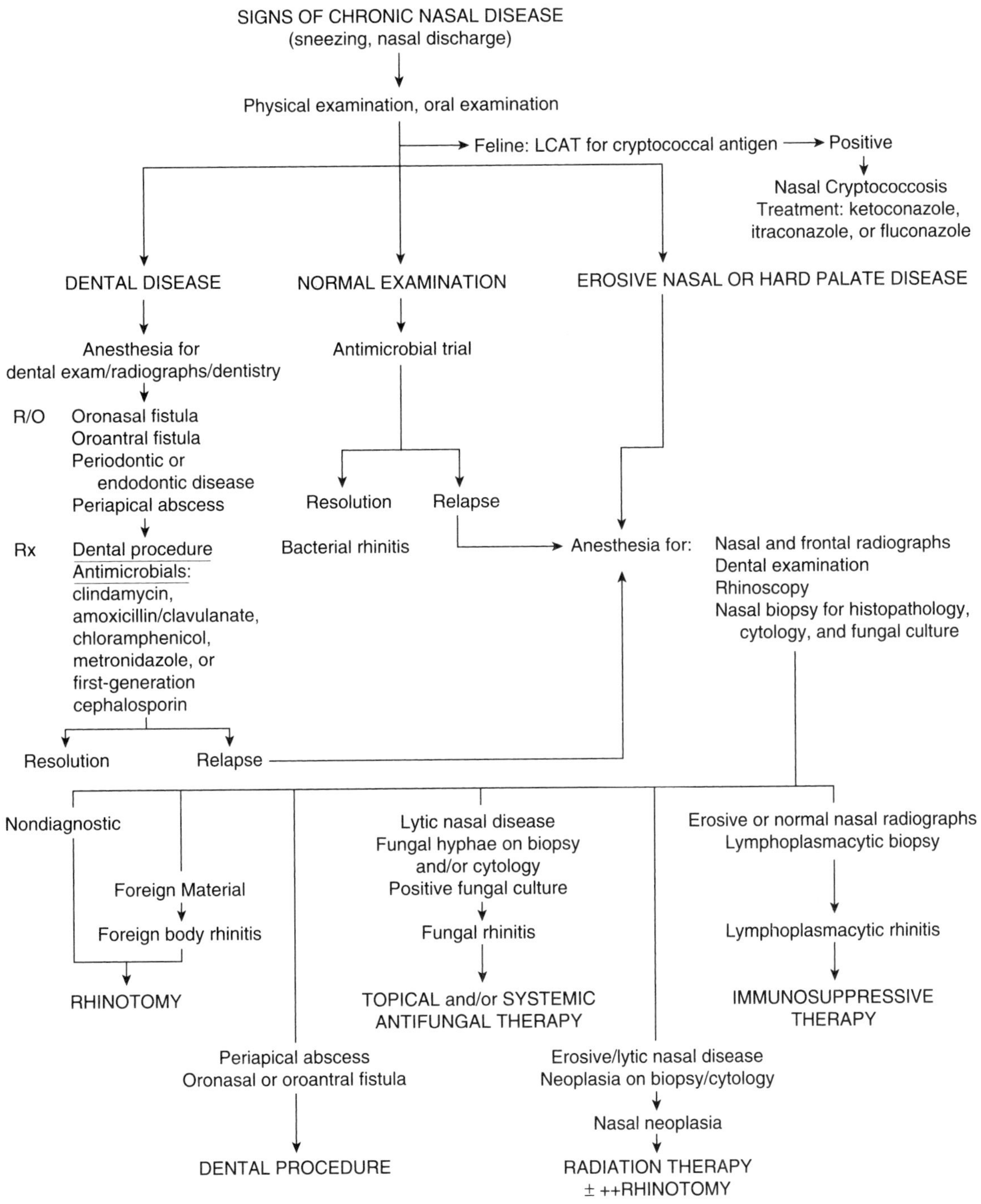

Figure 9-7. Diagnostic algorithm for nasal disease.

should be taken in all animals with laryngeal disease to rule out aspiration pneumonia, metastatic neoplasia, or pulmonary edema secondary to upper airway obstruction. The most important diagnostic test in the evaluation of the larynx is direct inspection via oropharyngeal laryngoscopy. The veterinarian should inspect the glottis for both anatomic and functional abnormalities. The animal must be sedated for satisfactory evaluation, but functional movements are suppressed by cortical or vagal depression. A light plane of anesthesia is, therefore, important for accurate evaluation of glottis function.[49] Laryngeal inspection should take place as soon as the animal is beginning to lose resistance to opening the mouth. The movement of the arytenoid cartilages and vocal folds should be correlated with respiration. The arytenoid processes and attached vocal folds should symmetrically abduct during inspiration and relax to form a relatively small glottic opening during expiration.

Laryngeal Diseases of the Dog

Laryngeal Paralysis. Laryngeal paralysis occurs most commonly as a slowly progressive disease in middle-aged to older dogs.[51] Laryngeal paralysis may be acquired or congenital,[48] but only the acquired form is of concern in the geriatric animal. Acquired laryngeal paralysis may be caused by central or peripheral vagal nerve lesions, recurrent or caudal laryngeal nerve lesions, intrathoracic masses, cervical trauma or masses, laryngeal trauma, previous surgery affecting the recurrent laryngeal nerve, mononeuropathies or polyneuropathies affecting the recurrent laryngeal, caudal laryngeal, or vagus nerve, or myopathies affecting the intrinsic laryngeal musculature.[51]

Idiopathic, acquired laryngeal paralysis occurs most commonly in older, male dogs of large and giant breeds. The mean age ranges from 7 to 12.2 years.[51] Labrador and golden retrievers, Afghan hounds, and Irish setters are seen most commonly.[51]

Respiratory distress and stridor are the most consistent clinical signs of idiopathic laryngeal paralysis. Gagging, coughing, cyanosis, phonation changes, exercise intolerance, and vomiting are also commonly seen. Syncope or collapse may be noted historically. Diagnosis is dependent on visual demonstration of decreased functional integrity of the glottis during inspiration. Most dogs with laryngeal paralysis are affected bilaterally, but unilateral disease is seen. A complete neurologic examination is important in all animals with laryngeal paralysis, because the paralysis may be the only sign of an underlying polyneuropathy.[52] Hypothyroidism should be ruled out as a potential cause of laryngeal paralysis.[53] However, the evidence linking laryngeal paralysis and hypothyroidism is tenuous at best.[54] Thyroid supplementation does not appear to resolve laryngeal paralysis.

Definitive treatment of laryngeal paralysis is dependent on surgical relief of the glottic obstruction. Initial medical treatment designed to stabilize the dog will depend on the severity of the clinical signs at the time of presentation. The animal in severe respiratory distress will require aggressive emergency therapy, whereas the animal presented with less severe, chronic dyspnea may require minimal initial medical therapy before surgical correction of the airway obstruction. Dogs with severe stridor may require endotracheal intubation or transtracheal intubation via tracheostomy.[55]

Surgical widening of the glottic opening is the definitive treatment of canine laryngeal paralysis.[56,57] Three procedures have been advocated: 1) partial laryngectomy (ventriculocordectomy and partial arytenoidectomy) performed either through the mouth or through a ventral laryngotomy incision[49-51,57,58]; 2) castellated (step-like) laryngofissure and vocal cord resection[51,59]; and 3) unilateral or bilateral arytenoid lateralization.[49-51,60-62]

All surgical procedures have been shown to open the glottis and improve airflow. Aspiration pneumonia is the most serious complication during the postoperative period. Partial laryngectomy has been shown to carry an exceptionally high incidence of aspiration pneumonia.[58] Other complications associated with partial laryngectomy include coughing, hemorrhage, hematemesis, failure to effectively alleviate the dyspnea and stridor, and obstructive scar tissue formation.[58] Because of the high incidence of complications and the greater success reported with arytenoid lateralization, partial laryngectomy is not recommended. Unilateral arytenoid lateralization is a proved technique that consistently provides relief from respiratory distress, improves oxygenation, and has a low complication rate.

During the first 48 hours after laryngeal surgery, the animal should be monitored closely for respiratory dysfunction secondary to laryngeal hemorrhage or edema and aspiration pneumonia. If a tracheostomy tube is used, postoperative care should include aseptic aspiration and cleaning of the tube at frequent intervals. To prevent postoperative aspiration pneumonia, food and water should be reintroduced slowly while the animal is closely monitored.

Laryngeal Neoplasia. Laryngeal neoplasia is a rare cause of upper airway dyspnea and stridor in the older dog.[63,64] Clinical signs of laryngeal neoplasia are caused by obstruction of the glottic opening. Early clinical signs include voice change, increased respiratory noise, and snoring. Hemoptysis and oral cavity hemorrhage is occasionally seen and is suggestive of neoplasia. Inspiratory dyspnea, stridor, cyanosis, exercise intolerance, coughing, and gagging are also signs that may be noted.

Laryngeal tumors include rhabdomyoma, undifferentiated carcinoma, adenocarcinoma, squamous cell carcinoma, mast cell tumor, osteosarcoma, melanoma, lipoma, chondrosarcoma, leiomyoma, fibrosarcoma, fibropapilloma, myxochondroma, undifferentiated myoblastoma, and oncocytoma.[63,65] Rhabdomyoma, carcinoma, and squamous cell carcinoma comprise almost half of the reported cases.[63] Invasive perilaryngeal or metastatic tumors occasionally cause upper airway obstruction and dyspnea in older dogs.[65]

Diagnosis of laryngeal neoplasia is dependent on visualization of a laryngeal mass and histologic conformation of neoplasia. Perilaryngeal tumors, such as thyroid carcinoma, may cause similar clinical signs but are usually obvious on physical examination.[66] Partial and total laryngectomy has been reported as a treatment option for small localized tumors.[67] Permanent tracheostomy must be maintained after surgery, and hypoparathyroidism is a likely complication.[68]

Laryngeal Diseases of the Cat

Laryngeal disease is much less common in older cats than in older dogs. The clinical signs, diagnostic evaluation, and management considerations are very similar, however.

Laryngeal Neoplasia. Laryngeal neoplasia in the cat is rare. Twenty-one laryngeal tumors have been reported.[63,64] Carcinomas and lymphosarcoma are most commonly seen. Squamous cell carcinoma, adenocarcinoma, epidermoid carcinoma, and undifferentiated carcinoma have also been reported.

Laryngeal Paralysis. Laryngeal paralysis is rare in the cat; 13 cases have been reported.[69-71] Of these cases, six were considered idiopathic, three were congenital, two were thought to be related to generalized neurologic disorder, and two were secondary to neoplastic involvement of the vagus nerve. Lymphosarcoma was reported to infiltrate the vagal nerve in an 11-year-old cat,[72] and a ceruminous gland adenocarcinoma involving the tympanic bulla was reported to cause compression and degeneration of the vagus nerve in a 4-year-old cat.[69]

Clinical signs of laryngeal paralysis in cats include voice change, change in purr, and inspiratory dyspnea. Cats are usually sensitive to stress and become severely dyspneic during examination or attempted radiography. Diagnosis is dependent on demonstration of laryngeal dysfunction. Failure of arytenoid abduction during inspiration, paradoxic arytenoid movements, and paramedian displacement of the aryepiglottic folds are diagnostic. Care must be taken to differentiate poor laryngeal function from laryngospasm.

Partial laryngectomy,[70,71] arytenoid lateralization procedures,[71] and castellated laryngofissure with vocal fold resection[73] have all been reported in the cat. Successful alleviation of dyspnea was reported with all three surgical procedures. Iatrogenic trauma to the recurrent laryngeal nerves—a potential postoperative complication in the surgical management of hyperthyroidism—may result in laryngeal paralysis.[74] Voice change without severe dyspnea is noted most commonly, but complete bilateral paralysis has resulted in severe stridor and death in a few cats.[75] The paralysis is usually temporary.

DISEASES OF THE TRACHEA

Tracheal disease is common in the geriatric dog but uncommon in the geriatric cat. Cough is the most common sign noted, usually being nonproductive and like a goose honk. Dyspnea may be seen if severe tracheal obstructive disease is present. The dyspnea is most pronounced on inspiration if the disease is affecting primarily the proximal trachea and may be most pronounced on expiration if the distal trachea is more severely involved.

Diagnostic Evaluation

A complete physical examination is warranted to identify abnormalities that may be concurrently or secondarily affecting the trachea. Thoracic and soft-tissue cervical radiographs are indicated. Extraluminal compression, tracheal stenosis, intraluminal masses, and tracheal collapse may be apparent radiographically. Expiratory and inspiratory radiographs are useful when evaluating the trachea for dynamic compression as may occur in tracheal collapse. Other dynamic airway studies include fluoroscopy and tracheoscopy. Tracheoscopy is useful in the evaluation of the trachea when obstructive or mucosal disease is suspected. A flexible pediatric bronchoscope (approximately 3.5 to 5 mm diameter) or a rigid arthroscope can be used to visualize the tracheal lumen (Figure 9-8).

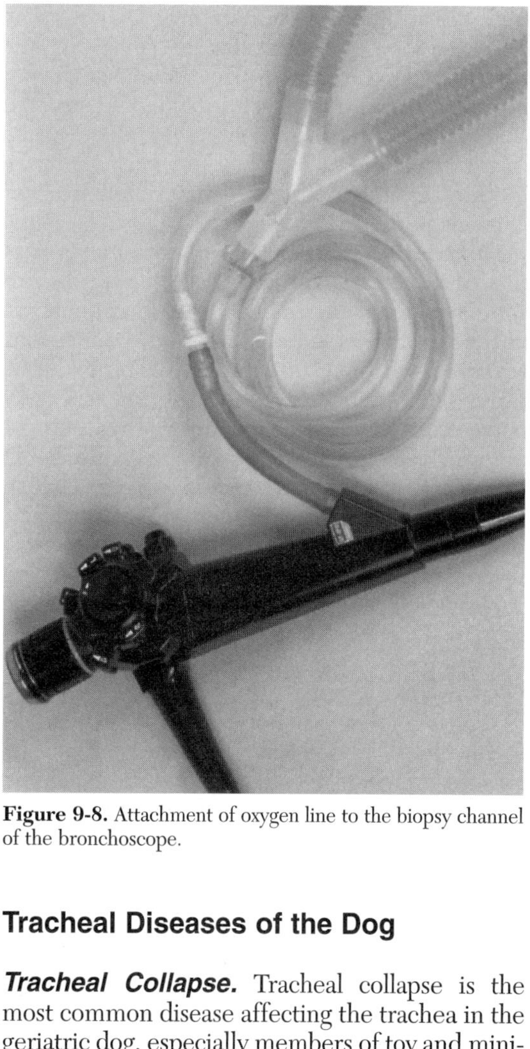

Figure 9-8. Attachment of oxygen line to the biopsy channel of the bronchoscope.

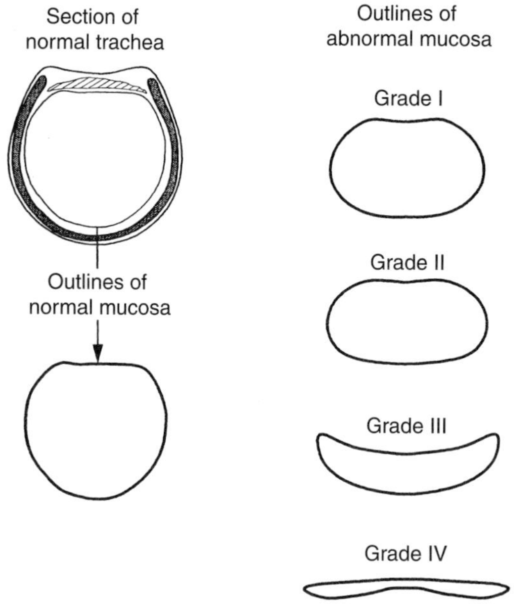

Figure 9-9. Classification of collapsed trachea by grade. *Grade I,* The tracheal lumen is reduced by approximately 25%. The tracheal membrane (trachealis muscle) protrudes slightly into the lumen, but the tracheal cartilage maintains a normal C shape. *Grade II,* The tracheal lumen is reduced by approximately 50%. The tracheal membrane is widened and pendulous, and the tracheal cartilages are partially flattened. *Grade III,* The tracheal lumen is reduced by approximately 75%. The tracheal membrane almost contacts the ventral surface of the trachea, and the tracheal cartilages are nearly flat. *Grade IV,* The tracheal lumen is nearly obliterated. The tracheal membrane contacts the ventral surface of the trachea, and the tracheal cartilages are flattened and may invert dorsally.

Tracheal Diseases of the Dog

Tracheal Collapse. Tracheal collapse is the most common disease affecting the trachea in the geriatric dog, especially members of toy and miniature breeds.[76,77] Pomeranians, miniature and toy poodles, Yorkshire terriers, and Chihuahuas are affected most commonly.[78] Although the disease is seen in dogs of all ages, the average age at diagnosis is 7.5 years.[77,79] The cause of tracheal collapse is not known. Dorsoventral flattening is typically seen, with the ratio of the width of the trachea to its height significantly increased compared with the tracheas of normal dogs.[80] Lateral collapse is rarely noted.

Diagnosis of tracheal collapse is usually based on the signalment, case history, and exclusion of other causes of dyspnea and cough. Some authors consider fluoroscopy the diagnostic test of choice,[77] but I feel that definitive diagnosis is best made by tracheoscopy. Both medical and surgical treatment have been advocated for the management of tracheal collapse.[77,79] Most dogs can be managed medically, especially during the initial stages. The goals of medical therapy include weight reduction, avoidance of stress and pressure on the trachea, minimizing inflammation of the tracheal mucosa, controlling cough, and treating concurrent or secondary conditions. Surgical treatment should be considered for dogs no longer responsive to medical management. Methods of surgical repair include dorsal tracheal membrane plication, the use of internal stents, tracheal ring transection, and external support with spiral or ring-shaped prostheses[78,79,81] (Figure 9-9). Surgery can be expected to lessen the dog's clinical signs but rarely eliminates them completely.

Tracheal Neoplasia. Tracheal neoplasia is extremely rare in the geriatric dog; osteochondroma, mast cell tumor, leiomyoma, chondrosarcoma, adenocarcinoma, osteosarcoma, chondroma, and undifferentiated carcinoma have been reported.[82] The median age in dogs is 8.6 years.[82] Clinical signs are related to tracheal obstruction and include dyspnea, wheezing, stridor, coughing, and cyanosis. Surgical treatment can be attempted.

Tracheal Diseases of the Cat

Tracheal disease in the geriatric cat is rare. Clinical signs are similar to those seen in the dog, although cough is a less consistent sign and respiratory distress and stridor are seen more commonly.

Tracheal Neoplasia. Tracheal neoplasia is extremely rare in the cat and includes lymphosarcoma, adenocarcinoma, undifferentiated carcinoma, squamous cell carcinoma, and seromucinous carcinoma. The median age is 8 years. Tracheal tumors are distinct intraluminal masses radiographically, but annular thickening may occur. Surgery should be considered for small, locally contained tumors.

Tracheal Collapse. Tracheal collapse is extremely rare[83] and is associated with chronic signs of dyspnea and inspiratory stridor. A cranial cervical obstructive lesion is noted.

DISEASES OF THE SMALL AIRWAYS AND LUNGS

Geriatric dogs and cats with lower airway disease usually have coughing and/or dyspnea. Varying degrees of both cough and dyspnea are typically seen.

History and Clinical Findings

Geriatric animals with disease affecting the small airways and lung parenchyma represent a diagnostic and therapeutic challenge to the veterinarian and animal owner. These animals tolerate stress poorly. Dogs and cats with bronchial disease typically have cough as a component of the history. Cats are less likely to be presented for cough, more commonly showing increased respiratory efforts when afflicted with chronic lower airway disease. Typically, dyspnea caused by lower airway disease is most pronounced on expiration but may also be noted during inspiration.

Both respiratory and cardiac disease should be considered when evaluating the geriatric animal because of cough or respiratory distress. A cardiac murmur or a rhythm abnormality might be noted with cardiac disease, whereas pulmonary diseases usually cause abnormal lung sounds. Evaluation of geriatric animals suspected of having lower airway disease may include thoracic radiography; bronchoscopy; cytology and culture (bacterial and fungal) of samples obtained by tracheal wash, bronchoalveolar lavage, or transthoracic aspiration; and histopathology of lung biopsy. Arterial blood gas analysis may be useful diagnostically as well as in predicting severity of disease and monitoring response to therapy. A heartworm test, fecal examination, and fungal or protozoal serology may be indicated.

Thoracic radiography is integral to the diagnostic evaluation of older animals with lower airway disease. Radiographs are helpful in localizing and determining the extent of disease, prioritizing differential diagnosis lists, and monitoring disease progression. Two views should always be taken (usually a lateral view and a ventrodorsal or dorsoventral view). The radiographic appearance of the lungs should be viewed for alveolar, interstitial, peribronchial, or vascular abnormalities (Box 9-1). Disseminated or diffuse interstitial pulmonary patterns are common in older dogs.[84] Calcification of small airways and small fissure lines between lung lobes are frequently seen.

Bronchoscopy is useful for evaluation of major airway diseases, allowing visual assessment of airway inflammation, structural abnormalities, and pulmonary hemorrhage, and is a valuable means of specimen collection for cytology and culture (see Figure 9-8). The bronchial mucosa of older dogs and cats with chronic airway disease appears erythematous with excessive mucus secretions that may plug or span the lumen of the airways.[85,86] The mucosa may appear thickened and have an irregular contour, with mucosal vessels appearing hyperemic. Dogs with chronic airway disease often have collapse of the dorsal tracheal membrane into the tracheal lumen or collapse of intrathoracic airways during passive expiration. Cats with chronic airway disease have collapse of the airways less commonly.

Bronchoalveolar lavage is useful for obtaining samples from the small airways, terminal bronchioles, and alveoli for cytology and culture.[87,88] It can be performed during bronchoscopy or via endotracheal intubation. Tracheobronchial lavage from the larger airways can also be performed in this way. Bronchoalveolar lavage samples are collected by instilling sterile 0.9% saline solution (25-ml aliquots in dogs or 10-ml aliquots in cats) through a bronchoscope that has been lodged snugly into a bronchus, followed by immediate retrieval via gentle suction. In general, total

BOX 9-1 Differential Diagnosis of Radiographic Abnormalities in the Geriatric Dog and Cat

Abnormal Vascular Pattern

Enlarged Arteries

Heartworm disease*
Thromboembolic disease*
Pulmonary hypertension

Enlarged Veins

Left heart failure*

Small Arteries and Veins

Hyperinflation of the lungs
- Allergic bronchitis*
- Feline asthma†
- Chronic bronchitis*
- Pulmonary emphysema

Hypovolemia
- Shock*†
- Dehydration*†
- Hypoadrenocorticism*†

Nodular Interstitial Pattern

Neoplasia

Metastatic*

Inflammatory

Pulmonary infiltrates with eosinophils
Lymphomatoid granulomatosis
Idiopathic granulomatous pneumonia
Fungal pneumonia
Parasitic pneumonia

Peribronchial Pattern

Allergic bronchitis*
Chronic bronchitis*
Feline asthma†
Bronchiectasis
Chronic bacterial bronchitis
Respiratory parasites

Mixed Interstitial and Alveolar Pattern

Neoplasia

Metastatic carcinoma
Lymphosarcoma

Inflammatory Disease

Infection
- Bacterial pneumonia*†
- Protozoal pneumonia
- Fungal pneumonia
- Parasitic pneumonia

Aspiration pneumonia*†
Pulmonary infiltrates with eosinophils
Lymphomatoid granulomatosis

Pulmonary Edema

Cardiogenic edema*
Neurogenic edema
Upper airway obstructive edema
Lymphatic obstruction

Pulmonary Hemorrhage

Thromboembolic disease*
Neoplasia
Systemic clotting disorders
Pulmonary contusions

*Common in the geriatric dog.
†Common in the geriatric cat.

nucleated cell counts from bronchoalveolar lavage solutions are less than 500/μl in healthy animals. The predominant cell type is the macrophage, with inflammatory cells occurring less frequently. Lymphocytes, neutrophils, and eosinophils should each constitute less than 5% to 10% of the total cell count in dogs.[87] Up to 25% eosinophils may be normal in cats.[88]

Tracheobronchial lavage samples can be collected with a through-the-needle type of jugular catheter via a transtracheal approach or with a 3.5 French male urinary catheter passed down the lumen of an endotracheal tube. When a transtracheal approach is used, the needle of the jugular catheter is placed into the tracheal lumen through the cricothyroid ligament in small or medium dogs or between tracheal rings in large dogs. The catheter is then passed to the level of the carina (fourth intercostal space), and 3 to 10 ml of sterile 0.9% saline solution is infused into the tracheal lumen, causing the animal to cough. Gentle suction is used to retrieve a sample of the solution. In small dogs or cats it is best to intubate the animal then pass a urinary catheter through the sterile endotracheal tube and instill saline solution as noted above for the transtracheal approach. Tracheal wash fluid from healthy dogs and cats contains primarily respiratory epithelial cells and a few macrophages; inflammatory cells are noted in diseases.

Cytologic and bacterial and fungal culture samples can be obtained by direct transthoracic aspiration of pulmonary tissue. The procedure is indicated in the evaluation of pulmonary or pleural mass lesions or in cases of diffuse pulmonary disease in which tracheobronchial and bronchoalveolar lavage have failed to yield a diagnosis. Lung aspiration can be performed with a 22-gauge needle and a 10- to 12-ml syringe. The needle should be inserted into the lung in the area of suspected disease. Spinal needles are useful if added length is required to reach the desired location. Multiple needle passes into the suspected disease should be attempted to maximize the diagnostic yield of the procedure. The animal should be manually restrained for transthoracic aspiration. Sedation is necessary in some animals, but general anesthesia is not recommended because hemorrhage potentially created by the procedure is not cleared as readily from the lungs.[76]

Lower Airway Diseases of the Dog

Chronic Bronchial Disease. Chronic bronchial disease is a complex, progressive, inflammatory disease of uncertain cause that involves the small airways. It is characterized by excessive secretion of mucus in the bronchial tree and frequent coughing, persisting for at least 2 months. Most dogs with chronic bronchial disease are older than 8 years.[77] Small and toy breeds, such as poodles, Shetland sheepdogs, Pomeranians, Pekingese, Chihuahuas, and Yorkshire terriers, are affected most often.[77] Cough and abnormal lung sounds are the most likely abnormalities noted on physical examination. Inspiratory and expiratory crackles are heard most commonly.

Diagnosis of chronic bronchitis is dependent on a history of chronic cough for which other causes have been ruled out (Box 9-2). The most helpful diagnostic tests include thoracic radiographs and tracheal or bronchial lavage for cytology and bacterial or fungal culture. Thoracic radiographs of most dogs with chronic bronchitis reveal a prominent bronchointerstitial pattern; thickened bronchial structures in an end-on and parallel orientation on radiographs have been described as "doughnuts" and "tram lines," respectively. Bronchiectasis (Figure 9-10) may be seen.[89,90] Excessive mucus with neutrophils and smaller numbers of lymphocytes and eosinophils characterize tracheal and bronchoalveolar lavage. Aerobic bacterial culture should be performed on all lavage samples. Positive cultures should alert the veterinarian to the possibility of bacterial infection, but it must be remembered that neither the lower airway nor lung parenchyma of healthy dogs is sterile.[91,92]

Bronchoscopic studies generally reveal a roughened airway surface, with loss of the glistening character of the normal airway mucosa, and excessive mucus secretions. The mucosa is often thickened and granular. Hyperemia of mucosal vessels is noted in most cases. Partial collapse of the mainstem or segmental bronchi may be noted during expiration and is generally considered a poor prognostic finding.[90]

BOX 9-2 Differential Diagnosis for the Geriatric Dog Presented for Chronic (2 Months' Duration) Cough

Common Diagnostic Rule-Outs
Heartworm disease
Chronic bronchial disease
Tracheal or mainstem bronchial collapse
Left-sided heart failure (chronic mitral valve insufficiency)

Uncommon Diagnostic Rule-Outs
Infectious bronchopneumonia (especially *Bordetella*)
Allergic or eosinophilic bronchitis
Bronchiectasis

Rare Diagnostic Rule-Outs
Bronchial foreign body
Parasitic bronchitis
Fungal pneumonia
Bronchopulmonary neoplasia
Eosinophilic or lymphomatoid granulomatosis
Pulmonary thromboemboli
Drug-induced cough (angiotensin-converting enzyme inhibitor)

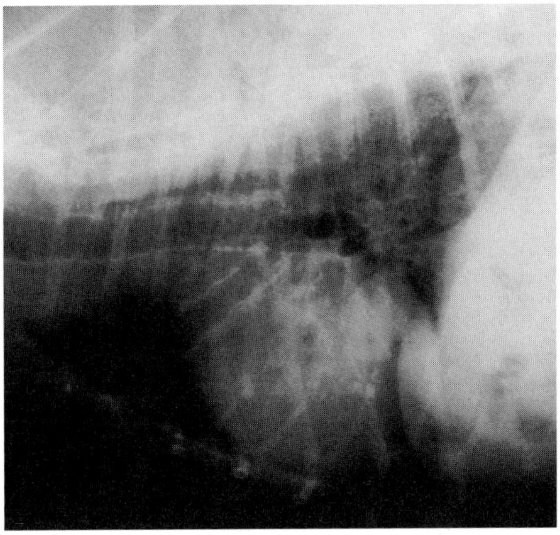

Figure 9-10. Lateral thoracic radiograph of a dog with bronchiectasis secondary to chronic bronchial disease.

Eosinophilic Bronchitis. Eosinophilic bronchitis is considered a pulmonary disease of potential allergic origin.[93] Its cause is usually unknown. The clinical signs, radiographic findings, and gross bronchoscopic findings can be identical to those seen in dogs with chronic bronchitis, but onset generally occurs at a younger age. The tracheal or bronchoalveolar lavage reveals excessive mucus and eosinophilic inflammation. Eosinophilia may be noted.[89]

Treatment of chronic bronchitis and eosinophilic bronchitis is similar. Symptomatic management for bronchoconstriction and cough as well as specific management of inflammation are important (Table 9-4). If bacteria are cultured from lavage samples, antimicrobial treatment should be based on appropriate sensitivity testing. Chloramphenicol, tetracycline, enrofloxacin, and amoxicillin-clavulanate combination are appropriate antimicrobial agents if *Bordetella* infection is suspected. Bronchodilators are used in the long-term management of dogs with chronic bronchial disease. Methylxanthines (salts of theophylline) may improve bronchial relaxation and

TABLE 9-4. DRUGS USED IN THE TREATMENT OF CANINE AND FELINE CHRONIC BRONCHIAL DISEASE

DRUG	DOSE	COMMENTS
Bronchodilators		
Sympathetic Amines		
Terbutaline	0.625 mg PO q12h (C) 0.04-0.1 mg/kg IV (C) 0.05-0.1 mg/kg PO q8h (D)	Long-term use is not recommended
Albuterol	0.02-0.04 mg/kg PO q8-12h (D)	Side effects include muscular tremors
Isoproterenol	0.1-0.2 ml SQ (C)	Tachycardia may occur
Epinephrine	0.5 ml of 1:10,000 dilution IM or SQ (C)	Use only in emergency situations and if isoproterenol is unavailable
Methylxanthines		
Aminophylline	4 mg/kg PO, IM, slow IV q8-12h (C) 6-11 mg/kg PO, IM, slow IV q8h (D)	
Sustained-release theophylline	25 mg/kg PO q24h (C)	
Dyphylline	4 mg/kg IM (C)	Neutral salt of theophylline; less painful
Corticosteroids		
Prednisolone sodium succinate	1-10 mg/kg IV, IM	
Dexamethasone	0.2-1 mg/kg IV, IM	
Prednisone	1 mg/kg PO q12h	Taper to lowest dose that controls signs
Methylprednisolone acetate	10-20 mg IM	Rule out infectious cause before administration
Triamcinolone	0.25-0.5 mg q24h	Taper to lowest dose that will control signs; once a week administration can often be achieved
Parasympatholytics		
Atropine	0.05 mg/kg SQ, IM (C)	May decrease mucociliary action
Sedatives		
Ketamine	0.1-1 mg/kg IV (C)	Intubate animal and administer 100% O_2 if necessary
Acepromazine	0.05-0.1 mg/kg IV (C,D)	Heart rate, pulse character, and perfusion should be monitored closely in geriatric dogs
Antitussives (Canine)		
Hydrocodone bitartrate	0.22 mg/kg PO q6-12h (D)	Use as needed; antitussives are most important in dogs with nonproductive cough or collapsing airway
Butorphanol	0.05-0.1 mg/kg PO, SQ q8-12h (D)	Use as needed
Antimicrobials*		
Amoxicillin-clavulanate	10-20 mg/kg PO q12h (C,D)	
Tetracycline	10-20 mg/kg PO q8h (C,D)	
Chloramphenicol	50 mg/kg PO IV q6-8h (D) 25 mg/kg PO IV q12h (C)	

*With efficacy against *Bordetella* and *Mycoplasma*.
C, Cat; *D,* dog; *PO,* oral administration; *IM,* intramuscular administration, *IV,* intravenous administration; *SQ,* subcutaneous administration.

contractility of fatigued diaphragm muscle.[94,95] Theophylline (11 mg/kg orally two to three times a day) should be used in dogs with exercise intolerance. Administration of β_2-adrenoceptor agonists such as albuterol and terbutaline results in excellent bronchial smooth muscle relaxation. It is appropriate to use these agents because airway smooth muscle in dogs is primarily innervated by the β_2 subclass of adrenoceptors alone. Albuterol is given at a dose of 0.02 to 0.04 mg/kg orally two to three times a day. Tremors and hyperactivity are dose-related side effects of the drug.

Cough suppression is indicated in some dogs with chronic bronchial disease. Judicious use of antitussive medication is recommended. Butorphanol (0.05 to 0.1 mg/kg orally two to three times a day) and hydrocodone bitartrate (0.22 mg/kg orally 2 to 4 times a day) are the cough suppressants most effective in dogs. The most effective drugs in ameliorating the signs of chronic bronchial disease are glucocorticoids. Before glucocorticoids are administered, airway infection should be ruled out. Prednisone is used at a dose of 1 mg/kg orally twice a day and tapered to the lowest effective alternate day dose.

Granulomatosis. Eosinophilic or lymphomatoid granulomatosis is a progressive condition of unknown cause that occurs in middle-aged and older dogs. The disease is usually slowly progressive, with cough, dyspnea, anorexia, and weight loss.[96-98] A diagnosis of lymphomatoid granulomatosis is difficult to make. Radiographically the disease is characterized by a diffuse interstitial and/or alveolar pattern with indistinct nodular pulmonary densities, lobar pulmonary consolidation, and hilar lymphadenopathy.[96] Bronchoalveolar lavage may reveal a suppurative, granulomatous, eosinophilic, or mixed inflammatory pattern. The definitive diagnosis is dependent on lung biopsy. Histopathologic findings have included angiitis, and angiocentric and angiodestructive granulomatous cellular infiltrates composed of mononuclear "lymphoreticular" cells, lymphocytes, plasma cells, macrophages, mast cells, and eosinophils. Affected dogs are usually not as responsive to corticosteroids. A few dogs have been treated with cyclophosphamide, vincristine, and prednisone with some response.

Thromboembolism. Pulmonary thromboembolism is increasingly being recognized in older dogs. The presenting signs include coughing, dyspnea, hemoptysis, tachycardia, lethargy, anorexia, and fever.[99] Physical examination may reveal a split S_2 sound, and distended jugular pulses due to pulmonary hypertension may be noted. The most common cause of pulmonary thromboembolism in dogs of all ages is dirofilariasis. Other causes include nephrotic syndrome, hyperadrenocorticism, immune-mediated hemolytic anemia, neoplasia, bacterial endocarditis, septicemia, surgery, trauma, hyperviscosity syndrome, polycythemia, vasculitis, disseminated intravascular coagulopathy, pancreatitis, hypothyroidism, and primary hypercoagulable states.[99-102] Thromboemboli may occur in the dog with hyperadrenocorticism resulting from a hypercoagulable state in which there are increased plasma concentrations of coagulation factors V, VIII, IX, X, ATIII, fibrinogen, and plasminogen.

The diagnosis of pulmonary thromboembolism is based on consistent radiographic changes in an animal, with arterial blood gases that suggest ventilation-perfusion mismatch. Blood gas findings include severe hypoxemia while the animal is breathing room air, with little improvement when the animal breathes 100% oxygen. Radiographic changes include increased alveolar densities that are usually fluffy and indistinct but may be lobar or triangular. Mild pleural effusion may occur in some cases.[103] Heartworm-induced thromboemboli are seen in animals with moderate to severe radiographic evidence of dirofilariasis, affecting primarily the caudal lung lobes. Selective angiography is the gold standard for the diagnosis of pulmonary thromboembolism but is invasive and requires general anesthesia. Ventilation-perfusion scintigraphy is technically easier to perform than angiography in the conscious animal and has been shown to have a high sensitivity when compared with angiography.[104]

Treatment of severe pulmonary thromboembolism is difficult and often unrewarding. Oxygen and bronchodilators are initially given but may have limited efficacy in animals with severe ventilation-perfusion mismatch. Glucocorticoids are important in the treatment of heartworm-induced disease but may be contraindicated in therapy of thromboembolism from other causes. If ongoing thrombosis caused by a hypercoagulable state is suspected, heparin is indicated to prevent further thrombus formation. Heparin at a dose of 200 units/kg IV followed by a continuous infusion of 15 to 20 units/kg/hour has been recommended.[105] Dissolution of existing thrombi can be accomplished using recombinant tissue plasminogen activator (rt-PA) at a dose of 1 mg/kg IV over 15 minutes.[106] Platelet inhibitors such as aspirin or dipyridamole are probably less effective than heparin. Cage rest is always recommended. If the underlying cause of thromboembolism can be determined, it should be treated specifically. The prognosis for heartworm-induced thromboembolism is good to excellent with strict cage confinement and corticosteroid, oxygen, and bronchodilator therapy. The prognosis for other causes is always guarded, especially if the underlying cause cannot be identified or resolved.

Pneumonia. Age-related changes in the pulmonary defense mechanisms predispose the geriatric dog to bacterial pneumonia. Pneumonia is especially prominent in dogs with bronchial disease in which the chronic degenerative process has resulted in bronchiectasis and decreased mucociliary clearance. *Klebsiella, Escherichia coli, Pasteurella, Enterobacter, Pseudomonas,* streptococci, and *Bordetella bronchiseptica* are common bacterial isolates.[107] Aspiration of food, gastric contents, or foreign material in dogs with diseases causing chronic vomiting, megaesophagus, laryngeal paralysis, or pharyngeal dysfunction also predisposes to bacterial pneumonia. Bacterial pneumonia should be suspected in any dog presented with fever and cough. Other clinical signs include lethargy, anorexia, dyspnea, exercise intolerance, and mucopurulent nasal discharge. Thoracic radiographs are generally characterized by alveolar and interstitial disease, most prominent in the cranial, middle, and ventral lung fields. If radiographic evidence is supportive of bacterial pneumonia, a tracheal or bronchoalveolar lavage should be performed and samples submitted for cytology, Gram staining, and aerobic bacterial culture and in vitro sensitivity testing.

Antimicrobials, airway hydration, and physiotherapy are the keys to successful management of dogs with bacterial pneumonia. Because the causative organisms and antimicrobial sensitivities of those organisms vary significantly, antimicrobial choice should be based on in vitro sensitivities, whenever possible. Trimethoprim-sulfonamide combination, amoxicillin-clavulanate combination, and first-generation cephalosporins are recommended for initial treatment while waiting for culture results in uncomplicated cases of bacterial pneumonia.[107] Enrofloxacin, cephalosporin-aminoglycoside combination, and chloramphenicol are recommended for life-threatening or nosocomial infections. Clinical improvement should be noted in 48 to 72 hours if an appropriate antimicrobial has been chosen. Radiographic improvement may lag behind clinical improvement. Antimicrobials should be continued at least a week beyond clinical and radiographic resolution.

After rehydration, physiotherapy for pneumonia is the process whereby mechanical attempts are made to promote coughing and facilitate clearance of exudate from the airways. Mild forced exercise and coupage are useful forms of physiotherapy. Coupage is generally safer in the severely compromised animal. In coupage a cupped hand should be used to forcefully strike the chest over the affected lung fields. The mechanical force induces coughing and helps to loosen secretions in consolidated areas.

If aspiration pneumonia is suspected, a thorough diagnostic evaluation looking for underlying diseases (usually related to esophageal or pharyngeal dysfunction) should be performed. Radiographic findings in aspiration pneumonia seen 12 to 24 hours after aspiration include consolidation and alveolar and interstitial infiltration of dependent lung lobes. Aspiration pneumonia should be treated similarly to other types of pneumonia. If the animal is seen shortly after aspiration has occurred, mechanical suction of the airways should be attempted. Bronchodilator therapy and a single dose of corticosteroids may reduce bronchoconstriction. Antimicrobials with efficacy against gram-negative and anaerobic bacteria should be used if secondary infection is suspected.

Neoplasia. Primary pulmonary neoplasia is rare in the dog, with mean age at diagnosis of approximately 9 to 11 years.[108-110] Cough (52%), dyspnea (24%), lethargy (18%), and weight loss (12%) are the most common clinical findings associated with primary lung tumors.[110] Reported paraneoplastic syndromes included hypertrophic osteopathy (3%), hypercalcemia (1%), and ectopic adrenocorticotropic hormone secretion (1%). Adenocarcinoma is the most commonly diagnosed primary lung tumor (75% of cases), followed by differentiated and anaplastic alveolar carcinomas (20% of cases), and squamous cell carcinomas and bronchial carcinomas (5% of cases).

Presumptive diagnosis of primary lung neoplasia is usually made radiographically.[109,111] The typical radiographic findings are a solitary nodular lesion involving a single lung lobe[111] and infrequently multiple nodules or diffuse involvement of one or more lung lobes. The right caudal lung lobe is most commonly affected (Figure 9-11). A single nodular lesion should suggest primary pulmonary neoplasia, whereas multiple nodules are more likely metastatic disease (Figure 9-12). Definitive diagnosis is dependent on cytologic or histologic confirmation of neoplasia. Surgical biopsy or fine needle aspiration is often necessary

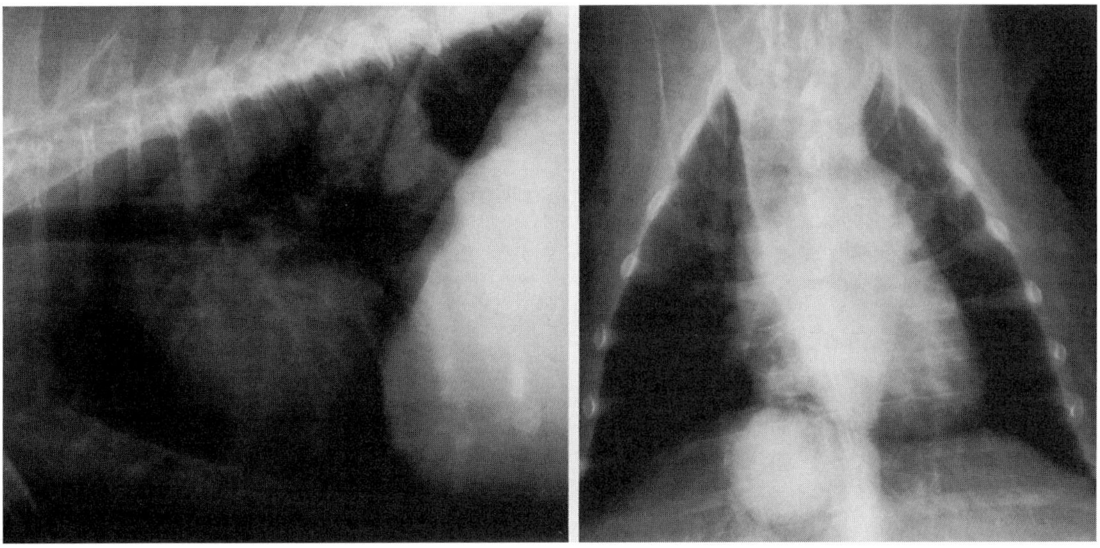

Figure 9-11. A, Lateral, and **B,** ventrodorsal radiographs of a dog with a primary lung tumor in the right caudal lung lobe.

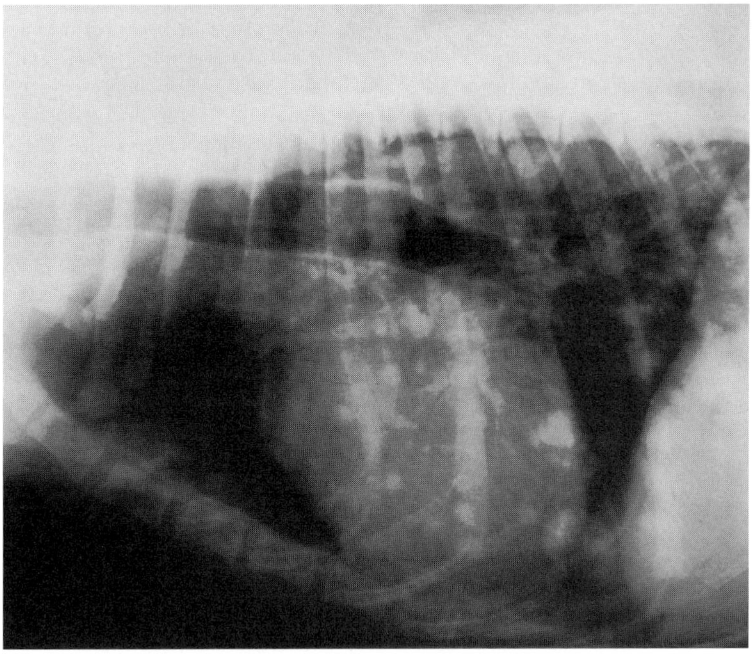

Figure 9-12. Lateral radiograph from a dog with metastatic neoplasia.

to confirm the specific neoplastic type. Wide surgical resection of the pulmonary mass is the treatment of choice for primary pulmonary neoplasia. The average survival is about 19 months postoperatively for dogs with adenocarcinoma and 8 months for those with squamous cell carcinoma.[112] Little information on the chemoresponsiveness of canine primary lung tumors is available. Improved survival has been reported in four dogs in which a combination of cisplatin and vindesine was used.[112] Cisplatin alone may be of benefit in some dogs.[113]

Lower Airway Diseases of the Cat

Neoplasia. Primary pulmonary neoplasia is rare in the cat. The clinical signs are usually nonspecific and include weight loss, lethargy, anorexia, and weakness.[109,114,115] The mean age of affected cats is 11 to 12 years. Adenocarcinoma is the most common tumor type (two thirds of primary lung tumors), followed by bronchoalveolar and anaplastic carcinomas (15%) and squamous cell carcinomas (14%). The most common radiographic pattern is focal, well-circumscribed solitary mass lesions or multiple poorly circumscribed masses. Adenocarcinoma affects all lung lobes equally, whereas squamous cell carcinoma tends to affect the middle and peripheral portions. Little is known about treatment of primary lung tumors in cats. Solitary mass lesions should probably be surgically removed, but metastasis is common, making the prognosis poor in most cases. Chemotherapeutic protocols for use in cats with pulmonary neoplasia have not been reported. It should be noted that cisplatin, a recommended agent in dogs, should not be used in cats because it produces severe, usually fatal pulmonary edema.[116]

Bronchitis and Asthma. Feline chronic bronchitis and feline asthma occur in young to middle-aged female cats. Siamese cats are predisposed to asthma.[117] Clinical signs include wheezing, gagging, dyspnea, tachypnea, coughing, and vomiting. A chronic history of coughing or respiratory difficulty may be present, but severe signs often occur acutely without a previous history that would support respiratory disease. Wheezes and increased breath sounds are heard on thoracic auscultation of most cats with chronic bronchial disease. Diagnosis is based on clinical signs and radiographic evidence of peribronchial interstitial infiltrates (Figure 9-13). Care should be taken not to stress affected cats. Severely affected cats should be initially treated based on clinical suspicion, rather than risk stressing them to take thoracic radiographs. Increased bronchial markings are the most common radiographic abnormality noted.[117] A tracheal wash should be performed on all stable cats with radiographic evidence of peribronchial disease. Bacterial bronchitis and aelurostrongylosis should be ruled out. Most cats have cytologic evidence of a nonseptic exudate. Eosinophilic, neutrophilic, granulomatous, and mixed infiltrates are all seen with about equal frequency.

Treatment of feline chronic bronchitis relies on antiinflammatory drugs, bronchodilators, and occasionally antimicrobials (see Table 9-4). Chronic outpatient therapy is usually sufficient, but overt cyanosis or status asthmaticus is occasionally seen and should be considered a medical emergency requiring quick therapeutic action. Dramatic response can usually be expected within 15 to 30 minutes of initiating therapy. Dexamethasone sodium phosphate or

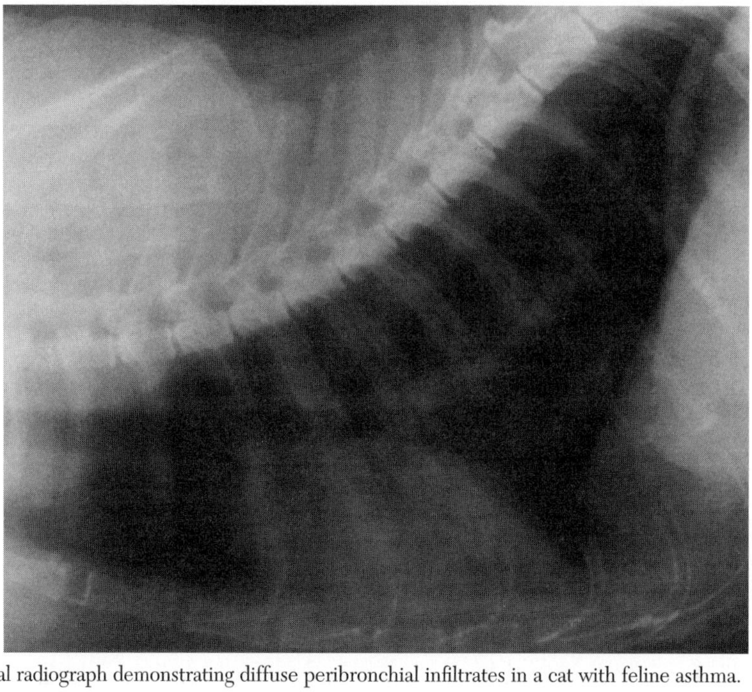

Figure 9-13. Lateral radiograph demonstrating diffuse peribronchial infiltrates in a cat with feline asthma.

prednisolone sodium succinate should be used initially, with bronchodilators such as the methylxanthine derivatives or the β_2-adrenoceptor agonist terbutaline used to augment the response. Less severely affected cats usually respond to oral glucocorticoids with or without augmentation from oral bronchodilator use. The dosage of the glucocorticoids should be tapered to the lowest possible dose that controls the clinical signs. Alternatively, long-acting steroids such as prednisolone acetate may provide better long-term management.

DISEASES OF THE PLEURA

Neoplastic pleural effusions are a primary concern in the geriatric animal (Table 9-5). Neoplastic pleural effusions can be of any type. Neoplastic involvement of the pleura may disrupt capillary integrity, allowing fluid and protein leakage into the pleural space and a resultant modified transudate. Protein and fluid accumulation can also be secondary to lymphatic obstruction. If the thoracic duct or other primary lymphatic structures are involved a chylous effusion may be seen. Hemorrhagic effusion can occur if vascular integrity is severely disrupted. Neoplasia should be high on the differential diagnosis list for any bloody effusion that is not due simply to hemorrhage. Lymphosarcoma often results in a pleural fluid containing many neoplastic cells. The diagnosis of lymphosarcoma can usually be confirmed via thoracocentesis and cytologic evaluation of the fluid.

Neoplastic diseases that may result in pleural effusion include metastatic disease, mesothelioma, lymphosarcoma (especially of mediastinal origin), thymoma, and tumors involving the right heart. Thymoma is derived from thymic epithelial tissue that frequently contains numerous lymphocytes. Thymoma may be either benign and noninvasive or malignant and invasive.[118] Diagnosis is based on radiographic evidence of a cranial mediastinal mass and cytologic or histologic conformation of thymoma. Thoracotomy may be necessary for definitive diagnosis.[119] Canine thymomas are locally aggressive, whereas feline thymomas tend to be less invasive.[118,120] Paraneoplastic syndromes are commonly associated with thymomas. Treatment of thymoma is dependent on the invasiveness of the tumor. Surgical resection is the treatment of choice in cats, in which the tumor is usually benign and well encap-

TABLE 9-5. DISEASES CAUSING PLEURAL EFFUSION IN THE DOG AND CAT

DISEASE	FLUID EVALUATION
Neoplastic disease Lymphosarcoma (mediastinal or diffuse pulmonary) Primary pulmonary neoplasia Metastatic neoplasia	Modified transudate, nonseptic exudate, chylous effusion, hemorrhagic effusion, and neoplastic effusion are all possible; reactive mesothelial cells in the effusion make definitive diagnosis of neoplasia difficult from cytology
Right heart failure	Transudate initially, then modified transudate when chronic
Hypoalbuminemia	Transudate
Diaphragmatic hernia	Modified transudate or nonseptic exudate
Lung lobe torsion	Modified transudate, nonseptic exudate, chylous or hemorrhagic effusion
Chylothorax Idiopathic Neoplasia Trauma Dirofilariasis Heart disease	Chylous effusion; triglyceride content is higher than serum, whereas cholesterol content is usually lower
Hemothorax Vitamin K–antagonist rodenticide toxicity Systemic coagulopathy Trauma	Hemorrhagic effusion
Pyothorax	Septic exudate
Pancreatitis	Modified transudate or nonseptic exudate
Pulmonary thromboemboli	Modified transudate or nonseptic exudate

sulated. However, the invasive nature of most thymomas in dogs makes surgical resection difficult.

Mesotheliomas are rare neoplasms that arise as papillomatous growths on the pleural, pericardial, and peritoneal surfaces.[121] Clinical signs are usually related to massive fluid accumulation in affected body cavities. Dyspnea, tachypnea, and weight loss are the primary clinical signs. Diagnosis is dependent on demonstration of the malignant cells in the pleural fluid or on biopsy. The effusion is usually characterized as a nonseptic, hemorrhagic exudate with numerous reactive or neoplastic mesothelial cells. Cytology of pleural fluid alone is unreliable as a method of confirming a diagnosis of malignancy because of the difficulty in distinguishing reactive mesothelial cells from those that are neoplastic. Therapy includes frequent thoracocentesis. Intracavitary chemotherapy with cisplatin (50 mg/m^2) infused into the pleural space has resulted in reduction or resolution of pleural effusion.[119] The combination of intracavitary cisplatin and systemic doxorubicin may prove to be the most effective treatment for mesothelioma in dogs.

References

1. Murray JF: Aging. In Murray JF: *The normal lung: the basis for diagnosis and treatment of pulmonary disease,* ed 2, Philadelphia, 1986, WB Saunders.
2. Mittman C, Edelman NH, Norris AH et al: Relationship between chest wall and pulmonary compliance and age, *J Appl Physiol* 20:1211, 1965.
3. Kundson RJ, Clark DF, Kennedy TC et al: Effect of aging alone on mechanical properties of the normal adult human lung, *J Appl Physiol* 43:1054, 1977.
4. Rea H, Becklake MR, Ghezzo H: Lung function changes as a reflection of tissue aging in young adults, *Bull Eur Physiopathol Respir* 18:5, 1982.
5. Georges R, Sauman G, Loiseau A: The relationship of age to pulmonary membrane conductance and capillary blood volume, *Am Rev Respir Dis* 117:1069, 1978.
6. Kronenberg RS, Drage CW: Attenuation of the ventilatory and heart rate responses to hypoxia and hypercapnia with aging in normal men, *J Clin Invest* 52:1812, 1973.
7. Ehrsam RE, Perruchoud A, Oberholzer M et al: Influence of age on pulmonary haemodynamics at rest and during supine exercise, *Clin Sci (Lond)* 65:653, 1983.
8. Ogilvie GK, LaRue SM: Canine and feline nasal and paranasal sinus tumors, *Vet Clin North Am Small Anim Pract* 22:1133, 1992.
9. Manfra Marretta S: Chronic rhinitis and dental disease, *Vet Clin North Am Small Anim Pract* 22:1101, 1992.
10. George TF, Swallwood JE: Anatomic atlas for computed tomography in the mesaticephalic dog: head and neck, *Vet Radiol* 33:217, 1992.
11. Moore MP, Gavin PR, Kraft SL et al: MR, CT, and clinical features from four dogs with nasal tumors involving the rostral cerebrum, *Vet Radiol* 32:19, 1991.
12. Ford RB: Endoscopy of the upper respiratory tract of the dog and cat. In Tams TR, ed: *Small animal endoscopy,* St Louis, 1990, Mosby.
13. Sullivan M: Differential diagnosis of chronic nasal disease in the dog, *In Pract* Nov:217, 1987.
14. Withrow SJ, Susaneck SJ, Macy DW et al: Aspiration and punch biopsy techniques for nasal tumors, *J Am Anim Hosp Assoc* 21:551, 1985.
15. Harvey CE: Surgery of the nasal cavity and sinuses. In Bojrab MJ, ed: *Current techniques in small animal surgery,* ed 2, Philadelphia, 1983, Lea & Febiger.
16. Ellison GW, Mulligan TW, Fagan DA et al: A double reposition flap technique for repair of recurrent oronasal fistulas in dogs, *J Am Anim Hosp Assoc* 22:803, 1986.
17. Manfra Marretta S: The diagnosis and treatment of oronasal fistulas in three cats, *J Vet Dent* 5:4, 1988.
18. Grove TK: Problems associated with the management of periodontal disease in clinical practice, *Probl Vet Med* 2:110, 1990.
19. Burgener DC, Slocombe RF, Zerbe CA: Lymphoplasmacytic rhinitis in five dogs, *J Am Anim Hosp Assoc* 23:565, 1987.
20. Sharp NJH, Harvey CE, Sullivan M: Canine nasal aspergillosis and penicilliosis, *Compend Contin Educ Pract Vet* 13:41, 1991.
21. Mortellaro CM, Della Franca P, Caretta G: *Aspergillus fumigatus,* the causative agent of infection of the frontal sinuses and nasal chambers of the dog, *Mycoses* 32:327, 1989.
22. Wolf AM: Fungal diseases of the nasal cavity of the dog and cat, *Vet Clin North Am Small Anim Pract* 22:1119, 1992.
23. Davidson A, Komtebedde J, Pappagianis D et al: Treatment of nasal aspergillosis with topical clotrimazole, *Proc Am Coll Vet Intern Med* 10:807, 1992.
24. Sharp NJH, Sullivan M, Harvey CE et al: Treatment of canine nasal aspergillosis with enilconazole, *J Vet Intern Med* 7:40, 1993.
25. Sharp NJH, Harvey CE, O'Brien JA: Treatment of canine nasal aspergillosis/penicilliosis with fluconazole (UK-49,858), *J Small Anim Pract* 32:513, 1991.
26. Sharp NJH: Nasal aspergillosis: treatment with enilconazole. *Proc Am Coll Vet Intern Med* 10:253, 1992.
27. Medleau L, Marks MA, Brown J et al: Clinical evaluation of a cryptococcal antigen latex agglutination test for diagnosis of cryptococcosis in cats, *J Am Vet Med Assoc* 196:1470, 1990.
28. Medleau L, Green CE, Rakich PM: Evaluation of ketoconazole and itraconazole for treatment of disseminated cryptococcosis in cats, *Am J Vet Res* 51:1454, 1990.
29. Madewell BR, Priester WA, Gillette EL et al: Neoplasms of the nasal passages and paranasal sinuses in domesticated animals as reported by 13 veterinary colleges, *Am J Vet Res* 37:852, 1976.
30. Patnaik AK: Canine sinonasal neoplasms: clinicopathological study of 285 cases, *J Am Anim Hosp Assoc* 25:103, 1989.
31. Smith MO, Turrel JM, Bailey CS et al: Neurologic abnormalities as the predominant signs of neoplasia of the nasal cavity in dogs and cats: seven cases, 1973-1986, *J Am Vet Med Assoc* 195:242, 1989.

32. Hahn KA, Matlock CL: Nasal adenocarcinoma metastatic to bone in two dogs, *J Am Vet Med Assoc* 197:491, 1990.
33. Gibbs C, Lane JG, Denny HR: Radiographical features of intranasal tumor lesions in the dog: a review of 100 cases, *J Small Anim Pract* 20:515, 1979.
34. Thrall DE, Roberton ID, McLeod DA et al: A comparison of radiographic and computed tomographic findings in 31 dogs with malignant nasal cavity tumors, *Vet Radiol* 30:59, 1989.
35. MacEwen EG, Withrow SJ, Patnaik AK: Nasal tumors in the dog: retrospective evaluation of diagnosis, prognosis, and treatment, *J Am Vet Med Assoc* 170:45, 1977.
36. Hahn KA, Knapp DW, Richardson RC et al: Clinical response of nasal adenocarcinoma to cisplatin chemotherapy in 11 dogs, *J Am Vet Med Assoc* 200:355, 1992.
37. Adams WM, Withrow SJ, Walshaw R et al: Radiotherapy of malignant nasal tumors in 67 dogs, *J Am Vet Med Assoc* 191:311, 1987.
38. Evans SM, Goldschmidt M, McKee LJ et al: Prognostic factors and survival after radiotherapy for intranasal neoplasms in dogs: 70 cases, 1974-1985, *J Am Vet Med Assoc* 194:1460, 1989.
39. McEntee MC, Page RL, Geidner GL et al: A retrospective study of 27 dogs with intranasal neoplasms treated with cobalt radiation, *Vet Radiol* 32:135, 1991.
40. Roberts SM, Lavach JD, Severin GA et al: Ophthalmic complications following megavoltage irradiation of the nasal and paranasal cavities in dogs, *J Am Vet Med Assoc* 190:43, 1987.
41. Thompson JP, Ackerman N, Bellah J et al: ^{192}Ir brachytherapy, using an intracavitary afterload device, for the treatment of intranasal neoplasms in dogs, *Am J Vet Res* 53:617, 1992.
42. Cox NR, Brawner WR, Powers RD et al: Tumors of the nose and paranasal sinuses in cats: 32 cases with comparison to a national database (1977 through 1987), *J Am Anim Hosp Assoc* 27:339, 1991.
43. Evans SM, Hendrick M: Radiotherapy of feline nasal tumors: a retrospective study of nine cases, *Vet Radiol* 30:128, 1989.
44. Anderson WI, Parchman MB, Cline JM et al: Nasal cavernous haemangioma in an American short-haired cat, *Vet Rec* 124:41, 1989.
45. Schrenzel MD, Higgins RJ, Hinrichs SH et al: Type C retroviral expression in spontaneous feline olfactory neuroblastomas, *Acta Neuropathol* 80:547, 1990.
46. Straw RC, Withrow SJ, Gillette EL et al: Use of radiotherapy for the treatment of intranasal tumors in cats: six cases, 1980-1985, *J Am Vet Med Assoc* 189:927, 1986.
47. Elmslie RE, Ogilvie GK, Gillette EL et al: Radiotherapy with and without chemotherapy for localized lymphoma in 10 cats, *Vet Radiol* 32:277, 1991.
48. Venker-van Haagen AJ: Diseases of the larynx, *Vet Clin North Am Small Anim Pract* 22:1155, 1992.
49. Aron DN, Crowe DT: Upper airway obstruction: general principles and selected conditions in the dog and cat, *Vet Clin North Am Small Anim Pract* 15:891, 1985.
50. Wykes PM: Canine laryngeal diseases. Part II. Diagnosis and treatment, *Compend Contin Educ Pract Vet* 5:105, 1983.
51. Greenfield CL: Canine laryngeal paralysis, *Compend Contin Educ Pract Vet* 9:1011, 1987.
52. Braund KG, Steinberg HS, Shores A et al: Laryngeal paralysis in immature and mature dogs as one sign of a more diffuse polyneuropathy, *J Am Vet Med Assoc* 194:1735, 1989.
53. Jaggy A: Neurologic manifestations of hypothyroidism to dogs, *Proc Am Coll Vet Intern Med* 8:1037, 1990.
54. Duncan ID: Peripheral neuropathy in the dog and cat, *Prog Vet Neurol* 2:111, 1991.
55. Taboada J, Hoskins JD, Morgan RV: Respiratory emergencies. In *Emergency medicine and critical care in practice,* Trenton, NJ, 1992, Veterinary Learning Systems.
56. Hedlund CS: Treatment of laryngeal paralysis. In Bojrab MJ, ed: *Current techniques in small animal surgery,* ed 3, Philadelphia, 1990, Lea & Febiger.
57. Petersen SW, Rosin E, Bjorling DE: Surgical options for laryngeal paralysis in dogs: a consideration of partial laryngectomy, *Compend Contin Educ Pract Vet* 13:1531, 1991.
58. Ross JT, Matthiesen DT, Noone KE et al: Complications and long-term results after partial laryngectomy for the treatment of idiopathic laryngeal paralysis in 45 dogs, *Vet Surg* 20:169, 1991.
59. Gourley IM, Paul H, Gregory C: Castellated laryngofissure and vocal fold resection for the treatment of laryngeal paralysis in the dog, *J Am Vet Med Assoc* 182:1084, 1983.
60. Bedford PG: Unilateral arytenoid lateralization in the dog. In Bojrab MJ, ed: *Current techniques in small animal surgery,* ed 3, Philadelphia, 1990, Lea & Febiger.
61. Gilson SD, Crane SW: Bilateral arytenoid lateralization by ventral midline approach in the dog and cat. In Bojrab MJ, ed: *Current techniques in small animal surgery,* ed 3, Philadelphia, 1990, Lea & Febiger.
62. White RAS: Unilateral arytenoid lateralisation: an assessment of technique and long term results in 62 dogs with laryngeal paralysis, *J Small Anim Pract* 30:543, 1989.
63. Carlisle CH, Biery DN, Thrall DE: Tracheal and laryngeal tumors in the dog and cat: literature review and 13 additional patients, *Vet Radiol* 32:229, 1991.
64. Saik JE, Toll SL, Diters RW et al: Canine and feline laryngeal neoplasia: a 10-year survey, *J Am Anim Hosp Assoc* 22:359, 1986.
65. Withrow SJ: Tumors of the respiratory system. In Withrow SJ, MacEwen EG, eds: *Clinical veterinary oncology,* Philadelphia, 1989, JB Lippincott.
66. Harari J, Patterson JS, Rosenthal RC: Clinical and pathologic features of thyroid tumors in 26 dogs, *J Am Vet Med Assoc* 188:1160, 1986.
67. Crowe DT, Goodwin MA, Greene CE: Total laryngectomy for laryngeal mast cell tumor in a dog, *J Am Anim Hosp Assoc* 22:809, 1986.
68. Henderson RA, Powers RD, Perry L: Development of hypoparathyroidism after excision of laryngeal rhabdomyosarcoma in a dog, *J Am Vet Med Assoc* 198:639, 1991.
69. Busch DS, Noxon JO, Miller LD: Laryngeal paralysis and peripheral vestibular disease in a cat, *J Am Anim Hosp Assoc* 28:82, 1992.
70. Hardie EM, Kolata RJ, Stone EA et al: Laryngeal paralysis in three cats, *J Am Vet Med Assoc* 179:879, 1981.
71. White RAS, Littlewood JD, Herrtage ME et al: Outcome of surgery for laryngeal paralysis in four cats, *Vet Rec* 118:103, 1986.
72. Schaer M, Zaki FA, Harvey HJ et al: Laryngeal

hemiplegia due to neoplasia of the vagus nerve in a cat, *J Am Vet Med Assoc* 174:513, 1979.
73. Cribb AE: Laryngeal paralysis in a mature cat, *Can Vet J* 27:27, 1986.
74. Birchard SJ, Bradley RL: Surgery of the respiratory tract. In Sherding RG, ed: *The cat: diseases and clinical management,* New York, 1989, Churchill Livingstone.
75. Meric SM: Therapeutic options for hyperthyroidism. In August JR, ed: *Consultations in feline medicine,* Philadelphia, 1991, WB Saunders.
76. Hawkins EC: Respiratory disorders. In Nelson RW, Couto CG, eds: *Essentials of small animal internal medicine,* St Louis, 1992, Mosby.
77. Padrid P, Amis TC: Chronic tracheobronchial disease in the dog, *Vet Clin North Am Small Anim Pract* 22:1203, 1992.
78. Nelson AW: Lower respiratory system. In Slatter DH, ed: *Textbook of small animal surgery,* Philadelphia, 1985, WB Saunders.
79. Hedlund CS: Surgical disease of the trachea, *Vet Clin North Am Small Anim Pract* 17:301, 1987.
80. Done SA, Drew RA: Observations on the pathology of tracheal collapse in dogs, *J Small Anim Pract* 17:783, 1976.
81. Fingland RB, DeHoff WD, Birchard SJ: Surgical management of cervical and thoracic tracheal collapse in dogs using extraluminal spiral prostheses, *J Am Anim Hosp Assoc* 23:163, 1987.
82. Carlisle CH, Biery DN, Thrall DE: Tracheal and laryngeal tumors in the dog and cat: literature review and 13 additional patients, *Vet Radiol* 32:229, 1991.
83. Hendricks JC, O'Brien JA: Tracheal collapse in two cats, J Am Vet Med Assoc 187:418, 1985.
84. Reif JS, Rhodes WH: The lungs of aged dogs: a radiographic-morphologic correlation, *J Am Vet Radiol Soc* 7:5, 1966.
85. Ford RB: Endoscopy of the lower respiratory tract of the dog and cat. In Tams TR, ed: *Small animal endoscopy,* St Louis, 1990, Mosby.
86. Padrid P: Chronic lower airway disease in the dog and cat, *Probl Vet Met* 4:320, 1992.
87. Hawkins EC, DeNicola DB, Kuehn NF: Bronchoalveolar lavage in the evaluation of pulmonary disease in the dog and cat, *J Vet Intern Med* 4:267, 1990.
88. Padrid PA, Feldman BF, Funk K et al: Cytologic, microbiologic, and biochemical analysis of bronchoalveolar lavage fluid obtained from 24 healthy cats, *Am J Vet Res* 52:1300, 1991.
89. Brownlie SE: A retrospective study of diagnosis in 109 cases of canine lower respiratory disease, *J Small Anim Pract* 31:371, 1990.
90. Padrid PA, Hornof WJ, Kurpershoek CJ et al: Canine chronic bronchitis: a pathophysiologic evaluation of 18 cases, *J Vet Intern Med* 4:172, 1990.
91. Lindsey JO, Pierce AK: An examination of the microbiologic flora of normal lung of the dog, *Am Rev Respir Dis* 117:501, 1978.
92. McKiernan BC, Smith AR, Kissil M: Bacteria isolated from the lower trachea of clinically healthy dogs, *J Am Anim Hosp Assoc* 20:139, 1984.
93. Taboada J: Pulmonary diseases of potential allergic origin, *Semin Vet Med Surg* 6:278, 1991.
94. Howell S, Roussos C: Isoproterenol and aminophylline improve contractility of fatigued canine diaphragm, *Am Rev Respir Dis* 129:118, 1984.
95. McKiernan BC, Neff-Davis CA, Koritz GD et al: Pharmacokinetic studies of theophylline in dogs, *J Vet Pharmacol Ther* 4:103, 1981.
96. Berry CR, Moore PF, Thomas WP et al: Pulmonary granulomatosis in seven dogs, 1976-1987, *J Vet Intern Med* 4:157, 1990.
97. Calvert CA, Mahaffey MB, Lappin MR et al: Pulmonary and disseminated eosinophilic granulomatosis in dogs, *J Am Anim Hosp Assoc* 24:311, 1988.
98. Fitzgerald SD, Wolf DC, Carlton WW: Eight cases of canine lymphomatoid granulomatosis, *Vet Pathol* 28:241, 1991.
99. LaRue MJ, Murtaugh RJ: Pulmonary thromboembolism in dogs: 47 cases, 1986-1987, *J Am Vet Med Assoc* 197:1368, 1990.
100. Dennis JS: The pathophysiologic sequelae of pulmonary thromboembolism, Compend *Contin Educ Pract Vet* 13:1811, 1991.
101. Green RA, Kabel AL: Hypercoagulable state in three dogs with nephrotic syndrome: role of acquired antithrombin III deficiency, *J Am Vet Med Assoc* 181:914, 1982.
102. Klein MK, Dow SW, Rosychuk RAW: Pulmonary thromboembolism associated with immune-mediated hemolytic anemia in dogs: ten cases, 1982-1987, *J Am Vet Med Assoc* 195:246, 1989.
103. Fluckiger MA, Gomez JA: Radiographic findings in dogs with spontaneous pulmonary thrombosis or embolism, *Vet Radiol* 25:124, 1984.
104. Koblik PD, Hornof W, Harnagel SH et al: A comparison of pulmonary angiography, digital subtraction angiography, and ^{99m}Tc-DTPA/MAA ventilation-perfusion scintigraphy for detection of experimental pulmonary emboli in the dog, *Vet Radiol* 30:159, 1989.
105. Wall RE: Respiratory complications in the critically ill animal, *Probl Vet Med* 4:365, 1992.
106. Schiffman F, Ducas J, Hollett P et al: Treatment of canine embolic pulmonary hypertension with recombinant tissue plasminogen activator, *Circulation* 78:214, 1988.
107. Stone MS, Pook H: Lung infections and infestations: therapeutic considerations, *Probl Vet Med* 4:279, 1992.
108. Madewell BR, Theilen GH: Tumors of the respiratory tract and thorax. In Theilen GH, Madewell BR, eds: *Veterinary cancer medicine,* ed 2, Philadelphia, 1987, Lea & Febiger.
109. Mehlhaff CJ, Mooney S: Primary pulmonary neoplasia in the dog and cat, *Vet Clin North Am Small Anim Pract* 15:1061, 1985.
110. Ogilvie GK, Haschek WM, Withrow SJ et al: Classification of primary lung tumors in dogs: 210 cases, 1975-1985, *J Am Vet Med Assoc* 195:106, 1989.
111. Miles KG: A review of primary lung tumors in the dog and cat, *Vet Radiol* 29:122, 1988.
112. Mehlhaff CJ, Leifer CE, Patnaik AK et al: Surgical treatment of primary pulmonary neoplasia in 15 dogs, *J Am Anim Hosp Assoc* 20:799, 1984.
113. Moore AS: Chemotherapy for intrathoracic cancer in dogs and cats, *Probl Vet Met* 4:351, 1992.
114. Barr FJ, Gruffydd-Jones TJ, Brown PJ et al: Primary lung tumors in the cat, *J Small Anim Pract* 28:1115, 1987.
115. Koblik PD: Radiographic appearance of primary lung tumors in cats: a review of 41 cases, *Vet Radiol* 27:66, 1986.
116. Knapp DW, Richardson RC, DeNicola DB et al: Cisplatin toxicity in cats, *J Vet Intern Med* 1:29, 1987.
117. Moise NS, Wiedenkeller D, Yeager AE et al: Clinical, radiographic, and bronchial cytologic features of cats

with bronchial disease: 65 cases, 1980-1986, *J Am Vet Med Assoc* 194:1467, 1989.
118. Bellah JR, Stiff ME, Russell RG: Thymoma in the dog: two case reports and a review of 20 additional cases, *J Am Vet Med Assoc* 183:306, 1983.
119. Moore AS: Chemotherapy for intrathoracic cancer in dogs and cats, *Probl Vet Met* 4:351, 1992.
120. Carpenter JL, Holzworth J: Thymoma in 11 cats, *J Am Vet Med Assoc* 181:248, 1982.
121. Madewell BR, Theilen GH: Tumors of the respiratory tract and thorax. In Theilen GH, Madewell BR, eds: *Veterinary cancer medicine,* ed 2, Philadelphia, 1987, Lea & Febiger.

CHAPTER 10

Cardiac Disease in Geriatric Dogs and Cats

ANTHONY P. CARR

Cardiac disease is frequently encountered in older dogs and cats. One of the goals of a senior care program is to identify those patients at risk for development of congestive heart failure (CHF) and to institute an appropriate monitoring and therapeutic plan. In older small-breed dogs, the predominant cause of CHF is valvular insufficiency as a result of mitral valve endocardiosis. Dilated cardiomyopathy (DCM) can occur in older dogs; however, many cases of DCM are seen in younger to middle-aged pets. In cats, primary cardiomyopathy can occur. Secondary cardiomyopathies caused by other diseases such as hyperthyroidism or hypertension are also not rare in cats. Early recognition of cardiac disease and monitoring of patients are vital to increase longevity and achieve a good quality of life.

Once cardiac disease has been identified in a geriatric patient a diligent effort must be made to identify concurrent health problems. It is not unusual for geriatric patients to have multiple health problems. One typical example is the dog with cardiac insufficiency and chronic renal failure. Because many of the medications used to treat CHF influence the kidney or are excreted through the kidney, toxicity can occur. Alternatively, the geriatric patient may have diseases that contribute to the progression of cardiac disease. An example of this is the dog with CHF and hyperadrenocorticism (HAC). Hypertension is frequently encountered with HAC and places undue strain on the heart by increasing afterload.

ASSESSING A GERIATRIC PATIENT FOR CARDIAC DISEASE

History and Physical Examination

The history is vital to establishing the possibility that cardiac disease may be present. Early signs of cardiac disease can include exercise intolerance, weakness, syncope, and breathing difficulties. The signs of CHF in dogs are usually quite easy to identify; unfortunately they are nonspecific and can be seen with other diseases, especially disease of the respiratory system. History taking and physical examination should attempt not only to establish if cardiac disease is present, but also to determine if any concurrent diseases might be present. Multiple historical complaints can occur with heart disease, though almost invariably cough is the most common in dogs. In cats cough is almost always related to respiratory disease and not to cardiac disease. Other signs that are common with CHF include weakness, exercise intolerance, weight loss, dyspnea, cyanosis, and syncope. With right-sided heart failure, ascites can develop in dogs, as well. Ascites is generally not a sign of heart failure in cats, although pleural effusion can develop.

On physical examination a murmur is almost always heard. If the heart is difficult to auscult, disorders such as obesity, pleural effusion, pneumothorax, and pericardial effusion need to be considered. The intensity, timing, and point of maximal intensity of any murmur should be noted in the medical record, although the intensity does not necessarily correlate to the severity of cardiac disease. The jugular vein should be inspected; distension or abnormal jugular pulses can be an indication of increased pressure in the right atrium, as is seen with right-sided heart failure and pericardial effusion. Often, dogs with CHF have evidence of muscle mass loss, especially if the problem has been chronic. This does not tend to occur in cats.

Electrocardiogram

In geriatric patients, changes in the electrocardiogram (ECG) can occur with cardiac and other disease. An ECG should be part of every cardiac exam and is needed if a definitive rhythm diagnosis is to be made. In geriatric patients a wide variety of abnormalities can be found; it is up to the clinician to decide if the ECG findings are significant and if specific therapy is indicated for any abnormalities detected. An ECG cannot determine if heart failure is present. An ECG can be indicative of heart enlargement, although the reliability of these findings is insufficient to make any therapeutic decisions.

Radiographs

Imaging studies are vital for the definitive documentation of heart failure in animals with appropriate signs. Good radiographs are usually adequate to achieve this goal. Both lateral and ventrodorsal (or dorsoventral) radiographs are needed if all chambers of the heart are to be assessed accurately. Radiographs also allow identification of any pulmonary abnormalities that may be present (e.g., chronic lower airway disease, metastatic disease). In almost all cases, the left atrium has to be enlarged for a dog with heart disease to be coughing (Figure 10-1). This is an important distinction to make, as dogs with a loud murmur can be well compensated and the cough may result from respiratory disease. In cats, radiographs will be of less value, because the predominant form of heart disease in cats, hypertrophic cardiomyopathy, involves concentric hypertrophy of the heart that makes cardiomegaly less obvious. It is, however, still possible to diagnose heart failure in cats via thoracic radiographs.

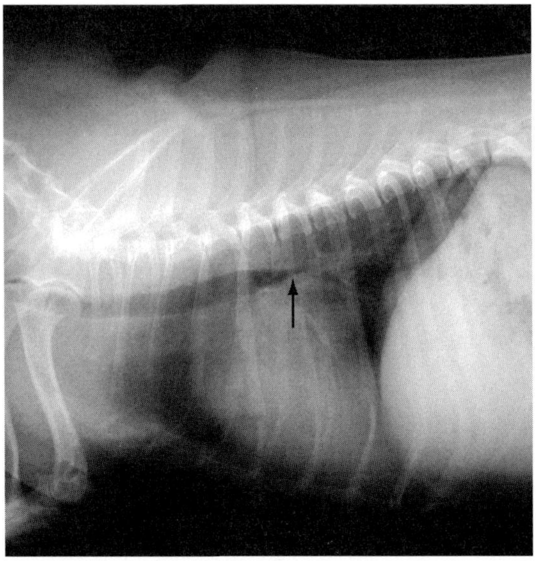

Figure 10-1. This radiograph shows cardiomegaly with compression of the mainstem bronchi *(arrow)* by the enlarged left atrium. Hepatomegaly is evident as well.

Ultrasound

Ultrasound can be a valuable tool in assessing for the presence of heart disease. Ultrasound is very useful in dogs, however, when radiographic findings are equivocal, when endocarditis is suspected, or in early cases of DCM. In those breeds in which CHF is rare (e.g., retrievers, setters) an ultrasound is usually recommended as well. In cocker spaniels an ultrasound is also advisable, as dogs of this breed can have a combination of DCM and valvular heart disease. In cats, ultrasound is vital for determination of the presence of cardiomyopathy and its form. This information is important with regard to devising an optimal therapy plan.

Ancillary Diagnostics

In general, if a patient has been identified as having cardiac disease, a complete laboratory workup is recommended, including complete blood count, serum biochemistry, T_4 levels, and urinalysis. This will help to establish a baseline for the patient and also identify underlying disorders that might complicate management. Blood pressure measurement should also be a routine part of a cardiac workup. This is especially true if cardiac medications are to be given. Many of the medications used to treat cardiac disease can have profound effects on blood pressure.

PATHOPHYSIOLOGY OF HEART FAILURE

In most instances heart failure results in decreased perfusion of organs. This decrease results in activation of compensatory mechanisms that try to maintain a normal blood pressure and thereby guarantee perfusion of vital organs such as the kidney. The same mechanisms are activated independent of the underlying cause of the heart failure. Activation of the renin-angiotensin-aldosterone system (RAAS) is a regular finding with heart failure. Renin is released by the kidney because of hypoperfusion. Renin then converts angiotensinogen to angiotensin I (AT-I). AT-I is converted to angiotensin II (AT-II) by the angiotensin-converting enzyme (ACE). This in turn leads to the increased secretion of aldosterone. The increased generation of AT-II and aldosterone leads to a vicious cycle in which fluid and salt are retained to increase volume and therefore preload. Increased preload does increase cardiac output; however, the increased volume stretches the heart, leading to eccentric dilation. Volume overload also leads to signs of congestion such as pulmonary edema. AT-II is also a potent vasoconstrictor. Vasoconstriction helps to maintain blood pressure and therefore perfusion of vital organs; this does, however, increase the pressure that the heart has to generate to pump blood out—that is, it increases afterload. With greater pressures being generated, compensatory hypertrophy of the ventricle occurs. Increased afterload is undesirable because it leads to decreased cardiac output.

Another major compensatory mechanism with heart failure is activation of the sympathetic nervous system with increased circulating levels of epinephrine and norepinephrine. These hormones increase heart rate. An increase in heart rate increases cardiac output. Contractility is also increased by the effects of sympathetic stimulation, again leading to an increase in cardiac output. Vasoconstriction also occurs, thereby maintaining blood pressure but increasing afterload. Activation of the sympathetic nervous system also leads to increased thirst and volume retention. Sympathetic activation predisposes to arrhythmias by increasing cardiac oxygen demand and increasing excitability.

SPECIFIC CARDIAC DISORDERS IN DOGS

Chronic Valvular Endocardiosis

Endocardiosis is an extremely common disorder in geriatric dogs and the most common reason for CHF. The mitral valve is predominantly involved, although the tricuspid can be affected as well. As a result of the myxomatous degenerative changes occurring, the valve leaflets lose proper apposition, resulting in regurgitation of some of the blood from the left ventricle into the left atrium. The left atrium begins to distend because of this. A certain portion of forward blood flow is lost. This results in activation of compensatory mechanisms to guarantee adequate perfusion. Initially, ventricular dilation with hypertrophy occurs. With chronicity, volume overload eventually leads to continued dilation with decrease in myocardial function. As the pressure in the left atrium rises, pulmonary edema results.

Clinical Features. Endocardiosis occurs more commonly in some breeds than others. It is very common in the Cavalier King Charles spaniel and manifests itself very early on. Most commonly affected are small to medium dogs. Progression usually is gradual. The first sign is often either exercise intolerance or cough. In many cases the cough is a result of airway compression by the enlarged left atrium rather than a result of pulmonary edema. Nocturnal cough is highly suggestive of heart-related problems. In those instances in which tricuspid involvement is present, ascites or pleural effusion can be seen. Syncope can occur as well, especially in association with coughing (cough-related syncope), although the exact mechanisms by which this occurs are unclear. Coughing can increase vagal tone, which would decrease heart rate, leading to decreased cardiac output. In addition, venous return may be compromised by increased intrathoracic pressure. With progression, breathing problems, including cyanosis, become more obvious. Weight loss with or without anorexia can occur as well.

With endocardiosis a variety of ECG changes can be seen. Cardiac enlargement patterns may be seen. Right atrial enlargement is suggested by an increased amplitude of the P wave. Prolongation of the P-wave duration is reflective of left atrial enlargement. Increases in R-wave amplitude and QRS duration can indicate left ventricular enlargement. Axis deviations can occur as well. Arrhythmias do develop on occasion, with both supraventricular and ventricular ectopic beats being possible, although they are seen less commonly than with DCM.

Radiographic changes vary according to which valves are affected and how advanced the disease is. Initially, ventricular enlargement will be seen, then atrial. The left atrium will be enlarged with advanced mitral valve disease. This is usually best seen on the lateral radiograph. It may also be possible to see compression of the mainstem bronchi by the left atrium, both in the lateral and ventrodorsal view. Right atrial enlargement is usually best judged on the ventrodorsal or dorsoventral view. Right atrial and right ventricular enlargement give a "reverse D" appearance. Right-sided heart failure can result in hepatomegaly from congestion and ascites. The pulmonary blood vessels are often also congested, the pulmonary vein with mitral valve disease and the pulmonary artery with tricuspid endocardiosis. In advanced cases, congestion in the form of pulmonary edema, ascites, or pleural effusion may be noted as well (Figure 10-2).

Echocardiography can be helpful with endocardiosis, although less so than with other cardiac disease. In those cases in which it is difficult to assess chamber enlargement on radiographs, echocardiography can be quite valuable. Thickening of the valves, abnormal motion of the valves (prolapse), or rupture of the chordae tendineae can be noted. The appearance of the valves can also help differentiate endocardiosis from endocarditis. In most cases of valvular insufficiency, measured contractility is normal to increased. With chronic volume overload in end-stage heart failure it is possible to see decreasing contractility.

Dilated Cardiomyopathy. DCM can occur in elderly patients. DCM results in decreased contractility and eccentric dilation of the ventricles. Many times with breed-related DCM, onset occurs at an early age. Generally, large-breed dogs are affected, although smaller dogs such as cocker spaniels can have the disease as well. Breeds with a high prevalence of DCM include Dobermans, Irish wolfhounds, Great Danes, and boxers. The etiology of primary cardiomyopathy is idiopathic. Some dogs have been identified as having deficiencies of certain nutrients such as L-carnitine (boxers) or taurine (American cocker spaniels), although in many instances even with supplementation the disease progresses to failure, albeit more slowly.

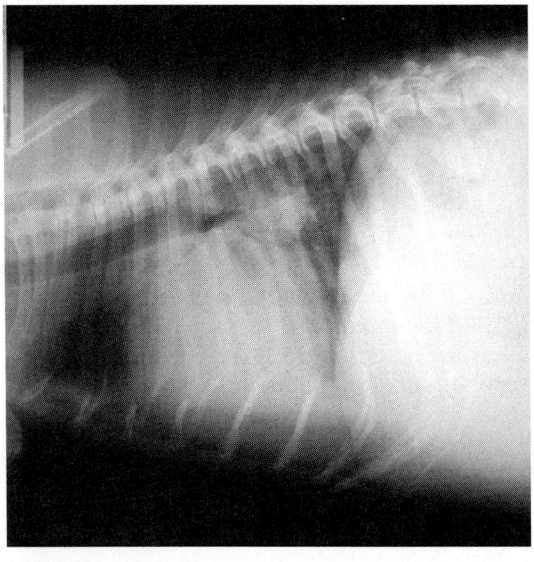

Figure 10-2. This radiograph shows generalized cardiomegaly with left atrial enlargement. There also is an interstitial and mild alveolar pattern in the perihilar region that is consistent with pulmonary edema. Abdominal detail is poor, a result of ascites.

Clinical presentation varies. Some breeds have arrhythmias as an important feature, and sudden death may be the only sign of DCM (e.g., in Dobermans and boxers). Initially, presenting complaints can be subtle—for example, exercise intolerance. Most patients, however, are presented for signs of CHF, either left or right sided. Some dogs have forward or low-output failure and can progress to cardiac shock. These patients have symptoms such as weakness, hypotension, cool extremities, poor capillary refill time, and hypothermia. Murmurs are often heard, although they may not necessarily be loud. A gallop can also be heard at times because of rapid ventricular filling into the dilated ventricle (S_3).

ECG abnormalities are very common with DCM, more so than with valvular heart disease. Most arrhythmias are tachycardias, both supraventricular and ventricular in origin. Atrial premature complexes can occur, and atrial fibrillation is also quite common (Figure 10-3). This can often be seen at initial presentation. The conversion to atrial fibrillation results in acute decompensation because of a marked increase in heart rate, compromising cardiac output. Ventricular ectopic beats and ventricular tachycardia can also occur (Figure 10-4). This can cause sudden death in some dogs and is especially prevalent in Doberman pinschers with DCM.

Imaging studies are necessary to assess dogs for the presence of DCM. In advanced cases, the presence of cardiomegaly and atrial enlargement make the heart failure evident. Pulmonary edema, ascites, or pleural effusion can all be present, depending on whether both sides or one side of the heart is predominantly affected. The diagnosis of DCM cannot, however, be confirmed without an echocardiogram. The stage of the patient's disease will determine which echocardiographic changes are seen. A decrease in contractility and an increase in left ventricular internal diameter will initially be detected. This is followed by progressive thinning of the ventricular walls and continued dilation of the ventricular chamber. Eventually this leads to stretching of the

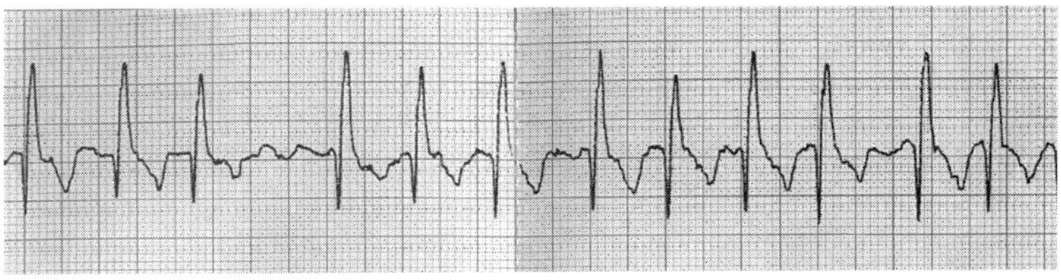

Figure 10-3. The electrocardiogram shows a rapid heart rate (260 beats per minute) with marked variation in the beat-to-beat interval, consistent with atrial fibrillation. Left ventricular enlargement is suggested by the prolongation in the QRS duration.

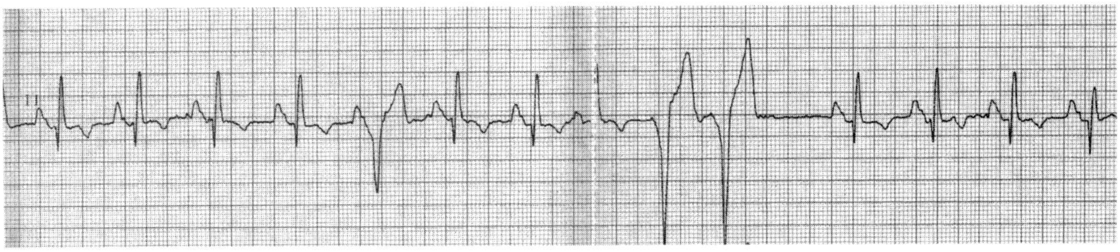

Figure 10-4. Ventricular premature complexes in a Doberman with dilated cardiomyopathy. Atrial enlargement is suggested by the wide and notched P wave.

atrioventricular (AV) valve annulus and regurgitation into the atria. The atria enlarge because of chronic volume overload and regurgitation.

Treating a Geriatric Patient with CHF

Once a patient has been diagnosed with CHF, an appropriate treatment plan needs to be made. A wide variety of agents are available for the treatment of heart disease (Table 10-1). Before therapy is initiated, it is important to be aware of the goals of therapy and what the therapeutic agents realistically can accomplish. Because pet owners can resort to euthanasia, it is vital that close attention be paid to how the owner perceives the situation. Although CHF is invariably fatal, painting too bleak a picture can lead to the owner giving up early in the disease process. It is important to transmit to the owner realistic expectations for the pet. Strenuous exercise is unlikely to be possible once CHF is present and is, in fact, not desirable, as it can destabilize a compensated patient. The therapies selected should seek to improve the patient's quality of life and if at all possible prolong it. They also should be used in a manner that limits toxicities from occurring. Factors that have been identified as leading to euthanasia by owners include weakness, recurrent episodes of acute CHF, and anorexia.[1] Therapy, of course, needs to be tailored to each patient and owner individually.

ACE Inhibitors. ACE inhibitors have proved to be one of the most significant breakthroughs in cardiac therapeutics for both human and small animal patients. Although there are many cardiac medications available, few have been shown to prolong life. ACE inhibitors not only prolong the lives of patients with heart failure, but they also improve quality of life. Quality of life is a vital issue in veterinary medicine, because owners can resort to euthanasia if the pet is perceived to be suffering or no longer living comfortably. Some vital issues practicing veterinarians need to be aware of are the indications for these medications, their side effects, the conditions under which it is advisable to start using them, and their efficacy in cats with CHF.

Mechanisms of ACE Inhibitor Action. ACE inhibitors have a variety of effects in heart failure. One of the hallmarks of heart failure is activation of the RAAS. This certainly does apply to dogs with DCM. It does not seem to be as uniform in dogs with valvular heart disease, however. The use of diuretics such as furosemide or marked salt restriction has been shown to lead to activation of the RAAS. AT-II is also thought to play a role in cardiac remodeling, a process that leads to progressive cardiac dysfunction. This may relate more to local concentrations of AT-II than to circulating blood levels. Recently attention has also focused on the ability of AT-II to activate the inflammatory cascade. Elevations in cytokines such as tumor necrosis factor–α are thought to

TABLE 10-1. COMMON CARDIOVASCULAR DRUGS, DOSES, AND SIDE EFFECTS

DRUG	INDICATIONS	DOSE	SIDE EFFECTS
Furosemide	CHF, edema formation	Dogs: 1-4 mg/kg sid-tid Cats: 0.5-2 mg/kg qod-bid	Dehydration, azotemia, hypokalemia
Enalapril	CHF	0.5 mg/kg sid-bid	Hypotension, renal insufficiency
Benazapril	CHF	0.25-0.5 mg/kg sid	Hypotension, renal compromise (rare)
Nitroglycerin	Pulmonary edema	1/8-1 inch transcutaneously	Hypotension, irritability, headache?
Digoxin	Myocardial failure, refractory CHF, supraventricular arrhythmias	Dogs: 0.011 mg/kg bid Cats: 1/4 of a 0.125-mg tablet qod	Vomiting, diarrhea, anorexia, depression, arrhythmias
Propranolol	Supraventricular or ventricular arrhythmias	Dogs: 0.2-2 mg/kg q8-12h Cats: 0.25-10 mg q8-12h	Worsening CHF, lethargy, bradycardia, bronchospasm
Atenolol	Supraventricular or ventricular arrhythmias	Dogs: 2.5-1 mg/kg bid Cats: 1/4 of a 25-mg tablet qod	Hypotension, bradycardia, worsening CHF
Amlodipine	Hypertension, afterload reduction	Dogs: 0.625-1.25 mg sid in small dogs, 1.25-2.5 mg in large dogs, titrate until desired blood pressure is achieved Cats: 0.625 mg sid-bid	Hypotension, renal compromise
Spironolactone	Diuresis, aldosterone antagonist	1-2 mg/kg sid-bid	Hyperkalemia, dehydration, azotemia
Hydralazine	Afterload reduction, refractory pulmonary edema, hypertension	Dogs: 0.5-2 mg/kg bid Cats: 0.5-0.8 mg/kg bid; start low, titrate until desired blood pressure is achieved	Hypotension, vomiting
Mexilitine	Ventricular tachycardias	Dogs: 5-8 mg/kg tid	Proarrhythmia, tremors, vomiting, ataxia
Sotalol	Ventricular tachycardias	Dogs: 1-2 mg/kg bid	Bradycardia, hypotension
Diltiazem	Supraventricular arrhythmias or hypertrophic cardiomyopathy	0.5-1.5 mg/kg tid	Hypotension, bradycardia
Lidocaine	Ventricular arrhythmias	1-4 mg/kg bolus: 40-80 µg/kg/min CRI	Vomiting, seizures, hypotension
Procainamide SR	Ventricular arrhythmias	Dogs: 6-20 mg/kg tid Cats: 62.5 mg tid	Hypotension, vomiting, agranulocytosis
Aspirin	Antithrombotic	Dogs: 5 mg/kg sid Cats: 1/4 of a 325-mg tablet PO q2-3day	Vomiting, GI ulceration

CHF, Congestive heart failure; *CRI,* continuous rate infusion; *GI,* gastrointestinal; *PO,* oral administration

be one of the ways in which cardiac cachexia develops. Research in dogs has shown that treatment with omega-3 essential fatty acids reduces cardiac cachexia, possibly by reducing cytokine levels.

Effects of ACE Inhibitors in CHF. A variety of studies have looked at the affects of ACE inhibitors in patients with symptomatic heart failure.[2-5] In dogs with marked heart failure from mitral valve disease, life expectancy more than doubled with ACE inhibitors when compared with placebo. This applies to both enalapril and benazapril. In dogs with DCM, enalapril had the same effect. Statistically it was not possible to show the same benefit with benazapril, although this may have related more to the small size of the group investigated rather than to any true differences between the medications. The ability to exercise was also significantly improved, as was the patient's overall well-being, when these medications were given.

There is little doubt that a dog with CHF should be placed on an ACE inhibitor unless it absolutely cannot tolerate the drug. This is especially true if diuretics are being used or if a salt-restricted diet has been prescribed. Adverse side effects are rare in dogs. The greatest concern is the development of azotemia. This usually occurs only when diuretics or salt restriction are concurrently being used and can often resolve when the diuretic dose is reduced. In fact, in some studies renal values improved in dogs that were receiving an ACE inhibitor in comparison with those given placebo.

When to Start a Patient on an ACE Inhibitor. The question arises as to whether to start using these medications in dogs with heart disease without clinical signs. The goal of starting these medications early would be to slow the progressive changes associated with heart disease and prolong the amount of time until heart failure develops. It appears that this does occur in humans; however, in humans one of the most common causes of heart failure is myocardial infarction, a disease in which progressive cardiac remodeling plays a significant role in future decompensation. Until recently few data existed regarding this effect in animals. A recent publication has looked at this important question in detail. The study was a prospective, placebo-controlled double blind study involving 229 Cavalier King Charles spaniels with mitral valve disease that had no evidence of heart failure.[6] The dogs were evaluated by physical examination, electrocardiography, and radiographs. The dogs were randomized to receive either placebo or enalapril at standard dosages. The study revealed that patients with cardiomegaly or louder murmurs progressed more rapidly to heart failure. The study, however, failed to show any preventive benefit from using enalapril in these asymptomatic dogs, whether or not cardiomegaly was present at enrollment. There are obvious limitations to this study in that only one breed and only one ACE inhibitor were studied. Nonetheless, given the scope of the study, similarity in progression of valvular endocardiosis in dogs, and the similar effects of various ACE inhibitors, it is likely that this study does apply to most dogs with mitral valve disease.

Unlike dogs with mitral valve disease, the situation in dogs with DCM may be dramatically different, in that an ACE inhibitor needs to be started at initial diagnosis. This may be because RAAS activation is more pronounced in DCM. A study in Dobermans tried to determine if early therapy was able to slow the progression of DCM and positively influence life span.[7] The study group consisted of dogs with evidence of DCM, defined as an increased left ventricular diameter, without having clinical signs of heart failure. Administration of enalapril in the occult phase resulted in a doubling of the life span and an increase in the time to onset of CHF. Overall it is recommended that an ACE inhibitor be started as early as possible in dogs suspected of having DCM, regardless of whether or not they have evidence of decompensation.

Diuretics. The mainstay of therapy is furosemide (1 to 2 mg/kg sid to bid; higher dosages possible in end-stage CHF). Furosemide is a potent loop diuretic that can rapidly diminish pulmonary edema. Diuretics should not be used as monotherapy, but should be combined with ACE inhibitors in virtually all patients other than those that absolutely cannot tolerate ACE inhibitors. Furosemide is used to keep congestion under control. Therefore, dosages should be reassessed frequently to achieve the lowest dose possible. A "newer" therapy is the use of spironolactone at low dosages, usually in combination with furosemide. The efficacy of this therapy has not been evaluated in veterinary medicine; however, the results in human trials are very promising. The dose is fairly low (1 mg/kg sid to bid), so diuretic effects are minimal. It may be that the spironolactone blocks aldosterone that is produced in spite of the use of an ACE inhibitor, thereby having a favorable influence on life span. Renal values and potassium levels need to be monitored 2 to 7 days after adding a diuretic or increasing the amount used.

Digoxin. Digoxin was once a medication commonly used in the treatment of CHF. In veterinary medicine there is no objective information available that allows us to definitively establish when digoxin should or should not be used. Digoxin can be very helpful in the management of supraventricular tachycardias such as frequent atrial premature complexes, atrial fibrillation (see Figure 10-4) or atrial tachycardia. Unlike many of the other medications used to control these arrhythmias, digoxin does not decrease cardiac output. Digoxin can, however, worsen ventricular premature complexes (VPCs) and needs to be used cautiously if this arrhythmia is present. It tends to be my preference to use digoxin sparingly in dogs with endocardiosis and no evidence of supraventricular arrhythmias. Toxicity is always a concern, and careful monitoring is needed. The owner also needs to be counseled with regard to the signs of toxicity so that continued overdosing does not occur.

Dietary Therapy. An area that is often neglected in the management of CHF is proper nutrition. Proper nutrition does not necessarily equate to a very-low-salt diet. It is important to remember that anorexia and weight loss are some of the signs that owners use to judge their pet's quality of life. Any dietary plan, no matter how good in theory it is for the dog, that results in anorexia or significant weight loss is risking the life of the patient. Generally, moderate salt restriction is considered to be beneficial once signs of CHF are present; severe salt restriction is needed only with very advanced heart failure. If the pet refuses the food chosen, then using a less-than-ideal diet may become necessary. Recent work has also suggested that the addition of omega-3 fatty acid supplements can reduce the signs of cardiac cachexia.[8] A variety of nutritional supplements have also been used with CHF. There certainly does seem to be a role for taurine (especially in American cocker spaniels with DCM) and carnitine in some, but not all, dogs with DCM. Coenzyme Q_{10} received some attention; however, there are no good clinical data available to prove whether this is effective or not.

Endocarditis

Bacterial infection of the lining of the heart generally is a devastating disease. Most often the valves themselves are affected. It does not occur frequently; however, the outcomes often are poor. Bacterial seeding throughout the body and immunologic response to the antigenic stimulus, as well as damage to the valves themselves, all participate in the clinical signs of this disorder. The source of the bacteria generally cannot be determined, although some cases probably relate to catheters and other invasive procedures. A variety of organisms have been implicated in endocarditis including *Staphylococcus* species, *Streptococcus* species, *Escherichia coli,* and occasionally *Erysipelothrix* species.[9] In recent years *Bartonella* has also been isolated from dogs with endocarditis.[10] Endocarditis tends to occur more frequently in large-breed dogs. Dogs with subaortic stenosis are also predisposed to endocarditis, probably because of turbulence resulting from this congenital lesion. Most commonly, aortic or mitral valves are affected. Diagnosis is ideally based on compatible clinical signs, echocardiographic changes compatible with endocarditis, and positive blood cultures (at least two).

Clinical signs are variable and at times vague. Fever is commonly seen. It can be intermittent or constant. Most patients are systemically ill, showing lethargy and anorexia. Polyarthritis can develop, leading to lameness. In rare instances bacteria will also seed to the joints. More frequently, bacterial embolization occurs in the kidney, spleen, and liver. Auscultation will often reveal a systolic or diastolic murmur. A diastolic murmur can be ausculted if the infection involves the aortic valve; suspicion of endocarditis should be high if this is found in a patient that has appropriate clinical signs. The ECG can reflect a variety of changes. Arrhythmias, especially ventricular premature beats and ventricular tachycardia, can occur. Conduction problems such as bundle branch blocks or AV blocks are also sequelae of endocarditis of the aortic valve. These valves are located close to the AV nodal tissue, and the infection can extend from the valve to this area of the septum. Echocardiography may show a vegetation on or near a valve. The valves may also appear brighter than normal in some cases (Figure 10-5). With severe valve damage, cardiac insufficiency can develop. Laboratory work can indicate signs of an active infection or inflammation with increased white blood cell counts, a left shift, or toxic changes. Urinalysis may document infection or proteinuria (antigen-antibody deposition in the glomeruli leading to glomerulonephritis). The chemistry panel may reflect damage to various organs, including kidney and liver.

Treatment for endocarditis consists of appropriate antibiotic therapy as well as treatment for cardiac insufficiency if this develops. The more severely the valves are damaged the poorer the prognosis. Ideally, antibiotic choice is guided by the results of the blood culture. Antibiotics should be chosen with a broad spectrum pending culture results, initially given parenterally if the patient is sufficiently ill. A good choice would be either an aminoglycoside (for initial therapy) or a fluoroquinolone together with a penicillin (amoxicillin or ampicillin). Fluoroquinolones have the advantage that they can be given orally, so they often are used for long-term therapy if needed. Antibiotic therapy is continued for 8 to 12 weeks. The combination of these antibiotics is also used if the culture is negative in a patient strongly suspected

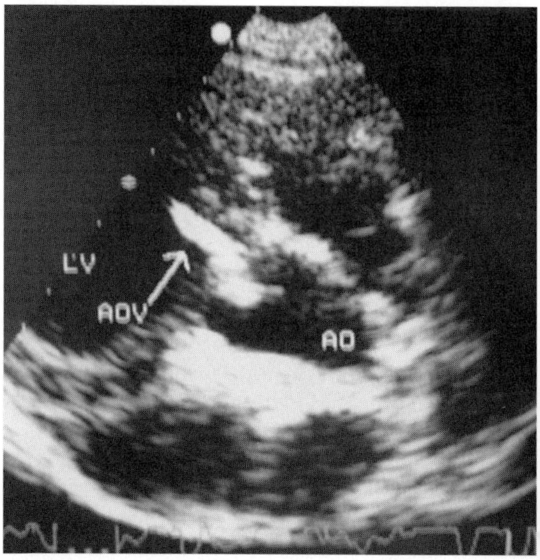

Figure 10-5. Short axis view of the heart at the level of the atria and aorta. Arrow shows a markedly thickened aortic valve in a dog with endocarditis.

to have endocarditis, because the antimicrobial spectrum is fairly extensive for this form of combination.

Cardiac Neoplasia

Neoplasms involving the heart are relatively rare. Diagnosis is usually made via echocardiography.[11] It is possible, of course, for any tumor to metastasize to the heart. There are, however, certain tumors that do have a predilection for the heart. Most commonly, tumors of the heart manifest because pericardial effusion develops. This is certainly the case with hemangiosarcomas. In most instances they involve the right atrium and lead to hemorrhage into the pericardial sac. Heart base masses and aortic body masses also occur and often cause pericardial effusion (Figure 10-6). These tumors tend to metastasize late in their course, so affected patients have a better prognosis, although effusion may need to be managed with repeated pericardiocentesis or pericardectomy. In most cases these cardiac tumors are amenable to neither surgery nor chemotherapy.

Pericardial Effusion

Pericardial disease occurs more commonly in older dogs, because one of the most common causes, neoplasia, occurs more frequently in older dogs. The most common tumors are hemangiosarcomas and heart base tumors. The metastatic potential with hemangiosarcomas is higher, and survival tends to be shorter. Other causes of effusion into the pericardial sac include infections and idiopathic hemorrhage.

Clinical signs often are dependent on how rapidly the pericardial sac is filled; the faster this occurs, the more compromised the patient will be. It is possible to see acute bleeds that result in death, especially in patients with atrial rupture. The presence of fluid in the pericardial sac leads to an increase in pressure in this space, eventually leading to tamponade. Jugular venous distension, jugular pulses, and a positive hepatojugular reflex can be seen in dogs with pericardial disease, although other causes of right-sided failure will cause the same signs. Heart sounds are often muffled, and the patient may be weak, hypotensive, or in shock, depending on the severity of the tamponade. With more chronic disease, ascites can develop, as can pleural effusion.

Definitive diagnosis can be achieved only via echocardiography (Figure 10-7). Echocardiography also allows documentation of tamponade and a search for a tumor that might be the reason for the effusion. Thoracic radiography can be helpful when there is much fluid present in the pericardial sac. The heart becomes globoid in shape. In addition, the margins of the heart become very clearly defined on radiographs

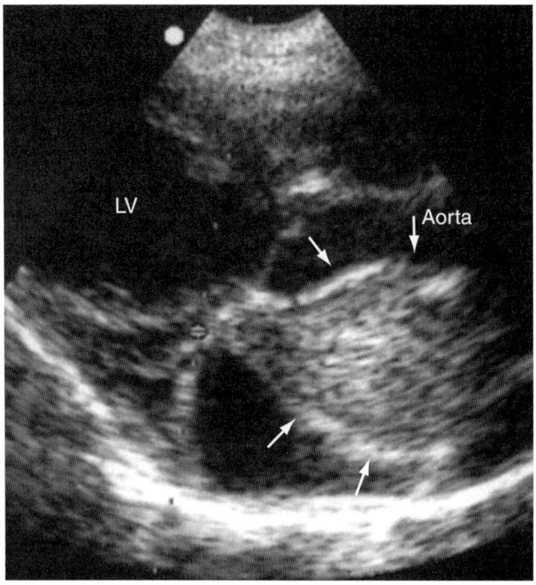

Figure 10-6. Long axis view of the heart showing a heart base mass *(arrows)* located next to the aorta in a dog.

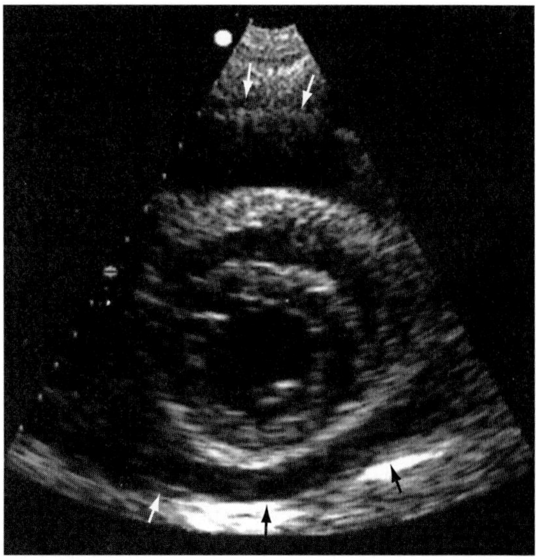

Figure 10-7. Short axis of the heart showing fluid in the pericardial space. The arrows outline the limits of the pericardial sac.

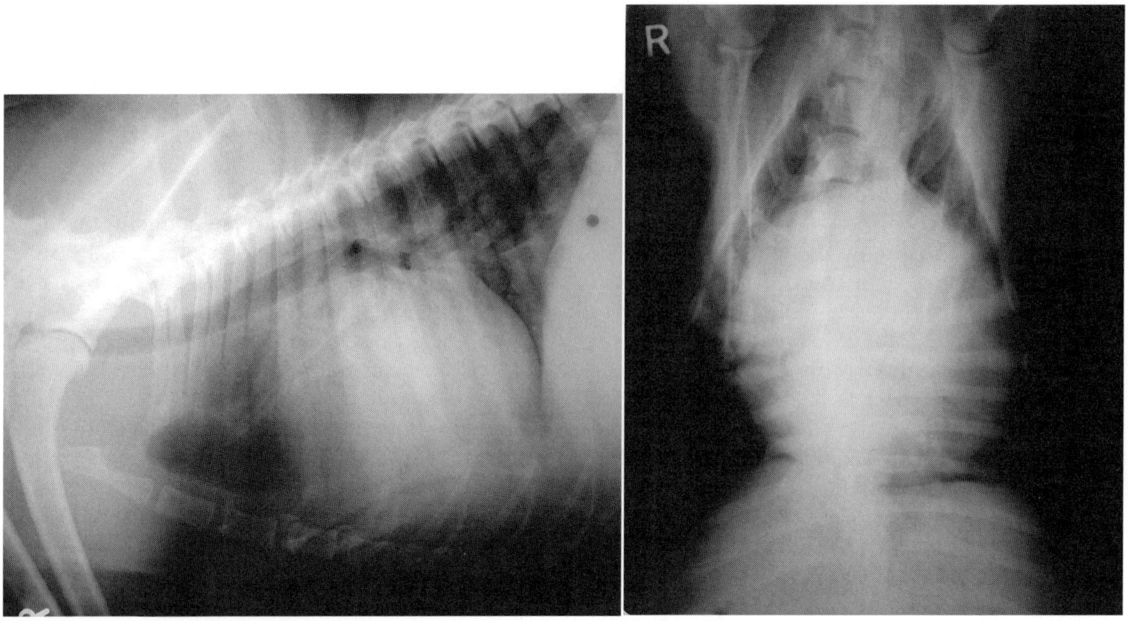

A B

Figure 10-8. Radiographs show crisp cardiac margins and marked cardiomegaly causing a globoid appearance without clear evidence of left atrial enlargement on the lateral radiograph.

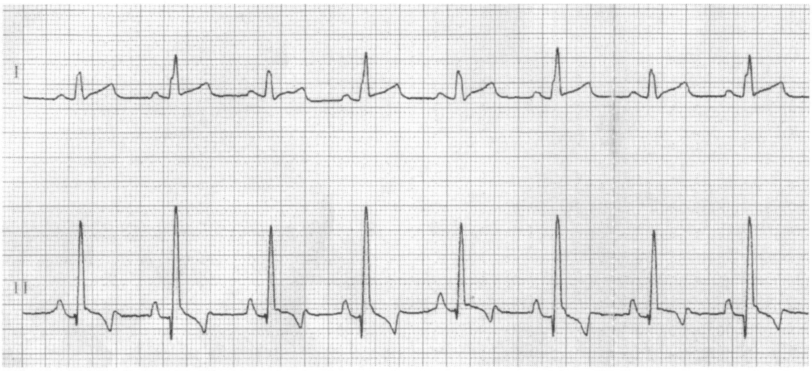

Figure 10-9. Electrocardiogram from a dog with pericardial effusion. Electrical alternans (alteration in R wave amplitude from beat to beat) is present in both lead I and lead II.

(Figure 10-8), because usually the heart is moving during radiography, which leads to blurring. When there is pericardial effusion, however, this motion occurs within the fluid-filled pericardium, which remains fairly static, leading to crisp cardiac margins. Electrocardiography can also be helpful; however, it is relatively rare that a "classic" ECG is seen with pericardial effusion. Electrical alternans (beat-to-beat variation in the amplitude of the QRS complex), ST segment depression or elevation, and low voltage complexes are potential changes noted (Figure 10-9).

Initial treatment for pericardial effusion usually depends on removing fluid via pericardiocentesis. This is best guided via an ECG; when the heart is touched by the needle of the catheter, VPCs will occur. As much fluid as possible should be removed, and some should be submitted for evaluation, although this rarely is of great diagnostic benefit. In those cases in which longer term management is indicated (e.g., no tumor found on echocardiography, slow growing tumor present) pericardectomy could be considered via a variety of surgical and thoracoscopic procedures.

Arrhythmias

A variety of arrhythmias can occur in dogs. The decision to treat these disturbances is often based on multiple factors. If clinical signs are associated with a rhythm disturbance, then treatment has a valid goal. In other instances it may be desirable to try to prevent premature death from a malignant arrhythmia. It is important that the medications being used are matched to the goal of therapy. In some instances a direct therapy of a rhythm may be necessary, for instance, in the context of a dog with heart failure. Often, initiating standard heart failure medications such as an ACE inhibitor, diuretics, and oxygen therapy can significantly improve the rhythm. Arrhythmias can also be caused by noncardiac disease such as that seen with splenic masses. In these situations, treating the underlying cause of the arrhythmias usually resolves the rhythm disturbance.

Tachycardias. Both ventricular and supraventricular tachycardias can occur. In most cases these arise because of underlying heart disease (e.g., endocardiosis, DCM). An important factor as to whether these tachycardias cause clinical signs is the rate at which the heart is beating. Generally, at rates over 170 beats per minute a compromise in cardiac output develops because of poor ventricular filling. At times differentiating supraventricular from ventricular rhythms can be difficult. If the QRS complexes are narrow, the origin of the tachycardia is supraventricular (Figure 10-10). In most instances a wide complex tachycardia is ventricular in origin; however, in patients with conduction problems (bundle branch blocks) supraventricular rhythms can have wide and bizarre looking QRS complexes (Figure 10-11).

Bradycardias. Slow heart rates often are seen with high vagal tone and are typical for well trained dogs. Bradycardias can also develop, however, through sinus nodal or atrioventricular (AV) nodal problems. The most common cause in aged dogs and cats is AV block resulting from fibrosis of the cardiac conduction system. First-degree AV block will not cause clinical signs, and the same holds true for mild second-degree AV block. With advanced second-degree (multiple P waves dropped before a QRS occurs) or third-degree AV block, clinical signs are common although not always present in dogs. In many cats, third-degree AV block does not cause overt clinical signs (Figure 10-12). Typical signs include weakness, lethargy, exercise intolerance, and syncope. With long-term bradycardia, heart failure can develop as well. Medical management may be possible and may help resolve signs. An atropine response test (0.04 mg/kg atropine intramuscularly, with the ECG repeated 30 minutes after the atropine is given) is useful in these cases. Atropine abolishes vagal tone and can improve some bradycardias. A lack of response to atropine usually indicates that medical therapy will not be effective. If it

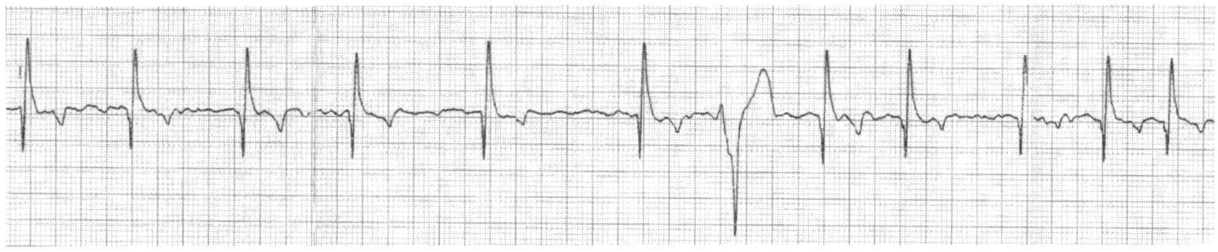

Figure 10-10. Electrocardiogram from a dog being treated for dilated cardiomyopathy. The rhythm is irregular, and P waves cannot be seen. Rate is slow because of use of digoxin and diltiazem to slow it. The majority of QRS complexes are short in duration because they are supraventricular in origin. A single ventricular premature complex is seen and is wide and bizarre in its morphology.

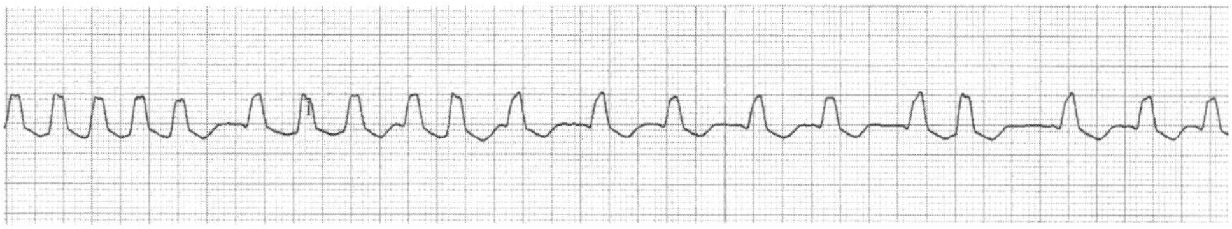

Figure 10-11. Lead I electrocardiogram from a dog with dilated cardiomyopathy. Note the very rapid heart rate (280 beats per minute) and markedly irregular rhythm diagnostic for atrial fibrillation. QRS duration is prolonged, consistent with a left bundle branch block

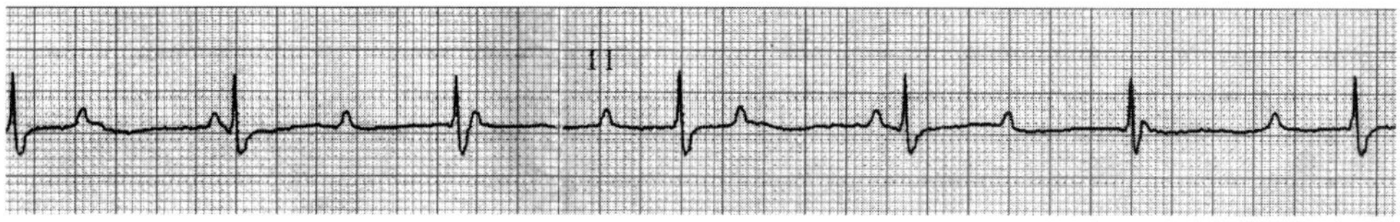

Figure 10-12. The electrocardiogram shows a ventricular rate of 120 beats per minute and a P-wave rate of 180 beats per minute. The P waves and QRS complexes are completely independent of each other, consistent with third-degree atrioventricular block.

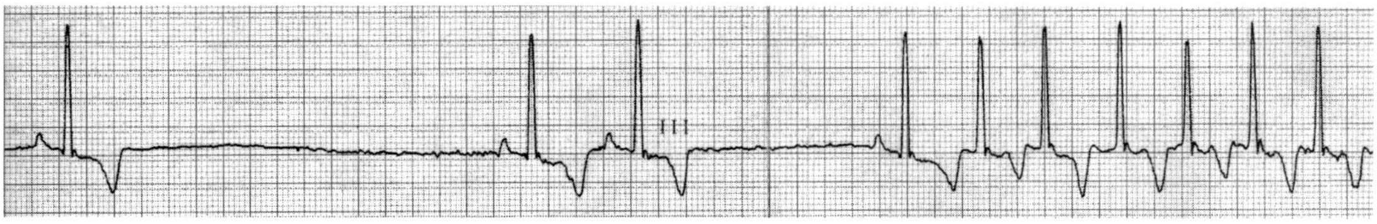

Figure 10-13. Prolonged pauses in the rhythm followed by atrial tachycardia at a rate of 240 beats per minute, consistent with sick sinus syndrome.

is not possible to control signs medically, a pacemaker may be needed to maintain a near normal heart rate.

Sick Sinus Syndrome. This rhythm disturbance in its simplest form consists only of problems with impulse generation. This manifests in the erratic generation of sinus beats so that prolonged pauses can occur. These pauses are, however, often so long that other pacemaker tissues should take over driving the heart. Because this does not happen there most likely is disease of the entire impulse generating system, not just the sinus node. An atropine response test is indicated in these patients as well, and medical therapy can be helpful, although often only temporarily. A pacemaker may be necessary. It is also possible to see tachycardias concurrently in this syndrome, usually supraventricular in origin (Figure 10-13). When bradycardia and tachycardia both are present, medical therapy is generally fruitless. Treating the bradycardia could make the tachycardia worse and vice versa. These patients are definitely in need of a pacemaker. The pacemaker prevents bradycardia so that aggressive medical management of the tachycardia is feasible.

CARDIAC DISORDERS IN CATS

Cardiomyopathies represent the most common heart diseases in cats.[12] By definition a cardiomyopathy is a disease involving the heart muscle. The change in the heart muscle leads to loss of function, and thereby clinical disease can occur. There are primary idiopathic forms as well as secondary forms that occur as a result of an underlying systemic-metabolic problem. Cardiomyopathies can be classified according to the structural heart changes that occur, usually diagnosed by ultrasound. In certain cats a familial predisposition to idiopathic hypertrophic cardiomyopathy has been identified. The secondary forms do occur commonly in cats, especially in geriatric patients. Good examples of secondary cardiomyopathies are DCM in association with taurine deficiency and cardiac hypertrophy that occurs in association with hyperthyroidism or hypertension.

Hypertrophic Cardiomyopathy

The most frequent form of cardiomyopathy is the hypertrophic form (HCM). In this disease the ventricular walls begin to hypertrophy and the heart muscle fibers become disorganized. With hypertrophy, the heart can no longer relax, and the ventricular lumen is decreased. Ischemia is also quite common with infarction. There is also a specific manifestation of HCM termed *hypertrophic obstructive cardiomyopathy,* or HOCM. In these cases there is dynamic obstruction of the aortic outflow tract during systole, leading to a situation similar to aortic stenosis. It is possible that this dynamic aortic stenosis leads to secondary generalized ventricular hypertrophy.

Restrictive Cardiomyopathy

Restrictive and intermediate cardiomyopathies are also recognized. Their classification does pose some challenges, as there is some inconsistency in nomenclature. The term *restrictive cardiomyop-*

athy (RCM) should probably be limited to those cases in which severe fibrosis of the endocardium and subendocardium has occurred. These hearts are stiff and noncompliant, and as a result diastolic dysfunction exists with an inability to fill the ventricle properly. Much of the normal cardiac architecture is deformed. This form of cardiomyopathy may be secondary to a previous bout of inflammation, although it may also represent an end stage form of cardiac disease in which ischemia and infarction have led to widespread scar-tissue formation.

The term *intermediate cardiomyopathy* (ICM) is somewhat more difficult to define. It usually refers to cardiomyopathy that has features of both dilated and hypertrophic cardiomyopathy, that is, hypertrophy of the ventricular walls is present, but with chamber dilation and normal to slightly decreased contractility. Whether this represents a discrete disease process or is a stage in the progression of cardiomyopathy from hypertrophic to dilated is uncertain.

Dilated Cardiomyopathy

With the advent of correct nutritional supplementation of taurine, DCM has become a relatively rare diagnosis in cats. There are still occasional cases seen, and taurine supplementation should be tried. Treatment focuses on relieving signs of CHF with diuretics and possibly ACE inhibitors. Arrhythmias occur frequently and may need to be addressed. With supraventricular tachycardias, digoxin becomes an attractive therapeutic option.

HISTORY AND GENERAL CLINICAL FINDINGS

History and clinical findings usually are not useful in differentiating among the various forms of cardiomyopathy, because they tend to be similar. Clinical manifestations, when present, are for the most part a reflection of heart failure, arrhythmias, or conduction abnormalities or a result of thromboembolism. In these situations presentation tends to be peracute and severe. Physical examination may raise the possibility of secondary cardiomyopathy by revealing a thyroid nodule (thyrotoxic cardiomyopathy), small kidneys (hypertensive cardiomyopathy), or retinal degeneration (taurine deficiency dilated cardiomyopathy).

The natural progression of these various heart muscle diseases is variable so that it is possible for cats to remain asymptomatic for prolonged periods of time. Many times heart disease is detected on routine physical examination without overt clinical signs having been noted. It is rare for cats to have a slowly progressive course as is seen with most dogs with CHF. It is also rare for cats to cough with cardiomyopathy, even when they have significant cardiomegaly or pulmonary edema. Sudden death can occur in some cases without prior signs of cardiac disease. In some instances owners detect decreased exercise tolerance and a tendency for a cat to breathe through an open mouth after minor exercise prior to development of CHF.

CARDIOVASCULAR EXAMINATION

Cardiovascular examination can reveal the presence of heart disease, although it, too, can rarely differentiate among the various forms of cardiomyopathy. Examination of the patient should begin with careful inspection of the cat at rest. Abnormal breathing patterns involving both respiratory rate and respiratory character may be present. The area of the jugular vein should be examined for evidence of distension or a jugular pulse. The neck should be palpated as well for the presence of a thyroid nodule. The femoral pulses should be palpated, and in most cases they should be fairly normal. With arrhythmias, of course, pulse deficits may occur. With low output heart failure and especially with DCM, pulses may be weak. If a thrombus is present, pulses to one or both rear legs are absent. In addition, the paw pads are pale or cyanotic. As previously mentioned, cats rarely cough or have ascites in association with cardiomyopathy.

The most important part of the cardiovascular examination is auscultation. Findings will depend heavily on whether or not heart failure is present. Without heart failure, at least a heart murmur should be present, usually with the point of maximal intensity near the left parasternal region. The murmur can be of variable intensity; it will be loudest when the cat is excited. This is typical for hypertrophic obstructive cardiomyopathy. Gallop rhythms are not uncommon with cardiomyopathy. They are a result of abnormal systolic filling such as occurs with DCM or atrial contraction in association with a stiff ventricle.

With heart failure, auscultation can reveal crackles with pulmonary edema, although this is the case less commonly in cats than in dogs. Even with severe dyspnea as a result of pulmonary edema, at times it can be difficult to auscult the sounds typically thought to be present with edema. Muffling of heart sounds in cats is almost always a result of pleural effusion. In dogs one would need to consider pericardial effusion, as well; in cats, however, most cases of pericardial effusion are also secondary to cardiomyopathy.

Diagnostic Testing

Electrocardiography. Electrocardiography can be helpful in the evaluation of a cat with suspected cardiac disease. The main findings that can point toward a cardiomyopathy are enlargement patterns on the ECG, conduction disturbances, and the identification of arrhythmias. As with most diagnostic tests routinely available, it generally is not possible to differentiate the various forms of cardiomyopathy based on the ECG.

Enlargement patterns in cats are mainly composed of two ECG changes. An R-wave that exceeds 0.9 μV suggests heart enlargement (Figure 10-14). Less commonly a prolongation of the QRS interval will be seen (>0.045 seconds). A cranial axis deviation pattern is also typical for cardiomyopathy. This is reflected in a positive R-wave in lead I and deep S-waves in leads II, III, and aVF. This may be an indicator of a left anterior fascicular block or may merely reflect a left ventricular enlargement pattern. If lead I is negative (deep S wave), along with leads II, III, and aVF, then this can be a sign of right ventricular enlargement, and heartworm disease needs to be considered.

A variety of conduction disturbances can be seen with cardiomyopathy. One of the more common is third-degree AV block. This may be caused by the pronounced thickening of the intraventricular septum in which the AV node resides. This must be suspected whenever a cat has a heart rate that is very slow (<120 beats per minute) and needs to be confirmed with an ECG. Generally cats do not show the signs typically shown by dogs with third-degree AV block, such as syncope or episodic weakness. This is because the intrinsic heart rate of the ventricle in cats is high enough to take over for the normal sinus rhythm and allow the cat to function without clinical signs even with this advanced conduction problem. Third-degree AV block will also be seen commonly in older cats as a result of fibrosis of the AV node.

Many arrhythmias can occur with cardiomyopathy. The most common by far are VPCs. Paroxysmal or sustained ventricular tachycardias are rarely seen. Supraventricular arrhythmias do occur, but are more rare. Atrial fibrillation will be seen and is associated with a poor prognosis. Atrial fibrillation usually develops only with massive left atrial enlargement. This tachycardia further compromises ventricular filling and also seems to be associated with a higher risk for thromboembolic disease.

Radiography. Radiography can be helpful in detecting evidence of heart enlargement and heart failure. It can also help to identify whether a cat is in respiratory distress because of heart disease or because of respiratory disease. Unfortunately, radiography cannot be used to differentiate the various forms of cardiomyopathy. Radiography is also not helpful in detecting the early forms of cardiomyopathy before significant cardiomegaly has occurred.

It is important to take the condition of the patient into consideration before obtaining radiographs. If the patient is markedly stressed and dyspneic, it may be advisable to allow the patient to stabilize first. The stress of restraint for radiographs can be too much for a cat that is in distress. It may be advisable to first place the cat in an oxygen-enriched environment (incubators for babies are ideal for this purpose in cats). The administration of a diuretic (furosemide intramuscularly) and a bronchodilator (aminophylline) should also be considered in these emergency cases before it is possible to differentiate whether the breathing problems are respiratory or cardiac in origin.

Radiographic findings are variable. Cardiomegaly may be detected. This can be localized or

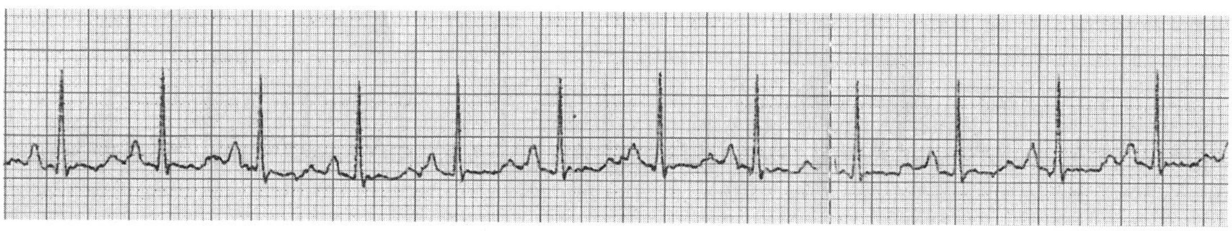

Figure 10-14. Electrocardiogram from a cat with hypertrophic cardiomyopathy. Normal R-wave amplitude should not exceed 0.9 μV (9 small boxes on the ECG grid). In this case, amplitude is 1.2 μV.

generalized. With left ventricular and left atrial enlargement the apex of the heart may shift off the midline to the right on ventrodorsal radiographs. This can result in the "valentine-shaped" heart that is seen with advanced cardiomyopathy (Figure 10-15). It is important to consider the body condition of the patient when assessing the heart for enlargement. Obese cats will have a large sternal fat pad that can overlap the heart on ventrodorsal radiographs, suggesting the presence of cardiomegaly. In some cats a tortuous aorta will be found, which some clinicians equate with hypertension, although this has not been proved. With DCM the heart tends to be extremely large, with biventricular and biatrial enlargement.

Heart failure can be reflected in a variety of ways on radiographs. Pulmonary edema in cats tends to be patchy in distribution. With dilated or restrictive cardiomyopathy a combination of pulmonary edema and pleural effusion is often seen. The pleural effusion can be severe enough that the heart silhouette cannot be seen. In these cases, thoracocentesis should be performed and radiographs repeated. This allows clearer visualization of the heart and cranial mediastinal region. It is important to view the cranial mediastinal region, because one of the other major causes of pleural effusion in cats is a cranial mediastinal mass such as lymphoma. Pericardial effusion also can occur with pericardial disease (pericarditis or tumor) as well as most commonly with heart failure secondary to cardiomyopathy. On radiographs, pericardial effusion is manifested as a large heart with very clear borders.

Echocardiography. Echocardiography must be considered a vital diagnostic test with cardiomyopathy. It allows differentiation of the various forms of cardiomyopathy through assessment of ventricular dimensions as well as contractility. The two-dimensional views taken can also document the presence of left ventricular outflow tract obstruction. Echocardiography can also reveal the presence of early or advanced heart failure by revealing the presence of atrial enlargement.

Advanced cardiac hypertrophy is easy to document on echocardiography. Septal or left ventricular free-wall measurements of greater than 5 mm in diastole are consistent with left ventricular hypertrophy. With hypertrophic cardiomyopathy, reduction of the size of the left ventricular lumen will be seen. Contractility will be normal or increased in most instances. The differential diagnoses for these findings include primary hypertrophic cardiomyopathy as well as hypertension and hyperthyroid heart disease. When hypertrophy is detected on an echocardiogram, a blood profile that includes thyroid testing is indicated. Because hypertension is almost always secondary to either hyperthyroid-

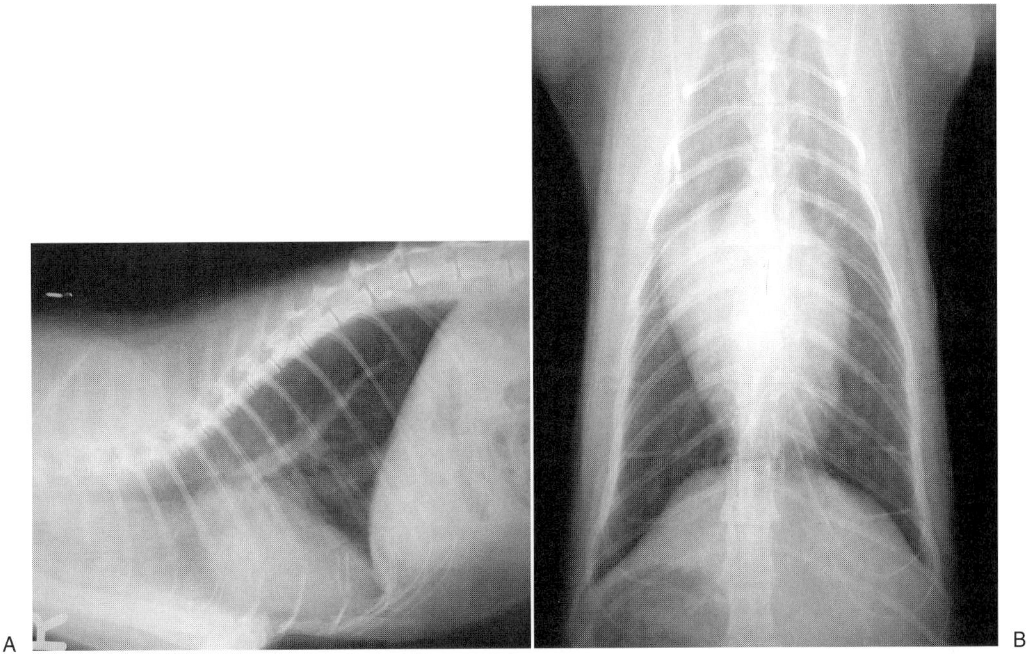

Figure 10-15. Marked cardiomegaly in a cat with hypertrophic cardiomyopathy. On the ventrodorsal radiograph ***(B)*** the valentine shape is easy to see.

ism or chronic renal failure in cats, the blood work will allow identification of risk factors for hypertension. Ideally, blood pressure should be measured using either Doppler or oscillometric technology.

Echocardiography also allows the diagnosis of HOCM as well as systolic anterior motion of the mitral valve. Assessment of the left atrium is vital. Left atrial enlargement is indicative of beginning congestion and can be a precursor to heart failure. In addition, thrombi can occasionally be seen in the left atrium and are a reason for great concern. Occasionally a swirling effect termed "smoke" can be seen in the left atrium. This is thought to be a sign of pooling of blood in the left atrium and may also be a marker of impending thromboembolism.

DCM is also relatively easy to diagnose with echocardiography. The disease tends to involve both the right and left ventricles. Both ventricles tend to be dilated with very poor contractility and thinning of the ventricular walls (Figure 10-16). Biatrial enlargement is commonly found, as is pleural effusion and sometimes pericardial effusion (Figure 10-17).

The more difficult diagnoses to make are restrictive and intermediate cardiomyopathy. These tend to have a combination of findings that are not consistent with the diagnosis of hypertrophic cardiomyopathy or DCM but are associated with significant atrial enlargement. Often the wall thicknesses of the left ventricle are near normal, or only mild thickening is present. The ventricular lumen tends to be mildly dilated. Contractility tends to be in the normal range. With restrictive cardiomyopathy, contractility can be quite reduced, and the endomyocardium can be quite bright on echocardiography. It is quite possible that these forms of cardiomyopathy represent a spectrum of changes so that they often do have features of both dilated and hypertrophic cardiomyopathy.

Treatment

Treatment should attempt to control the signs of clinical heart disease as well as, it is hoped, prolong the life of the patient. It is uncertain whether any of the treatments currently available prolong life. It is also uncertain whether asymptomatic patients benefit from early intervention with medications. Controlling the signs of heart disease does tend to be possible with a wide

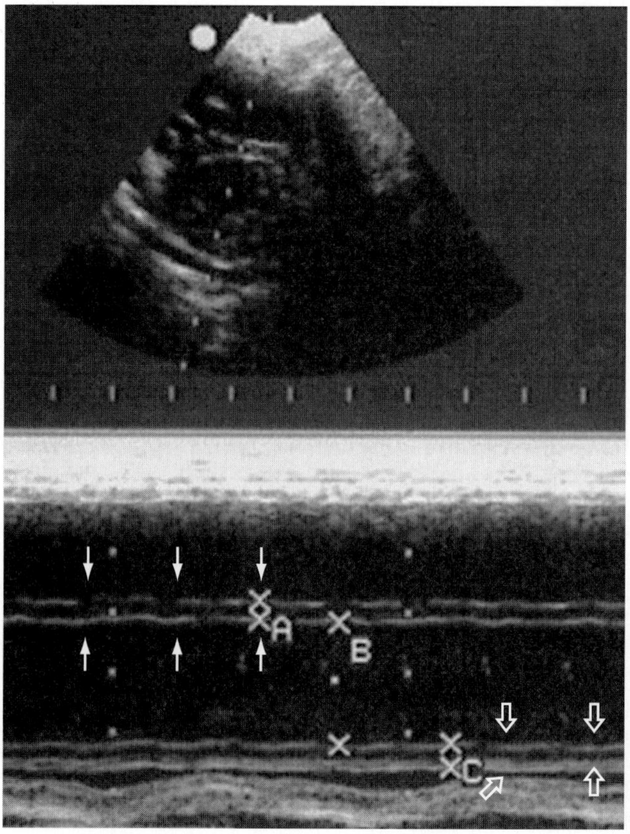

Figure 10-16. M-mode short axis of the ventricles of a cat with dilated cardiomyopathy. Wall motion of both the septum *(closed arrows)* and the left ventricular free wall *(open arrows)* is virtually nonexistent. The lumen of the left ventricle is markedly increased; a small amount of pericardial effusion is present.

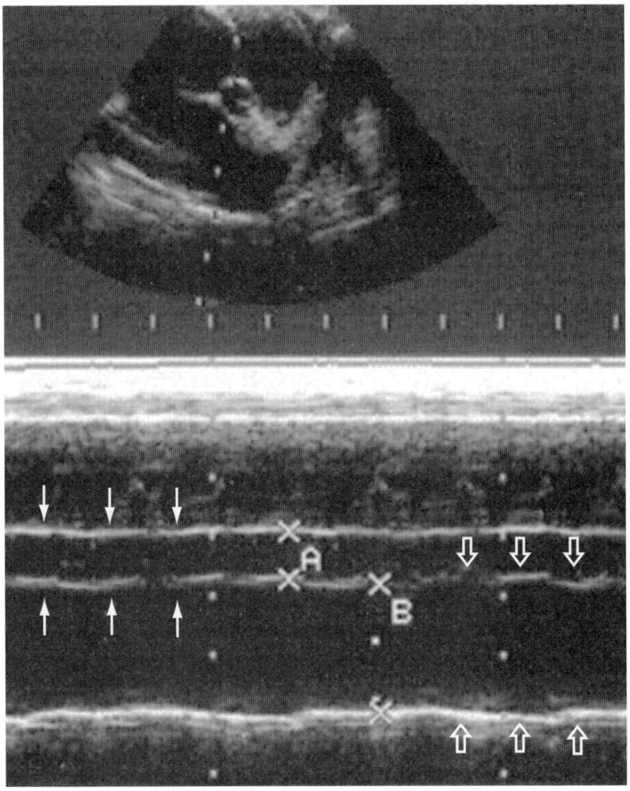

Figure 10-17. M-mode short axis of the atria *(closed arrows)* and aorta *(open arrows)*. The atrium and aorta should be roughly equal in diameter. In this case massive atrial enlargement is present.

variety of medications. Treatment for cardiomyopathy varies depending on the type of cardiac muscle disease present, at least with regard to maintenance therapies.

Acute Heart Failure. The treatment for acute heart failure tends to be independent of the form of cardiomyopathy present. Affected cats are often presented in severe respiratory distress and can very easily decompensate. Initial management focuses on managing dyspnea, which can result from pleural effusion, pulmonary edema, or a combination of the two. Minimizing stress in these patients is vital, and often too much early intervention by the veterinarian can have a negative effect on the patient's condition. Initially placing the patient in an oxygen cage is recommended to allow the animal to calm down from the trip to the veterinary office as well as to improve oxygenation. Oxygen cages also have the advantage that they tend to muffle typical upsetting noises found in a veterinary practice (e.g., barking dogs). If significant pleural effusion is present, thoracocentesis should be considered. Because these animals tend to be in very poor condition, it often is possible to perform this without sedation or local anesthetics.

Medications can often be started immediately on presentation. Furosemide (2 to 4 mg/kg) can be given. It should be administered either intramuscularly or intravenously, although the benefits of intravenous administration (more rapid onset of action) must be weighed against the risk associated with the restraint necessary to place an intravenous catheter. Nitroglycerin ointment (2%) can also be administered and is appropriate for emergency care. In most cats 1/4 inch of ointment is applied to an area with minimal hair (e.g., inside of an ear, inner thigh) every 6 to 8 hours. After 48 hours it is thought that patients become refractory to the effects of the ointment. The ointment should not contact the bare skin of people, as it will be absorbed (a glove should be worn when applying nitroglycerin ointment). Nitroglycerin ointment also has the advantage of having some antithrombotic effects, which can be helpful in cats with cardiomyopathy.

In cats it can at times be difficult to tell the difference between a patient suffering from acute heart failure and one suffering from an acute asthma attack. In those cases in which the two cannot be differentiated and in which it is considered too risky to the patient to take radiographs right away, use of furosemide, nitroglycerin, *and* medications for asthma should be considered. For asthma, treatment with injectable aminophylline (4 mg/kg intramuscularly) is usually adequate. Corticosteroids such as dexamethasone (0.25 to 1 mg/kg intramuscularly) are also commonly used to treat asthma; recent evidence, however, suggests that this could be deleterious to the heart in cats. The cat is placed in a cage (preferably with supplemental oxygen) to rest. *After* the cat's condition has stabilized, it is possible to perform diagnostic tests (radiographs, ECG, echocardiogram) as needed to establish a definitive diagnosis.

Chronic Therapy. Chronic therapy is directed at controlling signs of heart failure and ideally to slowing down progression of the disease. Therapy for heart failure is relatively the same, independent of the form of cardiomyopathy present. The therapies directed at slowing progression can vary among the various forms of cardiomyopathy.

Diuretics. Diuretics are needed to control the signs of congestion that occur with cardiomyopathy. The most commonly used diuretic is furosemide (1 to 2 mg/kg once to twice daily). Usually in cats a dose of 2 mg/kg twice daily should not be exceeded, as dehydration can easily occur. In addition, furosemide can lead to potassium depletion, so electrolyte and kidney values should be checked routinely. In those cases in which furosemide alone (with or without addition of an ACE inhibitor) cannot control congestion, the addition of a second diuretic should be considered. Consideration can be given to using spironolactone or spironolactone-chlorthiazide combinations. The dose is usually 1 to 2 mg/kg once or twice daily. These are potassium-sparing diuretics. They are probably not as potent as furosemide, but recent studies in humans suggest that this group of diuretics may extend life span in people with CHF. Diuretics are titrated to effect, that is, until signs of CHF are controlled.

ACE Inhibitors. ACE inhibitors have an important function in the treatment of heart failure. They are among the few medications that have been shown to prolong the lives of dogs and people with CHF. Their use in dilated, restrictive, and intermediate cardiomyopathy is usually not challenged. In hypertrophic cardiomyopathy there are theoretical drawbacks to use of ACE inhibitors. ACE inhibitors should be arterial and venous dilators. With the arterial dilation, pressure downstream from the heart should be reduced. In hypertrophic cardiomyopathy, especially if HOCM is present, this effect could worsen the prolapse of the mitral valve (less pressure downstream counteracts the tendency of the mitral valve to move into the outflow tract). However, a positive effect has been shown when ACE inhibitors have been used in cats with hypertrophic cardiomyopathy and refractory heart failure.[13,14] The dosage recommended is 0.25 to 0.5 mg/kg of enalapril or benazapril daily. Renal function should be monitored when these medications are used. Generally the blood urea nitrogen, creatinine, and potassium values should be checked 3 to 5 days after a patient starts receiving an ACE inhibitor and again 10 to 14 days later to make sure that azotemia has not occurred.

Beta-Blockers. Beta-blockers play an important role in the management of cardiomyopathies, especially hypertrophic cardiomyopathy and HOCM. Their role in DCM, restrictive cardiomyopathy, and intermediate cardiomyopathy is usually limited to control of arrhythmias, specifically supraventricular tachycardias (atrial fibrillation, atrial tachycardia, frequent atrial premature contractions) and ventricular tachycardia. In hypertrophic cardiomyopathy, beta-blockers slow the heart rate, which prolongs diastole, an important goal in management of this disease. This increases coronary blood flow and thereby reduces ischemia. Oxygen requirements are also reduced by reducing heart rate, contractility, systolic myocardial wall stress, and a variety of other factors. The arrhythmia control that is achieved also may prolong life (documented in humans), which is rare among antiarrhythmic drugs. In HOCM, beta-blockers reduce dynamic outflow tract obstruction. The predominant adverse side effect of these drugs is a result of decreased cardiac output, that is, exacerbation of heart failure or hypotension. This is less of a concern with hypertrophic cardiomyopathy, but needs to be considered in patients with other forms of cardiomyopathy. Using a low dose initially and then gradually increasing it is the preferred way to use this group of medications. Abrupt discontinuation should be avoided. Commonly used agents in veterinary medicine include atenolol (6.25 to 12.5 mg once to twice daily) and propranolol (5 to 10 mg two to three times daily). Atenolol is a selective β_2-blocker, which may decrease the likelihood of bronchoconstriction, as could in theory occur with nonselective beta-blocker therapy.

Calcium-Channel Blockers. The use of calcium-channel blockers is usually reserved for hypertrophic cardiomyopathy. In other forms of cardiomyopathy it is used as an antiarrhythmic drug, whereby it is most effective in managing supraventricular tachycardias (atrial fibrillation, atrial tachycardia). Calcium-channel blockers work to decrease heart rate, improve diastolic filling, and mildly decrease cardiac output (which decreases myocardial oxygen consumption). These are all positive effects in hypertrophic cardiomyopathy. A variety of preparations is available. Regular diltiazem (1 mg/kg three times daily) can be used but must be given frequently. Sustained-release products such as Dilacor XR (30 to 60 mg once daily in cats) or Cardizem CD (10 mg/kg once daily) are easier to use in cats because they need to be given less frequently.

Taurine. With the discovery of taurine deficiency as a cause of DCM, cat foods were altered to provide greater levels of taurine. Because of this, it is rare to see taurine deficiency DCM in clinical practice today. It still is advisable to try this supplement in cats that are diagnosed with DCM, because if it is taurine deficiency related, a cure for the cardiomyopathy can occur. Blood levels can be determined, but in most cases it is easier and often cheaper to try supplementation rather than running tests on taurine levels. The usual dosage is 250 to 500 mg twice daily. If this is the cause of DCM there will be marked improvement in 4 to 6 weeks.

Digoxin. Digoxin is used in some cases of dilated and restrictive cardiomyopathy (if right-sided heart failure is present). Unfortunately, toxicity with this drug is common and is especially pronounced if renal dysfunction or hypokalemia are present. It should not be used in cats that are anorectic or dehydrated. Dosage recommendations are as follows: cats weighing 2 to 4 kg receive 1/4 of a 0.125-mg tablet every 2 days; cats weighing 4 to 6 kg receive 1/4 of 0.125-mg tablet every 24 to 48 hours; and cats weighing >6 kg receive 1/4 of a 0.125-mg tablet every 24 hours, occasionally every 12 hours. It is best to use the lower dosages initially and recheck blood digoxin levels in 10 days (best at 8 hours after pill administration). Monitoring for signs of toxicity is vital. Any signs of anorexia or gastrointestinal problems warrant discontinuation of the drug and evaluating for toxicity by repeating a digoxin level determination.

Thromboembolism

Thromboembolism is a manifestation of cardiomyopathies that is of special interest in that it is associated with severe clinical signs as well as a very poor long-term prognosis.[15] In many cases the blood clot is the first clinical manifestation of heart disease. The signs are peracute and severe, with pain resulting in vocalization. Often the stress of the thrombus leads to decompensation and signs of CHF as well. Usually both rear limbs are affected. With large thrombi to the rear legs, the kidneys can also become involved, leading to acute renal failure. Rarely, a thrombus will lodge in a front leg or other organ (e.g., brain) (Figure 10-18).

A variety of factors predispose to the formation of thrombi in association with cardiomyopathy. In the area of the dilated atria, blood flow is severely decreased. This pooling of blood may allow clotting to be enhanced. In addition, the endomyocardial lining is often damaged in cats with cardiomyopathy, which is another factor that predisposes to formation of thrombi. Thrombi may be more common with restrictive cardiomyopathy. It is important to remember that thromboembolism in cats is taking place in a high flow situation, which is in the arterial system, and therefore platelet activation is the major factor in thrombus formation. This is unlike the situation with humans, where most thrombi are a result of deep vein thrombosis, in which activation of coagulation is the major component. This has important clinical implications with regard to therapy and prevention of thrombi in cats, and it helps explain why long-term prognosis is so poor with thromboembolism.

Prevention and treatment of thromboembolism in cats is frustrating. Aspirin therapy (81 mg every 3 to 4 days) has been recommended, but aspirin is not a very powerful platelet inhibitor. Warfarin has also been used in cats that are at high risk for thrombosis. Unfortunately, the drug is difficult to work with and frequent monitoring is indicated. The fact that the thrombosis that occurs in cats is an arterial clot makes warfarin less likely to be

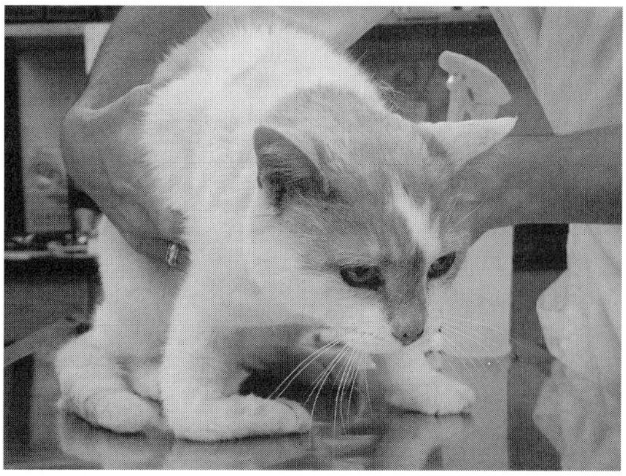

Figure 10-18. A cat with thrombosis of the right forelimb secondary to restrictive cardiomyopathy.

effective, because it is an anticoagulant that is more important in the prevention of venous thrombosis (for which it is commonly used in human patients).

Once a thrombus has developed, various treatments can be considered. Aspirin can be used if the cat is not already on this medication. Heparin has been recommended (200 units/kg intravenous loading dose, followed by 100 units/kg subcutaneously three times a day), although it is most effective in the management of venous thrombosis. This can lead to excessive bleeding. Lower dosages (75 to 100 units/kg subcutaneously three times a day) may have antithrombotic effects without being anticoagulatory. Monitoring of activated partial thromboplastin time levels is necessary to tailor heparin therapy. Clot lysis has been tried with streptokinase and tissue plasminogen activator, but this is an expensive therapy, and indications are that survival rates are no better than with more conservative management. Pain relief needs to be a part of the treatment protocol during the first 24 hours after the clot has formed, as it is a very painful process. Butorphanol (0.2 to 0.4 mg/kg intravenously, intramuscularly, or subcutaneously three to four times daily) is a good choice for analgesia. Use of phenothiazines (acepromazine, chlorpromazine) can be considered. These may establish collateral blood supply and help to sedate anxious cats. In addition, these medications also have desirable effects on platelets. It is important to not overly sedate animals with these medications, especially when an analgesic such as butorphanol is also being used.

Prognosis

Prognosis with cardiomyopathy is variable. It is possible for cats to have evidence of hypertrophic cardiomyopathy and yet remain free of signs for years. Once clinical signs develop, however, prognosis is generally poor. Although few studies have been done, one did look at survival. In those cats without clinical signs, survival was over 400 days; with those presented with CHF signs it was approximately 6 months; and in those with thromboembolism it was 2 months.[16]

HYPERTENSION

Measuring blood pressure is a valuable technique in veterinary practice. It is important to understand the various factors that can affect any reading obtained from a patient. In dogs, breed plays an important role in determining what the normal blood pressure range is. Sighthounds are known to have higher pressures than other breeds.[17] In both dogs and cats, blood pressure tends to increase with age. Blood pressure is also susceptible to stress-related changes, and it is therefore important to obtain readings in a manner that minimizes stress for the patient. There are a variety of ways in which blood pressure can be measured. It is important to realize that a reference range that is established for one device is often not directly transferable to a different blood pressure monitor. With appropriate blood pressure measurement protocols in place and sufficient experience it is possible to get diagnostically accurate readings.

Hypertension is a sustained elevated blood pressure. Some argument exists regarding what constitutes an elevated blood pressure, as well as when antihypertensive therapy should be initiated. If there are signs of end-organ damage such as retinal hemorrhage, then blood pressure that is considered indicative for hypertensive therapy will be lower than if no end-organ damage is present. Also, underlying kidney disease might constitute grounds for a more aggressive approach to therapy, because hypertension can exacerbate renal failure.[18] When evaluating blood pressure it is ideal to have both systolic and diastolic values in order to best assess blood pressure status. In general, a value above 160/95 mm Hg (either or both) needs to be considered elevated. Any decision to treat a patient without obvious end-organ damage should be based on repeated consistently elevated pressure readings, not a single measurement session. Readings can be repeated multiple times in 1 day or can be repeated over several days to see if pressure elevations are consistently recorded. If systolic pressure is above 200 mm Hg or diastolic above 120 mm Hg on repeated measurements, then antihypertensive therapy generally should be administered even if end-organ damage is not detected. The level of hypertension that can be tolerated in a patient heavily depends on what concurrent illnesses are present. Patients with underlying renal or cardiac disease will be less able to tolerate sustained elevations in blood pressure.

Most cases of hypertension are secondary to some other disease process. Primary hypertension, although the most common form of high blood pressure in humans, is rare in pets. Evidence supports the association between hypertension and hyperthyroidism in cats,[19] renal disease in dogs and cats,[20] HAC in dogs,[21] as well as other

TABLE 10-2. MEDICATIONS TO TREAT HYPERTENSION

DRUG	INDICATIONS	DOSE
Amlodipine	First-choice agent in cats with hypertension, especially secondary to renal disease	Cats: 0.625-1.25 mg/day Dogs: 0.05-0.1 mg/kg/day
Enalapril	Good choice if hypertension is a result of protein-losing kidney disease; often add-on drug	Cats: 0.25 -0.5 mg/kg once or twice daily Dogs: 0.5 mg/kg once or twice daily
Benazapril	Similar to enalapril in effects	Cats and dogs: 0.25-0.5 mg/kg daily
Ramipril	ACE inhibitor, potentially more marked reduction in blood pressure than other ACE inhibitors	Dogs: 0.125 mg/kg sid initially, can be increased to 0.25 mg sid if necessary Cats: 0.125 mg/kg sid
Atenolol	Good agent if hyperthyroidism is present, otherwise generally an add-on drug	Cats: 6.25 -12.5 mg twice daily Dogs: 0.25-1 mg/kg twice daily
Hydralazine	Need to monitor closely for hypotension; start low and titrate until effective; not an initial drug of choice	Dogs: 0.5 mg/kg bid, can gradually increase to 2 mg/kg bid if necessary Cats: 2.5 mg initially once daily, can be increased to bid if necessary
Nitroprusside	Only feasible if continuous blood pressure measurement is possible; severe hypotension can occur	1.5 μg/kg/min IV
Acepromazine	Use with caution, monitor blood pressure	0.05-0.1 mg/kg IV

ACE, Angiotensin-converting enzyme; *IV*, intravenous.

diseases. Prevalence of high blood pressure in these disease states can be quite high, exceeding 50% in some studies. Hypertension will resolve in the majority of patients with treatable disease conditions such as hyperthyroidism or HAC, but in some instances this will not be the case. Hypertension can cause end-organ damage such as retinal detachments and CNS hemorrhages. It also places excessive strain on the heart (increases afterload), leading to ventricular hypertrophy and on occasion heart failure. Of great concern in patients with renal disease is that hypertension leads to progressive renal injury. It has been shown that animals with renal disease have an impaired ability to autoregulate blood flow to the kidney, which normally would prevent excessive systemic arterial pressure from being passed on to the glomerulus.[22] Increased pressure in the glomerulus leads to injury that can lead to eventual loss of function.

When treating hypertension it is important to decide how rapidly blood pressure needs to be decreased and to what level. An animal that has been hypertensive for a prolonged period of time, especially with underlying renal disease, can have adverse effects from too aggressive an approach. With neurologic manifestations or retinal detachments a more rapid approach is warranted to prevent further end-organ damage. There are a wide variety of agents available to decrease blood pressure (Table 10-2). In most instances oral medications can be used and dosages adjusted upward to effect. In cats, amlodipine has proved to be the best agent for controlling hypertension. ACE inhibitors generally have a minor effect on blood pressure in cats when used at normal dosages. Beta-blockers can also be used, especially in those instances in which hyperthyroidism is present. In dogs, ACE inhibitors are most often the initial medication used because they seem to be more effective at decreasing blood pressure in this species. This is especially true if there is glomerular disease, as ACE inhibitors also tend to decrease proteinuria, independent of the effect on blood pressure. Additional agents such as amlodipine or a beta-blocker can be used if needed. In refractory cases, hydralazine can be of benefit as well, although careful dose titration is required.

References

1. Mallery KF, Freeman LM, Harpster NK, Rush JK: Factors contributing to the decision for euthanasia of dogs with congestive heart failure, *J Am Vet Med Assoc* 214:1201, 1999.
2. COVE Study Group: Controlled clinical evaluation of enalapril in dogs with heart failure: results of the cooperative veterinary enalapril study group, *J Vet Intern Med* 9:243, 1995.
3. Hamlin RL, Benitz AM, Ericsson GF et al: Effects of enalapril on exercise tolerance and longevity in dogs with heart failure produced by iatrogenic mitral regurgitation, *J Vet Intern Med* 10:85, 1996.
4. Ettinger SJ, Benitz AM, Ericsson GF et al: Effects of enalapril maleate on survival in dogs with naturally acquired heart failure, *J Am Vet Med Assoc* 213:1573, 1998.
5. BENCH Study Group: The effect of benazapril on survival times and clinical signs of congestive heart failure: results of a multicenter, prospective, randomized, double-blinded, placebo-controlled, long-term clinical trial, *J Vet Cardiol* 1:7, 1999.

6. Kvart C, Häggström J, Pedersen HD: Efficacy of enalapril for prevention of congestive heart failure in dogs with myxomatous valve disease and asymptomatic mitral regurgitation, *J Vet Intern Med* 16:80, 2002.
7. O'Grady MR, Home R, Gordon SG: Does angiotensin converting enzyme inhibitor therapy delay the onset of congestive heart failure or sudden death in Doberman Pinschers with occult dilated cardiomyopathy? *J Vet Intern Med* 11:138, 1997. (Abstract presented at the 1997 ACVIM Forum, Orlando, Fla.)
8. Freeman LM, Rush JE, Kehayias JJ et al: Nutritional alterations and the effect of fish oil supplementation in dogs with heart failure, *J Vet Intern Med* 12:440, 1998.
9. Sisson D, Thomas WP: Endocarditis of the aortic valve in the dog, *J Am Vet Med Assoc* 184:570, 1984.
10. Breitschwerdt EB, Atkins CD, Brown TT et al: *Bartonella vinsonii* subsp. *berkhoffi* and related members of the alpha subdivision of the Proteobacteria in dogs with cardiac arrhythmias, endocarditis, or myocarditis, *J Clin Microbiol* 37:3618, 1999.
11. Sisson D, Thomas WP: Pericardial disease and cardiac tumors. In Fox PR, Sisson D, Moise NS, eds: *Textbook of canine and feline cardiology,* ed 2, Philadelphia, 1999, WB Saunders.
12. Fox PR: Feline cardiomyopathies. In Fox PR, Sisson D, Moise NS, eds: *Textbook of canine and feline cardiology,* ed 2, Philadelphia, 1999, WB Saunders.
13. Rush JE, Freeman LM, Brown DJ et al: The use of enalapril in the treatment of feline hypertrophic cardiomyopathy, *J Am Anim Hosp Assoc* 34:38, 1998.
14. Amberger CN, Glardon O et al: Effects of benazapril in the treatment of feline hypertrophic cardiomyopathy: results of a prospective, open-label multicenter clinical trial, *J Vet Cardiol* 1:19, 1999.
15. Laste JN, Harpster NK: A retrospective study of 100 cases of feline distal aortic thromboembolism: 1977-1993, *J Am Anim Hosp Assoc* 31:492, 1995.
16. Atkins CE, Gallo AM, Kurzman ID, Cowen P: Risk factors, clinical signs, and survival in cats with a clinical diagnosis of idiopathic hypertrophic cardiomyopathy: 74 cases (1985-1989), *J Am Vet Med Assoc* 201:613, 1992.
17. Bodey AR, Michell AR: Epidemiologic study of blood pressure in domestic dogs, *J Small Anim Pract* 37:116-125, 1996.
18. Jacob F, Polzin DJ, Osborne CA et al: Association between initial systolic blood pressure and risk of developing a uremic crisis or of dying in dogs with chronic renal failure, *J Am Vet Med Assoc* 222:322, 2003.
19. Kobayashi DL, Peterson ME, Graves TK et al: Hypertension in cats with chronic renal failure or hyperthyroidism, *J Vet Intern Med* 4:58, 1990.
20. Bartges JW et al: Hypertension and renal disease, *Vet Clin North Am* 26:1331, 1996.
21. Ortega TM, Feldman EC, Nelson RW et al: Systemic arterial blood pressure and urine protein/creatinine ratio in dogs with hyperadrenocorticism, *J Am Vet Med Assoc* 209:1724, 1996.
22. Brown SA, Finco DR, Navar LG et al: Impaired renal autoregulatory ability in dogs with reduced renal mass, *J Am Soc Nephrol* 5:1768, 1995.

CHAPTER 11

The Oral Cavity and Dental Disease

JOHNNY D. HOSKINS

Oral pain, general malaise, and lack of activity are common signs noted in dogs and cats with advanced dental disease. The impact that severe dental disease has on a particular animal may not be evident until improvement is observed following treatment. Many owners are unaware that severe dental disease may cause systemic signs and attribute changes in their dog or cat to "old age" rather than to the dental disease.

THE EXAMINATION

When clinical signs suggest disease of the oral cavity, a complete examination of the oral cavity should be performed. Such signs include halitosis, changes in eating patterns, behavioral changes (e.g., reclusiveness or aggression), ptyalism, blood-tinged saliva, rubbing the face, nasal discharge, sneezing, facial swelling, and draining tracts.[1] Physical examination of the oral cavity should include evaluation of the lips, vestibule of the mouth, dentition, attached gingiva, hard and soft palate, tonsils, sublingual tissue, and tongue. External palpation of the mandible, maxilla, and local lymph nodes should also be included. The lips are retracted while the mouth is held closed to allow inspection of the labial and buccal tooth surfaces and to identify the occlusal pattern (Figure 11-1). A gloved finger can be used to examine the vestibule of the mouth (Figure 11-2). The mouth is then opened and the palatal and lingual aspects of the teeth are examined, followed by examination of the hard and soft palate, tongue, sublingual tissues, and tonsils. To examine cats, raise the animal's head vertically with one hand while holding the zygomatic arches and open the cat's mouth by pressing the mandible ventrally with a finger from the other hand (Figure 11-3). To examine the area under a cat's tongue, place a finger between the rami of the mandible and push dorsally (Figure 11-4).

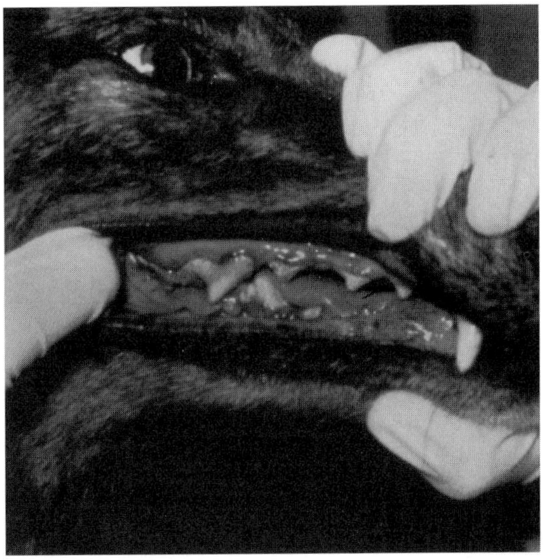

Figure 11-1. Retraction of the lips to allow for examination of the labial and buccal tooth surfaces.

PERIODONTITIS

Clinical Features

Plaque, bacterial by-products, and the resulting inflammatory response lead to periodontal disease.

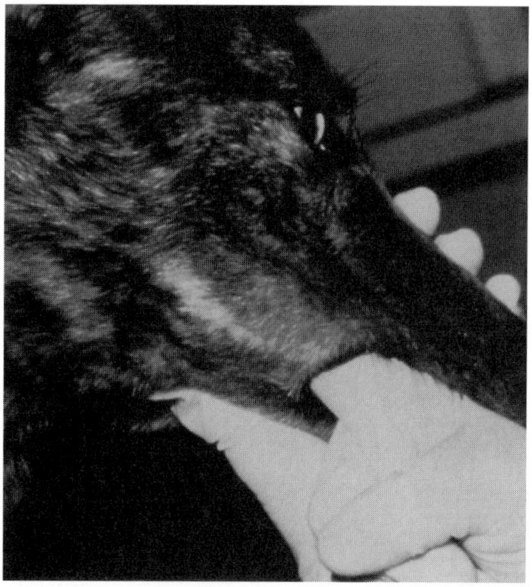

Figure 11-2. Examination of the vestibule of the mouth.

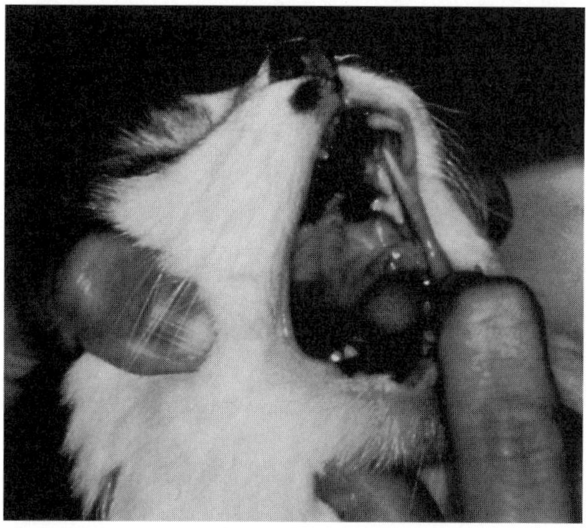

Figure 11-3. Examination of the cat's oral cavity.

The initial bacterial population is predominantly gram-positive in gingivitis, with gram-negative bacteria and spirochetes increasing as disease progresses to periodontitis.[2] Plaque tends to accumulate more readily on teeth that are crowded or have roughened surfaces (e.g., enamel hypoplasia or fractures). Diet may play a role, with soft, nonabrasive diets resulting in plaque buildup more rapidly than more abrasive diets.

The earliest stage of periodontal disease occurs when dental plaque accumulates on the tooth crown adjacent to the gingival margin. If supragingival plaque is not removed, it will progress subgingivally and result in gingival inflammation

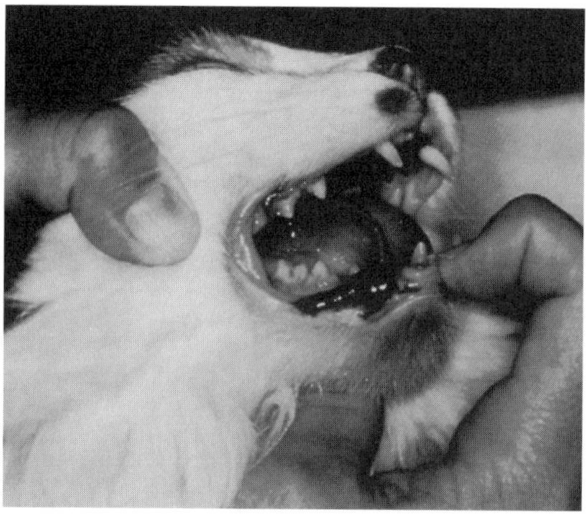

Figure 11-4. Examination of the sublingual area in a cat.

and progress beyond marginal gingivitis. Subgingival plaque and the associated inflammatory response may eventually lead to a breakdown of the epithelial attachment to the tooth, resulting in beginning pocket formation and periodontitis (loss of connective tissue and bone attachment).[3] Continued loss of tooth attachment results in advanced periodontitis, increased tooth mobility, and eventual tooth loss.

Normal gingival tissue is light pink in color with a sharp edge to the gingival margin. The gingival margin is closely opposed to the tooth crown. Gingival sulcus depth in dogs is normally 3 mm or less. Signs of periodontal disease vary and depend on the extent of disease that is present. Marginal gingivitis is the initial stage, with erythema of only the marginal gingiva. Established gingivitis is identified clinically by a rounding of the marginal gingival tissue from edema, erythema of the attached gingiva, and increased tendency to hemorrhage with gentle pressure on probing. In the absence of periodontitis, the epithelial attachment level is unchanged with gingivitis, and the depth of the gingival sulcus is normal unless gingival hyperplasia or edema results in pseudopocket formation. Clinical features of periodontitis include gingival recession, periodontal pocket formation, and increased tooth mobility, as well as signs of gingivitis. Nasal discharge, sneezing, and oronasal fistulas may be present with advanced periodontitis, especially when the maxillary canine tooth is involved. Uncommon signs of periodontal disease include severe hemorrhage of the gingival sulcus, pathologic jaw fracture, contact ulcers, intranasal tooth migration, and osteomyelitis.[1]

A complete dental examination is performed, with each tooth evaluated for clinical features of gingivitis or periodontitis. The depth of the gingival sulcus should be evaluated to determine the presence of periodontal pockets. Severe periodontitis may result in deep periodontal pocket formation on the palatal aspect of the maxillary canine tooth. The presence of periodontal pocket formation indicates loss of periodontal ligament and alveolar bone. An explorer is used to identify subgingival calculus and furcation exposure (which indicates alveolar bone loss). Periodontitis may occur without periodontal pocket formation if gingival recession occurs at about the same rate as alveolar bone loss. Dental radiographs are taken to verify the extent of periodontal disease and assist in treatment planning.[4,5] Common radiographic signs of periodontal disease include a rounding of the alveolar crest bone at the cementoenamel junction, increased width of the periodontal space, loss of integrity of the lamina dura, alveolar bone changes (e.g., increase or decrease in bone density), and loss of alveolar crestal bone. Horizontal bone loss is the most common type of alveolar bone loss (Figure 11-5). Vertical bone loss may also occur, resulting in infrabony pockets.

Management

The treatment should relieve oral pain, restore the mouth to a healthy condition, and maintain a healthy mouth following treatment. In determining the most appropriate treatment plan for an older animal, anesthetic risk versus the benefit of the dental procedure, the owner's commitment to regular dental treatments in severe cases, the owner's commitment and ability to perform home care, and the animal's temperament are to be considered.[6] It is best in some older animals to extract teeth with moderate to severe periodontitis rather than having the animal undergo repeated dental treatments.

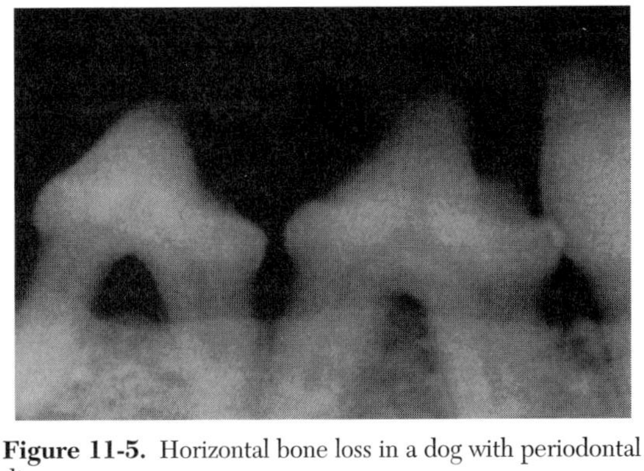

Figure 11-5. Horizontal bone loss in a dog with periodontal disease.

Antimicrobial administration before a dental procedure is recommended in the aged dog with any stage of periodontal disease if the dog is predisposed to a compromised immune system and is more susceptible to infections.[7] Adequate antimicrobial blood concentrations can be achieved by administration of a subcutaneous or intramuscular injection at the time of administration of preoperative medications or oral administration 24 hours before the dental procedure.[7,8] Amoxicillin-clavulanate and clindamycin are effective against the bacteria associated with periodontal disease. Depending on the severity of periodontal or oral disease, administration of antimicrobials is continued for up to 7 days after the procedure. The combination of amoxicillin and metronidazole is an alternative treatment for dogs with severe periodontitis. Dogs with chronic recurrent periodontitis may also benefit from long-term tetracycline administration.

A complete dental prophylaxis includes supragingival and subgingival scaling to remove all plaque and calculus, polishing of the teeth, and rinsing of the gingival sulcus.[9,10] Scaling may be done with mechanical and hand instruments. Mechanical instruments are used primarily on the crown to remove most plaque and calculus deposits. Newer ultrasonic scalers, however, such as the Vetrosonic Millennium (Summit Hill Laboratories, Tinton Falls, N.J.) and the Odontoson (Odonto-Wave, Fort Collins, Colo.), supply subgingival tips with improved water supply that work well and gently to disrupt the subgingival bacterial colonies and effectively treat periodontal infection.[10] Hand instruments are still necessary to remove remaining plaque and calculus deposits on the crown and to scale subgingivally. Scalers are used supragingivally, and curets are used supragingivally and subgingivally. Polishing the teeth is essential following scaling to decrease the rate of subsequent plaque accumulation by smoothing the irregular tooth surface left after scaling. Soft rubber prophy cup and fine prophy paste or flour pumice are used to polish the teeth. The gingival sulcus is irrigated with 0.1% to 0.2% chlorhexidine solution after polishing to remove polishing paste and debris that may have accumulated during the procedure; the teeth are then treated with fluoride.

When periodontitis is present and periodontal pocket depths are less than 4 to 5 mm, "closed" subgingival plaque and calculus removal and root planing can be performed.[9,10] Periodontal pockets greater than 5 mm in depth are difficult to treat conservatively.[6] When advanced periodontitis is present with periodontal pockets exceeding 9 mm in depth, with alveolar bone loss of 70% or greater, the tooth is best treated by extraction.

In older animals, extraction of moderately to severely periodontically diseased teeth is recommended. Simple extractions are those involving single rooted teeth excluding the canine tooth. Multirooted teeth, especially the maxillary fourth premolar, maxillary first molar, and mandibular first molar, are more difficult to extract. Difficult extractions usually include the canines, maxillary fourth premolar, first maxillary molar, and first mandibular molars. Complications that may occur when performing tooth extractions or following the extraction procedure include broken root tips, hemorrhage, jaw fracture, osteomyelitis, oronasal fistula, and oroantral fistula formation.[11]

Grade I and Grade II Periodontal Disease

Even though healthy gingivae show no evidence of disease, plaque still develops in the gingival sulci. If the plaque is not removed, acute gingivitis occurs (grade I periodontal disease), and advances from there. Periodontal disease progresses slowly over the course of 2 to 5 years before teeth loosen enough to exfoliate. However, the course can be markedly shortened in animals with compromised defense mechanisms and in cases of trauma-induced infection involving particularly virulent bacteria. This kind of infection can occur if the gingiva is penetrated by bones or wood that an animal chews and then is infected by bacteria such as *Bacteroides, Fusobacterium, Actinomyces,* hemolytic streptococci, and *Staphylococcus* species.

Grade I periodontal disease consists of marginal gingivitis and involves only the free edge of the gingiva. At this grade, periodontal disease is reversible with complete prophylaxis that includes supragingival scaling and polishing and subgingival root scaling, gingival curettage, and polishing. These procedures should be followed by flushing the resultant debris from the gingival crevice. After prophylaxis, home care should include brushing the animal's teeth at least three times a week. Owners of animals with grade I periodontal disease should be advised that annual teeth cleaning will now be necessary.

When periodontal disease progresses to grade II, the result is increased inflammation and gingival margins that glisten and are swollen, darker in color, and rounded. This is gingival edema, or chronic gingivitis. Complete dental prophylaxis will reverse the condition, but without proper home care, the periodontitis recurs. Because plaque begins to form within 20 minutes after a complete dental prophylaxis treatment and may begin to harden within 1 week, the owner should be advised to brush the animal's teeth three times a week. If any roots are exposed, the owner can desensitize the exposed surfaces by brushing the teeth with a 0.4% stannous fluoride gel. Professional cleaning once a year is recommended.

Grade III Periodontal Disease

Grade III periodontitis is the first stage of permanent damage. Suppuration and gingival recession often are present as sequelae to chronic gingivitis. Radiographs demonstrate a loss of cortical plate continuity next to the tooth at the alveolar crest. Treatment consists of prophylaxis including closed curettage, chlorhexidine treatment, placement of a biodegradable long-acting perioceutic periodontal packing (Doxirobe, Pfizer Animal Health, New York, N.Y.) to encourage soft-tissue reattachment for pockets of 4 mm or greater, and more aggressive home care. At home, the animal's teeth should be brushed every 1 to 2 days, and the mouth should be flushed with an antimicrobial solution such as 0.1% chlorhexidine gluconate (Chlorhexidine Rinse, Virbac Corporation, Fort Worth, Tex.) or zinc ascorbate and sulfur amino acids (Maxi/Guard Oral Cleansing Gel, Addison Biological Laboratory, Fayette, Mo.). Antibiotics and corticosteroids are used only for short-term therapy during acute exacerbations of periodontitis. Any underlying conditions present should be identified and treated appropriately.

Ancillary Therapy

Closed Curettage Procedure. Closed curettage is the sole subgingival treatment for grade I periodontal disease.[10] It may be combined with subgingival chlorhexidine therapy to treat grade II periodontal disease and is part of the treatment for grade III or more advanced periodontal disease. Closed curettage involves the complete removal of subgingival debris and includes root scaling, root planing, and subgingival curettage. Root scaling is the removal of plaque and calculus from the root, and root planing is the smoothing of roughened root surfaces. Débridement of the inner surface and fundus of the gingival sulcus is gingival curettage. These nonsurgical procedures are performed as part of dental prophylaxis in many dogs and cats admitted for routine care and are especially important in animals with grade II or worse periodontal disease. The goal of closed curettage therapy is to turn ulcerative gingivitis into a clean surgical wound.

Closed curettage requires anesthesia and is performed using subgingival curets. Some useful curets are size 3/4, 11/12, and 13/14 Gracey periodontal curets. The working end of the curet should be directed parallel to the tooth root so that the blunt end of the tip can be used to gently débride the fundus of the gingival sulcus of any fibrotic debris.

In root planing, crosshatch strokes are used and repeated, with application of less and less pressure until the root surface is smooth. Pressure is varied from firm to light as the transition is made from tooth scaling to root planing. Some bleeding is expected with adequate débridement. The gingiva should be reevaluated 2 weeks after this procedure to decide if further periodontal treatment is needed.

Fluoride Therapy. Any viable tooth with exposed dentin will be more sensitive, more susceptible to infection, and more likely to develop caries than a normal tooth.[10] Dogs and cats with grade II or worse periodontal disease will benefit from fluoride treatment. Fluoride hardens and desensitizes the tooth surface, increasing its resistance to infection. As acids in plaque dissolve enamel, trace amounts of topical fluoride act as a catalyst for the formation of more stable forms of calcium phosphate such as hydroxyapatite or fluorapatite. The damaged enamel crystals can be repaired by the surface coating of fluorapatite. In this way, enamel in etched areas becomes more caries-resistant than unaltered enamel, because the repaired crystals are larger and less reactive and have lost their most soluble carbonates and magnesium.

Fluoride therapy should follow prophylaxis in cases of grade II or worse periodontal disease. The materials needed include 1.2% fluoride phosphate gel, soft plastic tray foam liners (single disposable foam trays), and cotton swabs or soft small tooth brushes to apply the gel. The procedure is done while the animal is anesthetized and intubated, after the teeth have been scaled, curetted, polished, and flushed. The gel is applied to the crowns and exposed portions of teeth necks and roots, left on the teeth for 4 minutes, and then removed by wiping; do not rinse or flush it away. The gel's effect lasts about 6 weeks, as opposed to the 6-hour duration of a chlorhexidine dentifrice. The animal should not be allowed to swallow the fluoride gel. It has a pH of 3 and can irritate the stomach lining, causing nausea. Although little information is available on fluoride toxicity in dogs or cats, the clinical signs expected would be incoordination and depression. The fluoride gel that owners use on their animal's teeth at home should not be stronger than 0.4% and preferably should be a stannous fluoride product.

Gingivoplasty. Surgical treatment of periodontal disease may involve other areas of the gingiva besides the gingival sulcus.[10] Gingivoplasty is indicated in the animal with hyperplastic gingiva, a condition frequently seen in the boxer, English bulldog, and Great Pyrenees. Typical findings are infection and a pseudopocket created by gingival tissue overgrowing the crown of the tooth. Gingivoplasty involves reshaping and sometimes rearranging the attached gingiva to recreate the normal gingival structure. Small-loop electrosurgery works well for this procedure, because it decreases intraoperative and postoperative hemorrhage. Electrosurgery causes an extra 0.25 mm of gingival tissue loss because of sloughing; however, this tissue loss is acceptable, because excess tissue is being removed. A no. 15 scalpel blade can be used instead of electrosurgery, and a no. 12 blade, with its concave sharp edge, is useful interproximally. Suction is helpful in improving visibility if a scalpel is used.

The technique involves removing the excess attached gingiva by incising it at a 45-degree angle to the tooth. This recreates the normal gingival architecture with its scalloped effect. If an ossifying epulis is present, make a reverse beveled incision, beginning at the gingival margin and extending deeper to expose the abnormal alveolar crestal bone. Then retract the attached gingiva to remove the bony epulis, and suture the remaining superficial gingival tissue back in place. The gingiva heals very quickly after gingivoplasty. The animal should be fed soft food for 1 to 2 days after surgery. Daily application of a zinc ascorbate gel (Maxi/Guard) will help reduce plaque and bacterial by-products and so help the gingival tissue to heal.

Gingivectomy. Gingivectomy is indicated in those animals with true periodontal pockets that do not extend beyond the mucogingival line.[10] After gingivectomy, 2 mm of attached gingiva should remain. This procedure will reduce the pocket depth so that adequate home care can be administered. Procedurally, mark the depth and shape of the pocket by pushing a probe or hypodermic needle through the gingiva to create an outline of bleeding points. Remove the excess pocket with a no. 15 or 12 scalpel blade angled to recreate the knifelike appearance of the normal gingival edge and débride the subgingival walls and fundus with curets to remove any calculus or granulation tissue present. Attached gingiva should remain to provide periodontal support of the tooth.

Home Dental Care

Home care following the dental prophylaxis is necessary for optimal plaque control.[10] The success of home care depends on the owner's schedule and commitment and the animal's cooperation. Daily plaque removal is ideal but every 2 days is adequate.[12,13] Instruments used by owners to remove plaque should be designed to remove plaque without causing harm to the tooth surface. Suitable products for home care include children's or infant's soft toothbrushes, veterinary toothbrushes, finger toothbrushes, gauze pads, and other products designed for plaque removal. Oral hygiene products are available as toothpastes, liquids, gels, and sprays. Hard dog food and soft rubber chew toys may help to mechanically remove plaque. However, these are less likely to be successful in aged dogs that are missing some teeth and are more settled in their dietary and chewing habits. Dogs should not be allowed to chew on hard objects, as this may result in tooth fracture.

FRACTURED TEETH

Clinical Features

A tooth fracture extending into the dentin may cause pain from exposed dentinal tubules sensitive to heat, cold, or pressure.[14] Teeth that have been weakened by disease (e.g., feline odontoclastic resorptive lesions) may be fractured by normal occlusal forces.[15] An animal with an acute fracture involving the pulp may exhibit signs of pain or may show little evidence of discomfort.[16] Clinical signs may include refusal to chew or bite down on hard objects or food, refusal to carry objects in their mouths, chewing on one side of the mouth only, and constant licking. A fractured tooth crown may be identified by visual examination. Dental radiographs are necessary to identify root fractures. A dental explorer is used to determine if the pulp has been exposed by the fracture. If the fracture is new, the pulp tissue bleeds when probed. If the fracture is old, the pulp tissue appears as a dark spot in the center of the tooth.

Management

Specific treatment for a crown fracture is not required if pulp tissue is not exposed[17]; however, rough tooth edges that might lacerate the buccal mucosa should be smoothed.[14] Significant loss of the crown structure may require a crown build-up procedure with a restorative material to prevent gingival damage. Treatment to prevent periapical abscess of a fractured tooth with pulp exposure includes a root canal procedure or extraction. However, root canal treatment in older animals is more difficult because of the narrow diameters of the root canals.[9] The narrow root canal lumens are more difficult to locate and débride, and total débridement to the apex may not be possible. Conventional endodontic therapy may be successful even though radiographic evaluation demonstrates the obturation is 2 to 3 mm short of the apex. A surgical root canal procedure can be done to salvage the tooth if a conventional root canal fails.

In older animals, the typical choices for management of a recently fractured tooth are extraction or benign neglect. Horizontal root fractures occurring at the level of the alveolar bone crest and fractures that extend into the root of the tooth require extraction.[14] The root may be saved following crown extraction by treating it endodontically. A crown may be placed on the remaining root if a crown-lengthening procedure is done. A post-and-core crown restoration would be the preferred crown used for restoration. Horizontal root fractures that are below the alveolar crest may be sufficiently stabilized by surrounding bone and may not require treatment. If the crown is discolored—indicating pulpal trauma or death—the treatment options include extracting the entire tooth, performing root canal therapy, or leaving the tooth alone and periodically evaluating it for development of disease.

Root fractures occurring along the long axis of the root cannot be treated, and a tooth with this type of fracture should be extracted.[18,19] Root fractures in the coronal third of the root may be endodontically treated, followed by placement of a post in the endodontic system; however, the prognosis is poor with this type of fracture. Teeth should be extracted when root fractures occur in the middle third of the root. Treatment of root fractures in the apical third of the root may not be required. The apical segment may maintain its normal blood supply, and the coronal segment often receives adequate collateral circulation. If pulpal disease does develop, it is usually in the coronal segment, which can be treated with conventional endodontic therapy. The apical segment rarely becomes diseased; if it does, it should be removed and the coronal segment treated with conventional or surgical endodontic therapy.

PERIAPICAL ABSCESS

Clinical Features

Clinical signs may include avoiding chewing on hard food, excessive salivation, jaw chattering, constant licking, reluctance to carry anything in the mouth, and a general appearance of malaise.[18] Working dogs may be reluctant to bite down hard on objects used in training exercises. An apical abscess of the maxillary fourth premolar may lead to a soft-tissue swelling or draining fistula ventral to the medial canthus of the eye (Figure 11-6). These are usually painful until they rupture and drain. A fracture of the affected tooth with exposure of the pulp tissue may be noted on oral examination.

If the palatal root of the maxillary fourth premolar is affected, epistaxis or unilateral nasal discharge may be present. If the maxillary first molar has a periapical abscess, the animal may exhibit pain on opening the mouth. Exophthalmus and maxillary sinusitis may also be present. Periapical abscesses involving the maxillary canines usually cause facial swelling above the second premolar. A swelling below the mandible at the level of the second or third premolar is present with periapical disease of the mandibular canines. Mandibular canines with periapical abscesses may drain externally through the skin or into the oral cavity. The presence of a periapical abscess should be considered when a facial swelling develops over the apex of a tooth root. A dental radiograph is taken to confirm the diagnosis. A radiolucent area surrounding the apex of the tooth affected with a periapical abscess will be present.

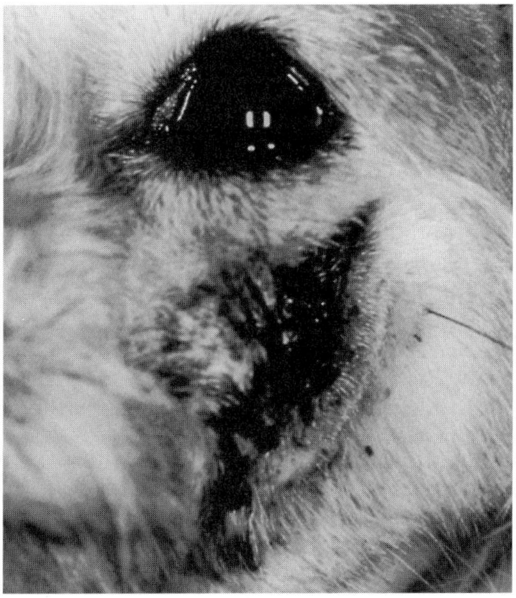

Figure 11-6. Draining tract from periapical abscess involving the maxillary fourth premolar tooth.

Management

If adequate alveolar bone remains the tooth may be successfully treated endodontically.[17] An alternative to root canal therapy is extraction. The procedure for surgical endodontics of the lateral rostral root of the fourth premolar tooth is as follows[10]:

- An elliptical incision approximately 2 to 3 cm is made at midroot level and extended equidistantly rostrally and caudally.
- The full-thickness mucoperiosteal flap is elevated apically, exposing the usually present fistula.
- The fistula is débrided with a suitable curet, exposing the apex. Extreme care must be exercised not to infringe on the infraorbital foramen just rostral to the apex of the upper fourth premolar.
- Approximately 2 mm of the apex is amputated with a tapered fissure bur and dental hand piece at a 45-degree angle to long access of tooth root. The amputation is tapered from apex to crown, medial to lateral, exposing pulpal canal, which will be quite evident by exposure of gutta-percha inside the canal.
- A no. 1 or ½ round bur is carefully introduced into the exposed root canal; exposed gutta-percha is removed and necrotic material débrided from around the walls of the canal to a depth of 2 mm. The canal is prepared with a slight undercut to retain the filling material. Care must be exercised not to overprepare the canal.
- The entire surgical site is packed with cotton balls (approximately 3 mm in diameter), saturated with epinephrine to provide hemostasis and isolation of the apex.

- Hand-triturated non–zinc alloy or newer cements are carried to the apex with the use of a retrograde alloy carrier and condensed with hand pluggers into the apical preparation until it is filled with alloy, or cement is condensed into the apical preparation.
- When alloy is used, the excess is removed by irrigation and suction. The same is done with cements. A periapical radiograph is taken to verify the fill.
- The flap is closed with 3-0 or 4-0 suture material.

NONINVASIVE MANDIBULAR FRACTURE REPAIR

There are many techniques currently used for mandibular fracture repair, ranging from simple tape muzzle placement to various forms of invasive surgical reduction. Surgical reduction techniques include intraoral wire cerclage or ligation, osseous plating, intermedullary pinning to extraoral fixation appliances, or combinations thereof. These various techniques require special instrumentation. They require longer surgical time to perform, with added trauma and subsequent postoperative discomfort for the animal. The major complication with invasive mandibular fracture reduction is postreduction dental malocclusion. Most surgical reductions, especially those that involve external fixation or plating, tend to displace the fracture segments when they are secured. The veterinarian must be able to evaluate the alignment and occlusion of the mandible throughout the procedure.[10] To ensure proper dental occlusion, mandibular fracture reduction must be performed with pharyngeal-tracheal intubation or intravenous anesthesia with appropriate monitoring and support, thus permitting occlusal evaluation during reduction without obstruction of the dental arcades by an endotracheal tube.

Mandibular fracture reduction can be accomplished without invasive procedures with the use of inexpensive dental materials, including forming wax or a similar boxing material such as caulking compound, orthophosphoric acid (enamel etching gel), dental acrylic, and nonexothermic temporary dental composite materials. The procedure is as follows:

- The entire oral cavity is flushed with a dilute chlorhexidine solution. Any open lesions are débrided, thoroughly flushed, and sutured.
- The lower dentition is scaled and polished with nonfluoridated pumice (flour pumice), rinsed, and thoroughly air-dried.
- The lower dentition is acid-etched with orthophosphoric acid for 1 minute, thoroughly rinsed with water, and air-dried.
- Forming wax or caulking compound is placed 0.5 to 1 cm below the marginal gingiva, forming a tightly adapted circumferential dam completely around the lower dental arch.
- The upper dentition is coated with a petroleum jelly. Care is taken not to contaminate the lower dentition with petroleum jelly, which would prevent retention of the acrylic.
- Dental acrylic such as repair acrylic is dispensed as powder and liquid (polymer and monomer) in the following manner. First the liquid is dispensed over the lower dentition and mucosa from a pipette or syringe, then the powder is dispensed, usually from a plastic dispensing bottle. This in effect mixes the acrylic directly over the dentition and mucosa, allowing the viscous mixture to flow into all possible undercuts and the etched surfaces of the enamel for retention.
- The placement of powder and liquid is repeated until the teeth and mucosa are covered with 3 to 4 mm of soft acrylic.
- The tongue is rolled back into the throat to remove the lateral borders of the tongue from dental interference. The mouth can then be closed with complete occlusal contact.
- The mandible is completely closed into a positive correct occlusal relationship while the acrylic is still soft. This position is held until the acrylic has polymerized, usually within 5 minutes. Flowing warm water over the acrylic can accelerate polymerization.
- After polymerization, the mouth is opened, the dam removed, and all rough edges of acrylic removed with an acrylic bur and slow-speed hand piece.

This procedure produces a very strong positive locking splint that ensures proper occlusal position throughout the reduction. The acrylic has received an exact indexing from the upper dentition while allowing for complete closure without premature contact from the acrylic splint. The animal is fed soft food for 5 to 6 weeks. Antimicrobial therapy is prescribed for 2 weeks. The acrylic cast is carefully removed with an acrylic bur or sectioned with a small hand-held blade. The teeth are polished with dental prophylactic paste and the soft tissue cleansed and flushed with a chlorhexidine solution. The acrylic split has formed a very rigid reduction mechanism that is noninvasive without postoperative malocclusion.

ORONASAL FISTULA

Oronasal fistulas are commonly associated with severe periodontal disease of the maxillary canines and fourth premolars (Figure 11-7).[10] These fistulas are often seen in members of smaller dog breeds, for example, dachshunds, Yorkshire terriers, and poodles. On extraction of these teeth, the nasal turbinates are visible through the socket as a result of the destruction of the thin plate of bone separating the alveolar socket from the nasal cavity. Oronasal fistula formation may also be a secondary result of careless teeth extraction, trauma, neoplasia, or infection. When turbinate exposure is encountered during tooth extraction, the fistula should be closed immediately. Sliding gingiva-mucoperiosteal flaps taken from the immediate area of the defect and extending into the alveolar mucosa are commonly used. The labial alveolar bone should be removed to eliminate the dead space in the alveolar socket. Oxytetracycline is packed in the remains of the socket, and the soft-tissue surfaces to be apposed are scarified. The full-thickness flap is then placed, without tension, and sutured with absorbable material. The periosteum must be included in the flap to provide strength to the repair. The failure of this flap and the subsequent development of a secondary fistula may be caused by a number of factors, including inadequate or inaccurate approximation of the apposing raw surfaces; inadequate scarification of apposing surfaces; suture line over the defect; flap tension (all flaps must be absolutely tension free); necrosis of part of the flap; careless suturing; infection; or traumatic disruption of the wound. Once a patent link between the oral and nasal cavities occurs, it is maintained and enlarged by the constant passage of food and fluid. Infection is inevitable. The fistulous tract develops an epithelial lining, ensuring its patency. The most effective closure of oronasal fistulas is in two layers, without tension or infection, with an adequate blood supply, proper suturing technique, and protection during healing.

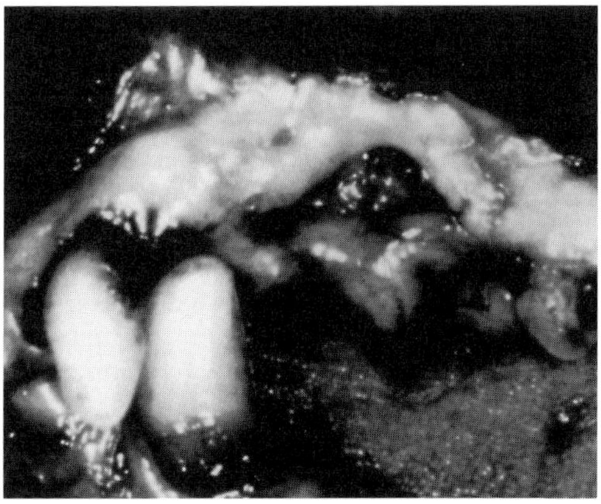

Figure 11-7. Dog with oronasal fistula secondary to severe periodontal disease involving the maxillary canine, which has been lost.

The double flap closure procedure is described as follows, using an upper left canine oronasal fistula as an example. First, determine the bacterial status of the fistula before surgery. The presence of bacteria, particularly hemolytic *Staphylococcus, Streptococcus,* or *Bacteroides* species, greatly impairs surgical remission. Bacterial culture and sensitivity are used to determine the most effective course of antimicrobial agents, administration of which may be required for several weeks before surgical closure to render the fistula as bacteria free as possible. A full-thickness mucoperiosteal flap is raised from the palate medial to the fistula. The incision line begins slightly rostral and medial to the defect, progressing to a medial point approximating the width of the defect. It is better to harvest too much than too little tissue. The incision turns caudally, parallel to the labial aspect of the fistula. At the level of the caudal extremity of the defect, the incision turns labially and runs to the caudal edge of the defect.

A sharp periosteal elevator is used to raise the full-thickness mucoperiosteal flap from the underlying palatal bone as far as the edge of the fistula. Do not push the elevator through into the fistula. The lateral margin of the fistula is scarified. The surface of the epithelium is scraped from a strip 2 to 3 mm wide, using a scalpel blade (or an abrasive disc, with care). The flap is turned upside down so that the oral epithelium is turned to face the turbinates. The flap should lie in place without tension. If it does not, further elevation is performed, ensuring that the flap is not punctured. A partial-thickness flap, approximately 1 mm thick, is raised lateral to the defect. The incision begins at the caudal edge of the fistula, 2 to 3 mm lateral to the defect, at the edge of the scarified strip. It runs parallel to the lateral margin of the fistula, 2 to 3 mm laterally, along the edge of the scarified strip, to a point rostral to the fistula. This determines the length of the flap, which must reach the most medial exposed area of the palate, without tension. Again, too much tissue is better than too little. The incision line is then taken laterally a distance equal to the width of the palatal donor site, then caudally, parallel to the lateral margin of the fistula, as far as the level of the caudal extremity of the fistula. The finger flap, 1 mm thick, is raised with a new scalpel blade, with great care taken not to puncture it. It is rotated medially over the upside-down palatal flap and its donor site, totally covering both. It is temporarily laid back on its donor site while the palatal flap is secured.

The primary, palatal flap is sutured in place, upside down, completely covering the fistula. Single simple interrupted sutures of absorbable material swaged onto a cutting needle are placed close together, totally closing the fistula. The lateral extent of the flap can be sutured to the labial plate of alveolar bone with two or three sutures for additional security if so desired. A tightly sutured, tension-free, primary flap that completely covers the fistula should be accomplished. The secondary partial-thickness finger flap is sutured over both the primary flap and the primary flap donor site with absorbable suture material. It is essential that all epithelial surfaces to be covered have been scarified and their epithelial surface removed. Tissue will not heal onto intact epithelium. The secondary flap donor site is closed by suturing the lateral and medial edges together with absorbable suture material. Continuation of the course of antibiotics is advisable. Soft food is recommended for 2 weeks postoperatively.

This technique produces a double flap closure in which the oral epithelium of the palatal flap is inside, adjacent to the nasal turbinates, and the lateral mucosal epithelium of the covering, secondary flap remains outside, in the oral cavity. Properly executed, this produces consistently effective fistula closure.

CARIES AND ODONTOCLASTIC RESORPTIVE LESIONS

Dogs and cats do not have serious problems with caries because most of their teeth are sectorial in design, built for shearing and tearing rather than grinding.[10] Unlike humans, they generally do not pack food between their teeth. Also, the average pH in a human's saliva is 6.5, whereas a cat or dog's saliva is 7.5. A pH of 7.5 discourages the growth of the cariogenic bacteria *Streptococcus mutans* and *Bacillus acidophilus*, which need an acidic environment to survive. A third reason that dogs have few problems with caries is that the urea content of their saliva is significantly higher than that of human saliva, so the teeth are constantly bathed by ammonium carbonate, an excellent acid-neutralizing agent. Despite their relative caries resistance, dogs do develop caries (defects on the lower third of the crown) (Figure 11-8) and cats do develop cervical line erosions. Exposed dentin is painful, and fluoride hardens the dentin as well as the enamel, reducing the tooth's sensitivity.

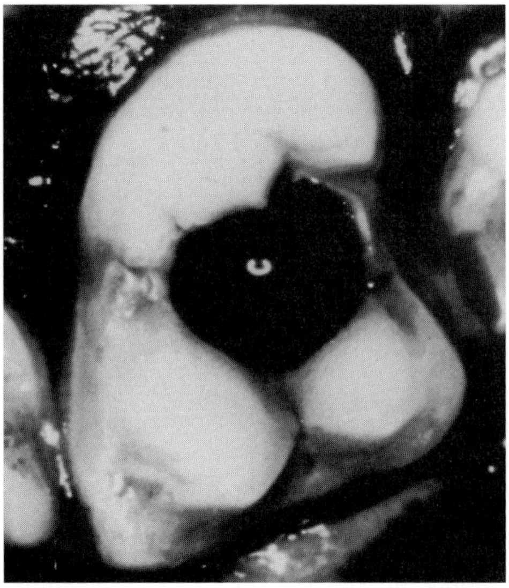

Figure 11-8. Caries on occlusal surface of the first maxillary molar.

Odontoclastic resorptive lesions are erosions in the tooth that begin at or near the cementoenamel junction. The underlying cause of these lesions has not been identified. Originally the lesions were thought to be caries; however, this is not the case. Odontoclastic resorptive lesions are a common problem in domestic cats. The prevalence rate has been as high as 67% of cats in some reports.[20] Siamese, Abyssinian, and Persian cats have been reported to have an increased incidence compared with other breeds. The buccal and labial surfaces of the premolar and molar teeth are most frequently affected. Clinical signs may be absent in cats with minor lesions. Cats with advanced lesions have significant oral pain and associated signs such as anorexia, changes in eating behavior, or changes in food preference (e.g., soft food versus dry food). Oral examination may suggest the presence of odontoclastic resorptive lesions. Proliferative gingival tissue will frequently cover a lesion (Figure 11-9), and the tissue usually bleeds very readily. Extensive tooth destruction may result in partial loss of a tooth crown or complete loss with retained root fragments. Gingivitis may be present in areas in which root fragments remain.

Odontoclastic resorptive lesions are classified into four stages based on the extent of the tooth resorption (Box 11-1). Stage 1 lesions are identified by using a dental explorer to locate the defect. Stage 2 lesions are painful, and the cat may

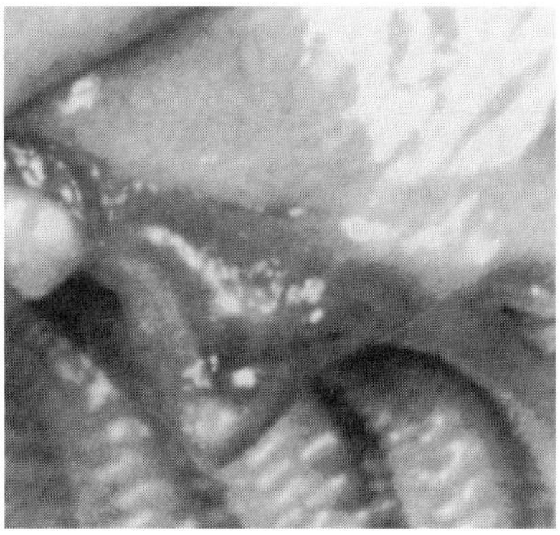

Figure 11-9. Proliferative gingival tissue covering an odontoclastic resorptive lesion.

BOX 11-1 Classification of Odontoclastic Resorptive Lesions

Stage 1	Early lesions with resorption involving enamel and cementum only
Stage 2	Lesions extend into the dentin but do not involve the pulp
Stage 3	Lesions are advanced and extend into the pulp
Stage 4	Chronic lesions with extensive tooth involvement

respond even under anesthesia when these are explored. In a light plane of anesthesia, the cat will typically exhibit a chattering motion with the jaw when the lesions are probed. Dental radiographs should be taken to determine that the pulp is not involved. In stage 3 lesions, tooth structure is compromised to a variable degree. Dental radiographs are taken to evaluate pulp involvement if there is any doubt. In stage 4 lesions the roots may be completely transformed by the resorptive process. The crown may be missing and gingival tissue may have closed over the root remnants. Radiographs may be required to identify retained root fragments. The tooth roots may be ankylosed to the alveolar bone as a result of periodontal ligament loss and cementum remodeling. Canine teeth typically have minimal evidence of disease on the tooth crown even when the root is totally destroyed (Figure 11-10). Dental radiographs should be taken of these teeth to diagnose the root resorption (Figure 11-11).

Treatment of odontoclastic resorptive lesions should be directed at resolving oral pain and returning the cat's oral cavity to a healthy, nonpainful condition. Stage 1 lesions are too small to require restoration. Treatment should include a complete dental prophylaxis followed by polishing with nonfluoridated flour-grade pumice.[21] A fluoride cavity varnish is applied to the clean, dry tooth and allowed to air dry. A fluoride gel should be applied to the tooth on a regular basis to slow plaque accumulation on the tooth. The treatment of stage 2 to 4 resorptive lesions in geriatric cats should be extraction. Treating stage 2 lesions by placing a restoration has been described but is not practical in the aged cat.

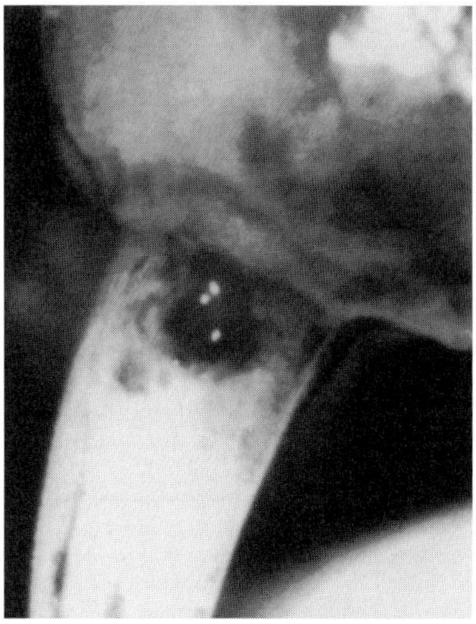

Figure 11-10. Feline canine tooth with evidence of an odontoclastic resorptive lesion at the gingival margin.

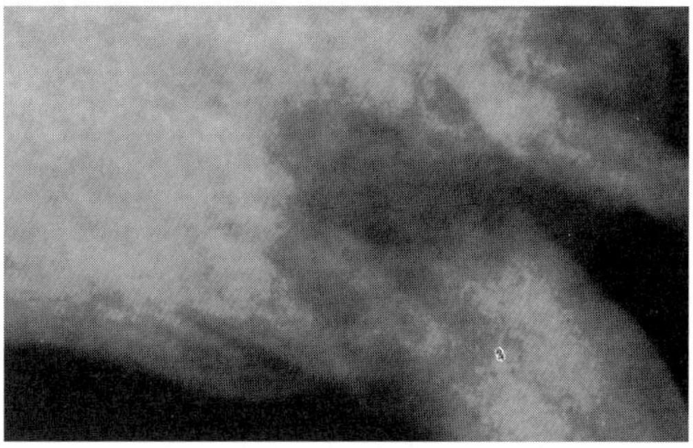

Figure 11-11. Dental radiograph of cat in Figure 11-10 demonstrating complete destruction of the maxillary canine tooth root.

ORAL TUMORS

The oral cavity is the fourth most common site of tumors in the dog (Table 11-1).[22] Malignant melanoma is the most common malignant oral tumor in dogs. Squamous cell carcinoma is the second and fibrosarcoma the third most frequently seen malignant oral tumors in dogs. Other malignant tumors may also be found in the oral

TABLE 11-1. COMMON ORAL TUMORS OF DOGS AND CATS

	CANINE				FELINE	
	SCC	FS	MM	DENTAL	SCC	FS
Frequency (%)	17-30	7.5-25	30-42	5	70	20
Age (yr)	8-10	7-8.3	10-12	9	10	10
Patient size	Larger	Larger	Smaller	None		
Site predilection	Gingiva; rostral mandible	Palate; gingiva; maxilla	Gingiva; buccal mucosa	Rostral mandible	Mandible; maxillary bone	Gingiva
Regional lymph node metastasis	Rare (except tonsil and tongue)	Rare	Common	Never	Occasional	Rare
Distant metastasis	Rare (except tonsil and tongue)	Occasional	Common	Never	Rare	Occasional
Prognosis	Good rostral; poor caudal	Poor-fair	Poor-fair	Excellent	Poor	Fair-good

Modified from Oakes MG, Hedlund CS, Lewis DD et al: Canine oral neoplasia, *Compend Contin Educ Pract Vet* 15:1, 15, 1993; Withrow SJ: Tumors of the gastrointestinal system. In Withrow SJ, MacEwen EG, eds: *Clinical veterinary oncology*, Philadelphia, 1989, JB Lippincott.
SCC, Squamous cell carcinoma; *FS,* fibrosarcoma; *MM,* melanoma.

cavity. Epulides are the most common benign oral tumors. Odontogenic tumors are benign and occur infrequently in dogs. Ameloblastomas are the most common odontogenic tumors in dogs.

Oral tumors occur relatively frequently in cats, and most tumors are malignant[23,24] (see Table 11-1). Squamous cell carcinoma is by far the most frequently found oral tumor in cats. Fibrosarcomas are the second most frequently reported feline oral tumor. Melanomas and other malignant tumors are much less frequently reported. Tumors of dental origin occur rarely in cats.[25] Benign oral tumors are less common than malignant tumors and have been infrequently reported.[26,27]

Clinical Features

Hemorrhage from the oral cavity, reluctance to eat or chew, drooling, loose teeth, and a foul oral odor may be associated with oral tumors. Frequently the tumors are large at the time of diagnosis and cause a facial deformity or are visible. Neoplasia should be suspected if a loose tooth is found in a focal area of inflammation or ulceration. The prognosis for long-term survival is poor for malignant melanomas because of local invasiveness and early metastasis.[22]

The diagnostic evaluation should allow for clinical staging according to the World Health Organization.[22] For affected dogs, a complete blood count, serum chemistry profile, and urinalysis should be performed, as well as specific diagnostic tests for evaluating the tumor. The tumor may be identified by fine needle aspiration cytology or biopsy collection with histopathologic evaluation. The local extent of tumor involvement may be determined by skull radiographs, computed axial tomography, or magnetic resonance imaging. Regional lymph node involvement and evidence of distant metastasis should also be determined.

Treatment

Surgical excision is generally the recommended treatment for most oral tumors.

CHRONIC ORAL INFLAMMATORY DISEASE

Inflammation involving the oral mucosa (stomatitis), pharynx, palate, tongue, and glossopalatine arches (faucitis) in older cats is common. Plasmacytic-lymphocytic gingivitis-stomatitis-pharyngitis has been described as a specific syndrome characterized histopathologically by an infiltrate of primarily plasma cells and lymphocytes. The cause of this inflammation in older cats is unknown. A group of cats diagnosed with plasmacytic-lymphocytic gingivitis have been evaluated for serum antibodies directed against known human periodontal pathogens.[28] An increased serum IgG titer against these pathogens suggests a bacterial component for the cause of plasmacytic-lymphocytic gingivitis-stomatitis-pharyngitis. An inappropriate or hypersensitivity response to oral bacteria has been suggested as a cause for chronic stomatitis. Inflammation, proliferation, and ulceration of tissue in the glossopalatine arch are the prominent features in some cats. Feline calicivirus causes acute gingivitis and faucitis, and it may play a role in chronic faucitis.[29] Calicivirus has been isolated from oropharyngeal swabs of the fauces in cats with chronic oral inflammation. Feline leukemia virus does not play a significant role as a primary pathogen of oral inflammatory disease.[30] Chronic gingivitis, periodontitis, and stomatitis are the most common clinical signs associated with feline immunodeficiency virus infection.[31] Cats with concurrent feline immunodeficiency virus and calicivirus infection are more likely to develop chronic faucitis.[32] The underlying cause of many cases of chronic oral inflammatory disease is undiagnosed at this time. The reason why some cats are more predisposed to developing chronic oral inflammatory disease is also unknown.

Chronic oral inflammatory disease with gingival and mucosal tissue proliferation and ulceration may cause clinical signs of halitosis, ptyalism, blood-tinged saliva, inappetence, anorexia, and oral pain. Oral examination, laboratory assessment, and history will help to rule out systemic disease, trauma, and neoplasia as underlying causes for oral inflammation. Oropharyngeal swabs may be collected for calicivirus isolation. Serologic tests to determine the presence of antibodies to feline immunodeficiency virus infection may also be indicated. A biopsy of the involved oral tissue should be collected for histopathology. Chronic inflammatory diseases usually show a predominance of neutrophils or plasma cells and lymphocytes.[33]

A complete dental prophylaxis should be performed on all cases to eliminate any inflammation secondary to plaque and calculus accumulation. Several medical treatments have been suggested for management of chronic oral inflammatory diseases; however, the response to therapy is generally poor. Antimicrobial agents may provide temporary relief, but generally the inflammation returns after antimicrobials are discontinued. Antiinflammatory doses of corticosteroids may also be beneficial in decreasing the inflammation. However, the frequency of administration required to alleviate clinical signs and the varied response to therapy make this a less desirable choice. Progestins, gold salt therapy, immunoregulin, cryotherapy, and laser therapy have been recommended with varying reports of success. Nonresponsive or severe cases may benefit from extraction of all the teeth behind the canines.

References

1. Manfra Marretta S: The common and uncommon clinical presentations and treatment of periodontal disease in the dog and the cat, *Semin Vet Med Surg (Small Anim)* 2:230, 1987.
2. Hennet PR, Harvey CE: Anaerobes in periodontal disease in the dog: a review, *J Vet Dent* 8:18, 1991.
3. Holmstrom SE, Frost P, Gammon RL: Dental prophylaxis; Periodontal therapy; Exodontics; Endodontics. In *Veterinary dental techniques,* Philadelphia, 1992, WB Saunders.
4. Smith MM, Zontine WJ, Willits NH: A correlative study of the clinical and radiographic signs of periodontal disease in dogs, *J Am Vet Med Assoc* 186:1286, 1985.
5. Zontine WJ: Dental radiographic technique and interpretation, *Vet Clin North Am* 4:741, 1974.
6. Harvey CE: Treatment planning for periodontal disease in dogs, *J Am Anim Hosp Assoc* 27:592, 1991.
7. Sarkiala E, Harvey C: Systemic antimicrobials in the treatment of periodontitis in dogs, *Semin Vet Med Surg* 8:197, 1993.
8. Manfra Marretta S: Current perspectives on periodontal disease in dogs and cats. In: *Veterinary exchange* (suppl), Trenton, NJ, 1992, Veterinary Learning Systems.
9. Harvey CE, Emily PP: Periodontal disease, oral surgery. In Harvey CE, Emily PP, eds: *Small animal dentistry,* Philadelphia, 1993, Mosby.
10. Holmstrom SE, Frost P, Eisner ER: Veterinary dental techniques, ed 2, Philadelphia, 1998, WB Saunders.
11. Manfra Marretta S, Tholen M: Extraction techniques and management of associated complications. In Bojrab MJ, Tholen M, eds: *Small animal oral medicine and surgery,* Philadelphia, 1990, Lea & Febiger.
12. Aller S: Basic prophylaxis and home care, *Compend Contin Educ Pract Vet* 11:1447,1989.
13. Aller S: Dental home care and preventative strategies, *Semin Vet Med Surg* 8:204, 1993.
14. Rossman LE, Garber DA, Harvey CE: Disorders of teeth. In Harvey CE, ed: *Veterinary dentistry*, Philadelphia, 1985, WB Saunders.
15. Wiggs RB, Lobprise HB: Dental diseases, Oral disease. In Norsworthy GD, ed: *Feline practice,* Philadelphia, 1993, JB Lippincott.
16. Williams CA: Endodontics, *Vet Clin North Am Small Anim Pract* 16: 875, 1986.
17. Harvey CE: Oral, dental, pharyngeal, and salivary gland disorders. In Ettinger SF, ed: *Textbook of veterinary internal medicine,* vol 2, Philadelphia, 1989, WB Saunders.
18. Emily P, Penman S: Periodontal disease, dental prophylaxis and minor periodontal surgery. In Emily P, Penman S: *Handbook of small animal dentistry,* New York, 1990, Pergamon Press.
19. Holmstrom SE: Feline endodontics, *Vet Clin North Am Small Anim Pract* 22:1433, 1992.
20. van Wessum R, Harvey CE, Hennet P: Feline dental resorptive lesion: prevalence patterns, *Vet Clin North Am Small Anim Pract* 22:1405, 1993.
21. Lyon KF: Subgingival odontoclastic resorptive lesions: classification, treatment, and results in 58 cats, *Vet Clin North Am Small Anim Pract* 22:1417, 1992.
22. Oakes MG, Hedlund CS, Lewis DD et al: Canine oral neoplasia, *Compend Contin Educ Pract Vet* 15:1,15, 1993.
23. Cotter SM: Oral pharyngeal neoplasms in the cat, *J Am Anim Hosp Assoc* 17:917, 1981.
24. Vos JH, van der Gaag I: Canine and feline oral-pharyngeal tumors, *J Vet Med* 34:420, 1987.
25. Abbott DP, Walsh K, Diters RW: Calcifying epithelial odontogenic tumours in three cats and a dog, *J Comp Pathol* 96:131, 1986.
26. Rothwell JT, Valentine BA, Eng VM: Peripheral giant cell granuloma in a cat, *J Am Vet Med Assoc* 192:1105, 1988.

27. Salisbury SK, Richardson DC, Lantz GC: Partial maxillectomy and premaxillectomy in the treatment of oral neoplasia in the dog and cat, *Vet Surg* 15:16, 1986.
28. Sims TJ, Moncla BJ, Page RC: Serum antibody response to antigens of oral gram-negative bacteria by cats with plasma cell gingivitis-pharyngitis, *J Dent Res* 69:877, 1990.
29. Reubel GH, Hoffmann DE, Pederson NC: Acute and chronic faucitis of domestic cats: a feline calicivirus–induced disease, *Vet Clin North Am Small Anim Pract* 22:1347, 1992.
30. Pederson NC: Inflammatory oral cavity diseases of the cat, *Vet Clin North Am Small Anim Pract* 22, 1323, 1992.
31. August JR: Feline immunodeficiency virus, *Vet Med Rep* 1:150, 1989.
32. Tenorio AP, Franti CE, Madewell BR et al: Chronic oral infections of cats and their relationship to persistent oral carriage of feline calici-, immunodeficiency, or leukemia viruses, *Vet Immunol Immunopathol* 29:1, 1991.
33. Harvey CE: Oral inflammatory diseases in cats, *J Am Anim Hosp Assoc* 27:585, 1991.

CHAPTER 12

The Gastrointestinal System

RETO NEIGER

The gastrointestinal tract of older dogs and cats is hardly affected by any classical age-related disease. In contrast to other body organs, it continues to run very smoothly despite having one of the fastest cell-turnover rates of all the body's organ systems. Reasons for this apparent immunity to the ravages of time are unclear. Besides significant changes in the gastrointestinal flora with an increase in *Clostridia* and a decrease in *Lactobacillus* and *Bacteroides* species,[1] there are no other discernible changes in gastrointestinal function in dogs. There is no information on any age-related changes in gastrointestinal function for cats.

In human medicine, the most important age-related changes seen in the gastrointestinal tract are dysphagia (despite normal saliva production), gastroesophageal reflux disorders, *Helicobacter pylori*–related gastritis, and functional colonic abnormalities (constipation, incontinence). Neoplasia (dog and cat), stomatitis (cat), idiopathic megaesophagus (dog), gastric motility disorders (dilatation-volvulus and gastroparesis) (dog), lymphocytic-plasmacytic enteritis (dog and cat), and idiopathic megacolon (cat) are the gastrointestinal diseases of major concern in small animal medicine (Box 12-1).

BOX 12-1 Age-Related Diseases of the Gastrointestinal Tract

	DOG	CAT
Pharynx	• Tumor • Infection (*Neospora*, tetanus) • Immune-mediated disorders	• Stomatitis or fasciitis • Periodontal disease • Tumors
Esophagus	• Megaesophagus • Foreign body • Tumors • Esophagitis • Esophageal stricture	• Tumors
Stomach	• Tumors • Ulceration • Gastritis • Gastric outlet obstruction • Motility disorders • Dilatation-volvulus	• Tumors • Gastritis • Hairballs
Small intestine	• Inflammatory bowel disease a) plasmacytic-lymphocytic enteritis b) eosinophilic enteritis • Tumors	• Inflammatory bowel disease a) plasmacytic-lymphocytic enteritis b) eosinophilic enteritis • Tumors
Colon, rectum, and anus	• Constipation • Tumors • Fecal incontinence	• Constipation • Megacolon • Tumors

LABORATORY EVALUATION

Generally, blood analysis is of little help in diagnosing a primary gastrointestinal abnormality in the older dog and cat. Hematology might reveal a nonregenerative, microcytic hypochromic anemia in cases of chronic gastrointestinal blood loss with subsequent iron deficiency. A peripheral eosinophilia can sometimes be found in dogs or cats with eosinophilic infiltration of the gastrointestinal tract mucosa (gastritis, enteritis, or colitis). Thrombocytopenia has been seen in dogs with idiopathic inflammatory bowel disease[2] or in association with various neoplasias. Hypoproteinemia (hypoalbuminemia and hypoglobulinemia) is the hallmark sign of animals with protein-losing enteropathy, whereas hypercalcemia of malignancy can point toward a neoplastic disorder (anal sac adenocarcinoma, rarely gastrointestinal lymphoma).

Serum folate and cobalamin concentrations have commonly been used in the diagnosis of small intestinal bacterial overgrowth. The measurement of these vitamins, however, has a low accuracy in dogs.[3] In cats, on the other hand, serum cobalamin concentration is often decreased in cases of small bowel disease (especially lymphoma), and substitution of cobalamin parenterally improves the recovery significantly.[4] Only recently, the measurement of serum unconjugated bile acids has been advocated to help in the diagnosis of small intestinal bacterial overgrowth,[5] and more studies are needed to show the usefulness of this test.

Fecal analysis is mandatory for all animals with clinical evidence of gastrointestinal problems. Besides egg count, zinc sulfate flotations to detect *Giardia* cysts or *Giardia*-specific antigen in feces are useful as well. Fecal culture should be used not only for *Salmonella* and *Campylobacter* species but also to find *Clostridia* and—in conjunction with molecular techniques—to analyze for enteropathogenic *Escherichia coli*.

DIAGNOSTIC IMAGING

Radiologic examination of the gastrointestinal tract in older dogs and cats continues to be an important clinical tool. Survey radiographs should be made of both the thorax and abdomen, especially in animals presented with a complaint of vomiting or regurgitation. It is surprising how often abnormalities such as megaesophagus, aspiration pneumonia, or unsuspected metastatic diseases can be seen in animals with signs of chronic gastrointestinal disease. Signs of gastrointestinal disease on survey films are listed in Box 12-2. Contrast radiographs of the gastrointestinal tract can be useful in animals with vomiting; however, they are of little diagnostic value in the animal with chronic diarrhea, because most lesions responsible for diarrhea are too small to be seen on abdominal radiographs. Lesions visible on contrast studies include intestinal obstruction, severe inflammatory changes, radiodense foreign bodies, or filling defects suggestive of neoplastic or ulcerative disease. Recently, barium-impregnated polyspheres (BIPS) have been shown to help in the diagnosis of gastric and small intestinal motility disorders (Figure 12-1).[6] Unfortunately, BIPS are not as useful in the diagnosis of functional gastrointestinal motility disorders as they are for diagnosis of mechanical abnormalities. Positive or negative contrast studies of the colon can be useful to delineate proximal colonic lesions.

Abdominal ultrasonography is regularly used in animals with gastrointestinal disease. Ultrasonography is especially useful in assessing

BOX 12-2 Helpful Findings in Abdominal Survey Radiographs in Dogs or Cats with Gastrointestinal Disease

Ileus	Ileus may be either paralytic or obstructive.
Peritoneal effusion	Fluid accumulation in the abdominal cavity is uncommon in gastrointestinal disease. The most common causes are 1) ascitic fluid seen in hypoproteinemia and some types of liver disease, and 2) the inflammatory exudate of peritonitis.
Radiopaque foreign objects	These will be visible on survey abdominal radiographs.
Abnormal soft-tissue shadows and/or displacement of the viscera	Displacement of the viscera can often be used as an indirect indication of a mass in a contiguous organ or structure. A displaced stomach, for example, suggests a tumor in that region of the abdomen. Gastric dilatation-volvulus is an obvious radiographic diagnosis. Lateral displacement of the duodenum may be seen in chronic pancreatitis or pancreatic tumors.
Pneumoperitoneum	Free gas in the peritoneal cavity may result from gas-forming bacteria (usually a result of rupture of some portion of the alimentary tract), a penetrating wound in the abdominal wall, or recent abdominal surgery.
Thickened or irregular intestine	An irregular mucosa suggests severe inflammatory or neoplastic intestinal disease. The "apple-core" intestine is virtually pathognomonic for intestinal lymphosarcoma.

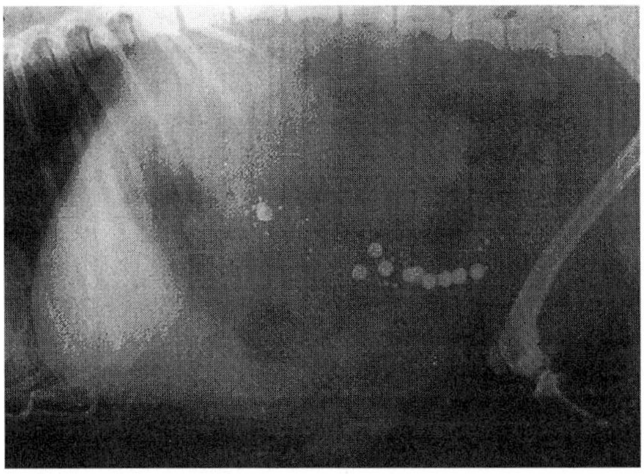

Figure 12-1. Barium-impregnated polyspheres study in a 9-year-old cross-breed with a 3-month history of chronic vomiting and suspicion of partial intussusception. Small and large spheres are seen in the colon, excluding an obstructive lesion.

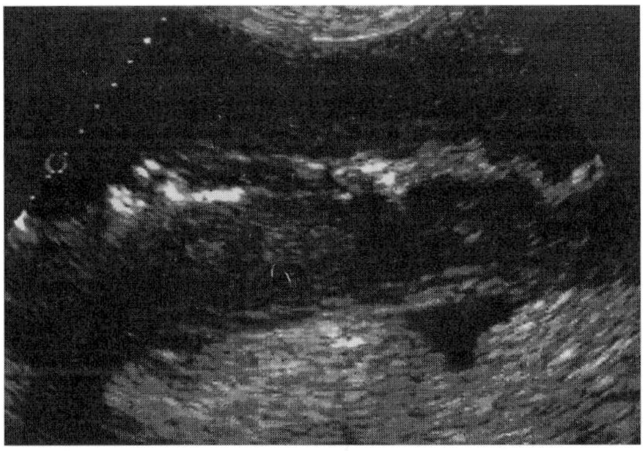

Figure 12-2. Ultrasonographic appearance of the markedly thickened intestinal walls in an 11-year-old cat with alimentary lymphoma. Ultrasound-guided fine-needle aspirate of the mucosa confirmed the diagnosis. (Courtesy of Dr. Chris Lamb, Royal Veterinary College, London.)

intraorgan parenchymal abnormalities external to the gastrointestinal tract but can also be used to measure intestinal wall thickness. Regional abnormalities such as neoplasia, regional enteritis, and intussusception can be better defined with ultrasonography than with radiography (Figure 12-2). In order for the stomach to be evaluated, it should be filled with water via gastric tube before the procedure is performed.

Functional motility disorders are difficult to evaluate with radiography or ultrasonography. Whereas fluoroscopy (barium swallow) is regularly used to assess pharyngeal and esophageal motility problems, this technique is less useful for gastric and intestinal motility disorders. The gold standard to evaluate these motility problems is scintigraphy; however, because of a lack of equipment and the radioactivity associated with the procedure, this technique is mainly used in large referral settings.

ENDOSCOPY

Endoscopy is one of the best and yet most fundamental methods of examining the gastrointestinal tract. However, despite the tremendous diagnostic advantages that endoscopy offers, it is still best used by the veterinarian as an adjunctive procedure in the evaluation of gastrointestinal diseases. Endoscopy is quick, is noninvasive, and carries a very low risk. Furthermore, it can be used to perform therapeutic interventions such as foreign body removal, dilation of esophageal strictures, and placement of percutaneous gastric feeding tubes. Finally, it is extremely important to remember that no endoscopy is complete unless multiple surface biopsies are obtained. Many extensive textbooks about veterinary endoscopy have been published recently for the interested reader,[7] and only a brief overview is given here.

A variety of new and used endoscopes are available at reasonable prices. For gastrointestinal endoscopy it is best to use a four-way tip deflected, flexible fiberoptic or video endoscope with a working length of at least 100 cm or greater and an outer diameter of 7.8 to 9.9 mm. The biopsy channel should be about 2.4 mm in diameter. Preparation of the animal for endoscopy is crucial. For upper gastrointestinal endoscopy, food must be withheld for 12 to 18 hours, and water withheld for 3 to 4 hours. Sucralfate and metoclopramide are discontinued about 12 hours before the procedure. The animal is anesthetized and placed in left lateral recumbency. The normal esophagus is normally empty except for a small quantity of saliva. Similarly, the stomach should contain nothing other than perhaps a small amount of bile-stained liquid. The gastric rugae are uniform in color and can be readily identified if the stomach has not been over-distended with air. The endoscope can be passed through the pylorus in most animals to allow examination and biopsy of the duodenum and proximal jejunum. Aspiration of duodenal juice for quantitative culture can be achieved by passing a sterile tube through the biopsy channel.

Colonoscopy can be performed in a sedated animal with a rigid colonoscope or, if the whole colon needs to be evaluated, in an anesthetized animal with a flexible endoscope. In both instances, it is crucial to prepare the colon appropriately; otherwise the mucosa cannot be evaluated adequately, and maneuverability in a sea of feces is virtually impossible. The animal should be fasted for at least 24 to 36 hours and should receive warm water enemas on the day of the procedure until the effluent is clear. Furthermore, two oral doses of colonic lavage solution (Golytly, Colyte, or Cleanprep) at a dose of 25 to 30 ml/kg 1 to 2 hours apart are given the night before.[8] In dogs the solution is best given by stomach tube, and in cats by a nasoesophageal tube. For flexible colonoscopy, the animal should be in left lateral recumbency. After a rectal examination to ensure that the distal rectum has no obstruction, the lubricated tip of the endoscope is advanced under direct observation. Normal colonic mucosa is pink with linear or circular folds. In the normal colon it is possible to see the network of submucosal vessels, which is an important criterion for normality. With practice, it is possible to navigate both the splenic and hepatic flexures and to evaluate the cecum and ileocolic junction. It is occasionally possible to pass the endoscope through the sphincter and examine the distal ileum.

LAPAROSCOPY OR EXPLORATORY LAPAROTOMY

For several reasons, the veterinarian may be unable to reach a diagnosis after conducting an endoscopic biopsy. Endoscopic biopsies normally include the muscularis layer but do not go deeper into the layers of the gastric and intestinal walls. Therefore, deeper lesions (neoplasia, lymphangiectasia) are usually not diagnosed by surface biopsies. In cases of very scirrhous mucosa, it might also not be possible to obtain adequate biopsies. In addition, most of the jejunum and the entire ileum cannot be reached by passage of an endoscope. If an endoscope is not available or unable to access the desired anatomic site, it might then be necessary to obtain full-thickness biopsies either during laparoscopy or exploratory laparotomy. In either procedure, biopsies should always be taken even if the gastrointestinal tract looks and feels normal, because the veterinarian's eyes and fingers are no substitute for a microscope.

ESOPHAGUS

Regurgitation is the typical clinical sign seen in dogs with esophageal disorders. It is important to differentiate regurgitation from vomiting, as the clinical assessment for these conditions is quite different. Regurgitation is an entirely passive process without the prodromal signs of nausea and retching. Hypersalivation is seen in both conditions, and the thrown-up material often is covered in mucus irrespective of the cause. Evaluating the regurgitated material is of little help to differentiate it from vomitus, as both can have a variable pH and both can have a "sausage-like" appearance. Regurgitation can be due to intraluminal obstruction, intramural abnormalities, and extramural obstruction (Box 12-3). Many animals with regurgitation can have secondary signs such as weight loss, polyphagia, weakness, dehydration, ballooning of the cervical esophagus, gurgling or burping sounds, coughing, and halitosis. The time between eating and regurgitation depends on the degree of dilation and the activity of the animal and can range from a few minutes to 24 hours or more. Esophageal disorders are rare in cats, the most common being esophageal tumors. Megaesophagus caused by feline dysautonomia (Key-Gaskell syndrome) is now seen only rarely.

Evaluation of esophageal disorders can often be achieved with the use of survey radiographs. However, it is important to remember that dilation of the esophagus can occur during sedation and anesthesia. Some free air in the cranial esophagus is frequently seen in anxious and stressed animals and does not mean that the animal has megaesophagus. Contrast studies with barium

BOX 12-3 Causes of Regurgitation in the Older Dog

Intraluminal Obstruction

Foreign bodies
Neoplasia of the esophagus

Intramural Abnormality

Megaesophagus
- Idiopathic
- Myasthenia gravis (focal or generalized)
- Systemic lupus erythematosus
- Hypoadrenocorticism
- Polyneuropathy
- Polymyositis
- Canine distemper
- Toxicity (lead, organophosphate, thallium)

Stricture (postanesthesia, following esophagitis)
Esophagitis (reflux, chemical, thermal)
Granuloma (*Spirocerca lupi*, fungal)
Diverticulum of the esophagus

Extraluminal Obstruction

Anterior mediastinal mass (lymphoma, thymoma)
Abscess
Hilar lymphadenopathy (fungal, tumor)
Hiatal disorders

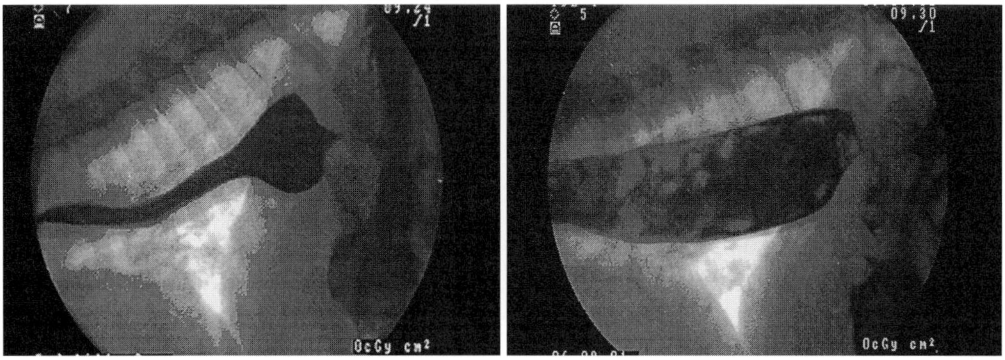

Figure 12-3. Fluoroscopic image of an esophageal obstruction in a 10-year-old Labrador retriever with 2-month history of regurgitation. **A,** Survey barium swallow. **B,** Barium mixed with food. Intraoperatively, a mass was found encircling the entire circumference of the cardia, which histologically was diagnosed as leiomyoma.

can help with the diagnosis of strictures as well as intraluminal and extraluminal obstructions (Figure 12-3). In all cases in which a megaesophagus has been reliably diagnosed on survey radiographs, giving barium to confirm the diagnosis is not indicated because these animals tend to be at increased risk for reflux and aspiration. In cases in which a diagnosis cannot be reached with a contrast study, the animal may need to have its esophageal peristalsis evaluated with fluoroscopy. Again liquid barium as well as barium mixed with food should be used. Research tools to assess esophageal abnormalities are endoultrasound, manometry, pH-metry, and scintigraphy.

Dysphagia

There are three major causes of dysphagia: 1) anatomic abnormalities of the oral cavity or pharynx; 2) pain associated with apprehension, mastication, or swallowing; and 3) neuromuscular dysfunction of cranial and pharyngeal muscles (Box 12-4).

History and Diagnosis. Dysphagia manifests itself as repeat attempts or inability to swallow, obvious difficulty or discomfort during swallowing, or aspiration and gagging when swallowing. It is imperative to first rule out rabies as a possible cause. Neuromuscular disorders are normally divided into three major categories. Lower motor neuron dysfunction resulting from masticatory myositis or deficits of cranial nerves (V, VII, XII) can prevent an animal from placing or keeping food in its mouth. Masticatory myositis is an immune-mediated disorder affecting muscles derived from the first branchial arch containing type 2M myofibers. Trismus and pain are frequent complaints. Presumptive diagnosis is based on typical clinical signs, elevated serum creatinine kinase levels, and absence of clinical or laboratory evidence of other systemic or muscular diseases (e.g., toxoplasmosis, polymyositis). The diagnosis is supported by histopathologic examination of frozen masticatory muscle sections demonstrating autoantibodies against type 2M myofibers and, clinically more relevant, circulating 2M antibodies. Tetanus can sometimes look very similar, with rigid jaw tone, although most animals have generalized muscle spasticity.

BOX 12-4 Causes of Oropharyngeal Dysphagia

Anatomic Problems

Neoplasia (squamous cell carcinoma, fibrosarcoma, melanoma)
Lymphadenopathy, lymphadenitis
Fracture (mandible, maxilla, hyoid)
Loss of anterior tongue (uremic, toxic)
Laryngeal and pharyngeal trauma

Pain

Stomatitis and glossitis
Foreign object (penetrating, linear)
Fracture
Temporomandibular joint disease
Tooth problem
Abscess (retrobulbar, soft-tissue)

Neuromuscular Cause

Rabies, pseudorabies
Masseter myositis
Myasthenia gravis
Oral dysphagia (cranial nerves V, VII, XII)
Pharyngeal dysphagia (cranial nerves VII, IX, X)
Cricopharyngeal dysfunction

The pharyngeal phase involves forming a food bolus at the base of the tongue and pushing it back to and through the cricopharyngeal sphincter. Assessing this part of the swallowing act can be assessed only with contrast fluoroscopy or cinefluorography. It is important to evaluate the swallowing of liquids (barium sulfate paste) as well as solids (barium mixed with food). Underlying problems, such as myasthenia gravis or systemic lupus erythematosus, should be evaluated. Finally, the cricopharyngeal phase involves coordinated relaxation of the cricopharyngeal muscle, allowing food boluses to pass into the esophagus, where primary esophageal peristalsis carries them to the stomach.

Megaesophagus

Moderate to severe esophageal dilation and ineffective esophageal peristalsis characterizes megaesophagus. Acquired megaesophagus may develop in association with a variety of conditions (see Box 12-3), with myasthenia gravis accounting for about 25% of the secondary canine cases. Sometimes myasthenia gravis can be a focal disease with no other clinical signs. However, most cases of adult-onset megaesophagus have no known cause and are referred to as *acquired idiopathic megaesophagus*. The syndrome occurs spontaneously in adult dogs between 7 and 15 years of age without sex or breed predilection. Acquired feline megaesophagus is a rare disorder. Recent studies in dogs have suggested a defect in the afferent neural response to esophageal distension. The responses of the upper and lower esophageal sphincters to swallowing appear to be intact, but esophageal distension does not initiate peristaltic contractions in affected animals. The exact site of this abnormality in the afferent neural response has not yet been determined.

Diagnosis. Hematology, serum chemistry profile, and urinalysis should be performed in all cases to investigate possible secondary causes of megaesophagus (e.g., hypoadrenocorticism, lead poisoning). Endoscopy may be performed and is useful in identifying concurrent esophagitis. A recent risk factor analysis suggests that esophagitis increases the risk for the development of megaesophagus in dogs.[9] It is unclear whether esophagitis is the cause or a consequence of megaesophagus. In acquired secondary megaesophagus, nicotinic acetylcholine receptor antibody testing to rule out myasthenia gravis and adrenocorticotropic hormone stimulation test to rule out hypoadrenocorticism are performed. Further ancillary tests may include antinuclear antibody testing, electromyography and nerve conduction velocity, and muscle biopsy. Although hypothyroidism has been cited repeatedly as a potential cause or complicating factor in the development of canine megaesophagus, hypothyroidism has not been identified as a risk factor in a case-control study, suggesting that hypothyroidism should be considered only on a case-by-case basis.[9]

Treatment. If identified, all underlying disease processes should be treated. Some cases of hypothyroidism and megaesophagus resolve when the animal is treated with thyroxin supplementation.[10] Animals with aspiration pneumonia are treated aggressively with antimicrobial agents. Ideally, a bronchial sample from the lung is obtained and submitted for bacterial culture and sensitivity testing. Until the results are available, broad-spectrum parenteral antimicrobial therapy with cephalosporin and gentamicin is initiated. Because many dogs with aspiration pneumonia are dehydrated, it is important to deliver adequate intravenous fluids. Only recently, bethanechol (2.5 to 5 mg/kg once to twice daily) has been advocated for dogs with megaesophagus; no long-term beneficial effects have been reported so far. Prognosis for idiopathic secondary megaesophagus is always guarded to poor. A few dogs do well if they are frequently fed small volumes from a height, with all food and water removed at night. The type of food should be determined by trial and error feeding of the affected animal. Some dogs do well with canned food mixed with water in a blender. Most dogs, however, appear to do better with dry food. Frequent and recurrent bouts of aspiration pneumonia are common and often result in extreme medical management or euthanasia. Some dogs can be maintained by inserting a gastrostomy feeding tube. Besides feeding, oral medications can be delivered through the feeding tube. Newer low-profile gastrostomy feeding tubes (e.g. Kimberly-Clark, Ballard Medical Products, Draper, Utah; Ross Feeding Device, Columbus, Ohio) make feeding management on a long-term basis even easier.

Esophageal Foreign Bodies

Esophageal foreign bodies are as commonly diagnosed in older dogs as they are in young dogs. Because of their fastidious eating habits, cats are less often presented with esophageal foreign bodies. Typically, a bony foreign body is found between the heart and the diaphragm in a West Highland white terrier.[11] Most owners suspect that an esophageal foreign body is causing the clinical signs when they present their dogs.

Diagnosis. Most commonly, a radiodense foreign body can be seen on a lateral thoracic radiograph (Figure 12-4). In cases of high suspicion but no clear diagnosis, a contrast study might help. However, barium in the esophagus will make endoscopy subsequently much more difficult. Removal is either achieved endoscopically or fluoroscopically.[11] I regularly use a long foreign-body forceps along the endoscope to grab the bone; the endoscope is then withdrawn and the bone slowly removed. One can also use a basket or alligator forceps through the working channel of the endoscope to grab the foreign object (e.g., coin, toy). Some foreign bodies can be pushed into the stomach. If the objects are nondigestible, either they can be left in the stomach in the hope that the pet will pass them, or they can be removed by means of elective gastrotomy. Surgical removal is indicated only when perforation or severe mucosal damage or perforation is suspected, in long-standing cases, if no endoscope is available, or if the owner refuses referral. After the object is removed the mucosa should be evaluated endoscopically, and follow-up thoracic radiographs should always be made to assess for pneumomediastinum.

Treatment. Severe esophagitis should be treated as follows. In some cases the esophagus should be rested for 7 to 10 days by feeding through a gastrostomy tube. Oral sucralfate suspension (Table 12-1) is indicated in all cases after foreign body removal. Parenteral antimicrobial agents (e.g., cephalosporin) should be given if pneumomediastinum is present. Antiinflammatory doses

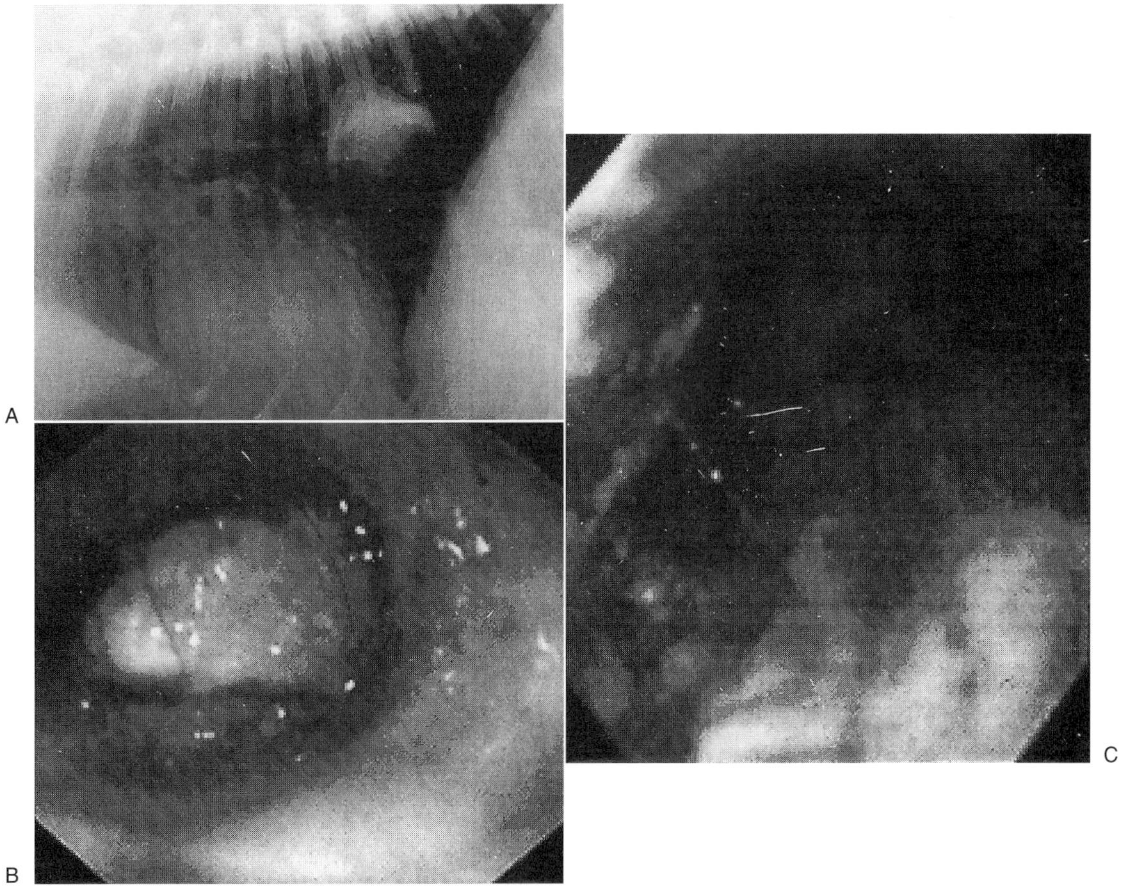

Figure 12-4. Bony foreign body in the esophagus of an 11-year-old West Highland white terrier. **A,** Thoracic radiograph showing the increased opacity caudal to the base of the heart. **B,** Endoscopic picture of the bone lodged in the esophagus. **C,** Marked esophagitis after foreign body removal. The dog was treated with a 4-day course of sucralfate and ranitidine and made an uneventful recovery.

TABLE 12-1. THERAPEUTIC AGENTS USED IN GASTRIC DISEASES

GENERIC NAME	CLASS OF DRUG	DOSAGES
Aluminum hydroxide	Antacid	Dogs: 100-200 mg PO q4-6h Cats: 50-100 mg PO q4-6h
Bismuth subsalicylate	Protectant	0.25-2 ml/kg PO q4-6h
Cimetidine	H_2-receptor antagonist	5-10 mg/kg PO or IV q8h
Famotidine	H_2-receptor antagonist	0.5-1 mg/kg PO or IV q12-24h
Misoprostil	Prostaglandin analogue	2-5 μg/kg PO q12h
Nizatidine	H_2-receptor antagonist	5 mg/kg PO q24h
Omeprazole	Proton-pump inhibitor	0.7 mg/kg PO q24h
Ranitidine	H_2-receptor antagonist	1-2 mg/kg PO or IV q12h
Sucralfate	Protectant	0.5-1 g PO q8h

IV, Intravenous administration; *PO*, oral administration.

of corticosteroids have not been reliably shown to prevent stricture formation and should not be used. Rarely, complications such as esophageal strictures or megaesophagus can occur weeks to months later. Pulsion diverticula and esophageal rupture are fortunately uncommon complications.

Esophageal Tumors

Tumors of the esophagus are very rare. Primary tumors include squamous cell carcinoma, adenocarcinoma, leiomyosarcoma, and plasmacytoma. In dogs *Spirocerca lupi* can induce primary esophageal tumors or granulomas in endemic areas. Metastatic tumors such as thyroid carcinoma, mammary carcinoma, and gastric carcinoma also occur. In addition, periesophageal tumors can invade by local metastatic spread. Signs are usually those of a stricture with orad dilatation and dysmotility. Primary esophageal tumors carry a poor prognosis, and little can be done for affected dogs or cats. Surgical resection may be considered as a palliative procedure, perhaps with transplantation of a length of small intestine in place of the resected segment. Percutaneous endoscopic gastrostomy (PEG) tube placement is often the best symptomatic treatment to allow feeding and medical management. *Spirocerca*-induced granulomas can be treated with doramectin (200 μg/kg subcutaneously at 14-day intervals for three treatments) with good success.[12]

Esophagitis

Esophagitis is most commonly seen as a complication of chronic reflux of acidic gastric contents into the esophagus (chronic vomiting), after removal of an esophageal foreign body, or after the ingestion of strong acid or alkaline solutions. Reflux of acid gastric contents into the esophagus can also occur during general anesthesia. The most common cause, however, appears to be a defective lower esophageal sphincter. Also, once esophagitis is present, the lower esophageal sphincter tends to become incompetent and perpetuate and exacerbate the problem. A history of recent anesthesia may be present.

Diagnosis and Treatment. Endoscopy is needed to confirm esophagitis; however, suggestive clinical and historical signs are often enough for treatment to be started (see Figure 12-4, *C*). Biopsy of the esophageal mucosa is very difficult and is indicated only in cases of signs of granuloma or neoplasia. Radiographic diagnosis is difficult, but contrast studies may occasionally reveal reflux or an anatomic defect such as hiatal hernia. Esophagitis is treated symptomatically by decreasing gastric acidity with H_2-receptor antagonists or proton-pump inhibitors (see Table 12-1). Sucralfate works best in an acidic environment, and its local effect in the esophagus has been questioned. However, as the local pH in an inflamed tissue normally is acidic, this reservation seems unwarranted, and sucralfate suspension should be given by syringe orally three times daily. In cases of chronic vomiting, metoclopramide, which has antiemetic as well as prokinetic properties, is indicated. Gastrostomy feeding tube placement may be needed to rest the esophagus in severe cases. Antimicrobial therapy is rarely needed.

STOMACH

In human medicine minor changes in motor and secretory function of the stomach are possible, but changes in gastric physiology attributable to age alone are rarely responsible for symptoms. *H. pylori* is almost invariably associated with type-

B gastritis and, in addition to the use of nonsteroidal antiinflammatory drugs (NSAIDs), is the most common cause of clinical signs in humans. In older animals, no information is available about the incidence of different diseases that affect the stomach. Irrespective of the problem, though, vomiting is the typical presenting sign. Besides the more common gastric problems, such as dietary indiscretion, gastric foreign bodies, tumors, defective gastric mucosal immune mechanisms, peptic ulcers, decreased motility, and abnormal acid secretion, there are many other differential diagnoses for animals presented with vomiting (Box 12-5). When the cause of vomiting cannot be elucidated, it may be necessary to treat some animals symptomatically with antiemetic drugs.

Acute Gastritis

Although many factors have been found to account for acute gastritis, the most common are dietary hypersensitivity and indiscretion. Acute gastritis has no age predilection and can occur in any dog or cat. It is most often a result of the ingestion of inappropriate food (spoiled, rotten, toxic) or foreign material (rock, bones, wood, weeds). Other possible causes in older animals are drugs (NSAIDs), chemicals (fertilizer, herbicide), or heavy metals (lead, zinc). Most often, only a tentative diagnosis is reached based on signalment, history, clinical signs, and physical examination findings. During endoscopy, superficial hemorrhage caused by erosions and edema can be seen.

BOX 12-5 Causes of Vomiting in Older Dogs and Cats

Dietary Problems (indiscretion, hypersensitivity)

Drugs (NSAIDs, cardiac glycoside, antineoplastic, or antimicrobial agents)

Metabolic Disorders
Diabetes mellitus
Renal disease
Hepatopathy
Electrolyte disorders (potassium, magnesium, calcium)
Acid-base disturbance

Disorders of the Stomach
Obstruction (foreign body, pyloric hypertrophy, external compression)
Chronic gastritis
Gastric ulcer
Gastric neoplasia
Motility disorder
Parasite (*Physaloptera* species, *Ollulanus* tricuspis)

Disorders of the Intestine
Inflammatory bowel disease (lymphocytic-plasmacytic, eosinophilic)
Intestinal neoplasia
Intraluminal obstruction (foreign body, intussusception)
Granulomatous diseases (fungal, *Pithium* species)
Obstipation

Abdominal Disorders
Pancreatitis
Peritonitis (including feline infectious peritonitis)
Inflammation elsewhere (prostatitis, pyometra, pyelonephritis)
Neoplasia

Neurologic Disorders (motion sickness, inflammation, edema, neoplasia)

Miscellaneous Causes
Hyperthyroidism
Feline heartworm disease

Treatment. Initially, dietary restriction by withholding food for 24 hours is all that is needed. Depending on the severity of the clinical signs (dehydration, continuous vomiting), the animal will need intravenous crystalloids (lactated Ringer's solution) but no oral water. Because most affected animals are hypokalemic, potassium often needs to be supplemented based on serum potassium measurement (generally 20 to 40 mEq potassium chloride per liter of fluids administered). A bland commercial diet (Waltham Digestive Tract Support, Hill's Prescription Diet i/d, Iams Low-Residue) or home-cooked diet (white fish or chicken and rice, cottage cheese) (Box 12-6) given in small amounts multiple times during the day is indicated. The regular food can then be slowly reintroduced over a 3- to 5-day period when vomiting has ceased.

In some animals, symptomatic treatment with antiemetics is needed. Because medical approaches to antiemetic therapy are based on the neurotransmitter-receptor interactions, it is important to understand these mechanisms. In the chemoreceptor trigger zone (CRTZ), several neurotransmitters and receptors have been found, including dopamine (D_2-dopaminergic), norepinephrine (2-adrenergic), 5-hydroxytryptamine (5-HT_3-serotonergic), acetylcholine (M_1-cholinergic), histamine (H_1 and H_2-histaminergic), and enkephalins (ENKδ-enkephalinergic). In the emetic center, the only receptors demonstrated so far are 5-hydroxytryptamine$_{1A}$ and α_2-adrenergic. The α_2-receptors in the emetic center and in the CRTZ may be antagonized by pure α_2-antagonists (e.g., yohimbine, atipamezole) or by mixed α_1/α_2-antagonists (e.g., prochlorperazine, chlorpromazine). In the vestibular apparatus, muscarinic M_1-receptors and acetylcholine have been demonstrated, and therefore mixed M_1/M_2-antagonists (e.g., atropine, scopolamine) and pure M_1-antagonists such as pirenzepine may inhibit motion sickness in dogs and cats. Many receptors are found in the gastrointestinal tract, but the 5-HT_3 receptors are likely to play the most important role in the initiation of vomiting. Cytotoxic agents cause the release of 5-HT from enterochromaffin cells in the gastrointestinal tract, which then activates the 5-HT_3 receptors on afferent vagal fibers. This vomiting induced by 5-HT_3-receptor activation can be completely abolished by treating the animal with 5-HT_3-antagonists, such as ondansetron, granisetron, or tropisetron. Another antagonist of 5-HT_3 is metoclopramide, but only in high concentrations.

Several antiemetic drugs have been formulated based on the neurotransmitter-receptor system just mentioned (Table 12-2). These antagonists are classified as α_2-adrenergic, D_2-dopaminergic, H_1-histaminergic, H_2-histaminergic, M_1-muscarinic

BOX 12-6 Home-Prepared Diets for Intestinal Disease in a Dog Weighing Approximately 10 kg

Highly Digestible, Low-Fat Hypoallergenic Diets (Single Source Protein)

Lamb	**Venison**	**Rabbit**
6 oz lean lamb	6 oz venison	6 oz rabbit
No corn oil	2 teaspoons corn oil	1 teaspoon corn oil
Add to:	10 oz boiled white rice	
	1 teaspoon dicalcium phosphate	
	1 teaspoon "lite" salt	
	1/2 capsule Centrum adult multivitamins or 1/2 to 1 tablet of Vitaline Total Formula	
Supplies 675 to 700 kcal	20% to 34% protein, 46% to 48% carbohydrate, 19% to 22% fat	

Highly Digestible, Moderate- and High-Fat Diets

Chicken (Moderate Fat)	Beef (High Fat)
6 oz chicken	6 oz hamburger (lean)
8 oz boiled white rice	5 oz boiled white rice
2 teaspoons corn oil	No corn oil
Add to:	1 teaspoon dicalcium phosphate
	1 teaspoon "lite" salt
	1/2 capsule Centrum adult multivitamins
Supplies 680 kcal	Chicken: 33% protein, 30% fat
	Beef: 33% protein, 43% fat

Ingredients for each diet should be well mixed and cooked in a microwave oven or casserole before serving

TABLE 12-2. ANTIEMETIC MEDICATION CLASSIFICATION AND DOSAGES

CLASSIFICATION	EXAMPLE	SITE OF ACTION	DOSAGE (MG/KG)	SIDE EFFECTS
α_2-Adrenergic antagonists	Prochlorperazine	CRTZ, emetic center	0.1-0.5 q6h-q8h SC, IM	Hypotension, sedation in all
	Chlorpromazine	CRTZ, emetic center	0.2-0.4 q8h SC, IM	
	Yohimbine	CRTZ, emetic center	0.25-0.5 q12h SC, IM	
	Atipamezole	CRTZ, emetic center	Unknown	
D_2-dopaminergic antagonists	Metoclopramide	CRTZ, GI muscle	0.2-0.4 q6h PO, SC, IM	Extrapyramidal signs
	Domperidone	GI smooth muscle	0.1-0.3 q12h IM, IV	None reported
	Trimethobenzamide	CRTZ	3 q8h-q12h IM	Allergic reaction
	Prochlorperazine	See above		
	Chlorpromazine	See above		
H_1-histaminergic antagonists	Diphenhydramine	CRTZ	2-4 q8h PO, IM	Sedation
	Dimenhydrinate	CRTZ	4-8 q8h PO	Sedation
	Prochlorperazine	See above		
	Chlorpromazine	See above		
M_1-cholinergic antagonists	Scopolamine	Vestibular, CRTZ	0.03 q6h SC, IM	Sedation, xerostomia
	Pirenzepine	Vestibular, CRTZ	Unknown	
	Prochlorperazine	See above		
	Chlorpromazine	See above		
5-HT_3-serotonergic antagonists	Ondansetron	CRTZ, vagal afferents	0.5-1 q12-24h PO	Sedation, head shaking in both
	Granisetron	CRTZ, vagal afferents	Unknown	
	Metoclopramide	See above		
5-HT_4-serotonergic antagonists	Cisapride	Myenteric neurons	0.1-0.5 q8h, PO	None reported

IM, Intramuscular; *IV*, intravenous; *PO*, oral; *SC*, subcutaneous.

cholinergic, 5-HT_3-serotonergic, and 5-HT_4-serotonergic. Some of these drugs have several mechanisms of action as antiemetics. The phenothiazines (e.g., prochlorperazine, chlorpromazine) are antagonists of α_1- and α_2-adrenergic, D_2-dopaminergic, H_1- and H_2-histaminergic, and muscarinergic cholinergic receptors. They are very potent but should be avoided in dehydrated or hypotensive animals without previous fluid support, and they are contraindicated in animals with known seizure history. Metoclopramide blocks receptors in the CRTZ, increases the threshold in the emetic center, and has an effect on the viscera (increased lower esophageal sphincter tone, decreased pyloric sphincter tone, increased gastric and duodenal amplitude and contraction). This makes metoclopramide useful in controlling vomiting from nonspecific gastritis or gastric motility disorder. Metoclopramide can be given orally, intravenously, or as a constant rate infusion.

Chronic Gastritis

The pathogenesis for chronic gastritis in dogs and cats is not fully understood. In some cases a cause such as parasitism or metabolic disorder (uremia, hepatopathy) can be identified. Several dog breeds are at risk for chronic gastritis, including the basenji, Drentse patrijshond, and Lundehund.[13] In most cases, however, an immune-mediated response is hypothesized to be responsible for inflammatory infiltrates within the gastric mucosa. Experimentally, chronic gastritis can be produced in dogs via mucosal irritants, systemic administration of gastric juice, or prenatal thymectomy. Each of these disturbs oral tolerance. Chronic idiopathic gastritis is probably a subset of the inflammatory bowel disease syndrome and may arise as an adverse reaction to food or bacterial antigens. The presence of gastric *Helicobacter* species in dogs almost certainly does not cause chronic gastritis. In cats the clinical role of gastric *Helicobacter* species is less clear. These bacteria can be seen in 70% to 95% of dogs and cats, depending on living conditions and if the animals were pretreated with antimicrobial agents. Dogs and cats can be infected with several *Helicobacter* species *(Helicobacter heilmannii, Helicobacter felis, Helicobacter bizzozeronii, Helicobacter salomonis)*, which complicates the investigation into the pathogenic role of gastric spiral organisms. Experimentally and naturally infected dogs have no change in morphology and function of their stomach when compared with uninfected dogs.[14] Cats experimentally infected with *H. felis* have only minor changes in gastric function. As mentioned previously, this finding is in contrast to effects seen in humans, in whom *H. pylori* is responsible for 70% of gastric ulcers and 90% of duodenal ulcers and is considered a carcinogen.

Clinical signs in dogs and cats with chronic gastritis are characterized by chronic persistent or intermittent vomiting of variable frequency and character. Because inflammation impairs motility and delays emptying, animals with chronic gastritis may retain food in the stomach for long periods of time. A definite diagnosis of chronic gastritis requires a mucosal biopsy. Histopathology then categorizes the forms into lymphocytic-plasmacytic gastritis, eosinophilic gastritis, atrophic gastritis, or hypertrophic gastritis.

Eosinophilic gastritis is an uncommon disorder of unknown cause that is characterized by diffuse eosinophilic infiltration in any combination of the distal stomach, small bowel, or colon. Gastric infiltration is usually restricted to the mucosa but in a few animals may extend through the muscularis to the serosa. Mucosal involvement causes enlargement of the rugal folds. The diseased mucosa may become ulcerated, which leads to bleeding or leakage of plasma protein into the gastric lumen. Peripheral eosinophilia is a common but a varied finding. Some pets also have a history of either urticaria or vomiting that may be associated with the ingestion of a specific diet.

Chronic hypertrophic gastritis is a rare disorder that appears either as a diffuse, generalized mucosal hypertrophy or, more frequently, as a localized hypertrophy of the antral mucosa that may cause intermittent or chronic pyloric obstruction. Causative factors that may lead to gastric mucosal hypertrophy include chronic inflammation, foreign bodies, or long-term drug (proton-pump inhibitors) administration. Neuroendocrine factors (e.g., hypergastrinemia) can have a trophic effect on the mucosa, as seen in chronic renal disease, chronic gastric distension, gastrin-secreting tumors (gastrinoma), and idiopathic hypertrophy of antral G cells. The diffuse form has a predilection for boxers and basenjis, whereas the localized form has a predilection for miniature and toy dog breeds (e.g., Lhasa apso, Shih Tzu, Pekingese, and Maltese). The hypertrophic mucosa is inflamed and causes delayed emptying, chronic vomiting, anorexia, and lethargy.

Atrophic gastritis is a rare disorder in which the gastric mucosa atrophies and loses its secretory function. The cause is unknown, but the condition occurs mainly in older dogs and may be mediated through immune mechanisms. It may also be a sequel to chronic reflux gastritis in dogs. The predominant complaint is chronic intermittent vomiting. Mucosal degeneration is thought to result in achlorhydria, which may predispose to bacterial overgrowth in the proximal small intestine. This can lead to malabsorption, chronic diarrhea, and loss of body weight and condition.

Treatment. If possible, the underlying mechanism should be managed first (e.g., removal of foreign body, cessation of drug administration). This, however, is rarely possible, and rational treatment options include dietary management, immunosuppressive therapy, inhibition or neutralization of gastric acid secretion (see discussion of treatment of gastric ulcers) or symptomatic antiemetic drug administration (see discussion of treatment of acute gastritis). Dietary management is based on the concept that antigens in foodstuffs are responsible for the immune-mediated problem. Feeding a novel protein and carbohydrate source, to which the animal has not been exposed, is the cornerstone of this concept. Although commercial "hypoallergenic" diets (e.g., Hill's Prescription Diet z/d; Iams Response FP; Waltham Hypersensitivity Control; Purina Limited Antigen brand Formula) are very useful, on rare occasions it is necessary to feed a home-cooked novel protein source (kangaroo, horse, and squirrel). Normally, some positive response should be seen after a 4-week strict dietary trial.

Immunosuppressive drug therapy is indicated in those dogs and cats that do not respond to dietary management alone (e.g., those with lymphocytic-plasmacytic or eosinophilic gastritis). Corticosteroids, in addition to their immunosuppressive and antiinflammatory properties, have regenerative effects on gastric parietal cells. The ulcerogenic property of corticosteroids is of concern only in dogs in which a marked synergistic ulcerogenic effect is present (e.g., because of NSAIDs or hypotension). Initially, prednisone is given at a dose of 1 mg/kg twice daily for 5 to 7 days. This dose is then gradually tapered in decremental doses of 50% over a period of several months. Other immunosuppressive drugs, such as azathioprine and cyclophosphamide, have been used only rarely in dogs with chronic gastritis and should not be used for this purpose in cats.

Hairballs (Trichobezoars) in Cats

Periodic "hairball" vomiting is considered normal for most cats, particularly the longhaired breeds, as long as no other signs of illness are present and it is not excessive. Sometimes cats will attempt to vomit up a hairball but are unsuccessful, producing a vomit of only bile and phlegm. A few cats develop hairball problems as a result of an underlying medical condition such as skin problems (e.g., flea allergy), intestinal disease, or neurologic disease. Cats that excessively groom themselves or other cats (sedentary behavior) are more likely to have hairballs. Hair is normally emptied from the stomach by powerful interdigestive aborally propagated gastric contractions (motor myoelectric complexes), and its accumulation to form a hairball suggests a potentially underlying defect in gastric motility. Gastric mucosal biopsy in cats with hairballs is unnecessary but would mostly reveal plasmacytic-lymphocytic gastritis with or without concomitant plasmacytic-lymphocytic enteritis.

Treatment. Removal of potential underlying problems is the first step. Nutritional control can be aided by using a high-fiber diet such as Hill's Prescription Diet Feline w/d in the young to middle-aged, normal-weight cat or Hill's Prescription Diet Feline r/d in the older, overweight cat. Lubrication of the gastrointestinal tract with petrolatum-based laxatives (e.g., Felaxin, Laxatone, Kat-A-Lax) can help in the short term.

Gastric Ulcers

By definition, an ulcer consists of damaged gastric mucosa to the level of the lamina muscularis mucosae or deeper. More superficial damage is called *erosion*. Such injury takes place when the "aggressive forces" (acid, pepsin, trauma) are more potent than the "protective forces" (mucosal microcirculation, epithelial turnover, gastric mucus, and prostaglandins). The epithelial cells have a rapid turnover and need an abundant blood circulation to ensure the transport of nutrients and oxygen and the removal of back-diffused hydrogen ions (H^+). The entire gastric surface is replaced every 2 to 3 days. Epithelial cells are produced in the crypts and migrate toward the stomach lumen, where they are shed. Gastric mucous neck cells produce a viscous gel of glycoprotein (5%) and water (95%), which adheres to the surface of the mucosa. This mucus protects against mechanical abrasion and acts as a barrier against digestive enzymes. In addition, bicarbonate is secreted actively into this layer. A pH gradient forms from lumen to epithelium, which neutralizes gastric acid. Finally, prostaglandins, which are derived from arachidonic acid via the enzyme cyclooxygenase (COX), have a protective role for the gut mucosa. They increase gastric mucus and bicarbonate secretion, maintain the mucosal blood flow by vasodilatation, and inhibit acid secretion. They may possibly stimulate mucosal cell turnover and migration by acting as an intercellular messenger. Prostaglandin-inhibiting drugs like NSAIDs can counteract all these mechanisms and lead to the formation of gastric ulcers.

Peptic ulcers of the gastric and duodenal mucosa are not commonly seen in dogs or cats. Several underlying mechanisms can lead to the ulcer formation (Box 12-7). NSAIDs (aspirin, flunixin, ibuprofen, indomethacin, ketoprofen, meloxicam, naproxen, phenylbutazone, piroxicam) inhibit the COX-1 enzyme, thereby limiting prostaglandin production. These drugs are by far the most common cause of peptic ulcers in dogs. Although eicosanoids produced by COX-1 are mainly responsible for the inflammatory and pain properties, those produced by COX-2 are mainly responsible for the protective role in the stomach.

BOX 12-7 Causes of Peptic Ulcers in Older Dogs and Cats

Drugs

NSAIDs
Corticosteroids (only if combined with other causes or with NSAIDs)

Infiltrative Disease

Gastric tumor
Pythiosis in endemic areas
Inflammatory bowel disease

Metabolic Diseases

Hepatopathy
Renal disease (common in older cats)

Hyperacidity

Gastrinoma
Mast cell tumor (rarely causes gastric ulcers)
APUDoma

Other Causes

Pancreatitis
Hypovolemia
Septic shock
Disseminated intravascular coagulation
Foreign objects (might worsen preexisting gastritis or ulceration)
Chemical toxins
Stress?

NSAIDs, Nonsteroidal antiinflammatory drugs; *APUDoma*, amine precursor uptake and decarboxylation tumors.

Unspecific COX inhibition increases the ulcerogenic risk dramatically. Newer NSAIDs are COX-2 specific (carprofen) and have a lower, although not abolished, incidence of peptic ulcers.

Corticosteroids decrease the production of protective eicosanoids, as well; nevertheless, they are responsible for peptic ulcers only in dogs with marked concurrent problems (e.g., severe hypotension) or if given together with NSAIDs. Mast cell tumors have long been thought to be responsible for peptic ulcers because of the histamine-containing granules, which can cause hyperacidity in the stomach. In multiple studies, however, no signs of gastric ulcers were found in dogs undergoing surgery for mast cell tumors, and their ulcerogenic role must be reevaluated. Finally, most dogs with acute intervertebral disk diseases have endoscopic signs of gastric erosions,[15] and surgical interventions with or without corticosteroids greatly increase the risk for peptic ulcers. Clinical signs of peptic ulceration are poorly defined. Chronic vomiting is probably the most frequent sign, with or without hematemesis. Unlike humans, the dog does not secrete acid continuously and blood in the vomitus does not, therefore, always appear digested. Melena and anemia may also be observed if bleeding is severe. Inappetence and anorexia are common. The history should also include specific questions about any medications the owner may be administering to the animal.

Diagnosis and Treatment. Although gastroscopy is by far the best tool to diagnose gastric ulcers, this is often not necessary if the history (NSAID administration, hematemesis) and clinical findings are indicative of the diagnosis. Diagnosis can also be made based on contrast radiographic studies or exploratory laparotomy. The latter has the disadvantage that the gastric mucosa is not easily evaluated from the exterior of the stomach. The goals of antiulcer therapy are to eliminate clinical signs, complications, and relapses (see Table 12-1). It is vital to avoid ulcerogenic drugs. Antacids work by neutralizing gastric acid. Calcium carbonate ($CaCO_3$), sodium bicarbonate ($NaHCO_3$), magnesium hydroxide ($Mg[OH]_2$) or aluminum hydroxide ($Al[OH]_3$) all contain an H^+-binding group. The neutralizing reaction with gastric acid produces water and a neutral salt. Antacids are also of benefit in that they bind to bile acids, decrease pepsin activity in the stomach, and stimulate the secretion of endogenous prostaglandins. However, frequent dosage and poor palatability make antacids an inconvenient drug for animals.

Histamine H_2-receptor antagonists block the secretion of stomach acid via their blockade of the gastric parietal cell histamine H_2 receptor. Cimetidine and ranitidine are used equally in veterinary medicine. Clinical trials comparing cimetidine and ranitidine showed no advantage of one drug over another. Ranitidine is 5 to 12 times more potent than cimetidine, has a longer half-life, and allows for a decreased frequency of administration. Famotidine and nizatidine are newer histamine H_2-receptor antagonists. In addition to their blockade of the gastric parietal cell histamine H_2 receptor, the histamine H_2-receptor antagonists increase luminal secretion of bicarbonate and mucus as well as raising mucosal blood flow. These effects may be related to a stimulation of prostaglandin synthesis. As another effect, cimetidine supposedly increases in vitro cell-mediated immunity by blocking the H_2 receptors on T lymphocytes. Cimetidine decreases liver perfusion and is recognized as an inhibitor of hepatic metabolizing P-450 and P-488 enzymes. Drugs metabolized via this mechanism may be cleared more slowly and reach a higher plasma level. Other histamine H_2-receptor antagonists do not show this interaction and may be preferred in animals receiving multiple drugs.

Omeprazole, a substituted benzimidazole, belongs to a newer class of drugs called *proton-pump inhibitors.* By blocking the H^+/K^+-APTase enzyme at the luminal membrane of the parietal cell, acid secretion is inhibited regardless of the secretagogue. Compared with cimetidine, omeprazole is about 20 times more potent and has a longer duration of action, because it accumulates in a pH-dependent manner. Newer proton-pump inhibitors include lansoprazole or pantoprazole.

Sucralfate is a gastromucosal protectant. It is a basic salt of a sulfate disaccharide with many aluminum hydroxide groups. It dissociates, after oral ingestion, to sucrose octasulfate and aluminum hydroxide and buffers H^+. Sucrose octasulfate reacts in the stomach with hydrochloric acid to form a paste-like complex that has greater affinity for damaged tissue than normal mucosa. Further damage by pepsin, acid, or bile will be prevented. Sucralfate may also have some cytoprotective effects, possibly because of stimulation of prostaglandin. Systemic absorption of sucralfate is minimal, and it is extremely well tolerated. Finally, misoprostil is a synthetic analog of prostaglandin E_1 (PGE_1). Although orally administered, it should be absorbed into the circulation to be effective. Its effect is the same as those of endogenous prostaglandins. Although the prophylactic effect of misoprostil in dogs receiving corticosteroids or undergoing spinal surgery is debatable, it is clear that this drug is not useful in dogs that already have a peptic ulcer.

Gastric Motility Disorders

Gastric emptying is a highly coordinated physiologic response to the presence of food in the stomach. This emptying can be impaired in several pathologic conditions. There are three general gastric motility disorders: accelerated gastric emptying, retrograde transit, and delayed gastric emptying. Delayed gastric emptying can be due to mechanical or functional obstruction. Causes of mechanical obstruction are pyloric stenosis, chronic hypertrophic pyloric gastropathy, foreign bodies, pyloric or duodenal neoplasia, chronic hypertrophic gastritis, or intraabdominal masses causing external compression of the pylorus. Functional disorders of gastric emptying result from one or more abnormalities in gastric motility. These motility disorders cause no morphologic changes. Inflammatory and infiltrative lesions, gastric ulceration, inflammatory bowel disease, altered electrolyte concentrations, acid-base disturbances, recent abdominal surgery, diabetes mellitus, and several drugs can affect gastric motility.

In normal monogastric animals the pylorus performs a sieving function during the postprandial period. Liquids pass easily and empty relatively rapidly from the stomach by first-order kinetics. The rate of liquid expulsion from the stomach is proportional to its volume: the greater the gastric fluid, the more rapidly it is expelled. Solids are handled differently, requiring reduction to small particles (<2 mm in diameter) before passage through the pyloric canal. In dogs, large food particles are normally retained in the stomach after feeding and pass into the duodenum only during the interdigestive period. During this period, called the *migrating motility complex* or *housekeeper contraction,* a special mechanism exists to expel these larger particles together with swallowed saliva, a small basal secretion of mucus and cellular debris. One migrating motility complex, which lasts about 2 hours, is divided in four phases, the third causing intense bursts of action potentials resulting in powerful distal gastric peristaltic contraction and emptying of larger particles. Abnormal gastric emptying is assumed to affect solid-phase gastric contents rather than liquids.

Diagnosis of mechanical obstruction is generally straightforward, whereas functional obstruction causing delayed gastric motility may be more difficult to confirm. Several methods are available for evaluating gastric emptying (Table 12-3). Contrast radiographic techniques are the most commonly available means for diagnosing gastric motility disorders in veterinary practice. Gastric emptying times for liquids, including barium suspension, are relatively short (about 1 hour in cats, up to 3 hours in dogs). Studies using barium mixed with food have shown gastric emptying times varying from 4 to 16 hours in the dog and 4 to 17 hours in the cat, depending on the composition of the food, thus making it difficult to diagnose an emptying disorder unless gastric emptying times are markedly prolonged. Furthermore, when solid meals are mixed with barium granules or suspension, the barium can dissociate from the food and redistribute into the liquid phase of the gastric contents. More recently, BIPS have been used to quantify gastric emptying in dogs and cats (see Figure 12-1). BIPS are produced in two diameters: 1.5 mm and 5 mm. The small BIPS are designed to empty with small particles, thereby mimicking solid-phase gastric emptying. Large BIPS tend to be retained in the stomach longer than small BIPS, often remaining after the test meal has passed into the duodenum and then leaving the stomach once the migrating motility complex begins. They should accumulate immediately orad to obstructing lesions. Interpretation of BIPS gastric emptying data has some of the same limitations as that of barium studies. The use of BIPS may be more helpful in documentation of mechanical than in documentation of functional obstruction.

TABLE 12-3. TECHNIQUES TO EVALUATE GASTROINTESTINAL MOTILITY DISORDERS

TECHNIQUE	INFORMATION GAINED	AVAILABILITY
Survey radiographs	+	+++
Contrast radiographs (barium)	+++	+++
Contrast radiographs (BIPS)	++	+++
Ultrasonography	+	++
Endoscopy	++	++
Breath test	++	+ - ++
Scintigraphy	+++	+ (referral institution)
Computed tomography	+	+ (referral institution)
Manometry	++	+ (referral institution)

BIPS, Barium-impregnated polyethylene spheres; + to +++ grades semiquantitatively from least to most the amount of possible information gained and the availability of each technique.

In humans, ultrasonography has been used as an alternative method of measuring gastric emptying times. Finding more than just a small amount of fluid in the stomach 18 hours after feeding provides evidence of delayed gastric emptying in the dog. Recently, gastric emptying has been evaluated by means of breath testing.[16] The main advantages of breath test technology are that no radiation is required; tests are noninvasive and non–operator dependent; and tests can be performed several times in the same subject without biologic hazard. Breath tracer studies of gastrointestinal transit involve detection of a gas or isotope produced in response to either the ingestion of a meal or administration of a labeled substrate. The substrate or meal is rapidly digested and absorbed at the site of interest by enzymatic degradation or microbial digestion, and the rate and appearance of the gas or isotope in breath is a direct reflection of the gastrointestinal transit of the substrate. The ^{13}C–octanoic acid breath test (^{13}C-OBT) is based on the administration of octanoic acid (a medium chain fatty acid) with a functional group containing ^{13}C. On leaving the stomach, the ^{13}C–octanoic acid is rapidly absorbed in the duodenum and metabolized in the liver. After oxidation, the resulting $^{13}CO_2$ is excreted into breath, which can be collected and measured by isotope mass spectrometry. Because gastric emptying is the rate-limiting step in the process of absorption and metabolism of the labeled substrate, the appearance of the ^{13}C in the exhaled breath is a direct reflection of the rate and pattern of gastric emptying. Finally, scintigraphy is considered the gold standard technique for measuring gastric emptying.

History and Clinical Signs. Affected animals appear normal except for intermittent postprandial vomiting. The vomitus is characteristically undigested or partly digested and occasionally mucoid and may have an acid pH; bile is absent. The precise interrelationships between pyloric stenosis and pylorospasm are unclear. Signs of gastric outlet obstruction vary with the degree of obstruction. Vomiting is the predominant sign and may occur at any time after a meal. The time for complete emptying of a normal meal from the stomach in the dog fed once daily is 7 to 8 hours. Vomiting of all or part of a meal at periods more than 10 hours after ingestion suggests delayed gastric emptying and the probability of a gastric, pancreatic, or proximal duodenal lesion.

Treatment. In addition to dietary therapy a prokinetic therapy is often needed. A low-fat, highly digestible blended or liquid diet with increased frequency of feeding may be helpful. Dopaminergic agonists (e.g., metoclopramide) have gastrointestinal prokinetic and antiemetic properties because they inhibit peripheral and/or central dopamine receptors. The exact mechanism of the prokinetic activity is not entirely clear but may be more due to other pharmacologic properties (e.g., 5-HT_3-receptor or 5-HT_4-receptor antagonism). Metoclopramide increases the amplitude and frequency of antral contractions, inhibits fundic receptive relaxation, and coordinates gastric, pyloric, and duodenal motility, all of which result in accelerated gastric emptying. Erythromycin, an antibiotic, has motilin-like action. It increases the pressure of the gastroesophageal sphincter and accelerates gastric emptying by inducing antral contractions similar to phase III of the migrating motility complex. The prokinetic dose is much lower than the antimicrobial dose. Some histamine H_2-receptor antagonists (ranitidine and nizatidine) have acetylcholinesterase-inhibiting properties, thereby stimulating gastric emptying and small-intestinal and colonic motility.

Cisapride was used to treat several gastrointestinal motility disorders in dogs and cats throughout the 1990s. Because of unexplained deaths in humans, cisapride has been taken off the market. Newer prokinetic drugs are tegaserod (Zelmac) and prucalopride (R093877, Janssen). Tegaserod is a potent partial nonbenzamide agonist at 5-HT_4 receptors and a weak agonist at 5-HT_{1D} receptors with known prokinetic effects in the canine colon. In vitro studies suggest that tegaserod does not delay cardiac repolarization or prolong the QT interval of the electrocardiogram as had been occasionally reported with cisapride. Clinical efficacy has been demonstrated in human motility disorders. Gastric and intestinal effects of tegaserod have not been reported in the dog, so this drug may not prove as useful as cisapride in stimulating proximal gastrointestinal motility. Prucalopride is a potent partial benzamide agonist at 5-HT_4 receptors but has no effect on other 5-HT receptors and lacks cholinesterase enzyme activity. Unlike tegaserod, prucalopride also appears to stimulate gastric emptying in the dog. Neither tegaserod nor prucalopride are commercially available.

The only effective treatment for hypertrophic disease in the stomach is pyloroplasty. In a few animals, outlet obstruction may be sufficiently severe that nutritional homeostasis cannot be sustained on any kind of diet, and enteral or parenteral feeding becomes essential.

Acute Gastric Dilatation-Volvulus

Acute gastric dilatation-volvulus is a sudden and often fatal gastrointestinal disorder that affects particularly large, deep-chested breeds (Great Dane, German shepherd, standard poodle, large mixed breed).[17] It has been estimated that there are as many as 60,000 cases in the United States each year, with an overall mortality of about 15% to 20% depending on the time from onset of signs to treatment. Although gastric dilatation-volvulus may occur at any age, there is a greater risk of occurrence in older dogs.[18] Gastric dilatation from rapid distention of the stomach with food, fluid, and especially gas (from swallowed air or fermentation) may progress to volvulus. This occurs because the forces exerted on the distended canine stomach cause it to rotate either to the right or left (most often to the left in a clockwise direction) on an axis at right angles to a line between the esophageal and pyloric sphincters.

A single causative agent in the pathogenesis of acute gastric dilatation-volvulus has not yet been identified. Several intrinsic physical risk factors (body size and thoracoabdominal dimension) and environmental risk factors (diet, accumulation of gastric gas, anesthesia, stress, being asleep) have been identified, and many more intrinsic anatomic (gastric ligament laxity, gastric volume and position, gastric hormones such as gastrin) and pathologic (gastric rhythm, motility and emptying) risk factors are suspected.[18] Feeding and exercise patterns did not alter the incidence of gastric dilatation-volvulus in a large population of military dogs.

History and Clinical Signs. The onset of clinical signs is usually acute or peracute. Abdominal distention is associated with progressive restlessness, unproductive retching, salivation, dyspnea, and gastric tympany, leading to severe pain and shock. Prolonged gastric distension markedly decreases the prognosis because mucosal ischemic changes may be irreversible. Death from hypovolemic and cardiogenic shock may occur within a few hours of the onset of signs. Rapid gastric distention adversely affects the function of the lower esophageal sphincter and appears to impair gastric motility and emptying. It has been postulated that distention occludes the gastroesophageal junction, precluding emptying by either eructation or emesis. Distention decreases gastric motility by impairing normal contraction and by reflex nervous inhibition. Following dilatation, the gastric mucosa and later the gastric smooth muscle undergoes potentially irreversible ischemic necrosis. There is also an accumulation and sequestration of gastric secretions. The distended stomach occludes venous return from the rear limbs and caudal abdomen and precipitates hypovolemic and cardiogenic shock. Lactic acid and other metabolic by-products accumulate in the poorly perfused hind limbs and viscera to cause severe metabolic acidosis, especially after relief of the gastric dilatation. Signs of reperfusion injury, endotoxemia, disseminated intravascular coagulation, and fatal cardiac arrhythmias may also occur. Splenic torsion with infarction and necrosis is a common sequel.

Diagnosis and Initial Treatment. Management of hypovolemia (to prevent or treat shock) is the primary goal of emergency treatment of gastric dilatation-volvulus. Fluid therapy should be started at a rate of 90 ml/kg intravenously through large-bore catheters with crystalloid solutions (e.g., lactated Ringer's solution) until the animal is stabilized. This fluid bolus is followed by high-volume crystalloid administration (20 ml/kg/hour) for maintenance of resuscitation. Gastric decompression is attempted only after correction of the hypovolemia is well under way. This can usually be achieved by orogastric intubation in unsedated animals using an equine nasogastric tube with large end and side holes. If orogastric intubation is unsuccessful, aseptically right- or left-sided gastrocentesis with a large-bore needle should be performed. Radiography is not necessary to diagnose gastric dilatation but is invaluable in diagnosing volvulus (Figure 12-5). When vital signs are stable, the dog should be taken to surgery for decompression and treatment of the volvulus. Small amounts of induction agents

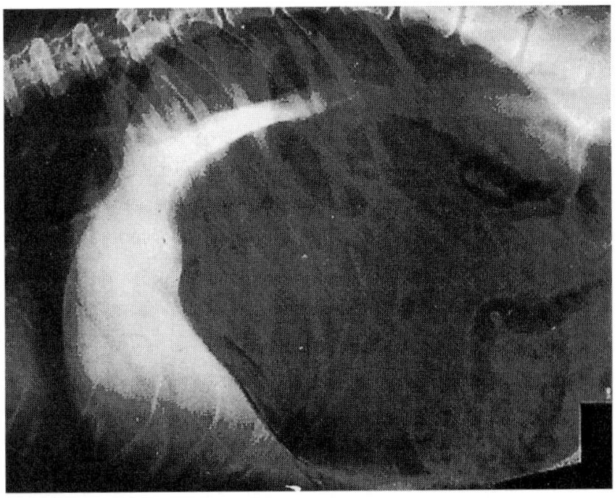

Figure 12-5. Typical radiographic picture of a gastric dilatation-volvulus ("double-bubble is trouble"). (Courtesy of Dr. Dan Brockman, Royal Veterinary College, London.)

(e.g., thiopental, propofol) are given to effect, and anesthesia should be maintained with halothane or isoflurane in oxygen. Nitrous oxide is not given until permanent gastric decompression is performed. Contemporary surgical experience suggests that the incidence of recurrence may be reduced by gastropexy. Cardiac arrhythmias, usually premature ventricular contraction or ventricular tachycardia, occur frequently up to 3 days after surgical correction and require treatment if there is evidence of poor cardiac performance. Follow-up management includes feeding of a meat-based, canned, highly digestible diet at least three times daily in conjunction with gastropexy as the best approach to the prevention of recurrence. Pyloroplasty does not influence the rate of recurrence.

Gastric Tumors

Primary gastric tumors are rare in the dog. Ninety percent are malignant, with adenocarcinoma (74%), lymphoma (8%), and leiomyosarcoma (4%) being the most commonly encountered. Leiomyoma and adenoma are the benign tumors. Adenocarcinomas are more likely in the antrum and lesser curvature, with a potential breed predilection for the Belgian shepherd, collie, and Staffordshire bull terrier. In cats, gastric tumors are even less common, with only 11% of all gastrointestinal tumors arising from the stomach. Lymphoma is by far the most common tumor in cats, with an average age at onset of 11 years. While *H. pylori* is clearly a risk factor for gastric adenocarcinoma and mucosa-associated lymphatic tissue lymphomas (MALTomas) in humans, there is no proven association of *Helicobacter* species and neoplasia in dogs. Only recently, however, MALT gastric lymphoma of the cat was thought to be potentially *Helicobacter* dependent.[19]

Gastric tumors are characterized by chronic vomiting of gradually increasing severity, inappetence or anorexia, and loss of body weight and condition. Anemia, diarrhea, and hematemesis may also be present. The time from onset of signs to presentation may vary from as little as 2 to 3 weeks to as long as 12 months. Signs may be subtler in some animals, with, for example, anorexia of sudden onset as the only presenting sign.

Contrast radiography may show delayed gastric emptying, mucosal filling defects, a rigid gastric wall, or ulcers. Ultrasound is often superior to radiography and may show a thickened wall of the stomach with potential loss of the normal layers, enlarged regional lymph nodes, or abdominal metastasis. Ultrasound-guided fine needle aspirates can be taken from a markedly thickened stomach wall.[20] Diagnosis is confirmed by gastroscopy and biopsy or by surgical biopsy. Gastric tumors often ulcerate and resemble peptic ulcers, so examination of a deep biopsy specimen is essential for diagnosis (Figure 12-6).

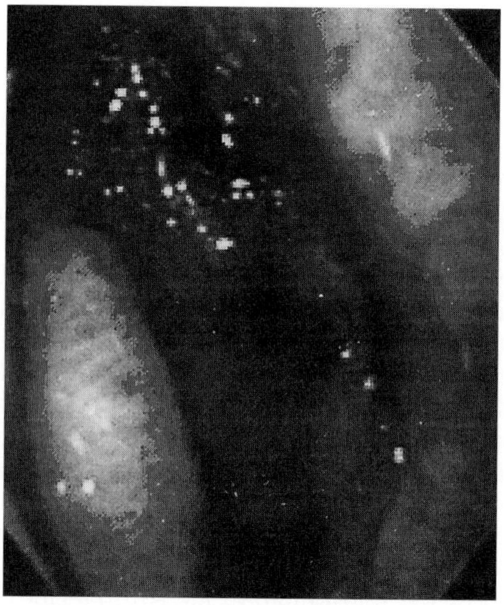

Figure 12-6. Endoscopic view of a peptic ulcer in a 9-year-old Staffordshire bull terrier with a gastric adenocarcinoma. The tumor was very hard, and no signs of malignancy were seen on endoscopic biopsies. Intraoperatively the entire lesser curvature including pylorus was involved.

Except for lymphomas, treatment is by wide surgical excision if clinically feasible. However, despite this, the prognosis is almost invariably grave.

SMALL INTESTINE

Malabsorption caused by bacterial overgrowth syndrome, chronic pancreatitis, or celiac disease is the most frequent problem encountered in the small intestine in geriatric human medicine.[21] With the possible exception of some types of neoplasia, there are no specific age-related small intestinal diseases of older dogs or cats. Acute small intestinal diarrhea—such as bacterial enteritis (salmonellosis, campylobacteriosis, yersiniosis, enteropathogenic *E. coli* infection), protozoal enteritis *(Giardia)*, enteritis caused by helminths, or diarrhea caused by ingestion of garbage or intoxicants—can also occur in older pets, but these conditions are less common than in younger animals.

Inflammatory Bowel Disease

The term *inflammatory bowel disease* broadly refers to a group of idiopathic gastrointestinal disorders characterized by the infiltration of the mucosa with varying numbers of inflammatory cells. Despite the high prevalence of ulcerative colitis and Crohn's disease in human medicine and inflammatory bowel disease in animals and a plethora of studies, no clear pathogenesis is known. Interactions among the mucosal immune system, host genetic susceptibility (e.g., basenji with lymphoplasmacytic enteritis or boxer with ulcerative colitis), and environmental factors are important. Inflammatory bowel disease is thought to result from either an abnormal immune response (e.g., host hypersensitivity precipitated by increased intestinal permeability, defective suppressor function of gut-associated lymphoid tissue, or other yet-to-be-defined primary immunologic event) or an appropriate immune response to an enteric pathogen.[22] Either way, cellular components (activated intestinal B and T lymphocytes) and molecular elements (cytokines, complement, eicosanoids) contribute to mucosal inflammation.

Lymphocytic-plasmacytic enteritis or enterocolitis (LPE) is the most common form of inflammatory bowel disease in cats and dogs. Some breeds, such as German shepherd dogs, Chinese Shar-Pei, soft-coated wheaten terriers, and possibly purebred cats, seem at increased risk for LPE. Basenjis and Lundehunds are subject to a particular form of severe immunoproliferative lymphocytic-plasmacytic enteritis.[23] *Eosinophilic enteritis*, which is considerably less common than LPE (and occurs more frequently in dogs than in cats) might be a variant of inflammatory bowel disease or an allergic manifestation to dietary or parasitic antigens. A severe form is hypereosinophilic syndrome, which exists in cats and rarely in dogs. German shepherd dogs and Irish setters might be predisposed to eosinophilic inflammatory bowel disease. Several inflammatory bowel disease variants, such as chronic histiocytic-ulcerative colitis, suppurative colitis, and granulomatous enterocolitis (regional enteritis), are occasionally diagnosed.

History and Clinical Signs. Animals with inflammatory bowel disease normally present with chronic small, large, or mixed diarrhea (depending on location of inflammation), vomiting, anorexia, lethargy, and weight loss. The animal may be cachectic if mucosal damage is severe, and edema or ascites may be detected if the disease process is sufficiently advanced to cause protein-losing enteropathy. Thickened intestinal loops may occasionally be palpated.

Diagnosis. Differential diagnoses of disorders resembling inflammatory bowel disease in older dogs and cats include intestinal neoplasia, lymphangiectasia, fungal infection, chronic parasitism (including giardiasis), feline infectious peritonitis, and feline hyperthyroidism. A definite diagnosis of inflammatory bowel disease can be made only from intestinal biopsies taken by endoscopy, laparoscopy, or laparotomy (Figure 12-7). Hematology might reveal thrombocytopenia in LPE[2] and eosinophilia in eosinophilic enteritis (more common in cats than dogs). The serum chemistry profile may show pan-hypoproteinemia in animals with protein-losing enteropathy caused by inflammatory bowel disease. Not uncommonly, cats have liver involvement with inflammatory bowel disease and increased serum liver enzymes activities. Serum folate concentration may be increased, suggesting bacterial overgrowth, or may be normal to decreased, suggesting severe proximal small intestinal disease. Serum cobalamin activity is either normal or decreased, suggesting distal small intestinal disease.[24]

Treatment. Management of inflammatory bowel disease may include controlled diets, dietary fiber supplementation, and administration of antimicrobial, antiinflammatory, and immunosuppressive drugs. No large trials have been conducted, and treatment remains largely empirical.

Dietary Therapy. Because dietary antigens are thought to play an important role in the pathogenesis of inflammatory bowel disease, the diet

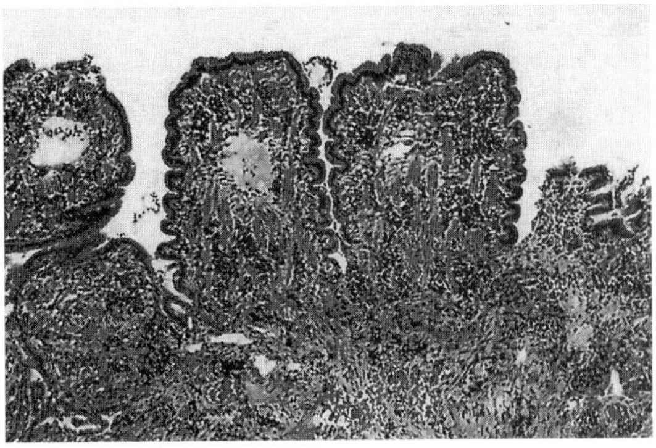

Figure 12-7. Blunted and fused villi with infiltration of lymphocytes and plasma cells of the duodenal mucosa from an 8-year-old German shepherd dog with marked inflammatory bowel disease. The dog responded to dietary management and corticosteroids.

is usually modified. Modified diets have a characteristic highly digestible protein and carbohydrate source and are relative hypoallergenic, gluten free, low in lactose and fat, nutritionally balanced, and highly palatable. Animals appear to benefit from a diet containing a protein to which they have not been previously exposed (novel proteins such as venison, rabbit, lamb, whitefish, or turkey). Only recently a "sacrificial protein" has been advocated for treatment of inflammatory bowel disease.[25] In this approach, a first novel protein is fed to animals in the early phase of therapy when the bowel is still markedly inflamed and the mucosal barrier porous. After 6 weeks or when the prednisone dose is decreased from immunosuppressive to antiinflammatory, the protein source is changed again, at which time it is hoped that mucosal inflammation has been controlled. The second dietary protein is less likely to result in acquired food hypersensitivity. Recurrence of signs after challenge with known allergens such as soya, beef, or gluten is essential to document the specific dietary sensitivity. Altering the dietary ratio of ω-6 to ω-3 polyunsaturated fatty acids might alter the inflammatory response in the gut, but controlled studies in animals with inflammatory bowel disease are not yet available.[21] Finally, increasing the fiber content of the diet might increase fecal consistency, bind potential colonic irritants, improve abnormal motility, and produce beneficial short-chain fatty acids.

Antimicrobial Therapy. On the premise that abnormal bacterial flora or enteric pathogens may be a cause or complicating factor, the use of antimicrobial therapy is reasonable (Table 12-4). Oral oxytetracycline appears to be effective and has the advantage of being inexpensive. Other choices include metronidazole and tylosin. Some owners find that they can reduce the antimicrobial dose to once daily and still effect a remission of signs. Experimentation with various antimicrobial agents and/or diets should show what combination works best for a particular animal.

Immunosuppressants. The initial drug for treatment of LPE and eosinophilic inflammatory bowel disease is prednisone or prednisolone at an initial dose of 1 to 2 mg/kg orally twice daily for 2 weeks and then tapered in 50% decrements every 2 weeks if signs improve. In mild to

TABLE 12-4. THERAPEUTIC AGENTS USED IN INTESTINAL DISEASES

GENERIC NAME	CLASS OF DRUG	DOSAGES
Azathioprine	Antiinflammatory, immunosuppressive	Dogs: 2 mg/kg q24h then q48h Cats: 0.3-0.5 mg/kg PO q48h
Cisapride	Prokinetic	0.1-1 mg/kg PO q8-12h
Clarithromycin	Antibiotic	5-10 mg/kg PO q12h
Docusate calcium	Emollient laxative	Cats: 50-100 mg PO daily
Docusate sodium	Emollient laxative	50-200 mg PO daily
Erythromycin	Antibiotic Prokinetic	10-20 mg/kg PO q8h 0.5-1 mg/kg PO q8h
Lactulose	Osmotic laxative	0.5-1 mg/kg PO q8-12h
Metronidazole	Antibiotic	10-20 mg/kg PO q8-12h
Mineral oil	Lubricant laxative	5-25 ml daily
Nizatidine	Prokinetic	2.5-5 mg/kg PO q24h
Olsalazine	Antiinflammatory, immunosuppressive	Dogs: 10-20 mg/kg PO q12h
Oxytetracycline	Antibiotic	20 mg/kg PO q8h
Prednisolone	Immunosuppressive	1-2 mg/kg PO q24h starting dose, then decrease slowly
Prucalopride	Prokinetic	0.5 mg/kg PO
Psyllium	Bulk-forming laxative	1-4 tsp PO as needed in food
Ranitidine	Prokinetic	1-2 mg/kg PO q12h
Sulfasalazine	Antiinflammatory, immunosuppressive	10-20 mg/kg PO q8h-q12h
Tegaserod	Prokinetic	0.05 mg/kg PO
Tylosin	Antibiotic	Dogs: 20-40 mg/kg PO q8h Cats: 5-10 mg/kg PO q12h
White petrolatum	Lubricant laxative	1-5 ml daily

PO, Oral.

moderate cases, drug administration on alternate days or every third day can often be achieved in 3 to 4 months and potentially discontinued after 6 months for both cats and dogs. In severe cases the reduction should be much more gradual, and a moderate dose (0.5 mg/kg daily) might be needed long term. Methylprednisolone acetate can be used in cats with mild to moderate inflammatory bowel disease as sole or adjunctive therapy. If remission cannot be maintained with corticosteroid use alone or in combination with metronidazole, or if the side effects of corticosteroids are intolerable, then the concurrent use of azathioprine is indicated. In dogs the dose is 2 to 2.5 mg/kg daily; azathioprine can also be used carefully in cats but in a markedly reduced dose of 0.3 mg/kg once every other day.[26] The owner should be advised about the possible side effect of azathioprine-induced pancreatitis in dogs and should be instructed to check the white blood cell count weekly (and stop the treatment if the white blood cell count falls below 4500/µl). Chronic colitis is better treated with sulfasalazine, which consists of 5-aminosalicylic acid linked by azo-bond to sulfapyridine. It is delivered relatively intact to the colon, where bacteria cleave the azo-bond. The 5-aminosalicylic acid moiety is poorly absorbed and has local antiinflammatory properties. On resolution of clinical signs, sulfasalazine can be gradually tapered by 25% at 2-week intervals and eventually discontinued as dietary management is maintained. The dose of sulfasalazine is much lower in cats (see Table 12-4). Newer immunosuppressive drugs such as cyclosporin or 5-lipoxigenase inhibitors (Zileuton) or newer 5-aminosalicylic acid preparations (enteric coated mesalazine, olsalazine) might be of some use in refractory cases of inflammatory bowel disease, but no information is available at present.

Supplemental Therapy. If weight loss and mucosal disease are severe, it is probable that secondary vitamin deficiencies may be present. Parenteral injection of cobalamin (750 µg/month) and oral folic acid administration (5 mg/day for 1 to 6 months) may be beneficial in dogs, because deficiencies of these vitamins may be due to impaired mucosal uptake. Diarrhea in hypoproteinemic animals may be exacerbated by decreased plasma oncotic pressure (<4 g/dl). Plasma transfusion or human albumin or hetastarch infusion in conjunction with other aggressive therapy often brings about dramatic resolution of signs. Ascites if present should not be treated by paracentesis, because it removes protein from the body and may exacerbate hypoproteinemia. Diuretic therapy using spironolactone is indicated if the ascites is sufficient to cause respiratory distress. Furosemide should only be used in emergency situations when rapid fluid loss is required.

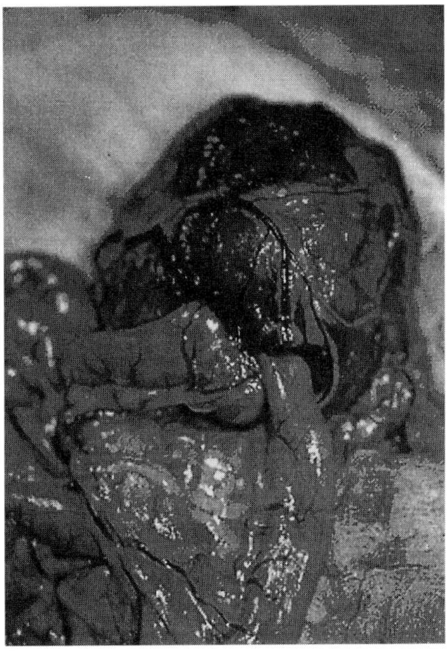

Figure 12-8. Intraoperative view of an alimentary lymphoma in a 13-year-old cat with chronic vomiting. After excision of the mass and end-to-end anastomosis, the cat was treated with chemotherapy and survived 13 months.

Small Intestinal Tumors

Adenocarcinoma, lymphoma, and leiomyosarcoma are the most common malignant intestinal tumors of dogs, whereas cats most frequently have lymphomas (Figure 12-8). All tumors are more common in older animals, but there is no breed or sex predisposition. Lymphoma in cats sometimes results from LPE, and affected cats are usually feline leukemia virus negative. Signs include vomiting, diarrhea, and weight loss and are related to malabsorption and protein-losing enteropathy secondary to infiltration of the intestinal wall. The presence of abnormal bacterial flora is not uncommon, especially if the tumor causes partial intestinal obstruction. Survey abdominal and contrast radiographs are rarely helpful in diagnosing intestinal tumors when no abdominal mass can be palpated. Abdominal ultrasound helps in localizing masses, shows irregular thickened mucosa with loss of the normal layers, and may show a lymphadenopathy or local spread. Ultrasound-guided fine needle aspirates or even true-cut biopsies can sometimes be obtained from an intestinal mass. Endoscopy is only helpful when the tumor is located in the descending limb of the duodenum. Exploratory laparotomy and intestinal and mesenteric node biopsy are confirmatory. Solitary tumors (even alimentary solitary lymphomas, because of the risk of obstruction) should be surgically resected. Lymphomas will then be followed-up with standard chemotherapy protocols. The prognosis for alimentary lymphomas in dogs is guarded, but cats respond moderately well to a combination protocol including doxorubicin and L-asparaginase.[27] Adenocarcinomas carry a poor prognosis in both species unless diagnosed very early, in which case resection of a localized lesion can produce marked clinical improvement. Leiomyomas and leiomyosarcomas are often slow-growing tumors with a good prognosis following complete surgical excision.

COLON, RECTUM, AND ANUS

Primary signs of colonic and rectal disorders are constipation, diarrhea, fecal incontinence, and rectal bleeding. None of these conditions is unique to older animals. In elderly humans diverticulosis, neoplasm, ischemic colitis, fecal incontinence, and constipation occur with increased frequency. In older dogs and cats colonic and rectoanal disease is relatively uncommon. Such animals do, however, occasionally suffer from colonic or rectal tumors and appear to have the same incidence of colonic inflammatory disease as younger animals. Infectious colitis (caused by helminths, bacteria, fungal organisms) occurs, but less commonly than in younger animals. The major large intestinal problem in older dogs and cats is obstipation or constipation.

Constipation

When feces are retained in the colon for a prolonged period of time, water will be absorbed, resulting in gradual impacted feces that become progressively harder and drier. Obstipation is a condition of intractable constipation in which colon and rectum become excessively impacted with hard feces, so that normal defecation cannot happen. *Megacolon* is a term that refers to a disorder, not a clinical sign, in which the colon becomes extremely dilated and hypomotile, usually irreversibly so.

There are a large number of predisposing factors for and underlying causes of constipation, which can be categorized into ingested foreign material, environmental factors, painful conditions, obstruction, neuromuscular disorders, fluid or electrolyte abnormalities, and drug-related effects (Box 12-8). In cats the most common form is idiopathic megacolon, of which the pathogenesis is poorly understood. The disorder may be due to a generalized dysfunction of colonic smooth muscles.

BOX 12-8 Causes of Constipation and Dyschezia in Older Dogs and Cats

Mechanical Obstruction
Colorectal mass
Healed pelvic fracture with narrowed canal
Perineal hernia
Intrapelvic mass (lymph node, tumor, inguinal testicular mass)
Strictures
Prostatomegaly

Neurologic Problems
Paraplegia
Cauda equina
Dysautonomia (Key-Gaskell syndrome)

Pain
Pelvic trauma
Anorectal problems
Anal sac abscess
Tumor
Perianal fistula
Hind limb musculoskeletal problems (hip dysplasia)

Ingested Material (bones, foreign material, cat litter)

Other Causes
Dehydration
Hypothyroidism
Electrolyte abnormalities (hypokalemia)
Drugs (opioids, anticholinergics)
Soiled or absent litter box

Idiopathic Megacolon

History and Clinical Signs. Constipated animals are usually presented with a history of tenesmus (defined as ineffective or painful straining to defecate) and dyschezia (defined as painful defecation) for a period of time ranging from days to weeks to months. Dry, hard feces can be seen around the anus or in the litter box (cats). Chronically constipated animals may have intermittent episodes of hematochezia or diarrhea caused by mucosal irritation. Long-standing problems can lead to anorexia, weight loss, and vomiting.

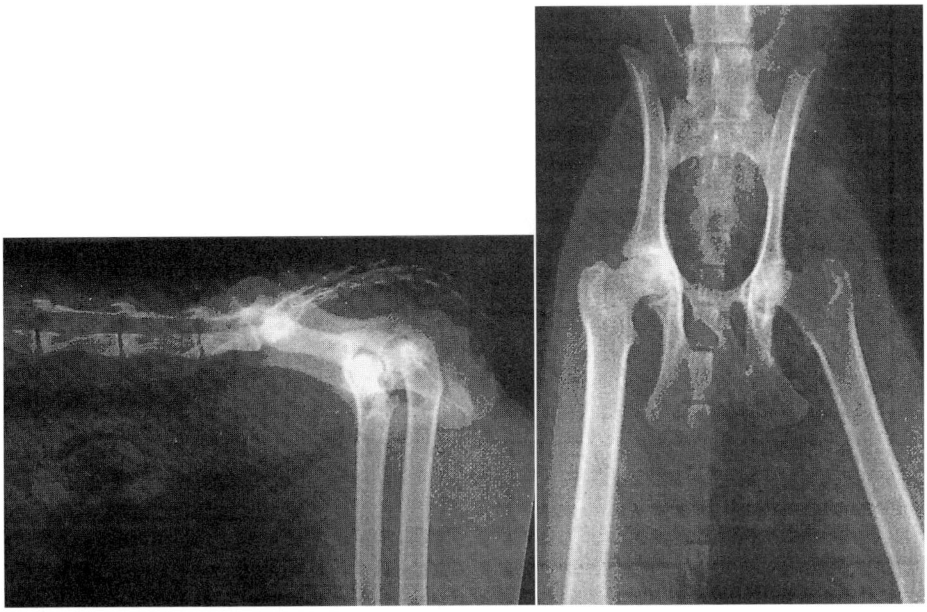

Figure 12-9. Abdominal radiographs of a 12-year-old cat with constipation. **A,** Lateral view shows a constipated colon. **B,** A narrowed pelvic canal can be seen on the dorsoventral view. The cat had been involved in a road-traffic accident several years previously.

Physical Findings and Diagnostic Studies. Depression and dehydration are not uncommon findings. Abdominal palpation may reveal a hard tubular mass. In a search for potential causes the tail should always be lifted and the perineum carefully examined and palpated for abnormalities. Digital anorectal examination might detect painful or obstructive lesions (prostatic enlargement, narrowed pelvic canal, lymphadenopathy) (Figure 12-9). If the rectum in a dog contains feces and the animal is frequently straining to defecate, a colonic motility defect should be suspected, because these signs imply that the marked colonic contraction, called a *mass movement,* is ineffective. Rectal sacculation or dilatation may also be identified by rectal examination even if obvious signs of perineal hernia are absent. Anal protrusion and some ventral breakdown of the pelvic diaphragm are to be expected in dogs with a long history of tenesmus. A thorough neurologic examination may reveal neuromuscular problems (cauda equina syndrome, feline dysautonomia). Blood analysis is indicated in recurrent constipation to search for underlying conditions and guide supportive therapy. Hypothyroidism should be ruled out by appropriate testing. Abdominal survey radiographs confirm the presence of colonic dilatation and impaction and in some instances may reveal the cause. Ancillary tests useful in selected cases are contrast studies, colonoscopy, myelography, and magnetic resonance imaging.

Treatment. Treatment is based on the degree of constipation. Dietary management and oral or suppository laxatives are sufficient in mild cases. Moderate constipation often requires multiple enemas with warm water (5 to 10 ml/kg), mineral oil (5 to 30 ml), lactulose (5 to 20 ml), or dioctyl sodium sulfate (5 to 30 ml). Sodium phosphate enemas should not be used, as they may cause hyperphosphatemia. In severe cases that are nonresponsive to enemas, the animal should first be rehydrated and then the constipated stool removed under anesthesia. Breakdown and removal of fecal masses impacted in the colon should be accomplished as slowly and gently as possible. It is less traumatic if the feces are softened and removed over 2 to 4 days than if complete removal is attempted at one time. Most specific treatments are surgical and range from castration in the case of prostatic enlargement or perineal hernia (along with hernia repair), to resection of colonic tumors or realignment of an old pelvic fracture.

Once the fecal concretions are removed and, if possible, the underlying cause identified and eliminated, attention should be directed to prevention of recurrence. Nondigestible items should be eliminated from the diet, regular grooming instituted, and the opportunity provided for regular defecation. In every case, the therapeutic goal should be to have the animal form soft feces and to defecate regularly. Laxatives promote evacuation of the bowel through stimulation of fluid and electrolyte transport or increases in propulsive motility. Laxatives are classified as bulk-forming, emollient, lubricant, hyperosmotic, or stimulant laxatives (see Table 12-4). Prophylaxis is done in a stepwise fashion. The first step involves adding fiber (e.g., bran) and/or emollient to the diet or giving the animal lubrication laxatives. In the next step, lactulose is added in a dose that results in two to three soft fecal motions daily. A prokinetic agent (nizatidine, cisapride, tegaserod) with effect in the colon can promote motility if all previous measures are not sufficient.

Surgery. Severe recurrent obstipation or megacolon that is unresponsive to medical therapy, especially in cats, requires surgical resection of the atonic colon. The procedure is technically simple and provides a successful and realistic alternative to the stress of repeated enemas and long-term laxative therapy. Colectomy with colocolic, ileocolic, and jejunocolic anastomosis may be performed, depending on the extent of the disease. The ileocolic junction should be preserved whenever possible.[28] Cats treated by total or subtotal colectomy usually maintain a soft or semisolid fecal consistency, which is acceptable to owners.

Colonic and Rectal Tumors

Colonic and rectal tumors are relatively uncommon in dogs and cats. Adenomatous polyps are the most common type in dogs, accounting for up to 50% of rectal lesions; lymphosarcoma and adenocarcinoma are the most common malignant tumors. Leiomyosarcomas, carcinoid tumors, anaplastic sarcomas, and mast cell tumors (in cats) also occur. Adenocarcinomas occur predominantly in older animals (average age 12.5 years for cats and 8.5 years for dogs), in males more frequently than in females, and have a high incidence in German shepherd dogs, West Highland white terriers, and poodles. Adenomatous polyps are benign and do not metastasize; they may, however, be a precancerous condition. Adenocarcinomas have been classified based on their gross characteristics as infiltrative, ulcerative, or proliferative. Whereas in dogs they have a low tendency to spread, in cats the incidence of metastasis at the time of diagnosis is above 75%. Although slow growing, the tumor can eventually spread through the rectal wall and result in stricture formation. Colonic and rectal lymphosarcomas are uncommon and occur either as a discrete mass or as diffuse mural infiltration along the length of the organ. Carcinoid tumors, although rare, occur in the small and large intestine. These tumors are associated with diarrhea, gastrointestinal hemorrhage, and, as a result of their secretion of serotonin, systemic vasomotor effects.

History and Physical Findings. Animals with large intestinal tumors usually have a history of dyschezia, hematochezia, tenesmus, and diarrhea and appear to be chronically ill and debilitated. Specific signs depend on the tumor location and type. Tenesmus tends to worsen as lesions develop, especially with proliferative or obstructive masses. Only a thin ribbon of feces may be passed with infiltrating adenocarcinomas, whereas hematochezia is a frequent complaint with ulcerating masses. Rectal examination reveals in over two thirds of dogs a painful ringlike mass or stenotic area, whereas a caudal abdominal mass can be palpated in about half of all affected cats. Infiltrative lymphosarcomas of the large intestine cause a chronic unresponsive diarrhea as seen in chronic histoplasmosis. Animals with colonic or rectal polyps are not as debilitated as those with malignant tumors. In these animals, tenesmus following defecation and perhaps a chronic, unresponsive bloody or mucoid diarrhea occurs. If tenesmus is severe, the tumor may prolapse through the anus.

Diagnosis and Treatment. Rectal examination is sufficient to confirm the presence of a rectal mass, and biopsy is usually diagnostic (Figure 12-10). Colonic tumors are diagnosed by colonoscopy. Colonoscopy may be difficult or impossible when the tumor causes rectal stenosis. Surgical resection of adenocarcinomas and carcinomas

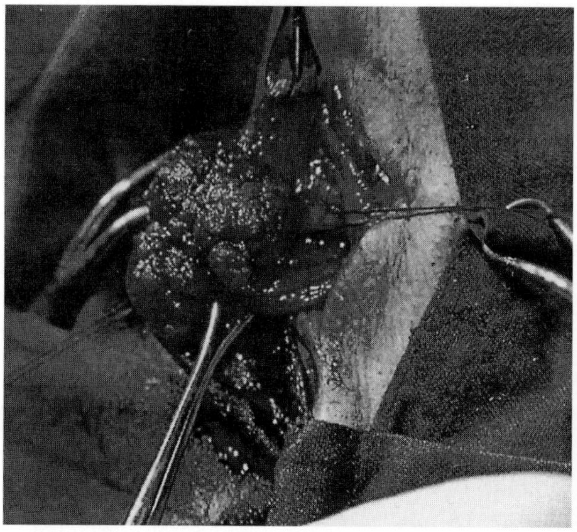

Figure 12-10. Pull-through technique to excise a rectal carcinoma in a 10-year-old mixed breed.

should be attempted. About 75% of polyps are removed by surgical excision or an electrocautery or laser procedure through the anus and are easily removed if the rectal mucosa is everted by gentle traction using a pull-through technique. Polyps located more proximally can be excised with an electrocautery snare passed through the colonoscope or, as a last resort, via a colectomy. The prognosis after polyp removal is good. Colonic lymphomas are treated with standard chemotherapy, with a median survival of 5 months in dogs and 3 months in cats.

Anal Tumors

Perianal tumors are common in male dogs but rare in female dogs and in cats. Perianal adenomas are the most common tumor of the anal region, accounting for 80% in male dogs. Other benign neoplasms occasionally found include lipomas, melanomas, and leiomyomas. Malignant anal tumors (e.g., squamous cell carcinoma, malignant melanoma, perianal gland adenocarcinoma, and anal sac adenocarcinoma) are rare.

Perianal gland adenomas arise from the perianal and circumanal glands of dogs and occur most often in intact males older than 6 years. In female dogs they occur almost exclusively in spayed animals. Cocker spaniels and fox terriers might have a higher incidence. Testicular tumors, mostly Leydig cell neoplasia, and hyperadrenocorticism are not uncommonly seen in conjunction with perianal adenomas. These tumors are benign but cause owner concern because of their tendency for ulceration and hemorrhage, their unsightliness, their interference with defecation, and the animal's excessive licking of the perineum. Perianal gland adenomas occur most often in the skin surrounding the anus but can be found anywhere on the perineum, tail-base area, or external genitalia. Diagnosis is confirmed by biopsy. Initial treatment for nonulcerated adenomas is castration. The tumor often regresses or stops growing without further need for treatment. If tumors are ulcerated or large or if the dog is female, surgical excision, laser excision, electrosurgery, or cryosurgery is indicated. The prognosis is favorable with all forms of treatment. Perianal carcinomas do not respond to castration alone; wide surgical excision is required, and the risk exists that fecal incontinence will occur. Adjuvant radiation therapy or chemotherapy should be used, but prognosis is often poor.

Squamous cell carcinoma of a distinct cloacogenic type has been reported to occur in the anal canal of the dog. Squamous cell carcinoma of the cutaneous portion of the anus may also be encountered infrequently. The tumor initially appears as a small, indurated ulcer that progresses to a cauliflower-like ulcerated mass with irregular edges. The tumor metastasizes readily, and early radical excision is essential if a cure is to be effected. The prognosis is fair if the tumor is excised early. A malignant melanoma occasionally occurs as a flat-to-round nodule on the anus, especially in breeds with heavily pigmented skin. An adenocarcinoma emanating from the apocrine cells in the anal sac occurs in aged female dogs. These tumors are an ectopic source of a parathyroid-like substance, which causes signs of pseudohyperparathyroidism. Malignant anal tumors cause extensive local invasion and metastasize to iliac lymph nodes, liver, and lungs. The prognosis is almost always poor.

References

1. Benno Y, Mitsuoka T: Effect of age on intestinal microflora of beagle dogs, *Microecol Ther* 19:85, 1989.
2. Ridgway J, Jergens AE, Niyo Y: Possible causal association of idiopathic inflammatory bowel disease with thrombocytopenia in the dog, *J Am Anim Hosp Assoc* 37:65, 2001.
3. Neiger R, Simpson J: Accuracy of folate, cobalamin and the hydrogen breath test to diagnose small intestinal bacterial overgrowth in dogs, *J Vet Intern Med* 14:376, 2000.
4. Simpson KW, Fyfe J, Cornetta A et al: Subnormal concentrations of serum cobalamin (vitamin B-12) in cats with gastrointestinal disease, *J Vet Intern Med* 15:26, 2001.
5. Melgarejo T, Williams DA, OConnell NC et al: Serum unconjugated bile acids as a test for intestinal bacterial overgrowth in dogs, *Dig Dis Sci* 45:407, 2000.
6. Robertson ID, Burbidge HM: Pros and cons of barium-impregnated polyethylene spheres in gastrointestinal disease, *Vet Clin North Am Small Anim Pract* 30:449, 2000.
7. Tams TR: Gastroscopy. In Tams TR, ed: *Small animal endoscopy*, ed 2, St Louis, 1999, Mosby.
8. Burrows CF: Evaluation of a colonic lavage solution to prepare the canine colon for colonoscopy, *J Am Vet Med Assoc* 195:1719, 1989.
9. Gaynor AR, Shofer FS, Washabau RJ: Risk-factors for acquired megaesophagus in dogs, *J Am Vet Med Assoc* 211:1406, 1997.
10. Plotnick AN: Megaesophagus and hypothyroidism in an English springer spaniel and response to thyroxine supplementation, *Canine Pract* 24:14, 1999.
11. Lüthi C, Neiger R: Esophageal foreign bodies in dogs: 51 cases, 1992-1997, *Eur J Comp Gastroenterol* 3:7, 1998.
12. Berry WL: *Spirocerca lupi* esophageal granulomas in 7 dogs: resolution after treatment with doramectin, *J Vet Intern Med* 14:609, 2000.
13. Davenport DJ, Remillard RL, Simpson KW et al: Gastrointestinal and exocrine pancreatic disease. In

Hand MS, Thatcher CD, Remillard RL, Roudebush P, eds: *Small animal clinical nutrition,* ed 4, Topeka, Kan, 2000, Mark Morris Institute.
14. Neiger R, Simpson KW: *Helicobacter* infection in dogs and cats: facts and fiction, *J Vet Intern Med* 14:124, 2000.
15. Neiger R, Gaschen F, Jaggy A: Endoscopically detectable gastric mucosal lesions in dogs with acute intervertebral disc disease: prevalence and effects of omeprazole and misoprostol, *J Vet Intern Med* 14:33, 2000.
16. Yam PS: New breath test to assess gastric emptying in the dog, *J Small Anim Pract* 41:376, 2000.
17. Brockman DJ, Washabau RJ, Drobatz KJ: Canine gastric dilation/volvulus syndrome in a veterinary critical care unit: 295 cases, 1986-1992, *J Am Vet Med Assoc* 207:460, 1995.
18. Brockman DJ, Holt DE, Washabau RJ: Pathogenesis of acute canine gastric dilation-volvulus syndrome: is there a unifying hypothesis, *Compend Contin Educ Pract Vet* 22:1108, 2000.
19. Marini RP, Fox JG, White H et al: *Helicobacter* spp. influences the development of primary gastric lymphoma in cats: a viable hypothesis, XIV International Workshop on gastroduodenal pathology and *Helicobacter pylori*, Strasbourg, Belgium, 6-8 Sept. 2001.
20. Lamb CR, Grierson J: Ultrasonographic appearance of primary gastric neoplasia in 21 dogs, *J Small Anim Pract* 40:211, 1999.
21. Rodrigues C: The small bowel. In Tallis R, Fillit H, Brocklehurst JC, eds: *Brocklehurst's textbook of geriatric medicine and gerontology,* ed 5, Edinburgh, 1998, Churchill Livingstone.
22. Jergens AL: Inflammatory bowel disease, *Vet Clin North Am Small Anim Pract* 29:501, 1999.
23. Ochoa R, Breitschwerdt EB, Lincoln KL: Immunoproliferative small intestinal disease (IPSID) in Basenji dogs: morphological observations, *Am J Vet Res* 45:482, 1984.
24. Burrows CF, Merritt AM: Assessment of gastrointestinal function. In Anderson NV, ed: *Veterinary gastroenterology,* ed 2, Philadelphia, 1992, Lea & Febiger.
25. Guilford G: Sacrificial proteins in inflammatory bowel disease. In Hand MS, Thatcher CD, Remillard RL, Roudebush P, eds: *Small animal clinical nutrition,* ed 4, Topeka, Kan, 2000, Mark Morris Institute.
26. Tams TR: Chronic diseases of the small intestine. In Tams TR, ed: *Handbook of small animal gastroenterology,* Philadelphia, 1996, WB Saunders.
27. Zwahlen CH, Lucroy MD, Kraegel SA et al: Results of chemotherapy for cats with alimentary malignant-lymphoma—21 cases, 1993-1997, *J Am Vet Med Assoc* 213:1144, 1998.
28. Washabau RJ, Holt D: Pathogenesis, diagnosis, and therapy of feline idiopathic megacolon, *Vet Clin North Am Small Anim Pract* 29:589, 1999.

CHAPTER 13

The Liver and Exocrine Pancreas

JOHNNY D. HOSKINS

THE LIVER

Normal function of the liver does not appear to change significantly as a result of age. Despite this, older dogs and cats are at greater risk for development of liver disease. The initial work-up for the older dog or cat with suspected liver disease should begin with a complete blood cell count, serum chemistry profile, and urinalysis (Box 13-1). These procedures may be followed by liver function test, radiographs, ultrasonographic imaging studies, hepatic fine-needle aspiration, and, ultimately, liver biopsy.

Evaluation of serum bile acids is the most practical method of assessing liver dysfunction in nonicteric dogs and cats. After a 12-hour fast, 1 ml of serum is obtained, and the animal is fed several tablespoons of a high-protein commercial diet; a second 1-ml serum sample is collected 2 hours after feeding. Fasting baseline and 2-hour postprandial bile acid concentrations will be increased in the presence of primary or cholestatic liver disease.[1]

Abdominal radiographs may show liver size by permitting evaluation of the position of the caudal portion of the liver and stomach. Abdominal radiographs may also be used to identify cholelithiasis. Hepatic ultrasonography is useful in the evaluation of hepatic parenchyma, for instance, helping to identify differences in echogenicity within the hepatic parenchyma that would suggest diffuse or localized liver diseases, dilated biliary ducts, and gallbladder diseases.[2]

Fine-needle aspiration of the liver is a relatively safe method of obtaining cells and fluids from the liver parenchyma and gallbladder for diagnosis of hepatic disease. Liver aspirates may be obtained from a conscious dog or cat placed in either dorsal or right lateral recumbency. Procedurally, an ultrasound-guided 1.5-inch, 22-gauge needle is advanced into the liver parenchyma or gallbladder. Gentle aspiration with a 6-ml syringe usually yields adequate numbers of cells or fluid for cytologic examination. Smears of the aspirated sample are made, and the slide is stained with Wright's-Giemsa or Diff-Quick stain for cytologic viewing.

Although easy to perform, ultrasound-guided aspirations cannot totally replace ultrasound-guided hepatic biopsy in the diagnosis of liver disease. A liver biopsy is required for definitive differentiation of types of liver disease. Liver biopsy may be performed in several ways: percutaneous biopsy via a transabdominal or transthoracic approach; ultrasound-guided transabdominal percutaneous liver biopsy; or keyhole, laparoscopic, and modified laparoscopic (using a sterile otoscope) techniques.[3] Laparotomy and surgical biopsy can also be performed, with the advantage of being able to visualize the entire liver and extrahepatic biliary system.[3,4] A veterinary pathologist well versed in hepatic diseases should perform histopathologic evaluation of any liver biopsy specimen.

HEPATOBILIARY DISEASES OF THE DOG

Chronic Inflammatory Hepatopathies

Infections, drugs, or copper accumulation can cause chronic hepatitis, or it can occur as an

BOX 13-1 Conditions that Increase Serum Hepatobiliary Enzyme Concentrations

Primary Liver Disease
Increased serum ALP, ALT, GGT, AST

Drugs
Corticosteroids (dogs): Increased serum ALP, GGT, ALT, AST
Anticonvulsants (phenobarbital, phenytoin, primidone): Increased serum ALT, ALP, AST, GGT
Cyclosporine: Increased serum ALP, GGT, ALT, AST

Endocrinopathies
Hyperthyroidism: Increased serum ALP and ALT
Hypothyroidism (dogs): Increased serum ALP
Diabetes mellitus: Increased serum ALP
Hyperadrenocorticism (dogs): Increased ALP, ALT, GGT, AST

Hypoxia or Hypotension
Congestive heart failure: Increased serum ALT, ALP, GGT, AST
Severe acute blood loss: Increased serum ALT, ALP, GGT, AST
Status epilepticus: Increased serum ALT, ALP, GGT, AST

Hypotensive Crisis
Surgery: Increased serum ALT, ALP, GGT, AST
Septic shock: Increased serum ALT, ALP, GGT, AST
Hypoadrenocorticism: Increased serum ALT, ALP, GGT, AST
Circulatory shock: Increased serum ALT, ALP, GGT, AST

Muscle Injury
Acute muscle necrosis or trauma: Increased serum ALT and AST
Malignant hyperthermia: Increased serum ALT and AST
Myopathies: Increased serum ALT and AST

Neoplasia
Adenocarcinomas (pancreatic, intestinal, adrenocortical, mammary): Increased serum AST, ALT, ALP
Sarcomas (hemangiosarcoma, leiomyosarcoma): Increased serum AST, ALT, ALP
Hepatic metastasis: Increased serum AST, ALT, ALP (unique enzyme induction: increased ALP and GGT)

ALP, Alkaline phosphatase; *ALT,* alanine aminotransferase; *AST,* aspartate aminotransferase; *GGT,* gamma-glutamyltransferase.

idiopathic process, possibly immune mediated. The pathologic process involved in chronic hepatitis often begins with necrosis, followed by infiltration of the liver with lymphocytes, plasma cells, or macrophages, which may lead to hepatic fibrosis and cirrhosis. Both acute and chronic hepatitis can be caused by viral infection (e.g., infectious canine hepatitis and canine acidophil hepatitis) and bacterial infection (e.g., canine leptospirosis). Although acute and chronic hepatitis tend to cause hepatic necrosis in their early stages, they may result in the same type of chronic injury seen with other chronic hepatopathies.

Almost any drug has the capacity to produce an idiosyncratic reaction in any given individual; some drugs are more likely to be associated with chronic hepatic inflammation in dogs, especially older animals. Administration of primidone, phenobarbital, clomipramine, oxibendazole-diethylcarbamazine, or nonsteroidal antiinflammatory drugs (NSAIDs) has been associated with periportal hepatitis and hepatic vacuolar change.

A familial predisposition to develop chronic hepatitis has been suggested in certain dog breeds. Breeds at increased risk for chronic hepatitis include the Bedlington terrier, West Highland white terrier, Doberman pinscher, American and English cocker spaniel, Skye terrier, Labrador retriever, standard poodle, and others (Box 13-2).

Abnormal hepatic retention of dietary copper and copper hepatopathy occurs in Bedlington terriers.[5] An autosomal recessive mode of inheritance is involved; only individuals homozygous for the recessive gene develop the excess copper

BOX 13-2 Dog Breeds with Increased Chronic Hepatic Disease and Associated with Copper Accumulation

Airedale terrier
Bedlington terrier*
Boxer
Bulldog
Bull terrier
Cocker spaniel, American and English
Collie
Dachshund
Dalmatian
Doberman pinscher*
Fox terrier, wirehaired
German shepherd dog
Golden retriever
Keeshond
Kerry blue terrier
Labrador retriever
Norwich terrier
Old English sheepdog
Pekingese
Poodle, standard
Samoyed
Schnauzer
Skye terrier*
West Highland white terrier*

From Rolfe DS, Twedt DC: Copper-associated hepatopathies in dogs, *Vet Clin North Am Small Anim Pract* 25:399, 1995.
*Hereditary mechanism for increased hepatic copper.

accumulation in hepatic lysosomes. Hepatic copper concentrations exceeding 2000 μg/g dry tissue are consistently associated with morphologic and functional evidence of the progressive hepatopathy that over time progresses to chronic hepatitis and cirrhosis.[5,6] Diagnosis of copper-associated hepatopathy in Bedlington terriers can be made by examination of hepatic tissue for excessive copper storage or by performing genetic tests on DNA samples collected from suspected dogs. The frequency of the recessive gene in Bedlington terrier dogs is estimated to be as high as 50% in the United States, with a similar frequency in England. This means that more than 25% of Bedlington terrier dogs are "affected" and another 50% are "carriers."

The DNA samples can be collected using a soft cheek brush that is provided by a commercial genetic laboratory.* When the inside of the dog's cheek is gently brushed, cells containing DNA are removed. The collected DNA samples then are analyzed to determine the genetic status of the suspect dog. Useful for dogs of any age, the DNA sample collection and analysis activities can be completed before puppies are purchased at 6 to 10 weeks. The results of the DNA testing also may be formally registered with the Orthopedic Foundation for Animals. For further information about the Orthopedic Foundation for Animal's Registry for Copper Toxicosis in Bedlington Terriers, contact the Orthopedic Foundation for Animals.*

Primary hepatobiliary disease associated with an increased accumulation of hepatic copper, albeit smaller amounts of tissue copper than in Bedlington terriers, has been described in Doberman pinscher, Skye terrier, West Highland white terrier, and American and English cocker spaniel dogs.[7-9] The chronic hepatitis associated with an increased liver copper content in Doberman pinscher dogs occurs primarily in middle-aged female dogs. A familial copper-associated liver disease occurs in West Highland white terrier dogs.[9] Hepatic copper concentrations in affected dogs have ranged as high as 3500 ppm, considerably lower than the maximum values recorded for Bedlington terriers. Liver disease has also been observed with unexpected frequency in American and English cocker spaniel dogs.[8] The liver disease appears to be progressive, and dogs dying of hepatic cirrhosis have had hepatic copper concentrations three to five times normal.

Primary copper hepatopathy as the inciting cause of liver disease should be considered in those breeds known to have an increased incidence of copper retention (Box 13-2). The diagnosis is confirmed by liver biopsy, revealing copper-containing granules in excess of what might be considered normal for the degree of cholestasis and fibrosis that is present.[10]

Dogs with chronic hepatitis from any cause usually have a slowly progressive onset of disease and are characterized by depression, weight loss, anorexia, and polyuria or polydipsia. Laboratory evaluation of dogs with chronic hepatitis can vary depending on the stage of disease. Initially, affected dogs will have marked increases in serum alanine aminotransferase (ALT) and aspartate aminotransferase (AST) activities, with little evidence of cholestasis or liver dysfunction. As the disease progresses, cholestasis develops, with increases in serum alkaline phosphatase (ALP) activity and

*VetGen, 3728 Plaza Drive, Suite 1, Ann Arbor, MI 48108. Phone: (734) 669-8440; toll-free phone: (800) 4-VETGEN; Fax: (734) 669-8441. Web site: www.vetgen.com.

*Orthopedic Foundation for Animals, 2300 East Nifong Boulevard, Columbia, MO 65201-3856. Phone: (573) 442-0418.

total bilirubin concentration. Liver function progressively decreases; the decrease is first seen in serum bile acid concentrations and later is obvious in serum albumin, urea nitrogen, glucose, and coagulation factor concentrations.

Abdominal radiographs are unremarkable except when a small liver or ascites accompanies advanced stages of the liver disease. Ultrasonography of the liver may be normal in the early stages of chronic hepatitis, or nonspecific changes in echogenicity may be detected. Potential ultrasonographic findings with hepatic cirrhosis include small liver, irregular liver lobe margins, focal lesions representing regenerative nodules, increased parenchymal echogenicity associated with fibrous tissue, and ascites. Splenomegaly may also be detected.

The histopathologic findings from liver biopsies include piecemeal necrosis, bridging necrosis (presence of inflammatory cells bridging the limiting plate between lobules), and active cirrhosis. Specimens should also be stained to detect copper, although the presence of excess copper in a liver with severe cholestasis and cirrhosis could represent secondary copper hepatopathy. If sufficient liver tissue is obtained, then copper concentrations within the liver should be determined.

If a probable cause of hepatic injury can be determined, then specific treatment is directed at removing the primary cause, such as replacing anticonvulsant primidone or phenobarbital therapy with potassium bromide therapy, treating for canine leptospirosis with antimicrobial agents, or chelating hepatic copper with penicillamine. In most cases, specific treatment is not available. Some of the drugs used in the treatment of chronic hepatitis are presented in Table 13-1.

Therapy for copper-associated hepatopathy includes reduction in dietary copper and chelation therapy. Currently, drugs used for copper chelation are penicillamine and trientine dihydrochloride. Penicillamine is effective at reducing hepatic copper concentrations, although the rate of hepatic "decoppering" is slow.[11] Trientine is as effective as penicillamine at reducing hepatic copper concentrations and is currently being used when penicillamine-associated vomiting occurs. It is likely that Bedlington terriers, West Highland white terriers, and possibly Doberman pinschers will benefit from the inclusion of copper chelation or oral zinc therapy in their therapeutic plans.

Other therapies that can be considered in dogs with chronic hepatitis include corticosteroids and antifibrotic drugs. Corticosteroids have immunosuppressive, antiinflammatory, and antifibrotic effects. Other antifibrotic agents such as colchicine can be used to prevent or treat hepatic fibrosis and cirrhosis. Free radicals may contribute to oxidative hepatocellular injury if not counteracted by cytoprotective mechanisms. Antioxidants, such as S-adenosylmethionine and vitamin E, are important in scavenging free radicals and preventing oxidative injury. Ursodeoxycholic acid is believed to be beneficial because it expands the bile acid pool and displaces potentially hepatotoxic hydrophilic bile acids that may accumulate in cholestasis. It also stimulates bile flow, stabilizes hepatocyte membranes, and has cytoprotective and immunomodulatory effects on the liver.

Chronic hepatopathies frequently cause alterations in plasma proteins (hypoalbuminemia) and vascular hydrostatic pressures, resulting in ascites or edema. Chronic hepatopathies increase resistance to blood flow in the liver (portal hypertension), which can lead to acquired portosystemic shunts, increased lymph formation, increased plasma volume, and ascites or edema. Liver-induced ascites can be diagnosed by physical examination and laboratory evaluation of peritoneal fluid, blood, and urine. Ascitic fluid of liver disease is usually a transudate or modified transudate, which is further substantiated by the presence of hypoalbuminemia. Peripheral edema may occur in end-stage liver disease. Similar mechanisms

TABLE 13-1. DRUGS USED IN THE MANAGEMENT OF CHRONIC HEPATITIS IN OLDER DOGS

DRUG	DOSAGE	INDICATION
D-Penicillamine	10-15 mg/kg q12h	Copper chelation; antifibrotic
Trientine	15-30 mg/kg q12h	Copper chelation
Zinc acetate	25-50 mg elemental zinc q12h	Decrease copper absorption
Prednisone	0.5-2 mg/kg q24-48h	Immunosuppressive; antiinflammatory; antifibrotic
Azathioprine	1 mg/kg q24-48h	Immunosuppressive
S-Adenosylmethionine	18 mg/kg q12-24h	Increase hepatic glutathione; antioxidant
Ursodeoxycholic acid	10-15 mg/kg q24h	Stimulates bile flow; cytoprotective; immunomodulatory effects
Vitamin E	200-800 IU q24h	Antioxidant

that trigger ascites may cause peripheral edema (e.g., distal legs, ventral abdomen and thorax, ventral neck region).

To reestablish the osmotic gradient in ascitic animals with hypoalbuminemia, administer intravenous colloids such as hetastarch or dextrans at 10 to 20 ml/kg over 1 to 2 hours, and repeat as needed after several infusions. Diuretics and a low-sodium diet are used in the management of ascites and edema.[12,13] Spironolactone is used to reduce ascites and edema without causing hypokalemia. If these measures are ineffective, furosemide may be substituted, although serum electrolyte concentrations should be frequently evaluated.

Hepatic Fibrosis and Cirrhosis

The liver can respond to severe damage and necrosis by either regeneration, mineralization, or fibrosis, depending on the severity of the challenge and the degree of damage to the supporting connective tissue structure. Loss of hepatocytes and connective tissue integrity caused by any disease can lead to hepatic fibrosis; thus, identification of hepatic fibrosis is not specific for any particular liver disease. When hepatic fibrosis is severe and leads to formation of small or large regenerative nodules limited by fibrous tissue, the term *cirrhosis* is used (Figure 13-1). Hepatic cirrhosis is considered an end-stage liver disease. Because hepatic cirrhosis is advanced, most affected dogs will have significant clinical and laboratory evidence of hepatic dysfunction. As cirrhosis progresses, portal hypertension develops, and many dogs with hepatic cirrhosis have ascites and acquired portosystemic shunts.[12] Most chronic hepatopathies progress slowly, and fibrosis occurs in concert with the progression of necrosis and inflammation. Radiographic evaluation may reveal a small liver, and ultrasonography shows an increase in hepatic echogenicity and possibly the presence of acquired portosystemic shunts. Liver biopsy is required for definitive diagnosis of hepatic fibrosis and cirrhosis.[3]

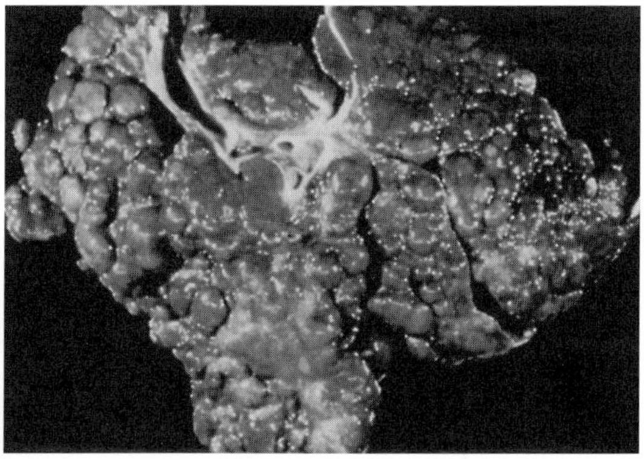

Figure 13-1. Severe hepatic cirrhosis in a dog.

Treatment for hepatic fibrosis is aimed at treating the underlying disease process and managing the complications of liver disease. Inhibition of collagen formation and lysis of excess hepatic fibrous tissue would be an additional goal of therapy for hepatic cirrhosis. When used for treatment of hepatic fibrosis in affected dogs, colchicine has produced improvement in clinical signs for several months.[14] Corticosteroids and azathioprine have antifibrotic properties. Other drugs for the treatment of hepatic fibrosis include penicillamine, which inhibits collagen polymerization secondary to its copper-chelating effects, and oral zinc, which decreases intestinal copper absorption and also has antifibrotic and hepatoprotective properties.

Chronic Infiltrative Hepatopathies

Alterations in hepatic structure and function may occur when hepatocytes are infiltrated with lipid, glycogen, amyloid, or other substances. Although hepatic lipidosis is a common histopathologic finding in dogs with diabetes mellitus, it seldom becomes a clinical problem associated with liver dysfunction. Other, less common infiltrative disorders include amyloid deposition and hemochromatosis.[3] Exogenous glucocorticoids and naturally occurring hyperadrenocorticism often lead to steroid hepatopathy in older dogs. Impairment of liver function can occur with severe steroid hepatopathy, but most dogs do not develop signs referable to hepatic dysfunction.[15]

Laboratory evaluation of dogs with steroid hepatopathy usually reveals a marked increase in serum ALP and gamma-glutamyltransferase (GGT) activity, occasionally up to a sixtyfold increase over normal values.[16] Values for hepatocellular enzyme activities (ALT and AST) will usually be increased, but not to the magnitude of serum ALP and GGT. Serum total bilirubin concentrations are usually normal, which supports the premise that serum ALP activity increase is secondary to steroid induction and not from cholestasis. If liver function tests are performed, there may be mild increases in fasting and postprandial serum bile acid concentration.[3] Liver biopsy is seldom performed, but expected changes of increased hepatic vacuolization are seen on histopathologic evaluation.

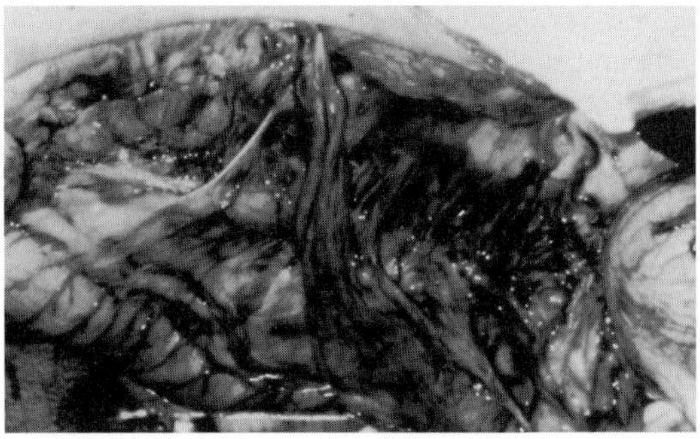

Figure 13-2. Multiple acquired portosystemic shunts in a dog. This dog had chronic hepatitis and severe portal hypertension.

Vascular Diseases of the Liver

The most common vascular disease of the liver in older dogs is acquired portosystemic shunts. Acquired portosystemic shunting occurs secondarily to portal hypertension, advanced liver disease, and hepatic fibrosis or cirrhosis (Figure 13-2). As portal pressures increase, small vessels routing the portal circulation to the systemic circulation increase in size and volume capacity, thus providing a "pop-off valve" for the increased portal pressures. Treatment of acquired portosystemic shunts is aimed primarily at treatment of the associated hepatoencephalopathy (HE). Attenuation of acquired portosystemic shunts is contraindicated, because this immediately results in extremely increased portal pressures, shock, and death.

Other vascular disorders of the liver include acquired arteriovenous (AV) fistulas and portal vein thrombosis. In dogs, acquired AV fistulas are usually the result of trauma.[17] The clinical signs associated with hepatic AV fistulas in dogs include ascites and hepatoencephalopathy. Diagnosis is based on contrast imaging studies, and surgical resection of the affected liver lobe usually results in resolution of clinical signs. In dogs, portal vein thrombosis occurs, resulting in altered laboratory parameters indicative of cholestasis, hepatocellular injury, and impaired liver function.[18] Thrombosis may be diagnosed based on mesenteric venography, but treatment is usually not attempted.

Hepatoencephalopathy

HE is the neurologic derangements that occur secondary to liver dysfunction.[19,20] Neurologic signs may be seen at any time, often being more prominent following ingestion of a high-protein meal or blood loss into the gastrointestinal tract. Initial signs of HE include depression, lethargy, and mild behavior changes ranging from increased docility to aggression. Aimless pacing or circling, apparent blindness, and head pressing may ensue, followed by stupor, seizure activity, or coma. The diagnosis of HE is based on identification of liver dysfunction and response to treatment. Fasting serum ammonia and serum bile acid concentrations are usually markedly increased in HE.

Medical management is directed toward minimizing the signs of HE and includes manipulation of dietary proteins and intestinal flora and avoidance of medications or substances capable of inducing encephalopathic signs. A restricted protein diet (2 to 2.5 mg/kg) composed of proteins rich in branched-chain amino acids with comparatively smaller amounts of aromatic amino acids is recommended. Foods containing milk protein (dried milk or cottage cheese) are best. The bulk of the caloric intake should consist of simple carbohydrates such as boiled white rice. Meals should be frequent and small to maximize digestion and absorption so that minimal residue is passed into the colon, where intestinal anaerobic bacteria degrade nitrogenous compounds to ammonia. Commercial diets formulated for use in the presence of liver or renal dysfunction or intestinal disease are used with success in most animals with encephalopathic signs.

Manipulation of intestinal flora with antimicrobial agents and lactulose also produces marked clinical improvement. For animals in encephalopathic crisis, intravenous isotonic electrolyte solutions supplemented with 2.5% or 5% dextrose solution and potassium chloride, cleansing enemas with warmed 0.9% saline solution, or enemas with added neomycin (15 to 20 ml of 1% solution three to four times daily), lactulose (5 to 10 ml diluted 1:3 with water three to four times daily), or Betadine solution (10% solution, rinse after 10 minutes with warm water) are recommended. For long-term medical management of encephalopathic signs, lactulose is given orally at a dose of 0.25 to 1 ml per 4.5 kg body weight; the dose is adjusted according to the frequency and consistency of the stools passed each day. Two to three soft or pudding-consistency stools indicate an optimal dose. Too great a dose may result in flatulence, severe diarrhea, dehydration, and acidemia. To further manipulate the intestinal flora, neomycin (22 mg/kg orally two to three times daily), metronidazole (7.5 mg/kg orally two to three times daily), ampicillin (5 mg/kg orally two to three times daily), or amoxicillin (2.5 mg/kg

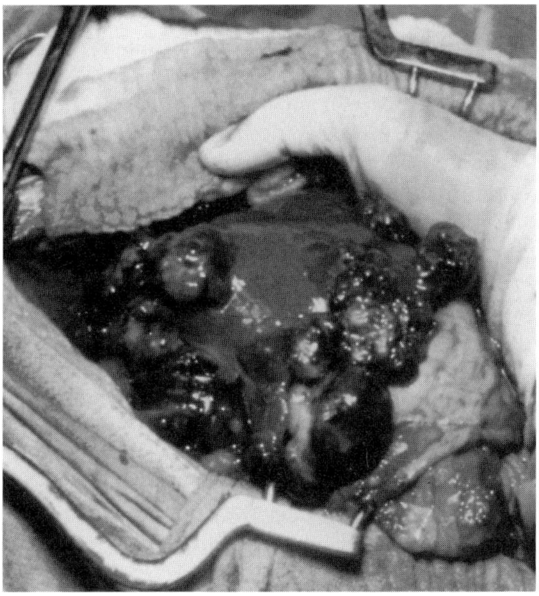

Figure 13-3. Surgical exploration of an 11-year-old Siberian husky with metastatic neoplasia in the liver. Multiple nodules are seen over the liver surface. Histopathologic evaluation identified the metastases as hemangiosarcoma.

orally two times a day) may be used intermittently for several weeks.

Hepatobiliary Neoplasia

Neoplasias involving the liver are primary hepatic tumors, metastatic carcinomas and sarcomas, and hemolymphatic tumors. In dogs, metastatic neoplasia is most common and can originate from the pancreas, spleen, mammary glands, adrenal glands, bones, lungs, thyroid glands, and gastrointestinal tract (Figure 13-3). Primary hepatic tumors may be epithelial or mesodermal in origin and either benign or malignant. Benign tumors of the hepatocytes are called *hepatocellular adenomas* or *hepatomas*, and malignant tumors are called *hepatocellular carcinomas*. Hepatocellular carcinomas are the most common primary hepatic tumors in dogs.[21] The cause of these spontaneous primary hepatic tumors in dogs is not known.

Primary hepatic tumors are most common in dogs that are 10 years of age or older. Dogs with hepatic tumors usually show vague, nonspecific signs of hepatic dysfunction that often do not appear until the more advanced stages of hepatic disease. The most consistent signs are anorexia, lethargy, weight loss, polydipsia, polyuria, vomiting, and abdominal distention. Other, less frequent findings include icterus, diarrhea, and excessive bleeding. Signs of central nervous dysfunction such as depression, dementia, or seizures can be attributed to HE, hypoglycemia, or central nervous system metastasis.

On physical examination, a cranial abdominal mass or marked hepatomegaly is commonly detected in dogs with primary hepatic tumors. Ascites or hemoperitoneum may contribute to abdominal distention. Tumor rupture and hemorrhage are most likely with hepatocellular adenoma, hepatocellular carcinoma, and hepatic hemangiosarcoma. Generally, laboratory evaluation shows mild to moderate increases in liver enzyme activities, with some dogs displaying abnormal liver function based on serum bile acid concentrations.[21] Hypoglycemia occurs in some dogs with hepatocellular carcinoma and other hepatic neoplasms. Abdominal radiographic findings include symmetric or asymmetric hepatomegaly or ascites. A right cranial abdominal mass causing caudal and left gastric displacement most often occurs. Thoracic radiographs should be obtained to determine whether pulmonary metastasis has occurred.

Potential ultrasonographic findings include focal, multifocal, or diffuse changes in hepatic echotexture. Primary or secondary hepatic neoplasia and nodular hyperplasia often appear as focal or multifocal hypoechoic or mixed echogenic lesions. The diagnosis of primary or metastatic hepatic tumors cannot be made on the basis of ultrasonographic findings alone. Definitive diagnosis of hepatic neoplasia requires liver biopsy and histopathologic examination. The procedure of choice for a single large hepatic mass is laparotomy, because the excision of the mass can be performed concurrently. Ultrasound-guided biopsy is useful for diagnosing focal or diffuse involvement, but the small size of the biopsy sample can make the differentiation of nodular dysplasia versus primary hepatic tumor difficult. A surgical wedge biopsy is often necessary.

Surgical removal of the affected liver lobe is the treatment of choice for primary hepatic tumors such as hepatocellular adenoma or carcinoma that involve a single lobe. Removal of a single mass lesion of hepatocellular carcinoma will typically allow 1 year of good-quality life after surgery. Therefore, early detection before metastasis to other liver lobes provides the best chance for surgical control. A complete evaluation of the abdominal cavity for the evidence of metastasis should be performed, and biopsy specimen of hepatic lymph nodes should always be obtained. When all liver lobes are affected, the prognosis is poor. Chemotherapy is not currently an effective treatment for control of hepatocellular carcinoma.

HEPATOBILIARY DISEASES OF THE CAT

Feline Inflammatory Liver Disease

Inflammatory liver diseases of older cats are probably best referred to as *feline cholangitis* or *cholangiohepatitis syndrome* (CCHS).[22] This syndrome can then be described as being either suppurative or nonsuppurative. Cats with suppurative CCHS usually are males. A history of vomiting and diarrhea of sudden onset is common. Affected cats are icteric, febrile, lethargic, and dehydrated on initial presentation. Less than 50% of cats have hepatomegaly. The most common organisms associated with suppurative CCHS are *Escherichia coli, Staphylococcus,* α-hemolytic *Streptococcus, Bacillus, Actinomyces, Bacteroides, Enterococcus, Enterobacter,* and *Clostridium* species.

Most cats with suppurative CCHS show a moderate increase in serum ALT, AST, ALP, and GGT activities. Some cats have left-shifted leukograms with an accompanying leukocytosis. On ultrasonography, severe ascending cholangitis associated with thickening of the extrahepatic biliary system and inflammation within the lumen of the intrahepatic bile ducts may be observed. Ultrasonography also may show coexisting extrahepatic bile duct obstruction (enlarged gallbladder, distended and tortuous common bile duct, and obvious intrahepatic bile ducts), cholecystitis (thickened, laminar appearance to gallbladder wall, adjacent fluid accumulation), and pancreatitis (prominent, easily visualized enlarged pancreas with adjacent hyperechoic fat). Cytologic evaluation of liver aspirates or imprints may reveal suppurative inflammation.

Most cats with nonsuppurative CCHS have been ill for several months.[22] Clinical signs are subtle and may include only episodic vomiting, diarrhea, and anorexia. Most cats have hepatomegaly, are icteric, and may have ascites. Concurrent disorders frequently include inflammatory bowel disease, low-grade lymphocytic pancreatitis, and cholecystitis. Cats with lymphoplasmacytic inflammation tend to have greater magnitudes of increased serum ALT, AST, ALP, and GGT activities than cats with only lymphocytic inflammation. Cats with lymphocytic inflammation may develop a lymphocytosis (total lymphocyte counts greater than 14,000/μl) without other evidence of malignant lymphoproliferative disease. As in cats with suppurative CCHS, abdominal radiographs rarely show important diagnostic information. In most cats with nonsuppurative CCHS, a multifocal hyperechoic pattern is recognized ultrasonographically, which represents peribiliary inflammation and fibrosis. In some cats, ultrasonography may fail to show any abnormalities. Cytologic preparations from liver aspirates may lack evidence of inflammation or may disclose only a few inflammatory cells. A wedge biopsy of the liver for histopathology is preferable for a definitive diagnosis because it more reliably demonstrates whole acinar units and portal triads.[22]

Treatment of suppurative CCHS incorporates appropriate antimicrobial therapy based on identification of infectious organisms (Box 13-3). If bacteria are cytologically observed, a Gram's stain facilitates selection of antimicrobial agents. Cats with extrahepatic bile duct obstruction should have the biliary occlusion decompressed, if possible. If biliary tract decompression cannot be accomplished, the biliary pathway may be rerouted by a cholecystoenterostomy. Biliary diversion is a vital early therapeutic intervention in the prevention or control of sepsis in obstructive suppurative cholangitis. Aerobic and anaerobic bacterial cultures should be collected from bile, tissue adjacent to any focal lesion, gallbladder wall, and liver tissue.

Any icteric cat suspected of having suppurative or nonsuppurative CCHS should be evaluated for coexistent extrahepatic bile duct obstruction,

BOX 13-3 Medical Management Used in Treatment of Feline Inflammatory Liver Disease

- Fluid therapy according to the cat's needs
- Prednisone (2 to 4 mg/kg orally once a day or divided twice daily with titration to the lowest effective dose over the next several months)
- Metronidazole (7.5 mg/kg orally two to three times daily), ampicillin (20 mg/kg orally three to four times daily), or chloramphenicol (50 mg/kg orally two times daily)
- At least 2-3 mEq daily of oral potassium gluconate (no matter what the serum potassium value is)
- Oral vitamin E (100 to 200 IU per day) or S-adenosylmethionine (18 mg/kg daily)
- Oral pancreatic enzymes supplementation
- Supplementation with L-carnitine 250 mg per day, water-soluble vitamins (two times the normal maintenance dose), and vitamin K_1 (0.5 to 1.5 mg/kg) subcutaneously or intramuscularly for three doses at 12-hour intervals and then once a week for 1 or 2 additional weeks may be provided
- Periodic oral lactulose as needed to control abnormal mental behavior
- Diet that the cat will eat well

pancreatitis, and inflammatory bowel disease, as well as for coexistent hepatic lipidosis. If lipid vacuolation is detected, nutritional support with a commercially prepared feline diet should be included in the treatment plan.

Immunosuppressive therapy for cats with nonsuppurative CCHS includes a combination of prednisone (initial dose of 2 to 4 mg/kg orally once a day or divided twice daily), with titration to the lowest effective dose over the next several months, and metronidazole (7.5 mg/kg orally two to three times daily).[22] Supplementation with L-carnitine 250 mg per day, water-soluble vitamins (two times the normal maintenance dose), and vitamin K_1 (0.5 to 1.5 mg/kg) subcutaneously or intramuscularly for three doses at 12-hour intervals and then once a week for 1 or 2 additional weeks may be provided. Oral *S*-adenosylmethionine (18 mg/kg daily) or vitamin E (100 to 200 IU daily) can also be added as a supplement to ensure adequacy as a free radical scavenger. Ursodeoxycholic acid (10 to 15 mg/kg orally per day) is given to all cats with CCHS once extra-hepatic bile duct obstruction is corrected and cholecystitis has resolved. Monthly serum liver enzyme activities and total bilirubin concentrations may be monitored to gauge response to treatment as well as to determine how well the cat is doing at home.

Pyogranulomatous Hepatitis (Feline Infectious Peritonitis)

Feline infectious peritonitis (FIP) virus (FIPV) can induce a multisystemic disease process, which may affect the liver by inducing pyogranulomatous hepatitis. Both effusive and noneffusive forms of FIP may affect the liver (Figure 13-4). Common clinical signs seen with pyogranulomatous hepatitis are anorexia, weight loss, fever, depression, icterus, and abdominal distention secondary to fluid accumulation. Laboratory evaluation of cats with FIPV-induced liver disease may reveal leukocytosis, nonregenerative anemia, and hyperglobulinemia. In addition, increased serum ALT, AST, and ALP activities and increased total bilirubin concentration may be present. Ultrasonography may confirm the presence of abdominal effusion and define nodular involvement of the liver secondary to the pyogranulomatous inflammation. Alternatively, fine-needle aspiration cytology of the liver may reveal pyogranulomatous inflammation. Liver biopsy is the most reliable method to confirm FIP of the liver. There is no specific treatment for FIPV-induced liver disease in cats.

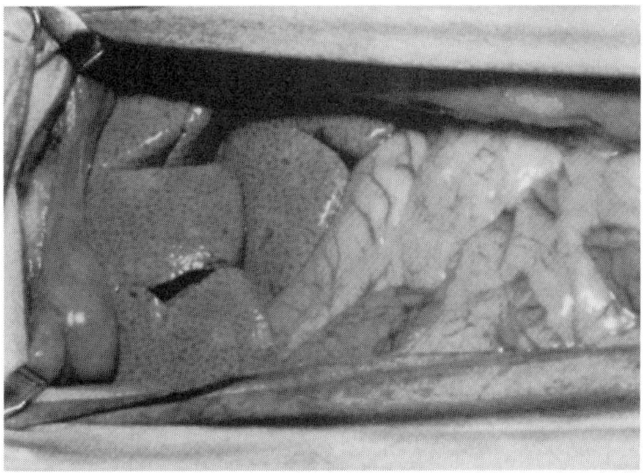

Figure 13-4. Hepatic disease associated with feline infectious peritonitis in a 13-year-old cat. Note the lighter colored granulomas in the liver.

Supportive measure can be used, along with good nutrition and nursing care.

Secondary Hepatic Lipidosis

Secondary hepatic lipidosis is characterized by progressive infiltration of hepatocytes with fat and concomitant hepatic dysfunction. The usual clinical findings include a period of anorexia in a previously obese cat, obvious weight loss, muscle wasting, icterus, and vomiting.[23] Icterus is usually seen in the later stages of disease, and some cats will have palpable hepatomegaly. Laboratory evaluation will show evidence of cholestatic liver disease. Ultrasonography shows a fine, diffuse increase in echogenicity.[24] Cytologic evaluation of fine-needle aspirates shows hepatocytes with marked vacuolar change[25] (Figure 13-5). Histopathologic evaluation of a liver biopsy specimen will reveal marked macrovesicular or microvesicular vacuolar change in most hepatocytes and evidence of bile stasis. Treatment is directed at restoring nutritional status and managing the underlying cause of the systemic illness. Enteral nutritional support by nasoesophageal, pharyngostomy, esophagostomy, or gastrostomy tube feeding is recommended.

Hepatobiliary Neoplasia

Primary neoplasia of the liver and biliary system is uncommon in older cats. Primary nonhematopoietic tumors of the liver include bile duct adenoma and adenocarcinoma, hepatocellular carcinoma, and hemangiosarcoma.[26] Metastatic lymphosarcoma occurs commonly in

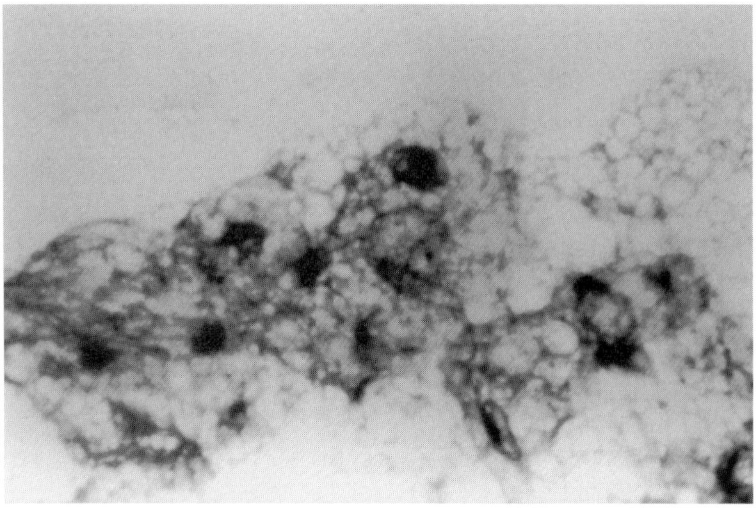

Figure 13-5. Cytologic specimen of a hepatic fine-needle aspirate from a cat with secondary hepatic lipidosis. Note the widespread vacuolization in all hepatocytes. (Wright-Giemsa stain; ×1,000).

cats, and other metastatic neoplasias seen in older cats include myeloproliferative diseases and mast cell tumors.[22] Clinical signs may include anorexia, lethargy, hepatomegaly, and icterus. If biliary obstruction is complete, clinical signs of extrahepatic bile duct obstruction will also be observed. Fine-needle aspiration for cytologic evaluation can be helpful with diffuse metastatic neoplasia, such as lymphosarcoma, mast cell tumor, or myeloproliferative disorders.[25] Treatment for primary hepatobiliary neoplasia is primarily surgical. Treatment of metastatic neoplasia is directed at the primary tumor.

GALLBLADDER DISEASES OF THE DOG AND CAT

Little is known about the effects of the normal aging process on the gallbladder and its function in older dogs and cats. The diagnosis of gallbladder disease is usually based on the case history, physical examination findings, and laboratory findings. Radiographic imaging, ultrasonographic imaging, serum bile acid determinations, fine needle aspiration of gallbladder for cytology and culture, and liver biopsy for histopathology may also be performed.

The CBC may show mild to moderate nonregenerative anemia, neutrophilic leukocytosis with a left shift, thrombocytopenia, or other morphologic changes. Increased serum liver enzyme activities such as increased serum ALT and AST are reliable indicators of hepatocellular damage or cholestasis. Serum ALP and GGT activities increase in cholestasis. In cats, any increase in serum ALP activity indicates cholestasis. Hyperbilirubinemia may occur with active hepatocellular damage and may also occur with cholestasis secondary to extrahepatic disease. Any degree of bilirubinuria in cats of any age is abnormal and suggestive of active liver disease.

The most practical method of assessing liver or gallbladder dysfunction in nonicteric dogs or cats is serum bile acid determinations (Table 13-2).[28] Fasting and 2-hour postprandial bile acid concentrations have the same normal range values irrespective of age and are increased with primary or cholestatic liver or gallbladder disease.

Survey abdominal radiography and ultrasonography may be helpful in diagnosing gallbladder diseases and may help in identifying distinct liver or gallbladder masses, mineralization, and cholelithiasis (Table 13-2). Ultrasound-guided fine-needle aspiration of the gallbladder for cytology is a relatively safe procedure for diagnosing some gallbladder diseases. Gallbladder aspirates may be obtained from a nonsedated animal placed in either dorsal or right lateral recumbency. The abdomen is clipped and prepared as for ultrasonography, and a 1- or 1.5-inch, 22-gauge needle is advanced into the gallbladder under guidance of the ultrasound beam. A single gentle aspiration with a 6-ml syringe usually yields adequate numbers of cells for cytologic evaluation and for bacterial culture. Smears of the gallbladder aspirate are then made, and the slides are stained with a cytologic stain such as Wright's-Giemsa. Exploratory laparotomy and surgical biopsy can also be performed, with the advantage of being able to visualize the liver lobes, gallbladder, and extrahepatic biliary system.

TABLE 13-2. BILE ACID AND ULTRASONOGRAPHIC FINDINGS ASSOCIATED WITH BILIARY TRACT DISEASE

DISEASE	BILE ACID FINDINGS	ULTRASONOGRAPHY
Hepatic disease (intrahepatic cholestasis)	Normal to increased	Normal liver parenchyma and/or biliary tract Hypoechoic Hyperechoic Focal to multifocal hypoechoic lesions (neoplasia, abscess)
Cholelithiasis	Normal to increased Highest concentrations with bile duct obstruction	Visible calculi (hyperechoic) ± Thickened gallbladder wall Dilated common bile duct Dilated intrahepatic biliary ducts Tortuous biliary ducts
Cholecystitis	Normal	± Visible calculi Thickened gallbladder wall
Necrotizing cholecystitis	Normal	± Visible calculi Thickened gallbladder wall
Parasitic gallbladder disease (flukes)	Normal to increased	Enlarged gallbladder Tortuous, dilated common bile duct Tortuous, dilated intrahepatic biliary ducts
Biliary neoplasia	Normal to increased	Mass visible in or associated with gallbladder
Pancreatitis with secondary common bile duct obstruction	Increased	Hypoechoic mass in area of pancreas Dilated common bile duct and intrahepatic biliary ducts
Trauma of lower biliary tract	Normal	± Abdominal fluid accumulation Absence of gallbladder

From Neer T: A review of disorders of the gallbladder and extrahepatic biliary tract in the dog and cat, *J Vet Intern Med* 6:186, 1992.

Cholecystitis and Cholelithiasis

Cholecystitis and cholelithiasis are considered by many people to be uncommon in older dogs and cats—a statement that is frequently quoted by many veterinarians and in veterinary textbooks and that is incorrect. Because of routine abdominal ultrasonography, more dogs and cats are now being diagnosed with acute and chronic gallbladder diseases. Cholecystitis often leads to vague signs of vomiting, fever, and abdominal pain. The usual cause of cholecystitis is thought to be a bacterial infection from ascending bacteria from the gastrointestinal tract or from hematogenous bacteria. When cholecystitis becomes severe, gallbladder necrosis and rupture may occur, with subsequent biliary peritonitis.[27] Ultrasonography shows increased gallbladder wall thickness and echogenicity; dilated, tortuous bile ducts; and concurrent cholelithiasis. Antimicrobial therapy based on bacterial culture and sensitivity test results is the optimal treatment for cholecystitis. Severe cases of cholecystitis, such as emphysematous or necrotic cholecystitis, may be treated surgically with cholecystectomy.

Choleliths are uncommon in older dogs as well. Choleliths are usually composed of cholesterol, bile acids, pigments, calcium, and protein. Diet and cholecystitis are predisposing causes for cholelith formation. The clinical signs of and diagnostic approach to cholelithiasis are similar to those associated with cholecystitis. Treatment of cholelithiasis may be either surgical or medical. Cholecystectomy can be performed for cholelithiasis, which will prevent recurrence. Medical therapy may include antimicrobial agents and commercial canine diet formulated for liver disease.

Extrahepatic bile duct obstruction can occur in older cats, usually secondary to cholelithiasis, inspissated bile, or parasitic infection. Choleliths in cats contain cholesterol, bilirubin derivatives, and calcium.[29] Occasionally, bile sludging secondary to increased mucosal uptake of bile fluid can result in overt inspissation of bile with biliary obstruction. Biliary obstruction and choleliths result in anorexia, vomiting, fever, icterus, and acholic (depigmented) stools in severely affected cats.

Cats of any age may be affected with a fluke infection of the biliary tract or pancreas.[29,30] Signs associated with a fluke infection are similar to those associated with other causes of biliary obstruction. Diagnosis of flukes is made by routine fecal sedimentation or use of formalin-ether sedimentation techniques to identify the typical-appearing fluke eggs. Occasionally, fluke eggs may be detected in abdominal fluid or liver cysts. Optimal treatment for liver and pancreatic flukes is praziquantel (20 to 30 mg/kg single time or daily for 3 days). Parasitized cats with severe liver disease secondary to biliary tract obstruction may have a guarded prognosis.

THE EXOCRINE PANCREAS

Exocrine pancreatic function most likely changes with advancing age in dogs and cats. The pancreas may be less likely to withstand stresses such as drastic dietary changes, extrapancreatic illness, or recurrent episodes of pancreatitis. The older dog or cat may then develop functional exocrine pancreatic insufficiency (EPI) secondary to severe stress and demands on gastrointestinal and pancreatic activities.

The Dog

Exocrine Pancreatic Diseases

Pancreatitis. Pancreatitis is caused by the activation of pancreatic digestion enzymes within the pancreas itself, resulting in severe inflammation, necrosis, and metabolic abnormalities. Acute pancreatitis may occur in a milder edematous form or a severe hemorrhagic form.[31] Repeated episodes of pancreatitis often lead to chronic pancreatitis, with fibrosis and subsequently EPI and/or diabetes mellitus.[32] Presenting signs include sudden onset of vomiting, anorexia, and depression. Physical examination may reveal cranial abdominal pain and fever. Chronic pancreatitis occurs in dogs that are predisposed to repeated episodes of pancreatitis, such as dogs receiving long-term immunosuppressive therapy or a high-fat diet, or dogs with persistent hyperlipemia. Exacerbations of chronic pancreatitis may resemble acute pancreatitis. Older dogs with chronic pancreatitis are often asymptomatic, and clinical signs develop only as severe pancreatic fibrosis ensues, possibly contributing to entrapment of the biliary tract as the bile duct courses to its duodenal opening.

Diagnosis of pancreatitis includes evaluation of laboratory values and diagnostic imaging of the cranial abdomen.[33] The most common laboratory findings include neutrophilia, azotemia, and increased serum ALT, AST, and ALP activities. The specific tests available for the diagnosis of pancreatitis in dogs are serum amylase and lipase activities and possibly serum canine pancreatic lipase immunoreactivity assay.[34] Serum canine pancreatic lipase immunoreactivity values greater than 82.8 μg/L (normal range, 1.9 to 82.8 μg/L) are consistent with pancreatic inflammatory disease. Abdominal radiographs may show loss of cranial abdominal detail, lateral displacement of the duodenum, and abdominal and/or pleural effusion.

The pancreas is identified ultrasonographically with some difficulty in older dogs, requiring high-resolution equipment and careful attention to transducer position.[35] In large, obese, or deep-chested dogs or those with signs of abdominal pain, it can be difficult to find an ultrasonographic window to the pancreas. The left lobe may be visible between the stomach and transverse colon from a ventral or left lateral approach. The right lobe is best visualized from a right lateral approach using the transducer to indent the abdominal wall to displace the small intestine and to bring the area of interest into the focal zone of the transducer. Once the duodenum is located, the right lobe of the pancreas may be visible dorsomedial to it. The right pancreatic lobe is normally hyperechoic when compared with the adjacent liver parenchyma. The pancreaticoduodenal vein passes through the right lobe and is visible in some instances, providing a useful landmark. Ultrasonography of the cranial abdomen may then show a visualized enlarged pancreas with adjacent hyperechoic fat, pancreatic mass formation (secondary to peripancreatic fat necrosis), pancreatic pseudocysts, and abscesses in the region of the pancreas.[31]

Therapy for dogs with moderate to severe pancreatitis, intravenous fluid therapy at doses calculated to meet rehydration, maintenance, and ongoing losses should be provided (Table 13-3). The fluid therapy should maintain normal blood pressure, replace losses induced by vomiting or exudation into body cavities, and maintain a blood flow through the devitalized pancreas.[36] To assist in stabilizing systemic blood flow, intravenous colloids such as hetastarch or dextrans may be administered at 10 to 20 ml/kg given over 1 to 2 hours. Food should be withheld until the dog has not vomited for 24 hours; then water is provided in small amounts, followed by small amounts of a bland diet. If no vomiting occurs, a bland diet (i.e., containing minimal fat and fiber, with moderate quantities of easily digestible carbohydrates and proteins) can be fed for several days before a gradual shift to an appropriate diet.

Other therapies used for pancreatitis include analgesic (butorphanol) and antimicrobial agents (ampicillin or a cephalosporin). Although pancreatitis itself is seldom a bacterial disease, the devitalized pancreas and peripancreatic fat, along with the localized peritonitis, can create a site for

TABLE 13-3. THERAPIES FOR ACUTE PANCREATITIS IN OLDER DOGS

TREATMENT	GOALS
Give nothing orally	Decrease pancreatic secretions
Intravenous fluid therapy	Replace gastrointestinal losses Maintain vascular volume Increase blood flow to pancreas
Dietary change	Decrease need for fat digestion Increase availability of carbohydrates for energy
Analgesic agents Meperidine Butorphanol	Relieve peritonitis-associated pain
Broad-spectrum antimicrobial agents	Minimize risk of bacterial infection
Peritoneal lavage	Reduce enzymatic effects in peritoneal cavity
Surgical débridement	Remove devitalized pancreas and fat Resect pancreatic abscesses Divert obstructed biliary system

bacterial growth. Ursodeoxycholic acid and antioxidants, such as vitamin E, may also be administered during clinical recovery from pancreatitis and in those dogs that have experienced recurrent episodes of pancreatitis. Severe pancreatitis may also require the use of peritoneal lavage to reduce the caustic effect of pancreatic enzymes within the abdominal cavity.[36]

Complications of severe pancreatitis can include pancreatic and peripancreatic mass formation (with the mass composed of necrotic pancreatic and omental tissue), pancreatic abscess formation, and biliary obstruction.[37] Surgical intervention for treatment of pancreatic masses or abscesses is often unsuccessful, and most dogs with these conditions die. Severe extrahepatic bile duct obstruction induced by fibrosing pancreatitis may also necessitate surgical intervention for a biliary diversion procedure.[32]

Exocrine Pancreatic Insufficiency. In older dogs, EPI is usually seen secondary to severe chronic pancreatitis. When more than 90% of enzyme production is lost, clinical signs of EPI become obvious. Clinical signs include small bowel diarrhea with steatorrhea, weight loss, and polyphagia. Dogs that continue to have pancreatitis in combination with EPI may have vomiting and a decreased appetite. Physical examination may reveal signs of weight loss and diarrhea. The diagnosis of EPI is made when a decreased serum trypsin-like immunoreactivity (TLI) concentration (serum TLI values consistently $<5\ \mu g/L$) in a fasted dog is detected.

Treatment of dogs with EPI depends mainly on dietary management and supplementation with pancreatic digestive enzymes.[38,39] Efforts to treat these dogs are usually rewarded with a favorable response. The most effective dietary management for EPI is a highly digestible, low-fiber, moderate-fat diet supplemented with pancreatic enzymes. Commercial diets formulated for gastrointestinal disease may be fed. The dog's daily food intake is divided into two or three feedings or is fed free choice. The dietary replacement of pancreatic digestive enzymes is given orally with each meal. Reliable commercial products are available in powder form. The usual effective dosage of the powder preparation is 1 to 2 teaspoons per meal for each 20 kg body weight. The pancreatic enzyme product is mixed with the commercially prepared canned or well-moistened dry dog food and fed without necessarily any preincubation time. When diarrhea is in remission and the animal is gaining weight, then titrate the pancreatic enzyme product to the minimum effective maintenance dose per feeding.

Antimicrobial agents may be a helpful adjunctive therapy for the bacterial overgrowth of the small intestine that often accompanies malassimilation in dogs with EPI.[40] Medium-chain triglycerides may also be added to the dog's diet if additional dietary energy is needed to increase weight or maintain condition in the dog that fails to respond otherwise. The medium-chain triglycerides can be used to provide up to 25% of the dog's caloric need and, when fully utilized, provide 8 kcal/ml.[39]

The dog's body weight, general condition, and stool character should be monitored weekly during the treatment of EPI. Stool volume should decrease precipitously, and gains in body weight should begin soon after initiation of dietary management and the supplementation of pancreatic digestive enzymes. The dietary replacement of pancreatic digestive enzymes is generally required for the rest of the dog's life.

Exocrine Pancreatic Neoplasia. Pancreatic adenocarcinoma may arise from the pancreatic acinar cells, disrupting normal pancreatic function. Dogs with pancreatic adenocarcinoma may have clinical signs of acute pancreatitis and will not respond to conventional therapy.[3,35] Pancreatic adenocarcinoma frequently metastasizes to regional lymph nodes, stomach, duodenum, and liver.[3] Diagnosis requires a surgical biopsy. Surgical resection of the tumor is difficult. Chemotherapy for pancreatic adenocarcinoma can be attempted, but the prognosis is poor.

The Cat

Exocrine Pancreatic Diseases. Diseases of the exocrine pancreas have been thought to occur much less commonly in senior-aged or geriatric-aged cats than in comparably aged humans or dogs. This belief is absolutely incorrect. The history and clinical signs of exocrine pancreatic disease are vague and nonspecific, which is probably the primary reason that exocrine pancreatic disease problems have been so infrequently diagnosed in the older cat.

Pancreatitis. Pancreatitis is characterized as either acute pancreatitis or chronic pancreatitis depending on the presence of fibrosis on histopathologic evaluation and duration of illness. Pancreatitis is most often exhibited as a component of *feline triad disease*, a term which refers to concurrent inflammatory liver disease, lymphocytic pancreatitis, and inflammatory bowel disease all occurring in the older cat at the same time. Acute pancreatitis is diagnosed in cats 4 weeks to 18 years old or older. Domestic shorthair and domestic longhair cats are affected most commonly. No sex predisposition exists. Both acute and chronic pancreatitis may be mild or severe, depending on whether systemic complications are present or not.

The underlying cause of pancreatitis in older cats is generally unknown. Some cases have been associated with severe abdominal trauma (caused by road traffic accidents or falling from heights), infectious diseases (feline panleukopenia, feline herpesvirus type 1 infection, FIP, toxoplasmosis, and *Amphimerus pseudofelineus* infection), acute and chronic inflammatory liver disease, and organophosphate or drug intoxication. However, most cases of pancreatitis in the older cat are immune mediated. As in other organs involved in feline triad disease, the exocrine pancreas is infiltrated with varying numbers of mature lymphocytes and an inappropriate neutrophilic response to the amount of inflammation present, indicating an immune-mediated disease.

The clinical presentation of most cats with acute or chronic pancreatitis is vague and nonspecific. The clinical signs may include lethargy, anorexia, dehydration, hypothermia, vomiting, abdominal pain, palpable abdominal mass, dyspnea, ataxia, and diarrhea. Hematologic abnormalities are uncommon and also nonspecific. Serum chemistry profile shows mild increases of serum ALT, ALP, total bilirubin, and total globulins, probably reflecting feline triad disease or secondary hepatic lipidosis. Azotemia is also frequently observed and is attributable to dehydration in most cases or chronic renal failure. The determination of serum lipase and amylase activities is unfortunately of no value in the older cat.

Radiographic abnormalities can be present but are often subtle and rather subjective. Decreased contrast in the cranial abdomen; dilated and gas-filled small intestines; transposition of the duodenum, stomach, and transverse colon; and hepatomegaly may be noted. On abdominal ultrasonography, a soft-tissue mass effect may be observed in the cranial abdomen. Other ultrasonographic changes may include pancreatic swelling, increased echogenicity of the pancreas, and fluid accumulation around the pancreas.

A radioimmunoassay for measuring feline serum TLI activity is available for cats of all ages and breeds. Normal control range for this radioimmunoassay is typically 17 to 49 μg/L. In cases of suspected pancreatitis the serum TLI values would be expected to be >49 μg/L. Still, a definitive diagnosis of feline pancreatitis can be made only by pancreatic biopsy via exploratory laparotomy or laparoscopy (Figure 13-6).

Initial management of pancreatitis usually begins with rehydration—administration of crystalloid fluids (lactated Ringer's solution) at a rate and via a route that will provide maintenance and replace both deficits and ongoing losses over a 24-hour period. Cats with signs of shock require more aggressive support. The volume deficit can be replaced with crystalloid fluids at an initial rate of 60 ml/kg per hour, and then this rate can be tailored to maintain adequate tissue perfusion and hydration. Colloid solutions can be used in shocked animals to reduce the amount of crystalloid fluids required (intravenous hetastarch or dextran 70 at 10 to 20 ml/kg daily). Other symptomatic therapy includes controlling vomiting when it is persistent. Prophylactic antimicrobial agents such as cephalosporins and ampicillin may be warranted in animals in shock and may help prevent bacterial translocation and pancreatic abscess.

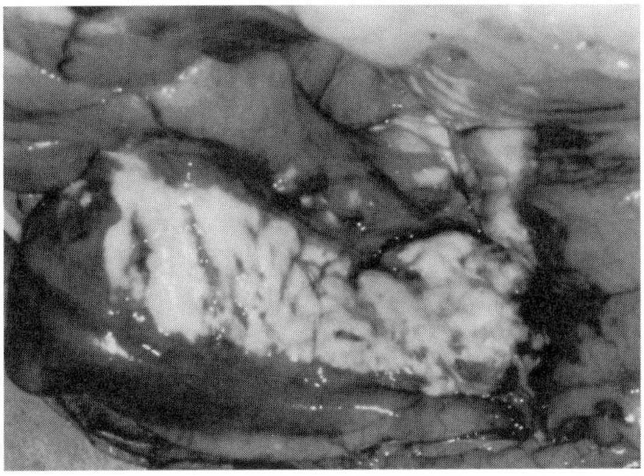

Figure 13-6. Surgical exploration of a 12-year-old cat with acute pancreatitis. Note the severe fat saponification and inflammation of the duodenum.

Maintaining adequate nutrition during a bout of pancreatitis may be difficult. The traditional recommendation for any animal suffering from pancreatitis is to give nothing orally for approximately 3 to 4 days. This recommendation is justified in cats with persistent vomiting, but there is little evidence to justify this strategy in other cats. The preferred routes of alimentation are a jejunostomy tube or total parenteral nutrition. These feeding strategies are impractical in most cases, and a gastrostomy tube, esophagostomy tube, or even a nasogastric tube is an acceptable alternative if the cat is not vomiting. If the cat has persistent vomiting and there is no evidence to support secondary hepatic lipidosis, the cat could be held off food for 3 to 4 days. After this time, water is slowly reintroduced, followed by small amounts of a commercially prepared cat food.

Corticosteroids may be needed to treat cats with concurrent inflammatory bowel disease, liver disease, and mild pancreatitis. It should also be remembered that many cats have a mild form of chronic pancreatitis and often benefit from daily administration of pancreatic enzyme supplementation therapy. Dried powdered extracts of bovine or porcine pancreas can be used—1 teaspoonful mixed into the meal given twice daily. If the cat refuses to eat the food with pancreatic extract included, raw beef pancreas can be used. One to three ounces (30 to 90 g) of chopped raw pancreas (which can be kept frozen for a long time without losing enzymatic activity) are given per meal initially. If the cat also refuses to eat raw pancreas, a fish-based liquid formulation of the enzyme supplement can be prepared; this preparation is readily taken by most cats.

Cats with suspected or confirmed pancreatitis should be carefully monitored to detect early forms of shock or other systemic abnormalities. Minimal monitoring for stable cats includes regular assessment of vital signs and fluid and electrolyte balance. In cats with systemic abnormalities, monitoring should be more aggressive and may include vital signs, packed cell volume, fluid intake and output, indirect blood pressure determination, serum electrolytes and glucose, acid-base status, total platelet counts, and coagulation status.

Exocrine Pancreatic Insufficiency. Cats affected with EPI may develop diarrhea and weight loss, with most cats displaying a good appetite. Diagnosis of EPI is based on ruling out other causes of weight loss with a good appetite in older cats (e.g., hyperthyroidism, diabetes mellitus, or intestinal malabsorption) and tests of pancreatic function. In cases of EPI, in which the exocrine pancreas is secreting insufficient amounts of digestive enzymes into the duodenum, serum TLI values will be <8 μg/L.[41–43] Response to therapy using pancreatic enzyme powder may be used as both a diagnostic and therapeutic trial, but improvement may be seen with diseases other than EPI. Treatment for EPI is similar to that in older dogs. Most cats with chronic pancreatic insufficiency also are severely cobalamin deficient. Initially, 100 to 150 μg of cobalamin is administered subcutaneously on a monthly basis.

Exocrine Pancreatic Neoplasia. Benign nodular hyperplasia, adenoma, and pancreatic adenocarcinoma have all been reported in cats.[44] Nodular hyperplasia and adenoma usually do not cause disease and are an incidental necropsy finding. In cats with adenocarcinoma of the pancreas, a palpable cranial abdominal mass may be the only significant finding.[44] Surgical resection of the mass may be attempted, but the overall prognosis is poor.

References

1. Center S, ManWarren T, Slater M et al: Evaluation of twelve-hour preprandial and two-hour postprandial serum bile acids concentrations for diagnosis of hepatobiliary disease in dogs, *J Am Vet Med Assoc* 199:217, 1991.
2. Biller D, Kantrowitz B, Miyabayashi T: Ultrasonography of diffuse liver disease, *J Vet Intern Med* 6:71, 1992.
3. Strombeck D, Guilford W: *Small animal gastroenterology*, Davis, Calif, 1990, Stonegate Publishing.
4. Bunch S, Polak D, Hornbuckle W: A modified laparoscopic approach for liver biopsy in dogs, *J Am Vet Med Assoc* 187:1032, 1985.
5. Hultgren B, Stevens J, Hardy R: Inherited, chronic, progressive hepatic degeneration in Bedlington terriers

with increased liver copper concentrations: clinical and pathologic observations and comparison with other copper-associated liver diseases, *Am J Vet Res* 47:365, 1986.
6. Twedt D, Hunsaker H, Allen K: Use of 2,3,2-tetramine as a hepatic copper chelating agent for treatment of copper hepatotoxicosis in Bedlington Terriers, *J Am Vet Med Assoc* 192:52, 1988.
7. Crawford MA, Schall WD, Jensen RK et al: Chronic active hepatitis in 26 Doberman pinschers, *J Am Vet Med Assoc* 187:1343, 1985.
8. Thornburg LP, Rottinghaus G: What is the significance of hepatic copper values in dogs with cirrhosis? *Vet Med* May:50, 1985.
9. Thornburg L, Rottinghaus G, Gage H: Chronic liver disease associated with high hepatic copper concentration in a dog, *J Am Vet Med Assoc* 188:1190, 1986.
10. Thornburg L, Rottinghaus G, Koch J et al: High liver copper levels in two Doberman pinschers with subacute hepatitis, *J Am Anim Hosp Assoc* 20:1003, 1984.
11. Brewer G, Dick R, Schall W et al: Use of zinc acetate to treat copper toxicosis in dogs, *J Am Vet Med Assoc* 201:564, 1992.
12. Johnson S: Portal hypertension. Part I. Pathophysiology and clinical consequences, *Compend Contin Educ Pract Vet* 9:741, 1987.
13. Johnson S: Portal hypertension. Part II. Clinical assessment and treatment, *Compend Contin Educ Pract Vet* 9:917, 1987.
14. Boer H, Nelson R, Long G: Colchicine therapy for hepatic fibrosis in a dog, *J Am Anim Hosp Assoc* 185:303, 1984.
15. Rogers W, Ruebner B: A retrospective study of probable glucocorticoid-induced hepatopathy in dogs, *J Am Vet Med Assoc* 170:603, 1977.
16. Badylak S, VanVleet J: Sequential morphologic and clinicopathologic alterations in dogs with experimentally induced glucocorticoid hepatopathy, *Am J Vet Res* 42:1310, 1981.
17. Hosgood G: Arteriovenous fistulas: pathophysiology, diagnosis, and treatment, *Compend Contin Educ Pract Vet* 11:625, 1989.
18. Willard M, Baley M, Hauptman J et al: Obstructed portal venous flow and portal vein thrombosis in a dog, *J Am Vet Med Assoc* 194:1449, 1989.
19. Tyler J: Hepatoencephalopathy. Part I. Clinical signs and diagnosis, *Compend Contin Educ Pract Vet* 12:1069, 1990.
20. Tyler J: Hepatoencephalopathy. Part II. Pathophysiology and treatment, *Compend Contin Educ Pract Vet* 12:1260, 1990.
21. Magne M: Primary epithelial hepatic tumors in the dog, *Compend Contin Educ Pract Vet* 6:506, 1984.
22. Center SA: The jaundiced cat, *Proc Feline Med Symp,* 1997.
23. Thornburg L: Fatty liver syndrome in cats, *J Am Anim Hosp Assoc* 18:397, 1982.
24. Meyer D, French T: The liver. In Cowell R, Tyler R, eds: *Diagnostic cytology of the dog and cat,* Goleta, Calif, 1989, American Veterinary Publications.
25. Post G, Patnaik A: Nonhematopoietic hepatic neoplasms in cats: 21 cases (1983-1988), *J Am Vet Med Assoc* 201:1080, 1992.
26. Church E, Matthiesen D: Surgical treatment of 23 dogs with necrotizing cholecystitis, *J Am Anim Hosp Assoc* 24:305, 1988.
27. Center S: Feline liver disorders and their management, *Compend Contin Educ Pract Vet* 8:889, 1986.
28. Neer T: A review of disorders of the gallbladder and extrahepatic biliary tract in the dog and cat, *J Vet Intern Med* 6:186, 1992.
29. Zawie D, Shaker E: Diseases of the liver. In Sherding R, ed: *The cat: diseases and clinical management,* New York, 1989, Churchill-Livingstone.
30. Schaer M: Acute pancreatitis in dogs, *Compend Contin Educ Pract Vet* 13:1769, 1991.
31. Matthiesen D, Rosin E: Common bile duct obstruction secondary to chronic fibrosing pancreatitis: treatment by use of cholecystoduodenostomy in the dog, *J Am Vet Med Assoc* 189:1443, 1986.
32. Schaer M: A clinicopathologic survey of acute pancreatitis in 30 dogs and 5 cats, *J Am Anim Hosp Assoc* 15:681, 1979.
33. Steiner J: Canine pancreatic lipase immunoreactivity (cPLI): a new test for pancreatitis. In Ruaux C, Steiner J, Williams D, eds: *GI Lab Newsletter, Texas A&M University,* November:1, 2000.
34. Lamb MA: Ultrasonographic imaging of endocrine organs, *Proc Am Coll Vet Intern Med* 15:57, 1997.
35. Mulvaney M, Feinberg C, Tilson D: Clinical characterization of acute necrotizing pancreatitis, *Compend Contin Educ Pract Vet* 4:394, 1982.
36. Edwards D, Bauer M, Walker Met al: Pancreatic masses in seven dogs following acute pancreatitis, *J Am Anim Hosp Assoc* 26:189, 1990.
37. Wiberg ME, Nurmi AK, Westermarck E: Serum trysinlike immunoreactivity measurement for the diagnosis of subclinical exocrine pancreatic insufficiency, *J Vet Intern Med* 13:426, 1999.
38. Lewis L, Morris M, Hand M: *Small animal clinical nutrition,* Topeka, Kan, 1987, Mark Morris Associates.
39. Simpson K, Batt R, Jones D et al: Effects of exocrine pancreatic insufficiency and replacement therapy on the bacterial flora of the duodenum in dogs, *Am J Vet Res* 51:203, 1990.
40. Lamb CR, Simpson KW, Boswood A et al: Ultrasonography of pancreatic neoplasia in the dog: retrospective review of 16 cases, *Vet Rec* 137:65, 1995.
41. Williams D, Reed S, Perry L: Fecal proteolytic activity in clinically normal cats and in a cat with exocrine pancreatic insufficiency, *J Am Vet Med Assoc* 197:210, 1990.
42. Steiner JM, Williams DA: Serum feline trypsin-like immunoreactivity in cats with exocrine pancreatic insufficiency, *J Vet Intern Med* 14:627, 2000.
43. Owens J, Drazner F, Gilbertson S: Pancreatic disease in the cat, *J Am Anim Hosp Assoc* 11:83, 1975.

Supplemental Reading

Rolfe DS, Twedt DC: Copper-associated hepatopathies in dogs, *Vet Clin North Am Small Anim Pract* 25:399, 1995.

CHAPTER 14

The Skin

SANDRA R. MERCHANT

No skin disease is found exclusively in the older animal. However, aging tends to predispose dogs and cats to various skin diseases. Impaired immunity, structural changes in the skin, and internal diseases with cutaneous manifestations (internal diseases found more often in the aged animal) all can increase the frequency of certain skin diseases in the aged animal.

As a general rule, decreased immune surveillance is believed to play a role in susceptibility to neoplasia. Endocrinopathies such as hypothyroidism, hyperthyroidism, diabetes mellitus, and hyperadrenocorticism are seen more often in older animals. Adult-onset demodicosis may also be associated with the aging process by way of its link to an underlying disease process (neoplasia, endocrinopathy, and so on). Many internal diseases that occur in aged animals may have specific or non-specific cutaneous manifestations. A catabolic or cachectic state occurring in an animal for any number of reasons may be reflected in the skin and hair by seborrhea and a dull, dry, brittle, sparse coat.

SENILE CHANGES OF THE SKIN

Much has been written concerning senile changes of human skin, but very little information is available concerning senile changes in the skin of domestic animals. The most comprehensive information is found in a study of the histopathologic changes seen in the skin of 14 aged dogs. The dogs ranged in age from 12 to 17 years.[1] Few histologic changes were observed except in extreme age. Epidermal and follicular hyperkeratosis was evident. Many follicles did not contain hair shafts, appeared flask-shaped, and were lined by a single layer of flattened epidermal cells. Atrophy of the epidermis and dermis was seen in extreme age (17 years). The epidermal cells were flattened with pyknotic nuclei, and the viable epidermis was often one cell thick. The dermis was almost cell-free.[1]

With increasing age, collagen bundles became granular and fragmented, and, in extreme cases, the dermis presented an eosinophilic hyaline appearance. There was an apparent decrease in reticulin tissue. Pigmented areas had a marked increase in dermal pigmentation.

Variable changes were seen in the glands of the skin. In some animals cystic dilation or hyperplasia of the apocrine glands was seen. Some apocrine glands contained large yellow refractile granules located in the secretory cells. The individual cells of the circumanal glands were reduced in size and contained pyknotic nuclei. Arrector pili muscles were more eosinophilic and fragmented, with vacuolization within individual fibers. In extreme age, all traces of these muscles sometimes disappeared. Changes in cutaneous blood vessels were not evident.

Clinically, the hair of some dogs became dull and lusterless, with areas of alopecia and callous formation over pressure points. Increased numbers of white hairs on the muzzle were frequently noted. The footpads were sometimes hyperkeratinized, and the claws malformed and brittle.

PATIENT EVALUATION

Dermatologic History

Whether the animal is presented for a routine geriatric examination or because the owner has noted a skin problem, a thorough dermatologic history and dermatologic examination are important parts of the minimum database.

The dermatologic history is the most important part of the evaluation of the skin and hair. The information derived from an in-depth and well organized dermatologic history often provides more diagnostic information than the physical or dermatologic examination or ancillary diagnostic tests.

The use of a dermatologic history questionnaire that can be filled in by the owner before the examination will save time and provides an effective format for the veterinarian to quickly gather information and clarify or complete the information as necessary. A standard dermatologic history questionnaire is therefore completed in all cases, and important questions are not forgotten (Figure 14-1). Other history-taking forms are published.[2-4]

Dermatologic Examination

The veterinarian who performs a thorough and in-depth dermatologic examination will gain valuable information and will be able to efficiently choose the few other specialized diagnostic tests needed to define the skin disease. Because recheck examinations are often necessary in dermatology, recording the dermatologic examination findings and test results at each visit are important for the documentation of the progression or regression of the disease. Having a standard figure in the record can be helpful for the systematic recording of location and severity of lesions (Figure 14-2).

ENDOCRINOPATHIES

Hypothyroidism

Hypothyroidism is a commonly diagnosed endocrine disorder in dogs and a rarely diagnosed endocrine disorder in the cat. There are myriad clinical signs associated with hypothyroidism, because thyroid hormones have an effect on almost every tissue of the body.

Pathophysiology. More than 95% of the cases of canine hypothyroidism are primary in nature, resulting from a destructive process involving the thyroid gland.[5] The remaining cases are secondary to hypothalamic or pituitary disease. Naturally acquired primary hypothyroidism has been documented in the cat. Reports have provided evidence for an autoimmune process.[6,7] Another study evaluated a congenital form of hypothyroidism in related Abyssinian cats.[8] Secondary or tertiary forms of hypothyroidism have not been documented in this species.

Primary hypothyroidism in the dog is usually a result of either lymphocytic thyroiditis or idiopathic thyroidal atrophy. Autoimmune mechanisms are thought to be involved in the initial attack on the thyroid gland in lymphocytic thyroiditis. Antibodies to thyroglobulin, microsomal antigen, CA-2 and a cell surface antigen have been documented.[5] Thyroid biopsies taken during acute stages of lymphocytic thyroiditis show a tissue infiltrate consisting of lymphocytes and plasma cells. Idiopathic thyroidal atrophy is characterized by loss of the normal thyroid parenchyma, which is replaced with adipose tissue. There is a lack of an inflammatory infiltrate. Hypothyroidism should be considered in any animal undergoing radiation therapy in which the thyroid gland is included in the radiation field.[9]

Clinical Features

Signalment. The onset of clinical signs occurs at varying ages but generally begins during middle age. Breeds that have been reported to be predisposed to hypothyroidism include the boxer, dachshund, Doberman pinscher, Great Dane, golden retriever, Irish setter, miniature schnauzer, poodle, and Old English sheepdog.[5,10] No sex predilection has been demonstrated. Familial lymphocytic thyroiditis has been reported in borzois.[11]

Spontaneous hypothyroidism in the cat is a rare clinical entity with no age, breed, or sex predilection. Bilateral thyroidectomy and overdose of radioactive iodine or antithyroid drugs in hyperthyroid cats are the most common causes of hypothyroidism and are most often seen in aged cats.

History. Hypothyroidism is usually insidious in nature. The owner or veterinarian may attribute many of the clinical signs simply to aging, or the signs may be completely overlooked, especially in the "nonworking" pet dog until late in the course of the disease. Because thyroid hormones affect most tissues in the body, the clinical signs are multisystemic, variable, and rarely pathognomonic for hypothyroidism. In addition, atherosclerosis secondary to hypothyroidism can cause

DERMATOLOGY HISTORY

NAME ______ CASE NO. ______

STREET ______

CITY, STATE, ZIP ______

PHONE: BUS ______ HOME ______

SPECIES ______ BREED ______ SEX ______

ANIMAL'S NAME ______ DATE OF BIRTH ______

COLOR-IDENTIFYING MARK ______

DATE:	CLINICIAN:	STUDENT:

CHIEF COMPLAINT(S) ______

______

______

Date (age) Problem First Noticed ______ Onset: Sudden ______ Slow ______

Is there a seasonal influence? No______ Summer ______ Fall ______ Winter ______

Where did problem begin? ______

What did it look like then? ______

Does animal itch? Yes ______ No ______ When? Constant ______ Sporadic ______ Night ______

Is there any exposure to other animals (neighbors, etc?) ______

Do other animals or people have skin problems, rash? ______

Describe animal's indoor environment, time (%): ______

______

Describe animal's outdoor environment, time (%): ______

______

What does animal sleep on? ______

What diagnostic tests have been performed? ______

What local treatment has been used? success? ______

______

What systemic treatment has been used? success? ______

______

Does owner have an idea of the cause? What makes it worse? ______

When did owner last see fleas? ______ Describe flea control ______

Animal's diet ______

Reproductive history: age of neutering? ______ Date, duration of last estrus ______

Breeding history (male or female) ______

Medical History: Previous diseases, treatments, results: ______

______

Is animal on any medication at present? ______

What other facts does owner think would be helpful? ______

______

______

Figure 14-1. Dermatology history form (Louisiana State University Veterinary Teaching Hospital and Clinic).

DATE:	CLINICIAN:	STUDENT:

NAME ____ CASE NO.
STREET ____
CITY, STATE, ZIP ____
PHONE. BUS ____ HOME ____
SPECIES BREED SEX
ANIMAL'S NAME DATE OF BIRTH
COLOR-IDENTIFYING MARK

PRURITUS?

PARASITES?

PRIMARY LESIONS (Circle)

Macule	Patch	Papule	Plaque
Vesicle	Bulla	Pustule	Wheal
Nodule	Tumor		

SECONDARY LESIONS (Circle)

Scale	Epidermal collarette	Scar	Ulcer
Erosion	Crust	Excoriation	Fissure
Comedone	Cyst	Abscess	Hypopigmentation
Hyperpigmentation	Erythema	Hyperkeratosis	Callus
Alopecia	Lichenification		

CONFIGURATION OF LESIONS (Circle)

Regional Linear Annular (Target) Grouped Irregular

QUALITY OF HAIR COAT

Epilation: + −
Pelage is: Dry,
Brittle, Dull, Oily

OTHER FACTORS

Footpads
Nails
Hyperhidrosis

LABORATORY TESTS

Scotch Tape: ____ Wood's Light + −
Skin Scraping: ____
KOH Digestion: ____
Direct Smear: ____
Fungal Culture: ____
Bacterial Culture: ____
Sensitivity: ____
Allergy: ____
Endocrine: ____
Immune:
D.I.T.: ____
I.I.T.: ____
ANA: ____
Other: ____
Biopsy: Site(s) ____ Path As. No. ____
RESULTS: ____

DISTRIBUTION OF LESIONS

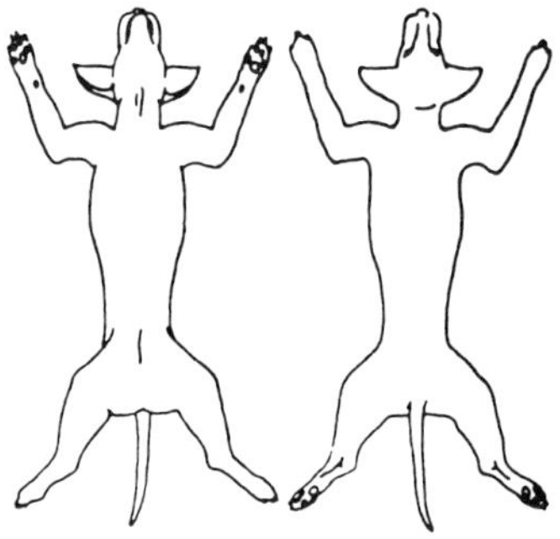

Ventral Dorsal

DIFFERENTIAL DIAGNOSIS:

COMMENTS:

SIGNED BY ATTENDING CLINICIAN

Medical Records—White
Clinician—Canary

Figure 14-2. Dermatology examination form (Louisiana State University Veterinary Teaching Hospital and Clinic).

BOX 14-1 Clinical Signs of Hypothyroidism in the Dog

Mental dullness
Lethargy
Exercise intolerance
Increase in weight
Seeking heat
Stiffness
Muscle wasting
Neuromuscular signs (lower motor neuron disease, peripheral vestibular deficits, megaesophagus, and laryngeal paralysis)
Constipation
Diarrhea
Vomiting
Ocular abnormalities (corneal lipid deposits, corneal ulcerative uveitis)
Reproductive dysfunction (female—infertility; prolonged interestrous intervals; failure to cycle; weak or silent cycles; prolonged estrual bleeding; and the birth of weak, dying, or stillborn puppies; male—lack of libido; testicular atrophy; hypospermia to azoospermia; and infertility)
Cardiac abnormalities (bradycardia, cardiac arrhythmias, impaired left ventricular function)
Dermatologic (dry scaly coat [Figure 14-3], bilaterally symmetrical nonpruritic truncal alopecia, rat tail)

Data from Jaggy A, Oliver JE, Ferguson DC et al: Neurological manifestations of hypothyroidism: a retrospective study of 29 dogs, *J Vet Intern Med* 8:328, 1994.

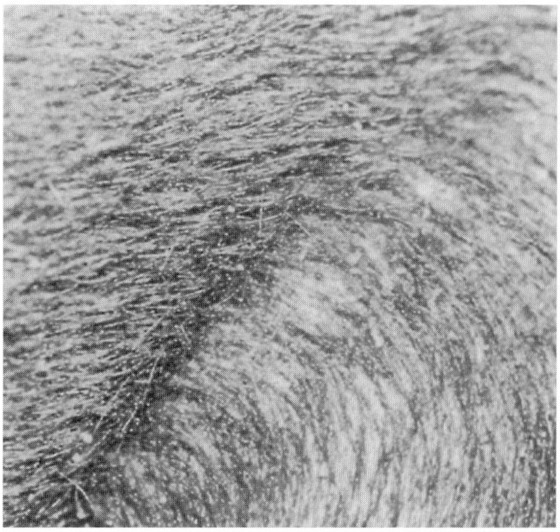

Figure 14-3. Dry, scaling skin and haircoat of a dog with hypothyroidism.

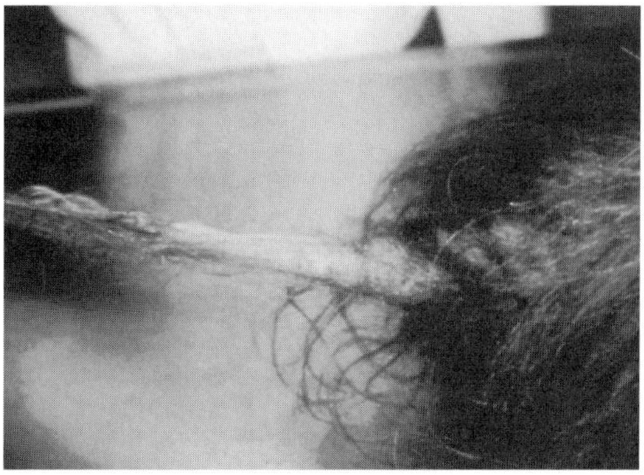

Figure 14-4. Hair loss on the tail of a dog with hypothyroidism.

multiorgan disease.[12] A complete list of clinical signs is found in Box 14-1. The following discussion focuses on the dermatologic manifestations of the disease.

Physical Examination. Most dogs (with the exception of working and breeding dogs) will be presented to a veterinarian when dermatologic abnormalities become evident. Early dermatologic manifestations of hypothyroidism include dryness, scaliness, and excessive shedding (Figure 14-3). Failure of hair regrowth secondary to cessation of the anagen hair phase leads to progressive symmetric alopecia. The pattern of hair loss is most often bilateral and symmetric, especially on the flanks, ventral neck, dorsal tail, and pressure points (Figure 14-4). The skin may be hyperpigmented and occasionally thickened secondary to myxedema (Figure 14-5). Pruritus may be seen with the occurrence of secondary dermatologic diseases such as seborrhea (Figures 14-6 and 14-7), *Malassezia* dermatitis, and staphylococcal pyoderma. The trauma from scratching the skin may also contribute to the lichenification and hyperpigmentation. Some animals may have recurrent staphylococcal pyoderma as the presenting sign. In very rare cases, hypertrichosis may be seen. A deficiency of thyroid hormone may also be a cause of insulin resistance.[13]

Clinical signs in the cat consist of profound apathy, inappetence, hypothermia, obesity, bradycardia, failure to cycle, dystocia, poor hair growth, severe seborrhea, dull haircoat, easily epilated hair, pinnal alopecia, lichenification, facial myxedema, poor wound healing, and decubital ulcers.[6,7,14]

Diagnosis. Once the veterinarian suspects hypothyroidism, further testing is required. Common laboratory tests in the dog include a complete

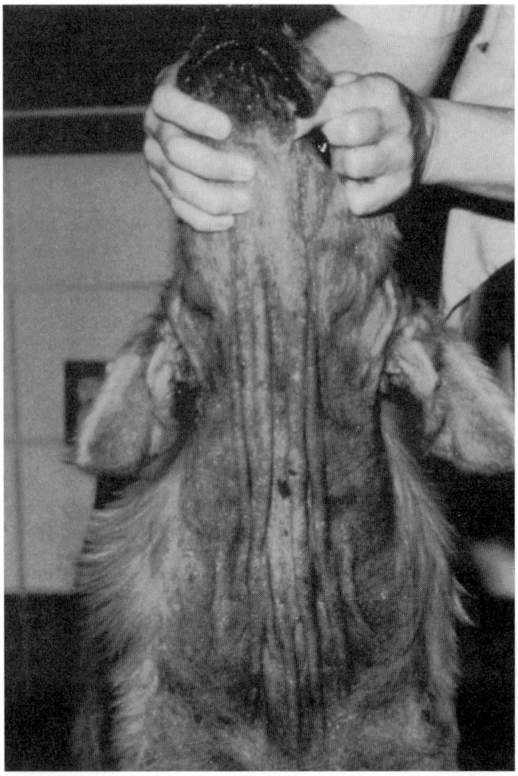

Figure 14-5. Extreme hyperpigmentation on the ventral cervical region of a golden retriever dog with hypothyroidism.

blood count, serum chemistry profile, and urinalysis. These not only may give supportive evidence to continue the search for hypothyroidism, but they may suggest other causes for the dermatologic signs (e.g., hyperadrenocorticism). Laboratory findings associated with hypothyroidism include hypercholesterolemia, hyperlipemia, and a normocytic, normochromic nonregenerative anemia. Results of urinalysis are usually normal.

Confirmation of hypothyroidism involves assessment of thyroid function. Many different tests for thyroid function in the dog have been reported in the literature. Measurement of basal serum thyroid hormone concentration is an often used initial test for diagnosing hypothyroidism in the dog. Thyroxine (T_4) is the primary hormone secreted by the thyroid gland and is present in higher concentrations in the serum than triiodothyronine (T_3). Basal serum T_4 is a more accurate indicator of thyroid status than basal T_3 concentration. Approximately 99% of thyroid hormones are bound to plasma protein. This bound fraction is unavailable to the tissues and acts as a reservoir. The unbound, free hormone is available to the tissues and is metabolically active. Measurement of basal hormone concentrations generally includes the measurement of both the bound and unbound fraction without separation.

Measurement of basal T_4 concentration should be viewed as a screening test. A total T_4 concentration that is well within the normal range should rule out hypothyroidism. The problem with the use of a basal T_4 concentration arises when the value is borderline. Overdiagnosis of hypothyroidism occurs often because of erroneous interpretation of borderline-to-low thyroid hormone levels. Numerous factors can influence thyroid hormone concentration (Box 14-2).

A very low serum T_4 concentration in the absence of any of the conditions mentioned in Box 14-2 in a dog with signs of hypothyroidism may be

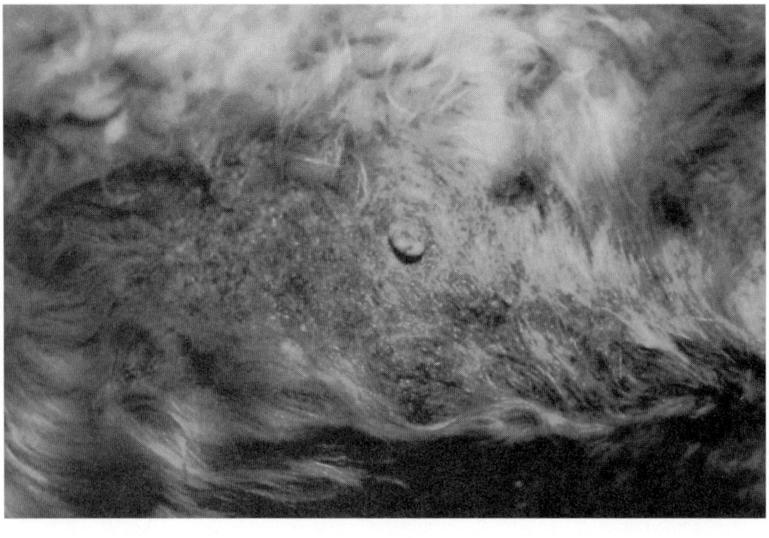

Figure 14-6. Seborrhea oleosa on the ventral abdomen of a cocker spaniel dog with hypothyroidism.

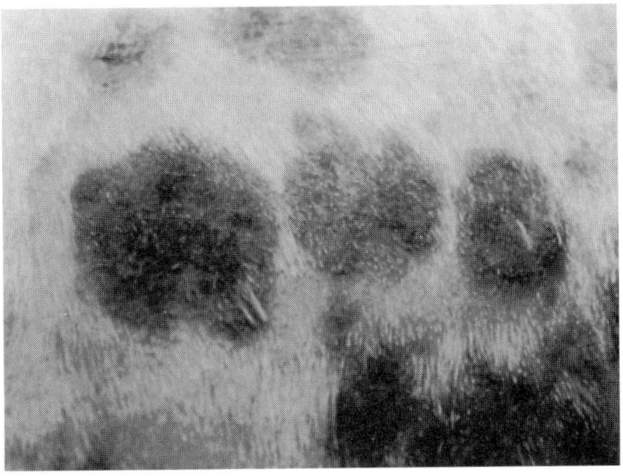

Figure 14-7. Plaques of seborrheic dermatitis on the ventral thorax and abdomen of a cocker spaniel dog with hypothyroidism.

BOX 14-2 Nonthyroidal Factors that Can Influence Basal T_4 Concentration in the Dog

Age:

Neonates: increased T_4 concentration
Adult dogs: decreased T_4 with age

Breed:

Tendency for increased T_4 concentration in small breed dogs, decrease in large breed dogs
Greyhound: Serum T_4 concentration is higher

Obesity:

Increased T_4

Hypoproteinemia:

Increase caused by decreased plasma protein binding

Drugs:

Glucocorticoids, anticonvulsants, some antibiotics (penicillin, trimethoprim-sulfa), androgens, phenylbutazone, quinidine, propylthiouracil, salicylates, sulfonylureas, carprofen, dopamine will decrease T_4
Insulin increases T_4

"Euthyroid Sick Syndrome"

Many acute and chronic illnesses will lower T_4 including renal disease, liver disease, diabetes mellitus, infectious disease, gastrointestinal dysfunction, hyperadrenocorticism, and demodicosis

Data from Feldman EC, Nelson RW: *Canine and feline endocrinology and reproduction,* Philadelphia, 1996, WB Saunders; Ferguson DC, Moore GE, Hoenig M: Carprofen lowers total T_4 and TSH, but not free T_4 concentrations in dogs, *Proc Am Coll Vet Intern Med Forum* 17:709, 1999; Beale KM: Techniques for evaluating thyroid function in the dog, *Vet Clin North Am* 20(6):1429, 1990b; Hall IA, Campbell KL, Chamber MD et al: Effect of trimethoprim/sulfamethoxazole on thyroid function in dogs with pyoderma, *J Am Vet Med Assoc* 202:1959, 1993; Kantrowitz LB, Peterson ME, Trepanier LA et al: Serum total thyroxine, total triiodothyronine, free thyroxine, and thyrotropin concentrations in epileptic dogs treated with anticonvulsants. *J Am Vet Med Assoc* 214:1804, 1999.

sufficient evidence for diagnosis. In a dog with appropriate clinical signs and a borderline value with or without factors affecting the basal thyroid hormone concentration, further testing is warranted. Evaluation of serum free T_4 by equilibrium dialysis may be chosen when the basal total T_4 concentration is borderline or when factors noted in Box 14-2 may be influencing the basal thyroid value in the animal. Free T_4 may be less affected by the factors listed in Box 14-2, but this value can still be falsely lowered by numerous factors listed. Evaluating free T_4 in conjunction with total T_4 may reduce the false-positive diagnosis of hypothyroidism. A recent study comparing total T_4, free T_4 by equilibrium dialysis, and thyrotropin hormone (TSH) concentration concluded that as a single test, measurement of free T_4 had the highest sensitivity, specificity, and accuracy.[15]

With the development of a canine-specific TSH assay, another test has been added to our armamentarium to diagnose hypothyroidism. Dogs with hypothyroidism should have an elevated TSH level as a response of the pituitary to decreased negative feedback from lowered blood levels of T_3 and T_4. In one study cited above, approximately 25% of hypothyroid dogs had TSH concentration in the normal range. Because of the lower sensitivity and accuracy, measurement of TSH concentration alone for the diagnosis of canine hypothyroidism is not recommended. The combination of measurement of serum free T_4 and TSH concentration was recommended for the diagnosis of canine hypothyroidism in this study.

Provocative function tests can be performed but have not been used as frequently since the validation of a canine-specific TSH assay. The most commonly used provocative function test is the thyrotropin hormone (TSH) stimulation test. Results of the TSH stimulation test can also be affected by nonthyroidal factors, and it is difficult to differentiate borderline TSH stimulation test results caused by nonthyroidal factors from those caused by early primary thyroid failure.

Other diagnostic tests that have been used for the diagnosis of thyroid function in the dog include thyrotropin releasing hormone (TRH) stimulation test, determination of serum free T_3, and measurement of circulating thyroglobulin antibodies or antibodies to T_3 and T_4. Injection of TRH causes an increase in TSH with a resultant release of T_4 and T_3. However, problems affecting the usefulness of this test are twofold. First, the increases in serum T_4 and T_3 are small and somewhat variable, and second, the influence of nonthyroidal factors on this response has not been determined. Serum free T_3 values can also be affected by nonthyroidal factors, and, in addition, the majority of free T_3 is located intracellularly, not extracellularly. A correlation has been found among circulating thyroglobulin antibodies, antibodies to T_3 and to T_4, lymphocytic thyroiditis, and hypothyroidism in the dog. However, the exact role that antibodies to thyroid antigen play in the development of canine hypothyroidism has yet to be defined. Antithyroglobulin antibodies are detected in approximately 50% of hypothyroid dogs by use of an enzyme-linked immunosorbent assay (ELISA) or chromic chloride hemagglutination (CCH). Unfortunately, antithyroglobulin antibodies have also been detected in normal pets and in dogs with nonthyroidal disease.[16] Therefore, their presence does not definitively indicate hypothyroidism. One potential use for the measurement of antithyroglobulin antibodies may be as a prognostic indicator for young dogs of breeds that are predisposed to the development of thyroiditis. A positive test result may indicate early thyroid disease, and a breeder can cull affected animals from a breeding stock.[16] The presence of autoantibodies to thyroid antigens may produce an erroneous elevation of thyroid hormone when some assays are used. Thus, in cases in which clinical signs suggest hypothyroidism but the basal thyroid hormone concentrations are elevated, testing for autoantibodies may be necessary to reconcile the problem. In a recent prospective study of 234 thyroglobulin antibody–positive dogs, 20% of dogs with laboratory test results that suggested subclinical hypothyroidism developed thyroid dysfunction within 1 year.[17]

In some situations, a therapeutic trial with thyroxine supplementation is warranted. However, response to therapy is nonspecific. Because of its anabolic nature, thyroid supplementation can create a positive effect in some dogs without thyroid dysfunction. In hypothyroid dogs that are supplemented appropriately, activity level should increase in 10 days, but complete hair regrowth may take as long as 4 to 6 months. Thyroid hormone causes increased hair growth to some extent in all dogs regardless of their thyroid status. If all clinical signs resolve completely and recur when the drug is stopped, then a diagnosis of hypothyroidism is probably appropriate.

As opposed to thyroid testing in the dog, thyroid testing in the cat is primarily for the diagnosis of hyperthyroidism. Measurement of baseline serum T_4 concentration is probably the best screening test for hypothyroidism in the cat. If the baseline serum T_4 is in the normal range, the cat most probably has normal thyroid function. In a cat with a low serum T_4 and lack of supportive clinical signs, such factors as euthyroid sick syndrome must be considered. As in the dog, measurement of serum free T_4 may also be helpful. TSH and TRH stimulation tests have been used in the cat, but these tests are seldom performed in this species. With tests that are seldom performed, it is important to follow the protocol established by the clinical laboratory being used to ensure accurate interpretation of results. TSH concentration levels have been reported to be elevated in a cat with hypothyroidism, and the validated results have been published.[14] As in the dog, the results of all of these tests can also be affected by nonthyroidal factors.

Therapy. Lifelong therapy should be initiated once hypothyroidism has been diagnosed. Synthetic levothyroxine is the initial therapy of choice. The plasma half-life of levothyroxine is probably between 12 and 16 hours, with a peak plasma concentration 4 to 12 hours after administration in the dog. Initially, a proprietary product should be used, as some dogs (like some humans) do not respond well to generic brands. I recommend a starting dose of 0.01 mg/lb every 12 hours. However, many veterinarians are using this dose beginning every 24 hours. Thyroid hormones have most of their effects through activation of nuclear receptors that induce gene transformation and protein production. Through this mechanism, thyroid hormones have a duration of activity that exceeds their half-life as measured in plasma, making once-daily administration successful in many cases.

Clinical signs should begin to resolve in a few weeks. Because of the variable pharmacokinetics of thyroid supplementation, after 3 to 4 weeks of treatment T_4 concentration should be measured before and 6 hours after pill administration if the thyroid supplementation is given every 12 hours, and before and 8 to 10 hours after pill administration if the thyroid supplementation is given every 24 hours, to avoid underdosing or overdosing an individual dog. Concentrations of T_4

both before and after pill administration should ideally be within the normal range. However, it is acceptable if the value before administration is within the normal range and the value after administration is slightly above the normal range, if the dog is not showing any signs of hyperthyroidism (e.g., weight loss despite a good appetite, personality changes, tachycardia). If the value before administration is very low and the value after administration is within the normal range, the supplementation should be adjusted upward, and the T_4 values both before and after administration should be reevaluated in 3 to 4 weeks. The opposite holds true for values that are too high. If continued low values are encountered, a problem with pill administration should be considered or a change to a different brand of T_4 may be tried to rule out poor bioavailability. If the thyroid supplementation is initially given every 12 hours and when the dog is in a stable state, it may be possible to change from twice-daily supplementation to once-daily supplementation. Once the T_4 value is stabilized, measurements before and after pill administration should be performed every 6 to 12 months for the remainder of the dog's life, and the dose adjusted as appropriate.

Measurement of serum TSH concentration to determine the appropriate therapeutic level of thyroid supplementation has not been extensively studied. In one report it was noted that when treating a hypothyroid dog, serum TSH should decrease by at least one third before any effect of exogenous thyroxine supplementation can be said to have influenced the serum TSH level.[18]

Therapy in the cat should be similar to that in the dog. The initial dose for cats is 0.05 to 0.1 mg of levothyroxine given once daily, with T_4 concentration both before and after pill administration assessed in 3 to 4 weeks. In one cat with documented hypothyroidism, clinical signs did not resolve, despite the fact that T_4 concentrations before and after pill administration were within the normal range, until the TSH concentration was decreased into the normal range.[19]

Hyperadrenocorticism

Canine Hyperadrenocorticism. The term *hyperadrenocorticism* or *Cushing's syndrome*, refers to the constellation of clinical and chemical abnormalities resulting from chronic exposure to excess glucocorticoids. These excessive glucocorticoids can be endogenously or exogenously supplied. Exogenous glucocorticoid excess is termed *iatrogenic hyperadrenocorticism*. Endogenous hyperadrenocorticism results from excess glucocorticoid secretion by the adrenal gland(s). The excessive glucocorticoid production may be secondary to increased release of adrenocorticotropic hormone (ACTH) from the pituitary gland (pituitary-dependent hyperadrenocorticism [PDH]) or may result from an autonomously secreting adrenal tumor (AT) or from adrenal dependent hyperadrenocorticism. Glucocorticoid administration is by far the most common cause of hyperadrenocorticism.

Pathophysiology. The underlying cause of 85% to 90% of spontaneous hyperadrenocorticism in dogs is excessive secretion of ACTH by the pituitary gland.[5] Excessive ACTH production causes bilateral adrenal gland enlargement, which results in increased cortisol release. The negative feedback mechanism normally controlling the hypothalamic pituitary adrenal axis is markedly reduced. PDH can result from tumors (adenomas or rarely carcinomas) or hyperplasia of the cells of the anterior pituitary lobe (corticotrophs) or intermediate pituitary lobe (A or B cells). The remaining 10% to 15% of the animals with spontaneous hyperadrenocorticism have a functioning glucocorticoid-producing adrenal adenoma or adenocarcinoma. Glucocorticoid treatment is the cause of iatrogenic hyperadrenocorticism in the dog and represents more than half of the total cases of Cushing's syndrome.

Clinical Features

SIGNALMENT. Spontaneous hyperadrenocorticism is largely a disease of middle-aged to older dogs. Dogs with PDH have a median age of 7 to 9 years.[5] Dogs with AT are older with a median age at the time of diagnosis between 9 and 13 years.[5] There is no sex predilection for dogs with PDH, but females seem to be over-represented with AT (3:1 ratio).[5] Dachshunds, Boston terriers, poodles, boxers, and beagles are breeds most commonly predisposed to PDH, with large breed dogs more commonly developing AT.

HISTORY. Spontaneous hyperadrenocorticism is insidious in onset and slowly progressive. Most owners, when questioned at the time of diagnosis, say they have been noticing the presence of some alteration indicative of hyperadrenocorticism for 1 to 6 years. It is common for owners to believe that most of these signs are simply due to aging. Common presenting clinical complaints include polyuria, polydipsia, polyphagia, weight gain, behavior changes including lethargy and reluctance to exercise, panting and skin disease including truncal hair loss. Some owners may report recurrent bacterial infections that were never seen when the animal was young. A lack of estrus may be noted in the intact female.

Physical Examination. A common physical examination finding is abdominal enlargement. This results from a combination of factors, including fat redistribution, hepatomegaly, muscle wasting or muscle weakness, and true obesity. Physical examination may reveal panting that is secondary to one or more of the following conditions; increased fat deposition over the thorax, muscle wasting and weakness of the respiratory muscles, increased pressure on the diaphragm caused by fat redistribution and hepatomegaly, and interstitial calcification. An increased incidence of thromboembolism may cause more acute respiratory distress. Obesity may be noted. Some animals will look heavier because of fat redistribution but some do gain weight because of polyphagia. Truncal obesity occurs at the expense of muscle and fat wasting from the extremities. Muscle atrophy may be evident, especially in muscles of the extremities and masseter muscles. On testicular evaluation in the intact male, the testicles are often small, soft, and spongy. Dermatologic abnormalities may be quite striking. Classic changes include hair loss, which is usually bilaterally symmetrical (Figure 14-8), although focal hair loss may also be seen. Comedones, especially on the ventral abdomen, and thin, inelastic skin are also usually seen (Figure 14-9). Other changes include hyperpigmentation, seborrhea sicca, telangiectasia, increased prominence of surgical scars, lack of hair regrowth after shaving, and adult-onset generalized demodicosis. One dramatic manifestation seen in 5% of dogs is calcinosis cutis (Figure 14-10).[20] Adult dogs that have never had bacterial skin disease may show a marked predisposition to recurrent staphylococcal skin infections (Figure 14-11).

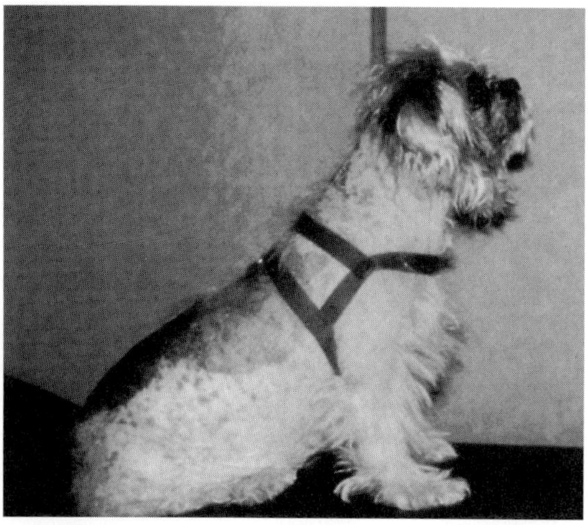

Figure 14-8. Truncal hair loss in a dog with pituitary-dependent hyperadrenocorticism. (Courtesy Dr. Joy Barbet, Archer, Fla.)

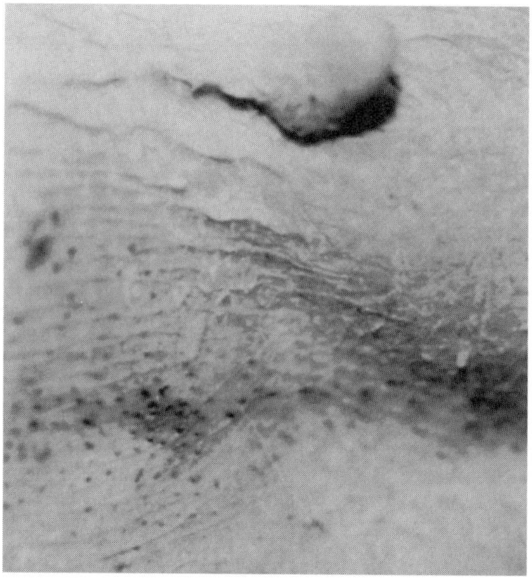

Figure 14-9. Thin, "crepe paper" skin with comedones on the ventral surface of a dog with pituitary-dependent hyperadrenocorticism.

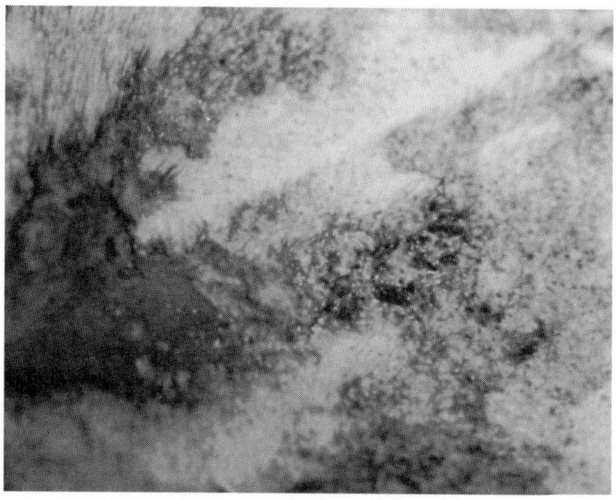

Figure 14-10. Plaques and ulcerated plaques of calcinosis cutis on the ventrum of a dog with iatrogenic hyperadrenocorticism.

Diagnosis. A presumptive diagnosis of canine hyperadrenocorticism can be made based on historical information, consistent physical examination findings, and supportive abnormalities in the complete blood count, serum biochemistry panel and urinalysis (Box 14-3). A complete evaluation of the skin disease should include a

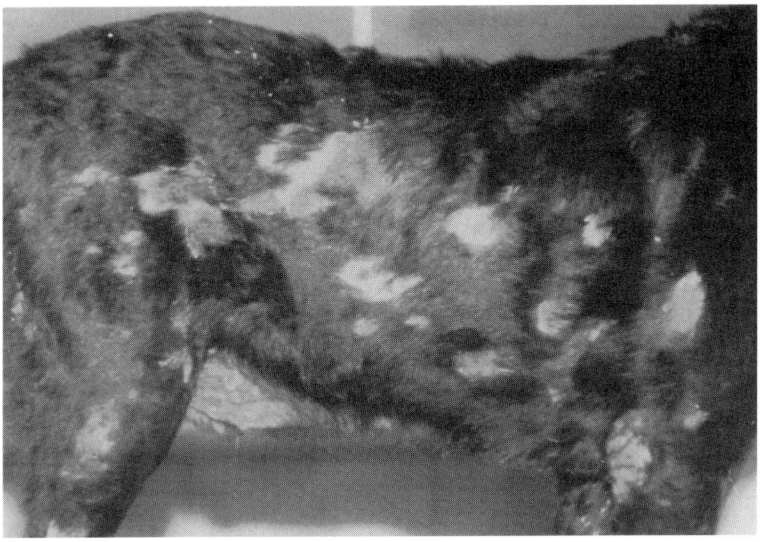

Figure 14-11. Multiple staphylococcal epidermal collarettes on the lateral thorax and abdomen of a dog with pituitary-dependent hyperadrenocorticism.

BOX 14-3 Hematologic, Serum Chemistry Profile, and Urine Abnormalities Consistent with Canine Hyperadrenocorticism

CBC Abnormalities

Mature leukocytosis
Neutrophilia
Lymphopenia
Eosinopenia*
Erythrocytosis
Nucleated red blood cells

Serum Chemistry Profile Abnormalities

Increased alkaline phosphatase*
Increased alanine aminotransferase
Increased cholesterol
Increased fasting blood glucose
Decreased blood urea nitrogen
Lipemia

Urinalysis

Specific gravity <1.015, often <1.008
Urinary tract infection (bacteriuria may be noted without inflammation)
Glucosuria if concomitant diabetes

*Most commonly seen abnormalities.

skin scraping for *Demodex,* dermatophyte fungal culture, and cytological examination. A bacterial culture and sensitivity testing may be performed if a pustular disease is present. Immunosuppressed animals are potentially predisposed to demodicosis and infectious skin disease. A skin biopsy may be helpful in differentiating an endocrine-induced alopecia from other causes of hair loss but will not be able to permit pinpointing the type of endocrine-induced alopecia.

If abnormalities are seen that are consistent with hyperadrenocorticism, then further evaluation is indicated to confirm the diagnosis and localize the cause. Water consumption should be monitored over a 3-day period at home to document polydipsia.

Additional laboratory investigation should proceed through two stages. The screening stage is to confirm (or exclude) the diagnosis of hyperadrenocorticism. Once the diagnosis is confirmed, the second stage is to differentiate PDH from that caused by AT.

Screening Tests

BASAL OR RESTING PLASMA OR SERUM CORTISOL. Basal resting plasma or serum cortisol levels are of minimal diagnostic value when attempting to distinguish normal dogs from dogs with hyperadrenocorticism. Single basal cortisol concentrations in dogs with hyperadrenocorticism overlap with cortisol concentrations in normal dogs. Only 10% of dogs with hyperadrenocorticism have an elevated plasma cortisol concentration on random morning sampling.[5]

URINARY CORTISOL/CREATININE RATIO DETERMINATION. Urinary cortisol/creatinine ratio may be used to screen for canine hyperadrenocorticism.[21-23] Two consecutive morning urine samples are collected, measured for concentrations of cortisol and creatinine and a cortisol/creatinine value is then calculated. This test is highly sensitive in that a dog with a normal cortisol/creatinine ratio is unlikely to have hyperadrenocorticism. On the other hand, the test has low specificity in that many diseases besides hyperadrenocorticism cause an abnormally high cortisol/creatinine ratio. Therefore, the test has value as a screening test to rule out hyperadrenocorticism.

ACTH Stimulation (Screening) Test. The ACTH stimulation test is a screening test for hyperadrenocorticism. This is the only test that will distinguish spontaneous hyperadrenocorticism from iatrogenic hyperadrenocorticism. This test is also used to monitor the response to medical manipulation of the adrenal gland.

Dogs with spontaneous (not iatrogenic) hyperadrenocorticism have enlarged adrenal(s) secondary to hyperplasia (PDH) or neoplasia (AT). Therefore, they have a large cortisol reserve and the potential for hyperresponding to a maximal ACTH stimulation. 0.25 mg of synthetic ACTH (Cortrosyn) is given via the intravenous (IV) or intramuscular (IM) route. For consistency between consecutive tests, either IM or IV administration of Cortrosyn should be chosen for an individual animal. Variability occurs with regard to when the peak cortisol response will be seen after IM or IV Cortrosyn administration. In my practice, for the first few ACTH stimulation tests, samples are taken before, 1 hour after, and 2 hours after administration. Once a consistent peak is seen at 1 or 2 hours, then the correct postsample time is chosen for subsequent tests.

Normal values will vary among laboratories. In our laboratory, a postadministration value above 20 μg/dl (550 nmol/L) is consistent with a diagnosis of hyperadrenocorticism in the dog. Values may be lower in the cat; this will also vary among laboratories. ACTH stimulation tests results are abnormal in 85% of the dogs with PDH, but only in 50% of the dogs with AT. Exaggerated responses to ACTH have also been documented in dogs with chronic illness. In dogs or cats with a recent history of glucocorticoids therapy, the ACTH stimulation test is the recommended initial screening procedure.

Low-Dose Dexamethasone Suppression (Screening) Test. Dogs with a normal pituitary adrenal axis will respond to the negative feedback from exogenously administered dexamethasone. Dogs with hyperadrenocorticism will be resistant to this negative feedback. A morning baseline serum or plasma sample is obtained; 0.01 to 0.015 mg/kg of dexamethasone is administered IV, and samples are taken 3 or 4 and 8 hours after injection. Approximately 90% to 95% of dogs with hyperadrenocorticism will fail to show normal suppression of cortisol at 8 hours. If the cortisol level of the 8-hour sample is less than 1 to 1.5 μg/dl (27 to 41 nmol/dl), then the test indicates that the dog is normal. This is also a screening test and does not distinguish PDH from AT with the exception of one pattern of suppression. If a dog suppresses at 3 to 4 hours (less than 1 to 1.5 μg/dl) and escapes the suppression at 8 hours (cortisol levels greater than 1 to 1.5 μg/dl), the dog probably has PDH, and further testing need not be performed. In all other instances a high-dose dexamethasone suppression test, abdominal diagnostic imaging, or blood ACTH concentration measurement needs to be performed to distinguish PDH from AT.

Differentiating Tests. The type of therapeutic intervention used on an animal depends on whether PDH or AT is present; therefore, it is important to differentiate these two problems.

Endogenous Plasma ACTH Levels. Plasma ACTH will be normal to high in dogs with pituitary-dependent disease but low in dogs with AT. Unfortunately some dogs have a value in the gray (nondiagnostic) zone, and several samples may need to be taken at different times to obtain a sample that truly reflects the underlying disease process. Proper handling of the specimen is paramount because ACTH is very labile. The addition of the protease inhibitor aprotinin to the ethylenediaminetetraacetic acid (EDTA)-containing blood collection tube (500 kallikrein inactivator units/ml blood) prevents breakdown of ACTH.[24] The use of aprotinin allows collection of blood into glass tubes and centrifugation at room temperature. Many laboratories do not perform this test, however, and laboratories that offer this service may have different recommendations concerning collecting and handling the sample.

High-Dose Dexamethasone Suppression Test. Dogs with a normal pituitary adrenal axis will respond to the negative feedback from exogenously administered dexamethasone. Most dogs with PDH will also respond to the negative feedback from this increased amount of dexamethasone. Dogs with AT will be resistant to this negative feedback. The protocol is the same as for the low-dose dexamethasone suppression test (LDDT) except that 0.1 mg/kg of dexamethasone is administered. If the dog suppresses at 8 hours, this is indicative of PDH. If the dog does not suppress at 8 hours, the test is inconclusive because 20% of dogs with PDH and 100% of dogs with AT do not suppress. If the 3- to 4-hour sample shows suppression but escapes at 8 hours, this finding is indicative of PDH. If the test results are inconclusive (nonsuppression at 3 to 4 and 8 hours), further evaluation is indicated.

Abdominal Diagnostic Imaging. Abdominal diagnostic imaging may be helpful in diagnosing AT and localizing which adrenal gland is involved. Radiographic documentation of a mass craniomedial to either kidney or calcification of the adrenal gland is supportive of a diagnosis of AT. Unfortunately, the tumor must be of a large size (or calcified) in order for the problem to be detected radiographically.

Ultrasonography of the Abdomen. Ultrasonography is a noninvasive method used to define location, size, and organ involvement of adrenal masses more precisely. Information gained will help to determine whether both adrenals are enlarged (probable PDH) or one adrenal is enlarged (probable AT). In addition, other organ involvement (e.g., hepatic) or vascular invasion or compression may be detected.[25] In a recent study, the use of both endogenous plasma ACTH concentration and adrenal ultrasonography were capable of discriminating between PDH and adrenal-dependent hyperadrenocorticism. The sensitivity and specificity of adrenal ultrasonography, combined with endogenous ACTH determination to identify the cause of hyperadrenocorticism, were demonstrated to be 100% and 95%, respectively, for adrenal-dependent hyperadrenocorticism.[26]

Computed Tomography. Computed tomography (CT) is currently considered to be the best approach for imaging of the adrenal and pituitary gland in animals with hyperadrenocorticism. It has proved successful in visualization of pituitary tumors and detection of unilateral and bilateral adrenal gland enlargement in the dog. This is very helpful in cases that have failed to suppress during the high-dose dexamethasone suppression test (HDDT). It is also helpful in cases of adrenocortical tumors to determine whether the tumor is on the left or right side and in cases of PDH to determine if a pituitary macroadenoma is present. Animals with macroadenomas have a greater chance of recurrence of the disease because of incomplete removal of the tumor, if the tumor can be surgically approached at all. In dogs with pituitary macroadenomas, radiation therapy may be considered. It is not possible to differentiate between malignant and benign adrenal masses on the basis of size.

Magnetic Resonance Imaging. Magnetic resonance imaging (MRI) offers superior soft-tissue contrast compared with CT and is used extensively in human medicine for visualization of both the adrenal glands and the pituitary gland. MRI is useful for imaging pituitary masses that cannot be seen on CT scans because of an x-ray beam hardening artifact.[27]

Therapy. Treatment depends on the cause of the hyperadrenocorticism. In all cases, a good rapport with the owner is essential in management of the disease. In general, treatment modalities include medical, surgical, and radiation therapy.

Pituitary-Dependent Hyperadrenocorticism

Medical management is the more common therapeutic modality for treatment of PDH. Therapy is aimed at decreasing cortisol production by the adrenal cortex. Drugs used for this purpose include mitotane (Lysodren), ketoconazole, aminoglutethimide, metyrapone, and deprenyl (Anipryl).[28] The most commonly used drug is mitotane.

Mitotane is adrenocorticolytic, causing severe progressive necrosis of the zona fasciculata and reticularis, which secrete cortisol. The zona glomerulosa, the zone responsible for mineralocorticoid production, is relatively resistant but can be affected.

Mitotane therapy is divided into two phases; loading and maintenance. The loading phase is initiated by giving 25 to 50 mg/kg/day of mitotane. In dogs that are polyuric and polydipsic, water consumption is monitored daily and drug therapy should be discontinued if water consumption drops precipitously. Unfortunately, 20% of the cases are not polyuric and polydipsic. In these cases medication is given for 5 to 14 days, and the animal is monitored for side effects of glucocorticoid insufficiency. If no side effects are seen after 10 to 14 days of therapy, the animal should be reevaluated with an ACTH stimulation test. Side effects caused by glucocorticoid insufficiency secondary to mitotane therapy include listlessness, decreased appetite, vomiting, and diarrhea. At the first sign of side effects (usually slight decrease in appetite), mitotane therapy should be discontinued. Some animals will experience vomiting as a direct effect of mitotane. This can be prevented by giving the medication with food or dividing the dose and giving it twice daily, or both. If severe side effects related to glucocorticoid insufficiency are seen by the owner, prednisone or prednisolone can be administered orally at a dose of 0.2 to 0.4 mg/kg until the dog can be evaluated. Generally, the signs will resolve within a few hours of glucocorticoid supplementation if the animal is not additionally mineralocorticoid deficient.

When an end point is reached, reevaluation of the pituitary adrenal axis is accomplished by performing an ACTH stimulation test. This test should be delayed for 24 to 48 hours if prednisone or prednisolone has been given. The goal of therapy is to have the post-ACTH cortisol value in the low-normal or slightly below-normal range. If there is a continued exaggerated response, then continued daily administration of mitotane is necessary. If the ACTH response is too low, prednisone or prednisolone therapy at the previously mentioned dose can be given if clinical signs of glucocorticoid insufficiency are seen. Intermittent ACTH stimulation tests should be used to monitor the dog until cortisol values rise to the low-normal to slightly below-normal range. In one study, mitotane decreased mineralocorticoid production in 5.5% of the dogs after a median of 4.6 months of therapy.[29] Affected dogs will not respond to glucocorticoid administration, and serum sodium and potassium levels should be evaluated for any abnormalities.

When cortisol levels after ACTH stimulation are in the appropriate range, maintenance therapy should be initiated. The dose to be given each week is equal to the daily loading dose. This total dose is usually divided in half and given twice weekly. An ACTH stimulation test should be repeated 1 month after initiation of maintenance mitotane therapy and subsequently every 3 to 4 months. It should be performed sooner if problems are noted. Approximately 50% of the treated dogs will relapse within 12 months and need to be reloaded or have their maintenance dose increased.

Ketoconazole decreases cortisol biosynthesis and is not adrenolytic. It is a safe and effective therapeutic agent for treatment of canine hyperadrenocorticism. Mineralocorticoid production is not affected. Enzyme inhibition is reversible, and cortisol concentration will return to its baseline value within 8 to 24 hours after drug discontinuation. Ketoconazole has been used as an alternative to mitotane therapy, particularly when mitotane is unsuccessful because of drug resistance or severe side effects. The initial dosage is 5 to 10 mg/kg given orally two times daily for 7 to 14 days. The animal is monitored as for mitotane therapy with an ACTH stimulation test repeated when water consumption decreases precipitously, when side effects are noted, or after 14 days of therapy. Higher doses may be required in some dogs. Direct side effects of the drug include anorexia, vomiting, diarrhea, and lightening of the haircoat. Lifelong, twice-daily therapy must be maintained. Reported incidence of lack of efficacy ranges from approximately 20% to 50% of the cases and is probably secondary to poor gastrointestinal absorption of the drug.

Surgical approaches include hypophysectomy and bilateral adrenalectomy. These procedures require a skilled surgeon, intensive monitoring, and lifelong hormone replacement therapy.

Radiation therapy has been used to treat pituitary tumors. Cobalt irradiation has been used successfully in cases of macroadenomas to reduce the size of the pituitary tumor.[30,31] Although cobalt therapy can reduce the size of the tumor and ameliorate neurologic complications, it does not appear to decrease pituitary ACTH secretion. Therefore, mitotane or ketoconazole therapy must be used concurrently.

L-Deprenyl (Anipryl) has been used successfully to treat canine PDH. In one study 71% of the dogs were treated successfully, with no untoward effects or laboratory abnormalities.[27] Other studies have failed to confirm this high success rate. Only 20% of dogs with PDH in a study published in 1999 showed improvement of clinical signs.[32] The effectiveness of this drug in large numbers of dogs and in long-term management of canine PDH is being questioned.

Other drugs that have been used to decrease cortisol synthesis are aminoglutethimide and metyrapone. Medical therapy directed toward the pituitary to decrease ACTH release includes cyproheptadine or bromocriptine. These drugs are not usually used because of their frequent side effects and infrequent success in dogs.

Adrenocortical Tumors

Surgery remains the treatment of choice for AT. Approximately 50% of the tumors are benign adenomas, and the animals are cured by adrenalectomy. Diagnostic imaging should be performed to check for metastatic disease before surgery. Intensive monitoring is needed during surgery and postoperatively to prevent acute adrenocortical insufficiency.

Medical therapy should be considered if there is metastatic disease, if the owner does not elect surgery, if the animal is a very poor surgical risk, or if a nonresectable tumor is found at surgery. Mitotane has the potential to destroy the cancerous tissue and all adrenal tissue, thus causing Addison's disease. Ketoconazole can also be used to block the cortisol synthetic pathway and decrease the signs associated with excess cortisol production. This treatment can also be used to stabilize the animal in preparation for surgery by placing the animal in a less catabolic state. Higher doses of mitotane and ketoconazole are usually needed to control dogs with AT when compared to dogs with PDH.

Feline Hyperadrenocorticism

Hyperadrenocorticism is a relatively rare disease in the cat as opposed to the dog.

Clinical Features. The average age of onset for this disease in the cat is 10.4 years. It is more frequently seen in females (78%),[33,34] and there is no apparent breed predilection. PDH accounts for 78% of reported cases of feline hyperadrenocorticism. Polyuria, polydipsia, polyphagia (usually secondary to diabetes) and a pendulous abdomen with hepatomegaly and muscle wasting and weight gain are the most common signs noted. Depression and weight loss are seen in less than 25% of the cases. Dermatologic abnormalities include truncal and abdominal alopecia, unkempt haircoat, thin skin, comedones, hyperpigmentation, bruising, and abscesses. In some cats, excessively fragile skin leads to tearing with normal manipulation or handling.[33,35]

Diagnosis. Approximately 81% of the cats with hyperadrenocorticism have overt diabetes. Complete blood count abnormalities include neutrophilia, eosinopenia, and lymphopenia in approximately two thirds of the cases. Serum biochemical abnormalities include hyperglycemia and hypercholesterolemia in over 75% of the cases, with increased alanine aminotransferase and serum alkaline phosphatase in approximately 50% of the cases.

Diagnosis of hyperadrenocorticism is difficult in cats. Diagnostic test results are often inconsistent, and testing has not been standardized. Cushingoid cats have a higher cortisol/creatinine ratio than healthy cats.[30] However, abnormal test results have been seen in cats with nonadrenal illness, making the cortisol/creatinine ratio useful only as a screening mechanism.[36] The ACTH stimulation test is probably the best test for diagnosis of hyperadrenocorticism in the cat. Cortisol concentration is measured before and 30 and 60 minutes after IM or IV injection of synthetic ACTH (Cortrosyn) at 125 μg/cat. It is important to obtain both post-ACTH samples because peak cortisol response is highly variable. It has been recently shown that 1.25 to 12.5 μg of synthetic ACTH administered to a cat will maximally stimulate the adrenal cortex.[37] If the smaller doses are given, it is important to realize that plasma cortisol concentration tends to peak earlier (30 minutes) and returns to baseline value more quickly. After reconstitution, a vial of Cortrosyn will be fully stable in 5 μg of saline solution/ml for at least 4 months.[38] Of cats with confirmed hyperadrenocorticism, 15% to 30% have a normal cortisol response to ACTH administration. In addition, stressed cats and those with nonadrenal illnesses may show an exaggerated response to ACTH in the absence of hyperadrenocorticism.

If the ACTH stimulation test is normal but hyperadrenocorticism is still suspected, an HDDT may be helpful at the dose of 0.1 mg/kg of dexamethasone given IV as in the dog. This procedure is used as a screening test in the diagnosis of feline hyperadrenocorticism, and not as a differentiating test as it is in the dog. It appears that a certain percentage of normal cats have an escape of serum cortisol suppression at the 8-hour sample. This test may not be as useful for the diagnosis of hyperadrenocorticism in the cat.

An HDDT with a dose of 1 mg/kg of dexamethasone given IV may be appropriate for distinguishing PDH from AT in cats. Normal-to-elevated plasma ACTH levels support a diagnosis of PDH, whereas low concentrations may require additional diagnostic testing.[34] ACTH levels should be used to distinguish PDH from AT only after hyperadrenocorticism has been confirmed by other screening diagnostics.

Because feline hyperadrenocorticism is an uncommon disease, more information is needed before firm recommendations can be made as to the best endocrine test to use for diagnosis of this disease. The veterinarian must realize the limitations of these tests and should consider clinical signs and laboratory abnormalities as well as results of adrenal function studies before making a definitive diagnosis of feline hyperadrenocorticism.

Therapy. Surgical, medical, and radiation therapies have been used to treat feline Cushing's syndrome. These therapies have met with varying degrees of success. Mitotane therapy, ketoconazole, cobalt irradiation, metyrapone therapy, and bilateral adrenalectomy have been used for the treatment of PDH. Bilateral adrenalectomy followed by mineralocorticoid and glucocorticoid replacement therapy has been a successful treatment for feline PDH. In contrast to dogs, cats do not appear to experience the reported complications from bilateral adrenalectomy as often. Transsphenoidal hypophysectomy for treatment of PDH has been performed successfully in the cat.[39] In spite of the feline sensitivity to chlorinated hydrocarbons, there have been several studies and cases of successful use of mitotane therapy in treatment of feline PDH.

Treatment for AT is surgical excision. A complete check for metastatic disease should be performed before surgery. Intensive monitoring is needed during surgery and postoperatively to prevent acute adrenocortical insufficiency.

In cats with extremely fragile skin that tears easily during manipulation, metyrapone should be initiated at 65 mg/kg every 12 hours until cortisol levels are normal and skin lesions have healed.[40]

Ketoconazole at a dose of 5 to 10 mg/kg every 8 hours may be used if the response to metyrapone is not adequate.[33]

Hyperthyroidism

Hyperthyroidism is the most common endocrine disorder of middle-aged to old cats. Functional adenomatous hyperplasia involving one or both thyroid lobes is the most common pathologic abnormality associated with feline hyperthyroidism. Approximately one half of affected cats have an unkempt haircoat with excessive shedding and matting of the hair. Changes in hair texture, partial hair loss, and increased nail growth also are features of feline hyperthyroidism. In cats with areas of complete alopecia, behavioral changes associated with excessive grooming have been documented. Medical therapy, radiation therapy, and surgery are treatment options. The reader is referred to Chapter 17 for complete information on diagnosis and treatment of this disease.

Diabetes Mellitus

Diabetes mellitus most commonly affects dogs between 4 and 14 years of age, with a peak incidence between 7 and 9 years. Females are affected about twice as frequently as males. Puli, cairn terrier, miniature pinscher, keeshond, golden retriever, poodle, beagle, miniature schnauzer, and dachshund are high-risk breeds.[5] Diabetes mellitus in cats is seen most commonly in cats that are 6 years of age or older and appears to be more common in males.

Cutaneous lesions associated with diabetes mellitus are uncommon. In one retrospective study, 16% of the dogs had dermatitis or otitis.[41] The most common dermatologic manifestations are pyoderma, seborrheic skin disease, demodicosis, thin skin, alopecia, and xanthomatosis. Necrolytic migratory erythema (also called *hepatocutaneous syndrome, superficial necrolytic dermatitis, or metabolic epidermal necrosis)* has been seen in dogs with diabetes mellitus. A complete clinical description of this condition can be found later in this chapter. The reader is referred to Chapter 17 for complete information concerning diabetes.

SKIN TUMORS

Papilloma

Cutaneous papillomas occur in older dogs and cats. They are not caused by a virus, in contrast to papillomas in younger dogs.

Clinical Features. Affected cats show no breed or sex predilection; in dogs, papillomas are more common in males and in cocker spaniels and Kerry blue terriers.[2] Cutaneous papillomas in both cats and dogs are usually solitary but may be multiple, occurring most commonly on the head, eyelids, feet, and genitalia.[42] They tend to be less than 0.5 cm in diameter, pedunculated or cauliflower-like, well circumscribed, alopecic, and varying from firm to soft (Figure 14-12). Although these masses are benign, they may be traumatized by the pet and on rare occasions have been reported to transform into squamous cell carcinoma.

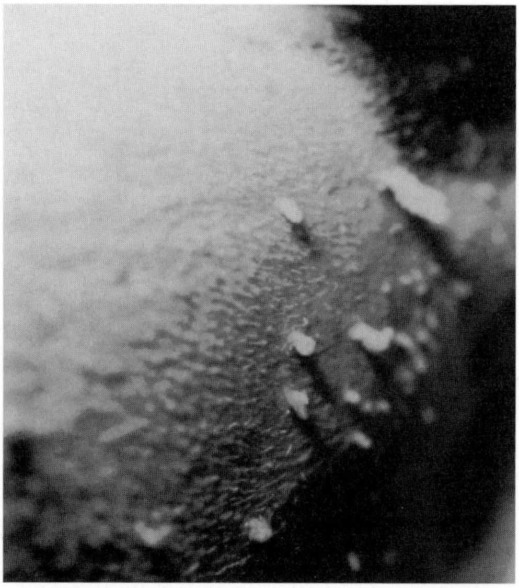

Figure 14-12. Multiple fibropapillomas on the abdomen of a dog. (Courtesy Dr. Carol Foil, DVM, Louisiana State University, Baton Rouge, La.)

Diagnosis. Diagnosis is by excisional biopsy. Histologically, papillomas are divided into two types. The most common type is the squamous papilloma, which is characterized by papillated epidermal hyperplasia and papillomatosis, with ballooning degeneration and basophilic intranuclear inclusion bodies as variable findings. The fibropapilloma is characterized by a fibroma-like proliferation of collagen with a hyperplastic epidermis.

Therapy. Clinical management of cutaneous papillomas may include surgical excision, cryosurgery, electrosurgery, or observation without treatment. Immune modulating drugs are without documented value.

Basal Cell Tumors

The term *basal cell tumors* has been used in the veterinary literature to describe a large group of neoplasms in the dog and cat that are derived from basal epithelial cells of both the epidermis and adnexa. Some authors reserve the term *basal cell tumor* for neoplasms that do not have any adnexal features and are completely benign.[43] These same authors use the term *basal cell carcinoma* to describe tumors of low-grade malignancy that arise from small, pluripotential epithelial cells within the basal cell layer of the epidermis and adnexa. The pluripotential nature of the basaloid epithelial cell is manifested by limited differentiation toward hair follicles, sebaceous glands, and sweat glands in some basal cell carcinomas.

In the older literature, when all basal cell and adnexal derived tumors were placed in one category, these "basal cell tumors" represented 3% to 12% of all skin tumors in dogs and 15% to 18% of all skin tumors in cats.

Clinical Features. Basal cell tumors in cats can occur anywhere on the body but show a predilection for the head and neck. There is no sex predilection, but Siamese and long-haired cats may be predisposed.[43] Affected cats have an average age of 7 to 10 years. The tumors are solitary, well circumscribed, firm, hairless, dome-shaped, elevated masses usually less than 2.5 cm in diameter and freely movable over underlying structures. Multicentric basal cell tumors have been seen. The tumors may be heavily pigmented and cystic. Ulceration may occur.

Basal cell tumors in the dog are usually solitary and are found most frequently on the head, neck, and shoulders. Basal cell tumors on the head are frequently located on the skin of the commissures of the lips, periocular tissue, pinna, and cheek. Tumors are usually less than 2.5 cm in diameter but can become as large as 10 cm or more. They are well circumscribed, encapsulated, and hairless, with a white glistening surface. They can be pigmented, appearing brown or black.

Diagnosis. Diagnosis is made by biopsy, following the classification scheme reported by Gross and coworkers.[43] The benign feline basal cell tumor is a well-circumscribed dermal nodule that generally has a fairly broad zone of connection to the overlying epidermis. Ulceration is common. The neoplasm is composed of small basaloid epithelial cells arranged in tightly packed lobules and trabeculae. Basal cell carcinomas can be subdivided into solid basal cell carcinomas, keratinizing basal cell carcinomas (basosquamous carcinomas), and clear cell basal cell carcinomas. The solid basal cell carcinoma is a circumscribed irregular dermal mass composed of multiple epithelial cell aggregates of varying size and shape. The boundaries of the neoplasm are not well demarcated from the adjacent dermis. The keratinizing basal cell carcinoma is an irregular dermal mass composed of epithelial cell aggregates that vary considerably in size and shape. A plaque-like configuration is common. The center of many of the epithelial islands displays abrupt squamous differentiation and keratinization. The clear cell basal cell carcinoma is structurally identical to the solid basal cell carcinoma. The cells are large and polygonal and have a characteristic water-clear, finely granular cytoplasm that gives the tumor its name.

The traditional classification of basal cell tumors involves histopathology that displays basal cells with prominent oval nuclei and relatively little cytoplasm. The cells are usually small and uniform and lack intercellular bridges. Some basal cell tumors can contain abundant amounts of melanin. They are subclassified on the basis of their histologic appearance into solid, cystic, ribbon, and medusoid. It is not uncommon to observe several different patterns within the same tumor.

Therapy. The treatment of choice for basal cell tumors is surgical excision. Cryosurgical treatment is an alternative approach.

Squamous Cell Carcinoma: Bowen's Disease

Multicentric squamous cell carcinoma in situ (Bowen's disease) has been reported in the cat[44,45] and in the dog.[43] It has been associated with *Demodex cati* in a few cases in the literature.[46]

Clinical Features. In the cat, there is no breed predilection for this disease. The median age of onset ranges from 11.5 to 13.5 years of age. This tumor is not solar induced. The lesions are located predominately on the head, digits, neck, thorax, shoulders, and ventral abdomen. The numbers of tumors on any individual cat range from two to more than 30. In some cases the skin becomes pigmented and then ulcerates in the center of the lesion. Lesions expand peripherally so that some lesions are greater than 4 cm in diameter. A scab may form over ulcerated areas. Removal of the scab is painful. The tumors may also appear as raised, red-crusted lesions that subsequently ulcerate and may intermittently bleed.

In the one case reported in the dog of multifocal intraepidermal carcinoma that histologically resembled Bowen's disease, the lesions were plaque-like, nodular, or verrucous and were sometimes covered with dark-brown or black scale. The lesions were seen on the glabrous skin of the abdomen and on the feet near the carpal and tarsal pads. The mucous membranes of the mouth and genitalia were also affected. Although lesions began in sun-exposed, glabrous skin, they progressed to hairy skin and to mucous membranes.

Diagnosis. Diagnosis is made by biopsy. Unlike solar-associated squamous cell carcinoma, the neoplastic epidermal cells do not penetrate the basement membrane into the surrounding dermis (carcinoma in situ) except late in the course of the disease in some cases. Two histologic subclasses of multicentric squamous cell carcinoma in situ have been identified; the irregular nonhyperkeratotic type and the verrucous hyperkeratotic type.[46] The lesions are characterized microscopically by proliferation of dysplastic, highly disordered keratinocytes, which replace normal epidermis and sometimes the follicular infundibula. Cats with invasive squamous cell carcinoma adjacent to lesions characteristic of multicentric squamous cell carcinoma in situ have been reported.

Therapy. Turrel and Gross reported successful treatment using radiation therapy with strontium 90 (^{90}Sr) to a total dose of 150 Gy in eight cats.[47] The sites healed in 4 to 6 weeks with no recurrence. New lesions requiring radiation therapy often developed at other sites. Successful surgical excision was performed in four cats. Miller and colleagues reported spontaneous remission in one of five cats. Plesiotherapy with ^{90}Sr resulted in partial regression of plaques but was not effective in treating larger, thicker plaques. Baer and Helton-Rhodes reported that during follow-up periods of 4 to 20 months, neoplasm did not recur locally after surgical excision, but similar lesions developed at new sites in 4 of 12 of the cases.

Sebaceous Gland Tumors

Sebaceous gland tumors are among the most common skin tumor in dogs, accounting for 6% to 35% of all skin tumors.[42] They are rare in the cat. Sebaceous gland tumors can be histologically classified as nodular hyperplasia, sebaceous adenoma, sebaceous epithelioma, sebaceous nevus, and sebaceous adenocarcinoma. These tumors are epithelial growths arising from sebaceous gland cells and their cause is unknown.

Clinical Features. Sebaceous gland tumors occur in dogs and cats at an average age of 9 to 10 years. There is no sex or breed predilection in cats. In dogs, the cocker spaniel, miniature schnauzer, shih tzu, Lhasa apso, malamute, Siberian husky, Irish setter, Kerry blue terrier, Boston terrier, poodle, beagle, dachshund, Norwegian elkhound, and basset hound are predisposed.[2] These tumors can be found on any area of the body but are found most often on the head, neck, legs, dorsal and lateral aspect of the trunk, and anus. They may occur singly or at multiple sites.

The lesions of nodular sebaceous hyperplasia are usually single or multiple, 2- to 10-mm diameter, firm, elevated, well circumscribed, alopecic, shiny, dome shaped, or papillated, pink to yellowish masses with a waxy to pearly quality (Figure 14-13). Sebaceous adenomas are solitary or multiple and tend to be larger (up to 2 to 3 cm in diameter) and less lobulated. The overlying skin is alopecic and sometimes ulcerated. Sebaceous nevi appear as alopecic, scaly plaques less than 2 cm in diameter with irregular or papillated surfaces. Sebaceous epitheliomas are clinically similar to basal cell tumors; they are usually solitary, firm nodular, or plaque-like masses ranging from several millimeters to several centimeters in diameter. Surface ulceration occurs frequently. Sebaceous adenocarcinomas are usually solitary, firm, poorly circumscribed nodules less than 4 cm in diameter. Alopecia and ulceration are common.

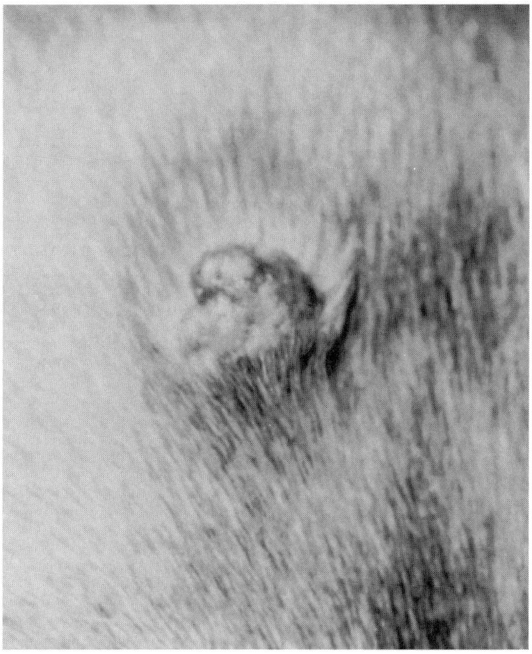

Figure 14-13. An epidermal pink, fleshy hyperplastic sebaceus gland mass on a dog. (Courtesy Dr. Carol Foil, DVM, Louisiana State University, Baton Rouge, La.)

Diagnosis. Diagnosis is made by biopsy. Animals with sebaceous hyperplasia display greatly enlarged sebaceous glands composed of numerous lobules grouped around centrally located sebaceous ducts. Sebaceous adenomas typically are composed of multiple large lobules of sebaceous cells that show normal maturation. In contrast to sebaceous hyperplasia, the lobules are not oriented around ducts or follicular infundibula. Sebaceous nevus is a plaque-like lesion covered by hyperplastic, hyperkeratotic epidermis that has a papillated configuration.[43] The sebaceous glands are large, numerous and randomly distributed through the superficial dermis. Sebaceous epitheliomas are composed of multiple lobules of basaloid epithelial cells. Sebaceous adenocarcinoma is an irregular, circumscribed, multilobular dermal neoplasm composed of islands of pleomorphic polygonal cells with atypia.

Therapy. Surgical excision, cryotherapy, electrosurgery, and observation without treatment are clinical management options for sebaceous nodular hyperplasia, sebaceous adenoma, sebaceous epithelioma, and sebaceous nevus. Sebaceous adenocarcinomas should be completely surgically excised. Reports of sebaceous adenocarcinomas metastasizing are rare.

Melanocytic Tumors

Benign and malignant melanomas together comprise 5% to 9% of all skin tumors in the dog.[48] Melanoma is rare in the cat, accounting for less than 2% of all feline tumors.[43] Although our understanding of the pathogenesis of canine melanoma is incomplete, alterations in expression or function of genes and proteins involved in cell cycle control and cell death may be of importance in the development of melanomas.[49]

Clinical Features. Melanomas occur in dogs and cats at an average age of 9 years. In cats there is no apparent breed or sex predilection. In dogs, Scottish terriers, Boston terriers, Airedale terriers, cocker spaniels, springer spaniels, boxers, Irish setters, Irish terriers, chow chows, Chihuahuas, golden retrievers, Pekingese-poodle mix, and Doberman pinschers are often affected.[50,2] Males may be affected more commonly than females, but not all studies have borne this out.

In the dog, the tumor is usually solitary, dome-shaped and pigmented, having a uniform, smooth appearance (Figure 14-14). The overlying epidermis is usually intact, but focal areas of ulceration can be found. The mass is usually alopecic. The tumors vary from 0.5 cm to several centimeters in diameter.[51] Some melanomas lack pigmentation and have a pale to dark-red color. Melanomas occur most commonly on the face, trunk, feet, and scrotum.[2] At the mucocutaneous junction the tumor appears as a pedunculated, pigmented, glistening nodule or mass measuring 1 to 4 cm in diameter.

In the cat, melanomas are hyperpigmented and occur most commonly on the head, especially the ears. They vary in color from gray to black, and they range in diameter from 0.3 cm to 2 cm.

Malignant melanomas in the dog are usually rapidly growing, larger than 2 cm in diameter, and frequently ulcerated. Most malignant melanomas are sessile, but occasionally they are polypoid or plaquelike. Eyelids, digits, and the trunk are the most frequent locations for cutaneous malignant melanomas in dogs.

In the cat, malignant melanomas are usually ulcerated, solitary, elevated, alopecic, intradermal masses, often red to red-brown in color. They range in diameter from 0.3 cm to 2.5 cm. The face and digits also appear to be preferential sites in cats.[44,51]

Diagnosis. Diagnosis is made by biopsy. Differentiation between benign and malignant lesions can be challenging. Important criteria that

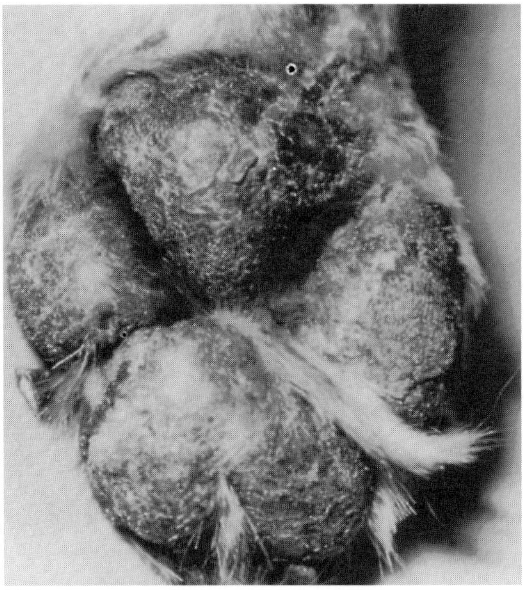

Figure 14-14. Small, round, pigmented melanoma on the central pad (upper right corner) of a dog. (Courtesy Dr. Carol Foil, DVM, Louisiana State University, Baton Rouge, La.)

suggest malignancy in the dog are metastasis, a mitotic index greater than or equal to 3 mitoses per 10 high power fields, nuclear and nucleolar pleomorphism, increased growth fractions as determined by immunostaining, and location of the melanoma. Malignant melanomas often arise from the mucocutaneous junction, oral cavity and subungual area. Melanomas are rare in the cat, and histologic evaluation to assign degree of benignity or malignancy has not been found to be an accurate predictor of clinical behavior.[52] Immunohistologic tests with antibodies that recognize lineage-restricted antigen may add support for a reliable definitive diagnosis of melanoma.[49]

Therapy. Wide surgical excision is the treatment of choice. Malignant melanomas often recur and metastasize via lymphatic and hematogenous routes. Regional lymph node metastasis is a common finding, with subsequent spread to the lungs. Other sites for metastasis include the brain, heart, liver, kidney, and spleen. Local recurrence is most frequently encountered with dermal tumors that are invasive and with tumors arising at mucocutaneous junctions. Prognosis for dogs with malignant melanomas is not influenced by age, sex, location, size, presence or absence of ulceration, or histologic cell type or other histologic features.[48]

Feline malignant melanoma often recurs at the surgical site (67%).[51] Metastases to regional lymph nodes occurs in 50% of cases. Metastatic lesions can be found in any organ, but lungs are the primary organ to which the tumor is likely to spread.

The use of cryotherapy has been reported but appears to have no benefits over conventional surgery. Malignant melanomas are generally radioresistant and there is no chemotherapy regimen that has consistently proved successful. Recent work has focused on immunotherapeutic approaches to treat canine malignant melanoma. One study used liposome-encapsulated muramyl tripeptide-phosphatidylethanolamine (L-MTP-PE), which stimulates secretion of proinflammatory cytokines and promotes strong tumoricidal activity of canine monocytes to macrophages as an adjunct treatment to surgery. This therapy was not helpful in dogs with advanced stage oral melanoma but did prolong survival time in dogs with early stage oral melanoma.[53]

Cutaneous Lymphosarcoma

Cutaneous lymphosarcoma is characterized by an infiltration of neoplastic lymphoid cells into the skin. The tumor may be primary to the skin, or skin involvement may occur in conjunction with disseminated disease. This section deals only with primary cutaneous lymphosarcoma. The reader is referred to Chapter 6 on neoplasia for discussion of noncutaneous lymphosarcoma.

Primary cutaneous lymphosarcoma can be classified as either epitheliotropic (tumor cells accumulating in the epidermal or adnexal epithelium) or nonepitheliotropic. The epitheliotropic cutaneous lymphomas are a subset of cutaneous T-cell lymphomas. Various forms of epitheliotrophic cutaneous T-cell lymphomas include mycosis fungoides and its leukemia (Sézary syndrome), and pagetoid reticulosis (Woringer-Kolopp and Ketron-Goodman types). Nonepitheliotrophic lymphosarcomas are lymphomas of the dermis and subcutaneous tissue and are almost equally likely to involve proliferation of B or T cells, with a small number being non–B-, non–T-cell lymphomas.[54] Recent immunohistochemic studies in the dog and cat have confirmed that the epitheliotrophic form is predominately a gamma-delta T-cell lymphoma.[54] In dogs, the cells uniformly express the CD3 marker, with 80% expressing the CD8 marker.

Primary cutaneous lymphosarcoma accounts for 5.2% to 8% of all canine lymphomas. Of all feline lymphomas, 1.7% are cutaneous.

Clinical Features. Clinical features of epitheliotrophic lymphosarcoma are highly variable. In humans there are three defined stages through which the tumor progresses. The first is a patch stage that consists of macular, erythematous lesions with scale. The patch progresses to a plaque stage consisting of firm, raised papules, pink to reddish purple-brown in color that coalesce to form smooth, solid erythematous scaling plaques. The tumor stage occurs late in the evolution of the disease. These tumors are firm and sessile and may be brightly erythematous. The tumors may regress spontaneously, or they may enlarge, ulcerate, and become secondarily infected. A unique variation is the "d'emblee" form, which begins in the tumor stage without progressing through the patch and plaque phases. Erythroderma may be present in any stage. When it is the most prominent feature, it has been termed *"l'homme rouge"* (red man).

In the dog, all of the clinical descriptions listed above have been seen. However, canine cases do not always easily separate into the stages that are recognized in humans. All three stages may be seen simultaneously in a dog. In one retrospective study, 80% of the cases had patchy to generalized erythema, 61.5% had plaques and scaling, 57.7% had nodules, 42.3% had ulcerations, and 38.5% had pruritus and crusting. Mucosal lesions were seen in 38.5% of the cases (Figures 14-15 and 14-16).[55] Peripheral lymphadenopathy is evident at presentation in 30.8% of the cases. Mucosal lesions or depigmentation may be the only clinical sign of epitheliotrophic lymphoma.

Woringer-Kolopp disease (pagetoid reticulosis) has been documented in the dog. It is a rare, focal to multifocal form of epitheliotrophic lymphoma that has minimal dermal infiltration and does not progress beyond the plaque stage.

Nonepitheliotropic lymphoma in the dog is similar to the epitheliotrophic form but more often takes the form of nodular masses of varying size that may be solitary but are more often multiple. Ulceration, erythema, scaling, and alopecia are common. In the study quoted above, no dogs displayed crusting, papules, or mucosal lesions. All dogs had nodules, with 55.6% displaying ulceration. An unusual presentation of multiple, firm, raised, erythematous, serpiginous, or branching cutaneous plaques that are bilaterally symmetrical has been reported.[16]

Papillomatous lesions associated with cutaneous lymphosarcoma have been reported in only one dog. The lesions originated on the pinna and spread to the entire body in several weeks.[51] Another unique presentation of cutaneous lymphoma in the dog is variably sized, firm, black, raised, exudative subcutaneous masses that fluctuate in size and frequently ulcerate. This is a cutaneous presentation of a vasoproliferative form of intravascular lymphoma in the dog.[56]

In the cat, cutaneous lymphosarcoma (epitheliotropic and nonepitheliotropic) can occur in the patch stage, plaque stage, or tumor stage. The tumor often begins as a single plaque with additional plaques appearing as the disease progresses. This progression is more common in the cat than in the dog.[51] Lesions also appear to be more pruritic in the cat, leading to self-inflicted trauma and ulceration. Solitary nodules are more common in the cat than in the dog.

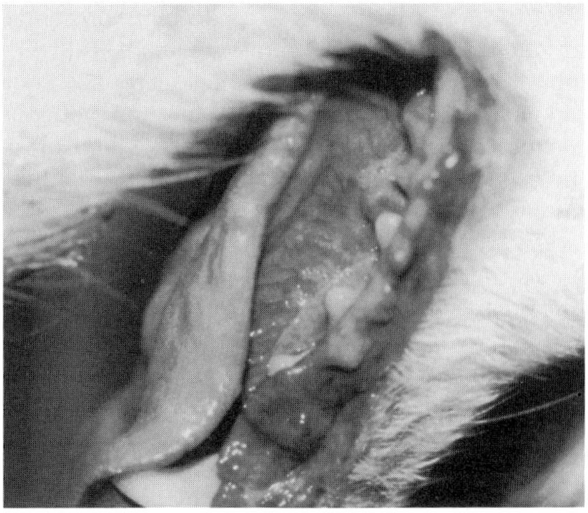

Figure 14-15. Ulceration at the mucocutaneous junction of the mouth in an 8-year-old Samoyed dog with cutaneous epitheliotrophic lymphoma.

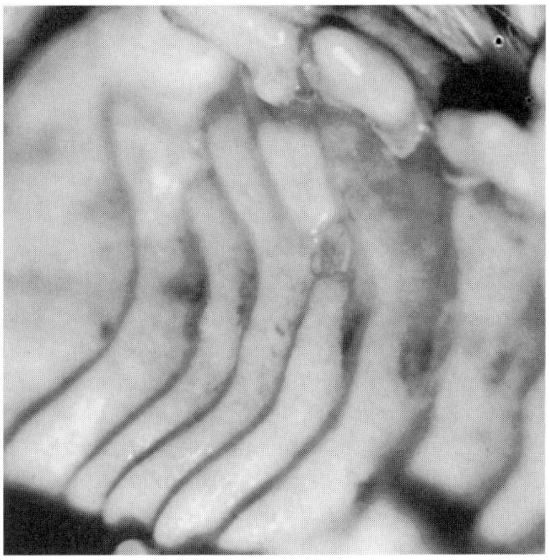

Figure 14-16. Ulceration on the hard palate of the dog shown in Figure 14-15.

Diagnosis. Diagnosis is made by microscopic examination of skin or mucosal biopsies. Non-epitheliotrophic lymphoma is characterized by a nodular to diffuse infiltration of homogeneous neoplastic lymphocytes in the dermis and often the subcutis. Neoplastic lymphocytes are infrequently noted within the epidermis. Dermal adnexa are usually effaced by tumor cells.

Epitheliotrophic lymphoma is characterized by progressive accumulation of neoplastic cells within the epidermis and adnexal epithelium. The histopathology varies depending on the stage of the disease. Early exfoliative lesions in the dog are characterized by small numbers of intraepithelial lymphocytes that are not overtly neoplastic.[43] In the plaque and nodule stages, lymphocytes increase in number and appear more malignant, being characterized by large, pale nuclei with a convoluted contour. It should be noted that the skin of cats tends to retain morphologically well-differentiated lymphocytes even in advanced stages of disease.[43] In the plaque and nodule stages, the epidermis becomes thickened and contains infiltrating lymphocytes. Groups of neoplastic lymphocytes in the epidermis are termed *Pautrier's microabscess*. The dermis contains similar neoplastic lymphocytes, and these frequently obscure the dermoepidermal junction. This phenomenon is referred to as a *lichenoid band* (cells hugging the dermoepidermal junction). As the disease progresses, the lymphocytes form dense infiltrates in the superficial dermis (plaque stage) or extend into the deep dermis and panniculus (tumor stage).

The d'emblee variant appears identical to the tumor stage lesions of the epitheliotrophic lymphoma. The Woringer-Kolopp variant is characterized by moderate to marked epithelial hyperplasia with the lower layers of the epithelium having a marked diffuse infiltration of neoplastic lymphocytes with a high mitotic index.

Therapy. Most cases of cutaneous lymphosarcoma in the dog and cat progress with the development of additional cutaneous lesions and finally metastasize to regional lymph nodes and internal organs. Several therapeutic regimens have been reported. Treatment trials in animals using systemic chemotherapeutic agents including prednisolone, prednisone, vincristine, cyclophosphamide, polyethylene glycol, L-asparaginase, mechlorethamine, and methotrexate have generally yielded poor results but some successes have been seen and treatment of these animals is encouraged. Many of these therapies are palliative and may help to control the erythema and scaling but do not appear to lengthen the survival rate of the animal. In addition, mechlorethamine (topical nitrogen mustard) can be a potent contact sensitizer and is itself potentially carcinogenic. Isotretinoin at 1 to 2 mg/kg has been used and seems to be well tolerated in both dogs and cats. This therapy is also only palliative; cure is not achieved, but the length and quality of life in treated animals is improved. In the dog, response to isotretinoin may be dose dependent, and a higher dose (3 mg/kg) may be more likely to produce a beneficial response.

Low-energy orthovoltage radiation was used in one case report, with histologic response seen after two fractions of 250 cGy each. However the dog became leukopenic and septicemic, and died shortly thereafter.[57]

TESTICULAR TUMORS

Dermatologic manifestations of testicular tumors are uncommon but have been seen in the dog. Three types of primary tumors of the testis occur in dogs: Sertoli cell tumors, interstitial cell tumors, and seminomas. Dermatologic manifestation occurs most commonly in the male feminization syndrome, which is seen most often with Sertoli cell tumors, but skin changes also occurs with seminomas and less often with interstitial cell tumors.[58]

Pathophysiology. Sertoli cell tumors arise from Sertoli cells and are slow growing. They are clinically important because of the potential for metastasis and the ability to produce excessive amounts of estrogen. Seminomas arise from the primitive gonadal cell of the testes, and interstitial cell tumors arise from the Leydig cells. The metastatic rate for seminomas is low, and metastasis does not occur with interstitial cell tumors.[42]

There is a much greater incidence of testicular neoplasia in cryptorchid testes than in normally descended testes. The right testis is more commonly cryptorchid; therefore, it has a higher frequency of neoplastic involvement. The location of the cryptorchid testis may dictate the type of tumor that develops. Sertoli cell tumors are more commonly associated with abdominally located testes, whereas seminomas appear to be more commonly associated with testes in the inguinal region. Interstitial cell tumors do not appear to be related to cryptorchidism.[5]

Clinical Features

Signalment. Testicular tumors usually occur in middle-aged to older dogs. The average age of occurrence varies: 9 years for Sertoli cell tumors, 11.5 years for interstitial cell tumors, and

10 years for seminomas.[59] Breed predispositions include boxers, Shetland sheepdogs, weimaraners, German shepherds, cairn terriers, Pekingese, and collies.[5,2]

Physical Examination. Dogs with male feminization display dermatologic signs of bilaterally symmetric alopecia that is nonpruritic. The alopecia usually begins in the perineal and genital regions and spreads to the ventral abdomen, thorax, flank, and neck (Figure 14-17). In chronic cases generalized truncal alopecia may be seen. In some cases, the alopecia is restricted to the flanks. The remaining haircoat may be dull and dry. The skin may become thin and hypotonic. Hyperpigmentation is variable but is usually present. Other signs of male feminization include gynecomastia, lactation, pendulous prepuce, attraction of male dogs, decreased libido, and standing in a female posture to urinate.[5,60]

Dermatologic abnormalities caused by excess androgens include tail gland hyperplasia, perianal gland hyperplasia, or neoplasia and benign prostatic hypertrophy.[60]

Other dermatologic manifestations of testicular tumors include seborrhea, ceruminous otitis externa, macular melanosis of the inguinal and perianal skin, and a linear erythematous or melanotic macular change along the ventral aspect of the prepuce extending to the scrotum (Figure 14-18).[2] Occasionally, a dog will be quite pruritic and have a papular eruption.

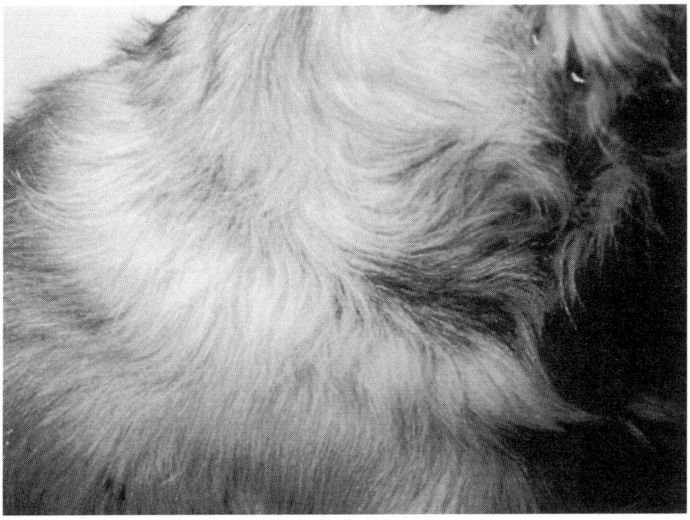

Figure 14-17. Neck alopecia in a golden retriever with a Sertoli cell tumor.

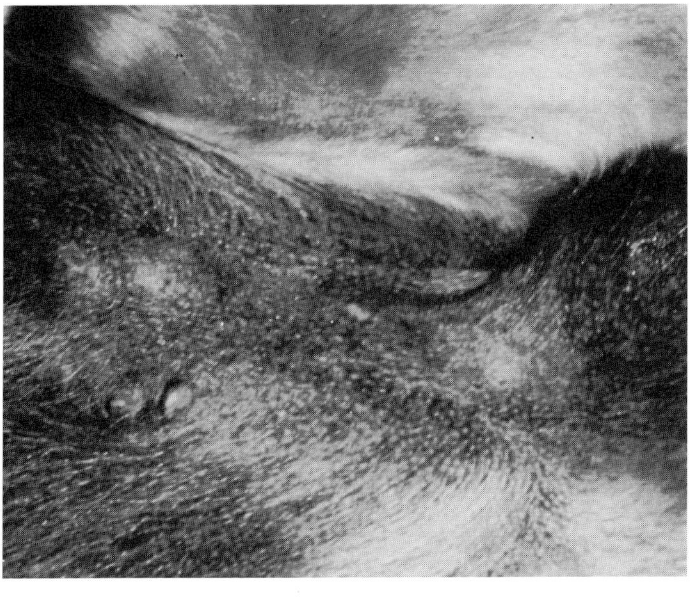

Figure 14-18. Linear preputial erythema in a dog with a Sertoli cell tumor.

Testicular examination may reveal testicular dyssymmetry, with the nontumorous testicle being soft and atrophic due to the effects of excess sex hormone production from the tumorous testicle. Occasionally, there is no palpable testicular abnormality.

Diagnosis. Clinical suspicion of testicular neoplasia is based on the presence of a combination of physical examination findings as listed above. Ultrasonic evaluation of the testes has become a method to assess testicular disease. Both scrotal and abdominal testes can be studied noninvasively. Ultrasonographic studies can reveal abnormalities in parenchyma density, distinguish focal from diffuse involvement, and help differentiate testicular from epididymal disease. Castration and submission of both testicles for histopathologic evaluation should be the diagnostic recommendation to the owner. If a testicular tumor is present, histologic examination of the testicle will confirm the type of neoplasia.

If the owner requests that other diagnostic tests be performed before the animal is castrated, serum samples can be submitted for the measurement of estradiol, progesterone, and testosterone. In most cases one of these three hormones will be abnormally elevated.[60] However, normal values for all three hormones do not rule out the presence of a testicular neoplasm. Also, information obtained from a fine needle aspiration for cytologic evaluation does not correlate with histologic classification or kinetic characteristics of testicular tumors.

Skin biopsies can be used to support the suspicion of a hormonally related skin disease, but the changes are not specific for testicular tumors. Histologic skin changes include orthokeratotic hyperkeratosis, epidermal atrophy with or without melanosis, follicular keratosis, follicular dilatation, follicular atrophy, predominance of telogen hair follicles, and sebaceous gland atrophy.

A complete blood count should be evaluated to determine if estrogen myelotoxicity is present. Abdominal and thoracic radiographs should be taken and examined for evidence of tumor metastasis. Although most testicular tumors are benign, they have the potential to metastasize to regional lymph nodes, liver, lungs, spleen, kidneys, and pancreas.[60] Sertoli cell tumors have the greatest potential for malignancy of all the testicular tumors, with metastasis occurring in approximately 10% to 20%.

Therapy. Castration is the treatment of choice. Dogs that have blood dyscrasia or bone marrow hypoplasia as the result of an estrogen-secreting testicular tumor will require additional treatment as an adjunct to castration. Advanced bone marrow suppression carries a grave prognosis for recovery.

Cutaneous improvement after castration will be seen within 3 months. If metastatic disease is documented by radiographs, histologic findings, or continuing signs of disease after castration, chemotherapy or radiation therapy may be attempted. Sertoli cell tumors are somewhat responsive to cyclophosphamide, vinblastine, or methotrexate therapy, and seminomas are radiosensitive and are also responsive to cyclophosphamide and vincristine.[5] The prognosis for metastatic testicular neoplasia is guarded to poor.

PHEOCHROMOCYTOMA

Pheochromocytomas are endocrine tumors arising from the adrenal medulla. These tumors are rare in dogs and extremely rare in cats. The clinical signs result both from the excessive production of catecholamines and by local invasive spread of the tumor.

Clinical Features. Pheochromocytomas occur most often in older dogs with a mean age of 10.5 years in one retrospective study, with no breed or sex predilection.[61] Because of the episodic pattern of tumor catecholamine secretion, clinical signs may not be present during the physical examination. Fifty percent of dogs will have no symptoms, with the mass seen on necropsy. The clinical signs associated with pheochromocytomas are quite variable and often subtle. Respiratory signs are common and include episodic panting or dyspnea and increased bronchovesicular sounds. Other common signs include weight loss, anorexia, and depression. Additional signs may include weakness, collapse, restlessness, seizures, paraparesis, exercise intolerance, cyanosis, abdominal distention, polyuria, polydipsia, epistaxis, diarrhea, constipation, vomiting, anxiety, and adipsia. The dermatologic manifestation is intermittent flushing of the pinna.

Diagnosis. There are no consistent abnormalities encountered in the routine laboratory evaluation of dogs with pheochromocytomas. Hypertension may be present intermittently. Thoracic radiology may reveal cardiac enlargement and pulmonary congestion or edema. Abdominal radiographs will show an adrenal mass in approximately one third to one half of the affected animals. A contrast intravenous urogram may aid in the diagnosis of pheochromocytoma. Vena caval venography should be performed in all suspect cases because it is common for tumor thrombus to invade the posterior vena cava. Ultrasonography, MRI, and CT are superior to radiography for examination of the adrenal areas in dogs. Determination of the urinary excretion of catecholamines or their metabolites is most reliable in the diagnosis of pheochromocytoma. However, the high cost, the lack of access to this technology, and the need for specific radioimmunoassay for protein chromogranin A released with catecholamines from storage vesicles in the adrenal medulla limit this type of testing. Metastasis to lung, liver, spleen, lymph node, heart, bone, kidney, skeleton, and eye have been documented.[62]

Therapy. Therapy for pheochromocytoma is surgical excision. Medical therapy is needed before surgery to stabilize the cardiovascular and metabolic status of the animal as well as to control blood pressure and cardiac arrhythmias. Surgical success is dependent on the invasive nature of the AT and presence or absence of metastatic disease. The majority of tumors are associated with only one adrenal gland.

NODULAR DERMATOFIBROSIS

Nodular dermatofibrosis is a syndrome in the German shepherd dog that was first reported in Switzerland in 1983.[63] Pedigree analysis suggests that the syndrome is inherited in an autosomal dominant fashion. Genetic mapping localizes the disease to a small region of chromosome 5.[64] Renal abnormalities (cysts, adenomas, and adenocarcinomas) and an increased frequency of uterine leiomyomas are associated with the cutaneous nodular disease. It has also been documented in a young golden retriever.[65]

Pathophysiology. Speculation concerning the connection between the cutaneous nodules and renal and uterine disease includes a possible role of an oncogenic virus.[66] The skin nodules and renal tumors may arise independently and be related only by a common hereditary mechanism, or growth factors produced by the renal tumor may somehow stimulate collagen synthesis, with the nodules being therefore a paraneoplastic syndrome.

Clinical Features. Nodular dermatofibrosis occurs in German shepherd or German shepherd mix dogs of middle age.[66] Age range has varied between 3 and 11 years. No sex predilection has been noted. Multiple collagenous nevi initially appear on the extremities and later develop on the head and trunk (Figure 14-19). The average age of development of dermatologic signs is 6.4 years.[67] The nevi are usually firm, well circumscribed, and 0.5 to 5 cm in diameter. The nodules may be pigmented, haired, alopecic, pitted, or ulcerated. Lesions usually cause no symptoms unless ulcerated or in an area that hinders locomotion. As the disease progresses, the nodules can proliferate and become locally infiltrative.

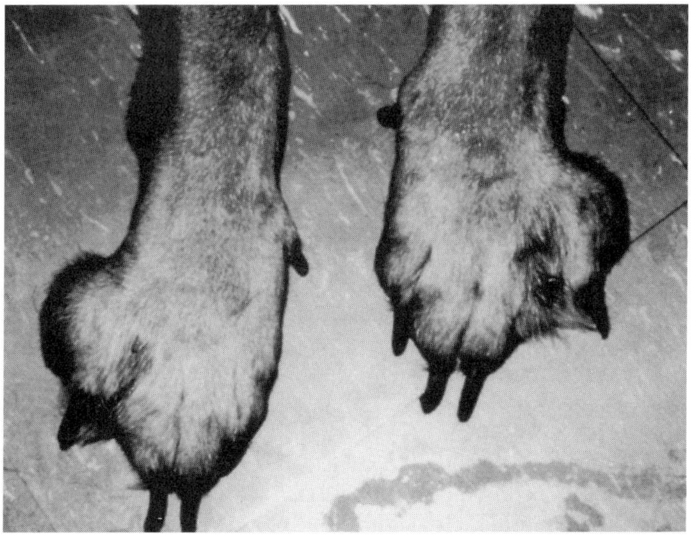

Figure 14-19. Nodules from dermatofibrosis on the legs of a German shepherd dog. (Courtesy Dr. Carol Foil, DVM, Louisiana State University, Baton Rouge, La.)

Clinical signs of renal failure may not be present in affected dogs, depending on the degree of renal impairment. Dogs with impaired renal function may have anorexia, polydipsia, vomiting, diarrhea, weight loss, abdominal distention, weakness, hematuria, and uremia.

Diagnosis. Multiple cutaneous nodules in a German shepherd breed dog should initiate a strong clinical suspicion of nodular dermatofibrosis. A diagnostic work-up should include a complete blood count, serum chemistry panel, urinalysis, radiographs, abdominal ultrasound, and dermal nodule biopsy.

Complete blood count, serum chemistry, and urinalysis abnormalities will vary depending on the degree of renal impairment.

Radiographs may reveal renomegaly, and abdominal ultrasound may document numerous renal cortical cysts of varying size. Skin biopsy reveals a subcutaneous nodule composed of irregular bundles of dense collagen fibers with few fibrocytes. Secondary inflammation with infiltrates of polymorphonuclear leukocytes and plasma cells is seen in some nodules. The uterine pathology consists of interlacing bundles of smooth muscle fibers with characteristic cigar-shaped nuclei. The renal adenomas show parenchymal compression associated with multilocular cystic masses with the absence of cellular atypia and mitotic activity. The adenocarcinomatous lesions consist of multifocal hyperplastic to highly malignant renal tubular epithelial cell proliferations.

Necropsy findings may include metastatic disease of lymph and blood vessels in the regional lymph nodes, liver, and lungs.

Therapy. Treatment of the dermal nodules may not be necessary, depending on their location and severity. Some cases may warrant surgical excision if they are ulcerated, infected, or in a location that is hindering locomotion. The progression of the disease is usually slow, but the long-term prognosis is guarded to poor because of tumor-induced renal failure, abdominal distention from the enlarging renal mass, and metastatic disease.

DEMODICOSIS

Demodectic mange of the dog is most often caused by *Demodex canis.* Demodectic mange of the cat is caused by *Demodex cati* and *Demodex gatoi.* It is a common skin disease in the dog but is uncommon to rare in the cat.

There are two types of demodicosis generally recognized; localized and generalized. It is important to differentiate these two forms because therapeutic intervention and prognosis is very different. Localized demodicosis is found more often in the juvenile animal, whereas generalized demodicosis is found in both the juvenile and the adult.

Pathophysiology. Follicular *Demodex* mites are normal inhabitants of hair follicles and sebaceous and apocrine glands. Each animal, including man, harbors its own host-specific mite species. Transmission of the follicular mite is thought to occur by direct contact with the bitch or queen during nursing in the first 2 or 3 days of neonatal life.[68] Stillborn puppies or puppies delivered by cesarean section and hand raised do not harbor mites.[69]

The follicular mite spends its entire life cycle on the host and cannot persist free in the environment for more than a few hours. Follicular demodicosis is not considered to be a contagious disease among nonneonatal healthy animals. The pathogenesis of the disease state associated with the proliferation of *Demodex* mites is not completely understood. There is evidence of hereditary predisposition in dogs for juvenile-onset generalized demodicosis. Adult-onset canine generalized demodicosis is most likely caused by suppression of the immune system. Several factors have been suggested or documented as initiating canine generalized demodicosis. These factors include administration of immunosuppressive drugs; serious systemic disease to include hyperadrenocorticism; hypothyroidism; diabetes mellitus; blastomycosis and other deep mycoses; lymphosarcoma; hemangiosarcoma and mammary adenocarcinoma. In addition, estrus, whelping, heartworm disease, and intestinal parasite infestation have all been associated with canine generalized demodicosis.

Because most cases of demodectic mange in the cat have occurred in the adult, immunosuppression as a result of an underlying disease has been proposed as the initiating factor. Generalized demodicosis has been seen in cats with diabetes mellitus, respiratory infectious, feline leukemia virus infection (FeLV), systemic lupus erythematosus, toxoplasmosis, feline endocrine alopecia, feline immunodeficiency virus (FIV), hyperadrenocorticism, feline infectious peritonitis (FIP), and neoplasia. Immunosuppressive drugs (glucocorticoids and progestational compounds) should also be considered potential initiating factors.

Clinical Features

Canine Localized Demodicosis. Localized demodicosis is usually seen as one to several patches of circumscribed alopecia with varying degrees of follicular plugging, erythema, scaling, and hyperpigmentation (Figure 14-20). The lesions tend to be seen on the head, neck, and forelimbs, but are not always confined to these areas. Occasionally, *Demodex* mites will be confined to the ear only. If a secondary bacterial infection is present, papules or pustules will be seen.

Canine Generalized Demodicosis. Generalized demodicosis can be seen on any area of the body, many times beginning cranially and progressing caudally (Figure 14-21). Generalized patchy or diffuse alopecia with erythema, scaling, crusting, and follicular plugging is seen. Some animals have prominent hyperpigmentation in affected areas. Secondary bacterial infection is common in dogs with generalized demodicosis (Figure 14-22). The infection may be superficial and characterized by pustules or papules, or it may be deep and characterized by furunculosis, which can progress to painful cellulitis. Pruritus and peripheral lymphadenopathy are seen most often in dogs with demodicosis complicated by a

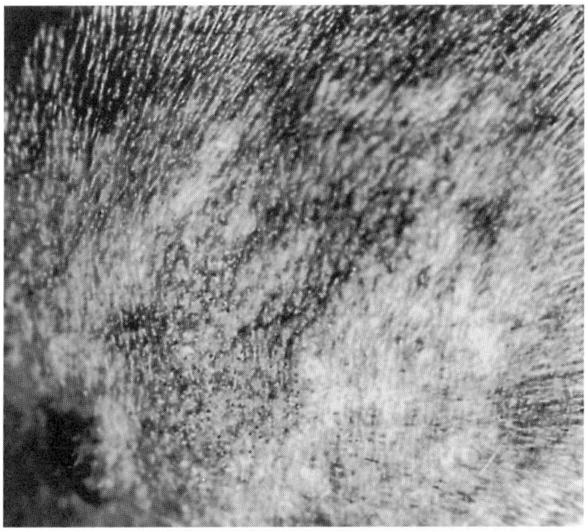

Figure 14-20. Area of alopecia, erythema, and follicular plugging (comedones) associated with demodicosis on a dog.

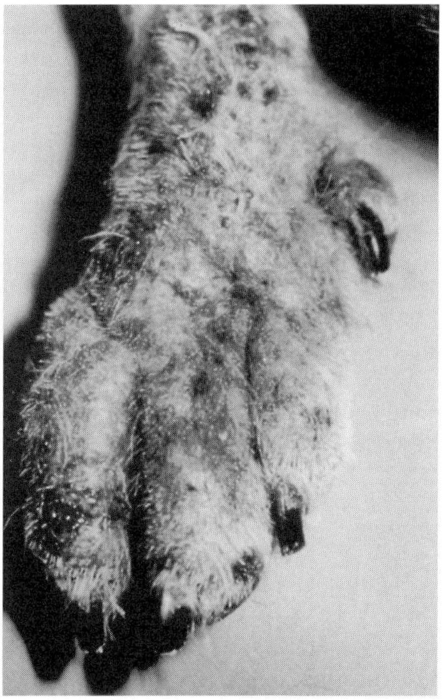

Figure 14-22. Chronic demodicosis on the foot with erythema alopecia, hyperpigmentation, and a secondary deep bacterial infection.

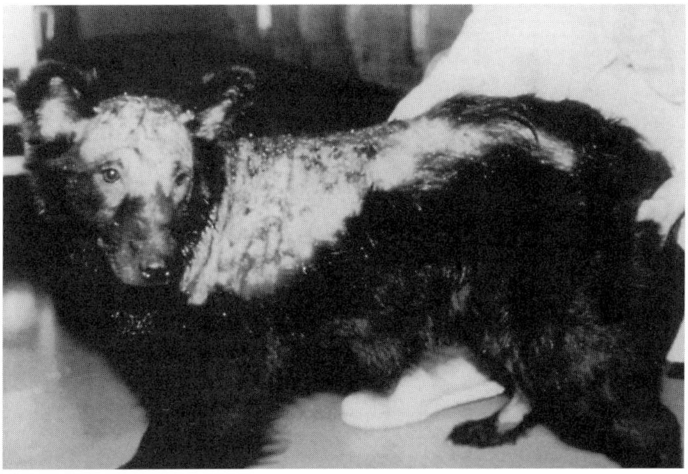

Figure 14-21. Chow chow dog with generalized demodicosis that began on the head and has progressed caudally down the back.

secondary bacterial infection. The more extensive and deep the bacterial disease, the more likely that systemic signs (fever, anorexia, lethargy) will be exhibited by the animal.

In some cases the *Demodex* infection is confined to the feet only. These cases should still be considered generalized for therapeutic purposes because the treatment and prognosis are more closely aligned with generalized demodicosis than with those for localized demodicosis.

Feline Demodicosis. Localized *Demodex* infection can be seen as a single area of alopecia and scaling of the eyelids, periocular area, head, and neck. Localized ceruminous demodectic otitis externa has also been described. Signs of generalized demodicosis secondary to *D. cati* include multifocal to generalized patches of alopecia with variable scaling, macules, papules, erythema, hyperpigmentation, crusting, and symmetric alopecia of the head, neck, legs, and trunk. Pruritus when present is either intermittent or mild. Clinical signs associated with *D. gatoi* include more severe pruritus, mild erythema, broken hairs, and alopecia of the hindlimbs, flank, and ventral abdomen. In some cats, mild clinical signs and patterns of involvement have been such that the condition could mimic psychogenic alopecia.

Diagnosis. Differential diagnosis for demodicosis in the dog and cat includes any other reason for hair follicle infection or infestation (folliculitis). The most important differential diagnoses include bacterial infection and dermatophytosis. Because of the highly variable nature of the clinical signs of demodicosis in the cat and the high incidence of the disease in the dog, all animals with significant skin disease should have skin scrapings performed to look for *Demodex* mites. The follicular mite in the dog and cat is best found by taking concentrated deep skin scrapings with a dull number 10 blade. Hair should be clipped from the affected areas, the skin squeezed to help extrude mites from the hair follicle, mineral oil placed on the lesion and on the slides, and the lesion scraped until capillary oozing is noted. If red blood cells are not seen, the scraping is probably not deep enough (Figure 14-23). It may be necessary to sedate fractious animals or animals that are difficult to restrain to obtain the appropriate skin scrapings. Care should be taken not to skin scrape in areas that are so severely damaged that the hair follicles have been destroyed. A minimum of 3 to 5 areas should be skin scraped to diagnose the disease and differentiate between localized and generalized demodicosis. Sites that should be surveyed include lesions, lip area, and interdigital spaces. If the scrapings are performed as outlined above, the diagnosis should be obvious except in some cases of *Demodex* infection in the Chinese shar-pei or in cases of severely scarred interdigital demodicosis with severe pyoderma. A biopsy may need to be performed in these cases to make the diagnosis. A substantial number of live adult mites or immature forms and eggs are needed to confirm the diagnosis. An occasional mite, especially from the face, may be a normal resident.

In the cat, *Demodex gatoi* lives in the stratum corneum, whereas *Demodex cati* occupies hair

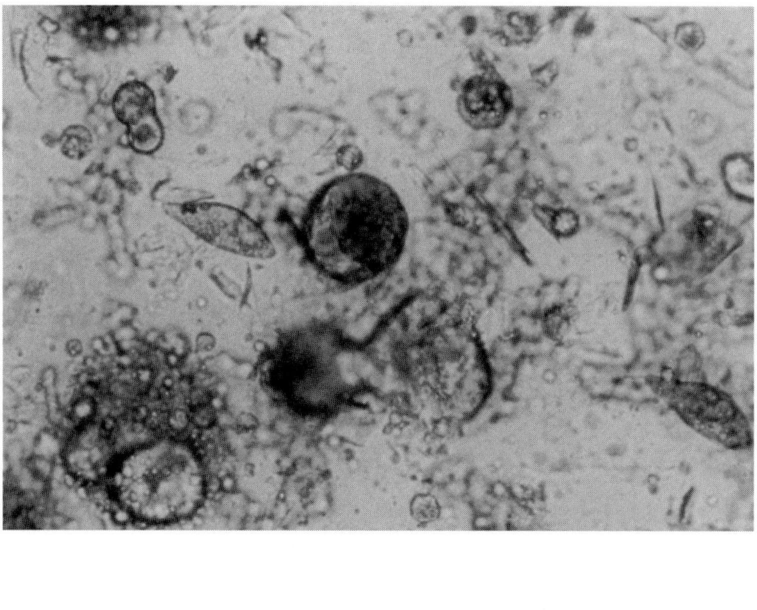

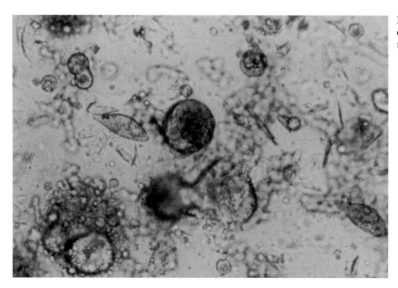

Figure 14-23. Skin scraping displaying *Demodex* mite eggs with red blood cells in the background.

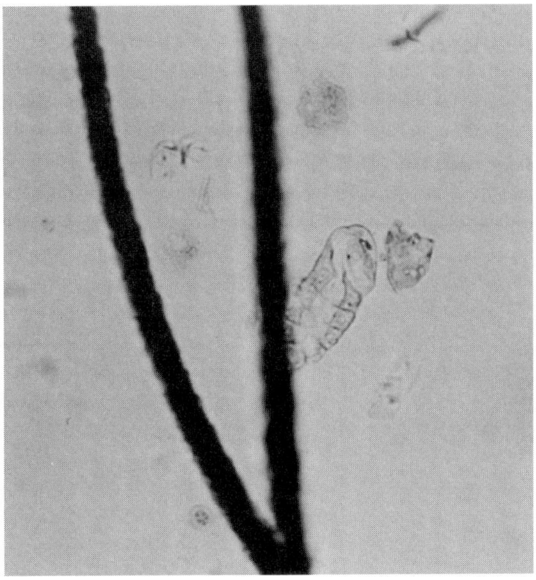

Figure 14-24. Superficial stratum corneum *Demodex gatoi* mite of the cat.

follicles. The dog also has several *Demodex* species (*D. canis*—most common follicular mite; a second, longer abdomen follicular mite; and a short abdomen demodectic mite found more superficially in the stratum corneum). Therefore, broad, superficial skin scrapings (over a large area) as well as deep, concentrated skin scrapings should be taken. Careful examination of the skin scraping slide is necessary, since *D. gatoi* in my opinion is more transparent and easily overlooked (Figure 14-24).

If mites are found in more than one body region (region one—head, neck, front legs; region two—trunk; region three—rear area), or extensive disease exists in one region, then the demodectic mange is considered generalized.

When a diagnosis of canine adult-onset generalized follicular demodicosis has been made, the veterinarian should begin a thorough search for any predisposing factors or underlying immunosuppressive or serious metabolic disease. Factors that can potentially predispose an animal to generalized demodicosis include administration of immunosuppressive drugs and underlying systemic disease. Hypothyroidism, hyperadrenocorticism, diabetes, blastomycosis and other deep mycoses, lymphosarcoma, hemangiosarcoma, and mammary adenocarcinoma have all been implicated.

In all cases of generalized demodicosis and preferably in all cases of adult-onset localized demodicosis in the dog, a complete medical evaluation should be performed. A thorough physical examination, complete blood count, serum chemistry panel, fecal test, heartworm test, and urinalysis should be the minimum evaluation performed. An evaluation for possible Cushing's disease or hypothyroidism should be considered in a dog with any evidence of an endocrinopathy. Any animal with deep pustular disease associated with the demodicosis should undergo a bacterial culture and sensitivity test.

Factors that can potentially predispose the cat to generalized demodicosis include diabetes mellitus, FIV, FIP, FeLV, systemic lupus erythematosus, hyperadrenocorticism, and toxoplasmosis. Medical evaluation of the cat with generalized demodicosis should include a complete blood count, serum chemistry panel, fecal, urinalysis, FeLV test, and FIV test. Endocrine evaluation should be considered.

Therapy

Localized Demodicosis. Localized demodicosis in the young animal will resolve spontaneously 90% of the time. If there is a concurrent bacterial infection, it is most important to treat with antimicrobial agents. Localized demodicosis in the adult or aged animal is a cause for greater concern. It is prudent to look for underlying factors that may predispose the animal to the onset of the disease (see recommendations for generalized demodicosis). Minimally, concern should be voiced to the owner, and lesions should be watched closely for continued progression.

Localized demodicosis will either spontaneously regress or progress to generalized demodicosis. There is no evidence that treatment of localized demodicosis will prevent generalized disease from occurring. Amitraz liquid is efficacious for localized demodicosis. However, there is currently questionable availability of this drug in the formulation approved for small animal use. In addition, because mites are capable of developing resistance to the insecticidal agent, the use of amitraz in treatment of localized demodicosis (which may undergo spontaneous remission) is a questionable practice. Topical therapies that may be used once daily on localized lesions include 1% rotenone ointment (Goodwinol), or benzoyl peroxide gel (Oxydex Gel, Pyoben Gel). Pustular localized demodicosis should be treated with an appropriate antibiotic for 2 weeks beyond resolution of the infection.

Adult-onset Generalized Canine Demodicosis. Owner education is extremely important when one undertakes the task of treating a case of adult-onset generalized demodectic mange.

Treatment of generalized demodicosis is a lengthy and costly undertaking. Many cases can be controlled but not "cured." Treatment should proceed only after the owner understands the disease and the economic and medical ramifications.

The only drug approved by the Food and Drug Administration for treatment of generalized demodicosis is amitraz (Mitaban). However, there is currently questionable availability of this drug in the formulation approved for small animal use. It is approved for biweekly use at 0.025%, but weekly amitraz dips appear to be more efficacious than dips every 2 weeks. No significant difference was noted when weekly single strength (0.025%) dipping was compared to weekly double strength (0.05%) dipping. To achieve maximal results with amitraz, I recommend following the guidelines in Box 14-4.

Alternative Therapeutic Protocols for Use of Small Animal Approved Amitraz. In a clinical trial,[70] application of a 12.5% amitraz solution (Taktic) diluted to a 0.125% solution (1 cc of Taktic/100 ml water) applied daily to half of the body on an alternating basis was studied. One investigator also applied the diluted dipping solution daily to the feet of dogs with pododemodicosis. An overall resolution rate of 79% was obtained. The overall average duration of treatment was 3.7 months. Dogs previously unresponsive to amitraz therapy had a resolution rate of 75% with the daily amitraz treatment. No serious toxic reactions were seen. Follow-up periods varied from 4 months to 1 year.

Alternate Therapeutic Options. Because of the labor-intensive nature of treatment with amitraz, many studies have been performed to document the efficacy of ivermectin and milbemycin given orally for treatment of generalized canine demodicosis.

Several studies have found the effectiveness of milbemycin to range from 42% to 86% using dosages varying from 1 mg/kg to 2 mg/kg. The higher-end dosage tended to have a higher cure rate.[71-73] Rare side effects of transient ataxia, lethargy, and vomiting have been noted and are reversible on drug discontinuation. Side effects may be seen more often in avermectin-sensitive collies given doses at or over 5 mg/kg.[74] I use milbemycin at 1 mg/kg once daily initially. If decreased mite counts are not seen within 4 to 8 weeks, the dosage is increased to 2 mg/kg once daily. Use of milbemycin is often limited by its cost.

Several studies have proven the efficacy of ivermectin in treatment of canine generalized demodicosis. Typically, daily oral doses of ivermectin at 300 to 600 μg/kg were used in these studies, with ivermectin found to be effective in up to 83.3% of dogs with generalized demodicosis.[75] It is much less expensive than daily milbemycin oxime. In a study using ivermectin every other day at 450 to 600 μg/kg, 8 of 12 dogs achieved a negative skin scraping.[76] Ivermectin is potentially toxic and should not be used in breeds such as collies, Australian shepherds, Old English sheepdogs, Shetland sheepdogs, their crosses, and possibly not in any other herding breed of dog. Side effects are most often seen in the breeds mentioned above and include ataxia, behavior disturbances, tremors, mydriasis, weakness or recumbency, apparent blindness, hypersalivation, depression, and, in severe cases, coma and death. If side effects are seen in dogs from nonsensitive breeds, they are more likely to develop mydriasis and mild ataxia, which usually subsides on drug discontinuation or on institution of a lower dosage. In a study to determine how commonly toxicities occur in breeds other than collies, only two of the 222 animals given ivermectin daily for treatment of generalized *Demodex* infection or weekly for the treatment of sarcoptic mange infestation showed side effects consisting of lethargy and slight ataxia.[77] For treatment of generalized *Demodex* infection in this study, the initial ivermectin dose was gradually increased from 50 μg/kg to the final dose of 300 μg/kg over a 5-day period. I currently use 600 μg/kg daily orally in non–ivermectin-sensitive breeds. If the health status or lineage is questionable and ivermectin is still chosen, an initial dose of 100 μg/kg is given daily orally with a daily increase of drug by 100 μg/kg to an end point of 600 μg/kg. If side effects are seen at doses less than 300 μg/kg, an alternative therapy is given. If the dog can tolerate 300 to 400 μg/kg, the ivermectin therapy is continued at this dosage. However, in my opinion, this lower dose has resulted in prolonged treatment in some but not all animals so treated.

Feline Generalized Demodicosis. Several treatment regimens have been used to treat cats with feline generalized demodicosis. However, there is not one widely accepted successful treatment regimen. Previous treatments have included weekly dips of lime sulfur, phosmet or fenchlorphos, 0.0125% amitraz (half strength) carbaryl shampoo, malathion dips, or one part rotenone in three parts mineral oil for the ears. One author recommends 2% lime sulfur dips for six to eight treatments as the initial therapy, with a malathion dip chosen next diluted to 0.25 ounces per gallon and applied weekly. Amitraz is the third choice, with

BOX 14-4 Guidelines in Treatment of Canine Generalized Demodicosis

1. A total body clip is necessary and the hair coat must be kept very short throughout the entire treatment period. This usually requires clipping the coat every 3 to 4 weeks.
2. Bathe the dog 12 to 24 hours before the dip in a follicular-flushing benzoyl peroxide shampoo. If the dog is bathed immediately before the dip, towel dry the animal completely so as not to dilute the dip.
3. Train in-hospital personnel to dip appropriately. Dip procedure should consist of a good 10 to 15 minutes of dip contact time, with continual gathering and repouring of the dip that has dripped off of the coat. The animal should be standing in the dip pooling in the bottom of the bathtub or dipping area. Most owners will not dip appropriately or for the appropriate length of time.
4. The dip must be made fresh and the solution used immediately. The dipping solution quickly loses its efficacy and degrades to compounds potentially more toxic. For this reason, once the bottle of amitraz has been opened, the whole bottle should be used immediately.
5. Allow the animal to drip dry without toweling.
6. Monitor for any side effects. In my opinion, all dogs that have been clipped and dipped appropriately will have some degree of side effects after the first dip. The side effects may be mild and will usually disappear with subsequent dips. The most common side effect is sedation or lethargy. This is usually transitory and lasts for 24 to 48 hours. Other side effects include anorexia, vomiting, diarrhea, pruritus, seizures, ataxia, hyperexcitability, personality change, hypothermia, appetite stimulation, bloat, polyuria, edema, erythema, and other varying degrees of skin irritation. Yohimbine (Yobine) will reverse the side effects of amitraz therapy. This drug can be given subcutaneously until effective (intravenously if acute problems are seen). The pretreatment dose is 0.03 mg/kg and the posttreatment dose is 0.01 mg/kg. The subcutaneous dose will usually last for 4 to 6 hours.
7. The dog should be kept dry between applications. Powdered products should be used instead of liquid solution between dips (e.g., flea powders vs. flea sprays).
8. Aggressively treat any secondary bacterial infection.
9. Monitor therapeutic success by serial skin scrapings every 2 to 4 weeks and record total mite counts. Note number of mites that are live, dead, mature (adult and nymphs), and immature (larvae and eggs). Continue to take skin scrapings from the five sites scraped for the original diagnosis. When one site is negative on two serial skin scrapings, stop using that site and add another affected site to the areas monitored.
10. A positive therapeutic response is initially a decreased number of immature forms and eventually a decreased number of mature and live adults.
11. Continue to dip for 1 month (2 to 4 treatments) after the first negative skin scraping. Rescrape 1 month after the last dip. Follow through with skin scrapings every few months for 1 year.
12. If clinical or skin scraping improvement is not seen after 4 to 8 dips, increase dipping to once-weekly (0.025% or 0.05%) strength.
13. Additional therapy that may be used along with the amitraz dip is Goodwinol shampoo (in addition to benzoyl peroxide shampoo) pre-dip and/or 400 IU of vitamin E given four times daily.
14. If scrapings from the feet or lips continue to be positive, daily application of 1 ml of amitraz in 29 cc propylene glycol or mineral oil to the lesions may be helpful. This solution should be made weekly (if dipping weekly) or every other week (if dipping biweekly). Be sure to decrease the amount of water that the dip is diluted with if the 1 ml of amitraz was removed from the bottle to make the painting solution.
15. If the animal is clinically normal but still skin-scrape positive after 8 to 10 dips, consider a maintenance dip protocol or change to a different treatment (see text).
16. A maintenance dip protocol will vary by individual animal. Most dogs will need to be dipped every 2 to 4 weeks for the rest of their lives to remain asymptomatic. Unfortunately, long-haired dogs should remain closely clipped.
17. If the animal is still symptomatic after the dipping procedure described in number 12, consider a different treatment or different dipping protocol.
18. All adult-onset generalized *Demodex*-infected intact female dogs should be spayed once the mite counts have decreased significantly because the stress of estrus may trigger a relapse of the disease. If the animal is being dipped on a biweekly schedule, then the spay should be done during the nondipping week. If the animal is being dipped weekly, then she should not be dipped during the week of the spay.

0.0125% dips started weekly. If the cat tolerates the 0.0125% amitraz well, but a cure is not achieved after 8 to 10 dips, then a 0.025% dip is applied weekly. Amitraz, fenchlorphos, and malathion are not approved for use in the cat. Organophosphate toxicity is a concern when the latter two dips are used. Side effects of amitraz therapy in the cat are anorexia, depression, diarrhea, hypersalivation, and hiding under furniture.

In the largest collection of published cases to date, all cats with either *Demodex cati* or *Demodex gatoi* were successfully treated with 2% lime sulfur dip given every 5 to 7 days for six treatments.[78] An Elizabethan collar is recommended until the dip has dried on the body to prevent ingestion of the lime sulfur from grooming.

There have been articles published noting several cats in two households infected with *Demodex gatoi*. This suggests that contagion between adult cats is possible.[79,80]

Generalized demodicosis in cats seems to be much more responsive to therapy than generalized demodicosis in dogs. This may be a reflection of the more superficial location of the mites in many cases or a different pathophysiologic mechanism and host immune response.

MISCELLANEOUS

Necrolytic Migratory Erythema

Necrolytic migratory erythema (diabetic dermatopathy, hepatocutaneous syndrome, superficial necrolytic dermatitis, metabolic necrolytic dermatopathy, or metabolic epidermal necrosis) has been seen in dogs with diabetes mellitus and glucagon secreting tumors of the pancreas, but is most often associated with hepatic disease (hepatopathy of unknown origin, hepatopathy secondary to ingestion of mycotoxins, hepatopathy secondary to phenobarbital or phenytoin administration, and hepatopathy possibly associated with primidone or phenobarbital administration). Older dogs are most likely to be affected, with an average age of 10 years. Animals of either sex may be affected, but an almost 2:1 male-to-female ratio is reported.[81]

Clinical Features. Necrolytic migratory erythema is an ulcerative dermatosis associated with erythema, crusts, and alopecia. It occurs most frequently periorally, periocularly (Figure 14-25), on the legs, feet, and external genitalia, and often in the groin region (Figure 14-26). The foot pads are usually hyperkeratotic (Figure 14-27) and may be fissured and ulcerated. Lesions may follow a waxing and waning course. The lesions may be mildly pruritic or painful. These lesions are commonly complicated by secondary infections with bacteria and yeast. Cutaneous signs may precede evidence of internal disease by weeks or months.[81]

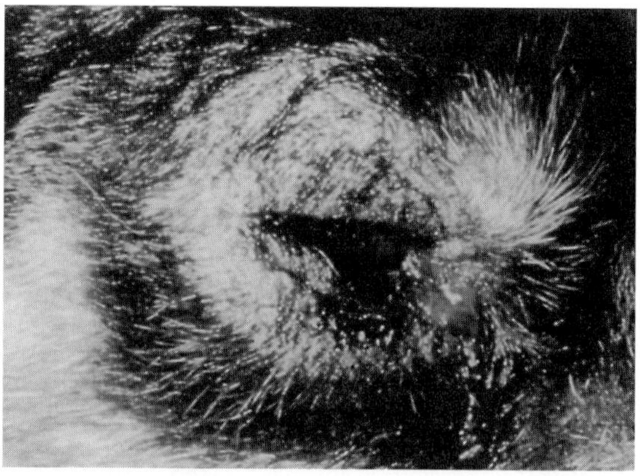

Figure 14-25. Periocular crusting on a miniature pinscher with necrolytic migratory erythema.

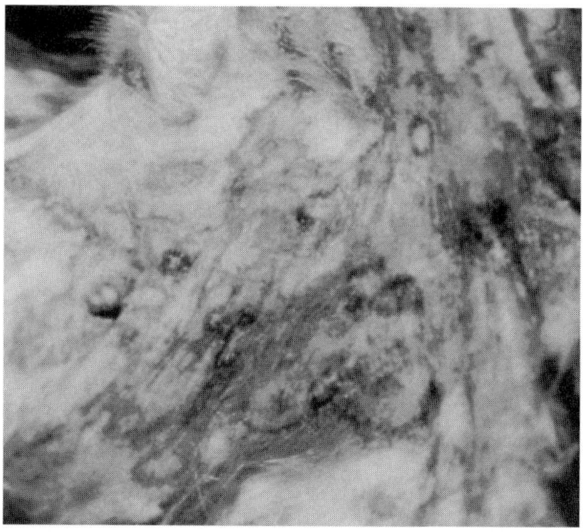

Figure 14-26. Circular ulcerations on the groin of a dog with necrolytic migratory erythema. (Courtesy Dr. Carol Foil, DVM, Louisiana State University, Baton Rouge, La.)

Diagnosis. The disease should be suspected on the basis of the history and physical examination. Affected animals typically are middle-aged or older dogs with a progressive crusting dermatitis affecting the face, distal extremities, and external genitalia.

Examination of skin biopsies of lesions on affected dogs reveals a unique combination of diffuse parakeratotic hyperkeratosis, epidermal necrosis, marked superficial epidermal edema, irregular epidermal hyperplasia, and mild superficial perivascular dermatitis. The epidermal edema is both intercellular and intracellular and is localized to the upper half of the epidermis (Figure 14-28). Severe edema may result in intraepidermal clefts and vesicles.

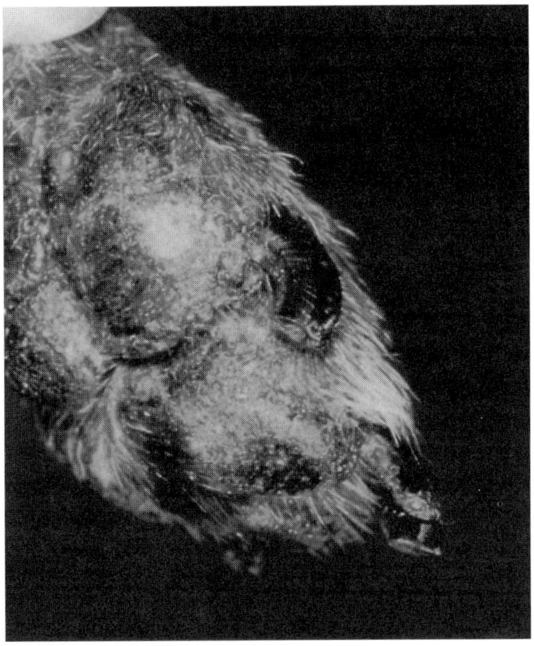

Figure 14-27. Footpad crusting on a miniature pinscher with necrolytic migratory erythema.

In dogs with hepatic disease associated with necrolytic migratory erythema, a unique "honeycomb" pattern is found on ultrasonographic evaluation of the liver. This pattern consists of variably sized hypoechoic regions surrounded by highly echogenic borders. These hypoechoic regions correspond to regenerative nodules bounded by severely vacuolated hepatocytes, numerous bile ductules, and a network of reticulin and fine collagen fibers representing remnants of collapsed hepatic lobules.[82]

Clinicopathologic abnormalities vary, depending on the specific inciting organ system and the progression of the disease. Complete blood count abnormalities include anemia, neutrophilic leukocytosis, and toxic neutrophilic changes. Serum biochemical abnormalities may include increased liver enzymes, total bilirubin, and bile acids. Hypoalbuminemia is a common finding, and many dogs develop hyperglycemia as the disease progresses. Glucagon concentrations are increased in some cases. In dogs with liver disease, severe, profound hypoaminoacidemia is often seen.

Therapy. Treatment is aimed at correcting the underlying metabolic disease. If the dog is diabetic, insulin therapy is indicated. In most cases, however, regulation is difficult. Surgical excision of a glucagon-secreting tumor of the pancreatic alpha cells may be possible. Unfortunately, most cases are associated with irreversible chronic liver disease and hepatic cirrhosis, making treatment largely unrewarding.

Therapy for dogs with severe hypoaminoacidemia (commonly seen in dogs with hepatic diseases) is nutritional support to include IV amino acid supplementation. The diet should consist of a good-quality protein diet. Fatty acid, zinc, and niacin supplementations have been used with some success. Intravenous amino acid supplementation regimens vary from 250 to 500 ml IV of

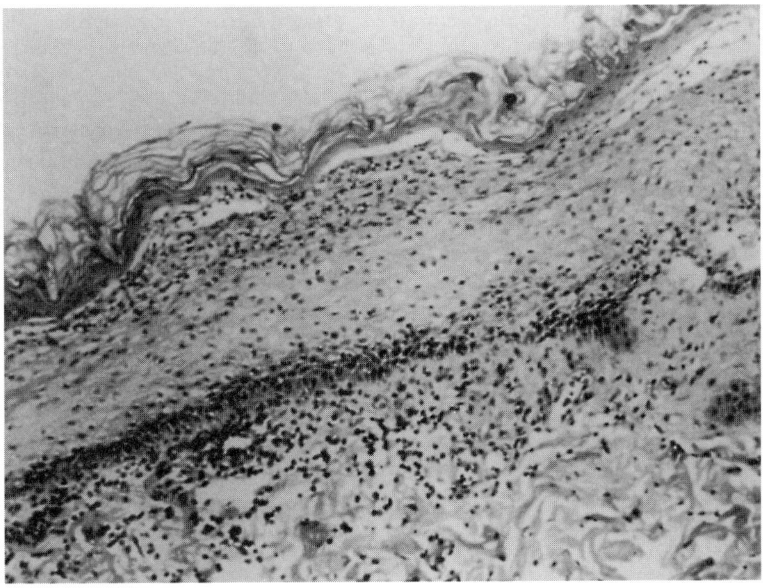

Figure 14-28. Magnification of the epidermis displaying intracellular and intercellular edema in the stratum granulosum and stratum spinosum, characteristic of necrolytic migratory erythema (× 400).

an 8% to 10% amino acid supplement given daily until dermatologic signs improve, to these doses given weekly for an extended period of time. Intravenous amino acid supplements are readministered in many animals when dermatologic signs return.

Antibiotics or antifungal agents should be used to treat secondary skin infections. Hydrotherapy and shampoo therapy can help remove crusts and lessen the pruritus and pain that may be present. Glucocorticoid therapy has been associated with improvement in cutaneous signs but should be used with caution as it may worsen the underlying metabolic disease.

Paraneoplastic Syndromes

Paraneoplastic syndromes consist of clinical signs that are associated with malignancies but not directly related to tumor invasion. The mechanism by which tumors produce paraneoplastic syndromes is not completely understood. Three general mechanisms are theorized: production of substances such as cytokines that directly or indirectly cause the dermatosis; depletion of substances by the tumor that results in the paraneoplastic syndrome; and a normal or aberrant host response to the tumor, which then causes the paraneoplastic disorder. Only rare paraneoplastic dermatoses have been associated with internal malignancies in dogs and cats. In the dog, these include the crusting or fissuring dermatosis associated with necrolytic migratory erythema; nodular skin disease (nodular dermatofibrosis) seen with renal and uterine tumors; paraneoplastic pemphigus vulgaris associated with a thymic lymphoma; suspect paraneoplastic pemphigus foliaceous from a Sertoli cell tumor and one from a mammary carcinoma; and necrotizing panniculitis associated with pancreatic carcinoma. In the cat these paraneoplastic dermatoses include the skin fragility syndrome seen with feline adrenal neoplasia; exfoliative dermatosis associated with feline thymoma; and a unique bilaterally symmetric, ventral glistening paraneoplastic alopecia associated with pancreatic carcinoma and bile duct carcinoma. Most often, these animals are geriatric animals because the underlying neoplastic disease is seen in the aged animal.

Feline Paraneoplastic Alopecia

Recognized in the 1990s, feline paraneoplastic alopecia is a condition that involves an alopecic dermatitis associated with internal malignancy, including pancreatic adenocarcinoma, bile duct carcinoma, and thymoma.[2,83-86] Affected cats have a 2-week to 5-month history of inappetence, lethargy, weight loss, and progressive alopecia.

Clinical Features. The alopecia seen primarily involves the ventrum and the leg, with pinnal and periocular alopecia seen less commonly. The alopecic skin has a unique smooth, glistening appearance. The footpads may become shiny, smooth, soft, and occasionally crusted and fissured. In some cases, because of pain associated with pad disease, cats are reluctant to walk.

Diagnosis. The disease should be suspected based on history, physical examination findings, and the unique dermatologic presentation. Hematologic and biochemical results are not indicative of underlying neoplasia. Skin biopsies show telogenization, marked atrophy, and miniaturization of hair follicles. Focal areas of epidermal hyperplasia with orthokeratotic and parakeratotic hyperkeratosis are seen. Areas of hypokeratosis have also been noted. Adnexal atrophy may be prominent. Radiology and ultrasonographic studies may fail to reveal thoracic or abdominal masses, and the diagnosis may be made during an exploratory surgery.

Therapy. The prognosis is usually grave, and many cats are euthanized when the neoplastic disease is confirmed. However, reports of surgical excision of the primary neoplasia have resulted in complete recovery. A case of surgical excision of a pancreatic mass resulted in complete hair growth, and although there was not evidence of metastasis seen at the time of surgery, the alopecia recurred 18 weeks later and metastasis was confirmed at necropsy.[2]

"Old Dog" Erythema Multiforme

Erythema multiforme is a cutaneous reaction pattern of multifactorial etiology seen uncommonly in the dog and rarely in the cat. An immunologic basis for the syndrome has been hypothesized. Erythema multiforme has been seen in older dogs without a history of drug hypersensitivity or concurrent disease in many cases.

Clinical Features. There is no breed or sex predilection for old dog erythema multiforme. Lesions are acute in onset and appear as erythematous macules and papules. Crusting commonly occurs as the lesions spread peripherally and form arciform patterns. Epidermal collarettes may be present. Annular target lesions with central clearing are seen in some stages of the syndrome. Widespread ulcers may evolve from urticarial or plaquelike lesions. The lesions are exudative and tend to be more proliferative than other subsets of erythema multiforme and often predominately involve the face and ears. Occult leukemia, pseudomonal otitis externa, staphylococcal folliculitis, anal sacculitis, pancreatic endocrine tumors, and *Pneumocystis* pneumonia have been identified in several old dogs.

Diagnosis. Diagnosis is made by histopathologic examination of a skin biopsy. For the biopsy, it is best to use areas of erythema without crusting or ulceration. An intact epidermis is necessary for the diagnosis of this syndrome. Individual cell necrosis of epidermal cells is the most characteristic histologic lesion of erythema multiforme. Acanthosis is present, and lymphocytes may closely surround the necrotic epidermal cells. Superficial follicular epidermal necrosis may be prominent.

Therapy. A search for an underlying disease is warranted, as there is no specific treatment for the skin disease. Correction of the underlying disease can possibly reverse the cutaneous signs. Symptomatic treatment for ulcerative skin disease and secondary bacterial infections, hydrotherapy, antibacterial shampoos, and antibiotics are probably also indicated. The use of glucocorticoids and other immunosuppressive drug therapy in treatment of this disease remains controversial and probably should be reserved for those cases in which other interventions have failed and clinical signs are worsening.

References

1. Baker KP: Senile changes of dog skin, *J Small Anim Pract* 8:49, 1967.
2. Scott DW, Miller WH, Griffin CE: *Muller and Kirk's small animal dermatology*, Philadelphia, 2001,WB Saunders.
3. August JR: Taking a dermatologic history, *Compend Contin Educ Pract Vet* 8:510, 1986.
4. Smith EK: Planning the workup for dermatologic patients, *Vet Med* 83:35, 1988.
5. Feldman EC, Nelson RW: *Canine and feline endocrinology and reproduction,* Philadelphia, 1996, WB Saunders.
6. Schumm-Draeger PM, Langer F, Caspar G et al: Spontaneous Hashimoto-like thyroiditis in cats, *Verh Dtsch Ges Pathol* 80:297, 1996
7. Rand JS, Levin J, Best SJ et al: Spontaneous adult-onset hypothyroidism in a cat, *J Vet Intern Med* 7:272, 1993.
8. Jones BR, Gruffydd-Jones TJ, Sparkes AH et al: Preliminary studies on congenital hypothyroidism in a family of Abyssinian cats, *Vet Rec* 131:145, 1992.
9. Kramer RW, Price GS, Spodnick GJ: Hypothyroidism in a dog after surgery and radiation therapy for a functional thyroid adenocarcinoma, *Vet Radio Ultrasound* 35:132, 1994.
10. Kemppainen RTJ, MacDonald JM: Canine hypothyroidism. In Griffin CE, Kwochka KW, MacDonald JM, eds: *Current veterinary dermatology; the science and art of therapy*, St Louis, 1993, Mosby.
11. Conaway DH, Padgett GA, Nachreiner R et al: Clinical and histological features of primary, progressive, familial thyroiditis in a colony of borzoi dogs, *Vet Pathol* 22:439, 1985.
12. Zeiss CJ, Waddle G: Hypothyroidism and atherosclerosis in dogs, *Compend Contin Educ Pract Vet* 17:1117, 1995.
13. Ford SL, Nelson RW, Feldman EC et al: Insulin resistance in three dogs with hypothyroidism and diabetes mellitus, *J Am Vet Med Assoc* 202:1478, 1993.
14. Daigle JC, Foil CS, Wolfsheimer K: Primary hypothyroidism in a cat, *Vet Dermatol* 11(suppl 1):43, 2000.
15. Peterson ME, Melian C, Nichols R: Measurement of serum total thyroxine, triiodothyronine, free thyroxine and thyrotropin concentrations for diagnosis of hypothyroidism in dogs, *J Am Vet Med Assoc* 211:1396, 1997.
16. Beale KM, Halliwell RE, Chen CL: Prevalence of thyroglobulin autoantibodies in dogs detected by enzyme-linked immunosorbent assay, *J Am Vet Med Assoc* 196:745, 1990a.
17. Graham PA, Lundquist RB, Refsal KR et al: A 12 month prospective study of 234 thyroglobulin antibody positive dogs which had no laboratory evidence of thyroid dysfunction, *Proc Am Coll Vet Intern Med Forum* 19:863, 2001.
18. Iversen L, Jensen AL, Hoier R et al: Biological variation of canine serum thyrotropin (TSH) concentration, *Vet Clin Pathol* 28:16, 1999.
19. Dr. Jenise Daigle, Davie, Florida, personal communication 2000.
20. White SD, Ceragioli KL, Bullock LP et al: Cutaneous markers of canine hyperadrenocorticism, *Compend Contin Educ Pract Vet* 11:446, 1989.
21. Jensen AJ, Iversen L, Koch J et al: Evaluation of the urinary cortisol:creatinine ratio in the diagnosis of hyperadrenocorticism in dogs, *J Small Anim Pract* 8:99, 1997.
22. Feldman EC, Mack RE: Urine cortisol:creatinine ratio as a screening test for hyperadrenocorticism in dogs, *J Am Vet Med Assoc* 200:1637, 1992.
23. Smiley LE, Peterson ME: Evaluation of a urinary corticol:creatinine ratio as a screening test for hyperadrenocorticism in dogs, *J Vet Intern Med* 7:163, 1993.
24. Kemppainen RJ, Clark TP, Peterson ME: Preservative effect of aprotinin on canine plasma immunoreactive adrenocorticotropin concentrations, *Domest Anim Endocrinol* 11:355, 1989
25. Barthez PY, Nyland TG, Feldman EC: Ultrasonographic evaluation of the adrenal glands in dogs, *J Am Vet Med Assoc* 207:1180, 1995.
26. Gould SM, Baines EA, Mannion PA et al: Use of endogenous ACTH concentration and adrenal

ultrasonography to distinguish the cause of canine hyperadrenocorticism, *J Small Anim Pract* 42:113, 2001.
27. Widmer WR, Guptill L: Imaging techniques for facilitating diagnosis of hyperadrenocorticism in dogs and cats, *J Am Vet Med Assoc* 206:1857, 1995.
28. Bruyette DS, Ruehl WW, Entriken T et al: Management of canine pituitary dependent hyperadrenocorticism with l-deprenyl (Anipryl), *Vet Clin North Am* 27:273, 1997.
29. Kintzer PP, Peterson ME: Mitotane (o,p'-DDD) treatment of 200 dogs with pituitary-dependent hyperadrenocorticism, *J Vet Intern Med* 5:182, 1991.
30. Goossens MM, Meyer HP, Voorhout G et al: Urinary excretion of glucocorticoids in the diagnosis of hyperadrenocorticism in cats, *Domest Anim Endocrinol* 12:355, 1995.
31. Mauldin GN, Burk RL: The use of diagnostic computerized tomography and radiation therapy in canine and feline hyperadrenocorticism, *Probl Vet Med Endocrinol* 2:557, 1990
32. Reusch CE, Steffen T, Hoerauf A: The efficacy of L-deprenyl in dogs with pituitary-dependent hyperadrenocorticism, *J Vet Intern Med* 13:291, 1999.
33. Zerbe CA, MacDonald JM: Canine and feline Cushing's syndrome. In Griffin CE, Kwochka KW, MacDonald JM eds: *Current veterinary dermatology: the science and art of therapy,* St Louis, 1993, Mosby.
34. Myers NC, Bruyette DS: Feline adrenocortical diseases. Part I—hyperadrenocorticism, *Semin Vet Med Surg (Small Anim)* 9:137, 1994.
35. Helton-Rhodes K, Wallace M, Baer K: Cutaneous manifestations of feline hyperadrenocorticism. In Ihrke PJ, Mason IS, White SD, eds: *Advances in veterinary dermatology* 2: Proceedings of the Second World Congress of Veterinary Dermatology, New York, 1993, Pergamon Press.
36. Henry CJ, Clark TP, Young DW, et al: Urine cortisol:creatinine ratio in healthy and sick cats, *J Vet Intern Med* 10:123, 1996.
37. Peterson ME, Kemppainen RJ: Dose-response relation between plasma concentrations of corticotropin and cortisol after administration of incremental doses of Cosyntropin for corticotropin stimulation testing in cats, *Am J Vet Res* 54:300, 1993.
38. Dickstein G, Scechner C, Nicholson WE et al: Adrenocorticotropin stimulation test: effects of basal cortisol level, time of day, and suggested new sensitive low dose test, *J Clin Endocrinol Metab* 72:773, 1991.
39. Meij BP, Voorhout G, Van Den Ing H et al: Transphenoidal hypophysectomy for treatment of pituitary dependent hyperadrenocorticism in 7 cats, *Vet Surg* 30:72, 2001.
40. Daley CA, Zerbe CA, Schick RO et al: Use of metyrapone to treat pituitary-dependent hyperadrenocorticism in a cat with large cutaneous wounds, *J Am Vet Med Assoc* 202:956, 1993.
41. Hess RS, Saunders HM, Van Winkle TJ et al: Concurrent disorders in dogs with diabetes mellitus: 221 cases (1993-1998), *J Am Vet Med Assoc* 217:1166, 2000.
42. Vail DM, Withrow SJ: Tumors of the skin and subcutaneous tissues. In Withrow SJ, MacEwen EG, eds: *Small animal clinical oncology,* Philadelphia, 2001, WB Saunders.
43. Gross TL, Ihrke PJ, Walder EJ: *Veterinary dermatopathology: a macroscopic and microscopic evaluation of canine and feline skin disease,* St Louis, 1992, Mosby.
44. Miller WH, Affolter VK, Scott DW: Multicentric squamous cell carcinomas in situ resembling Bowen's disease in five cats, *Vet Dermatol* 3:177, 1992
45. Baer K, Helton-Rhodes K: Multicentric squamous cell carcinoma in situ resembling Bowen's disease in cats, *Vet Pathol* 30:535, 1993.
46. Guaguere E, Olivry T, Delverdier-Poujade A et al: Demodex cati infestation in association with feline cutaneous squamous cell carcinoma in situ: a report of five cases, *Vet Derm* 10:61, 1999.
47. Turrel JM, Gross TL: Diagnosis and treatment of multicentric squamous cell carcinoma in situ (Bowen's Disease) of cats, *Proc Vet Cancer Soc October 27-29,* Minneapolis, Minn, 1991.
48. Aronsohn MG, Carpenter JL: Distal extremity melanocytic nevi and malignant melanomas in dogs, *J Am Anim Hosp Assoc* 26:605, 1990.
49. Modiano JF, Ritt MG, Wojcieszyn J: The molecular basis of canine melanoma: Pathogenesis and trends in diagnosis and therapy, *J Vet Intern Med* 13:163, 1999.
50. Ramos-Vara JA, Beissenherz ME, Miller MA et al: Retrospective study of 338 canine oral melanomas with clinical histologic and immunohistochemical review of 129 cases, *Vet Pathol* 37:597, 2000.
51. Goldschmidt MH, Shofer FS: *Skin tumors of the dog and cat,* Oxford, England, 1992, Pergamon Press.
52. Luna LD, Higginbotham ML, Henry CJ et al: Feline non-ocular melanoma: a retrospective study of 23 cases (1991-1999), *J Feline Med and Surg* 1:173, 2000.
53. MacEwen EG , Kurzman ID, Vail DM et al: Adjuvant therapy for melanoma in dogs: results of randomized clinical trials using surgery, liposome-encapsulated muramyl tripeptide, and granulocyte macrophage colony-stimulating factor, *Clin Cancer Research* 5:4249, 1999.
54. Moore PF, Affolter VK, Olivry T et al: The use of immunological reagents in defining the pathogenesis of canine skin diseases involving the proliferation of leukocytes. In Kwochka KW, Willemse T, Tscharner C von, eds: *Advances in veterinary dermatology,* vol 3, Oxford, England, 1993, Butterworth-Heinemann.
55. Beale KM, Bolon B: *Canine cutaneous lymphosarcoma: epitheliotropic and non-epitheliotropic, a retrospective study,* Proceedings of the Second World Congress of Veterinary Dermatology, Montreal, Quebec, Canada, 1992.
56. Vangessel VA, McDonough SP, McCormick HJ et al: Cutaneous presentation of canine intravascular lymphoma (malignant angioendotheliomatosis), *Vet Derm* 11:291, 2000.
57. DeBoer DJ, Turrel JM, Moore PF: Mycosis fungoides in a dog: demonstration of T cell specificity and response to radiotherapy, *J Am Anim Hosp Assoc* 26:566, 1990.
58. Rosychuk RAW: Cutaneous manifestations of endocrine disease in dogs, *Compend Contin Educ Pract Vet* 20(3):287, 1998.
59. Cooley DM, Waters DJ: Tumors of the male reproductive system. In Withrow SJ, MacEwen EG, eds: *Small animal clinical oncology,* Philadelphia, 2001, WB Saunders.
60. Rosser EJ: Sex hormones. In Griffin CE, Kwochka KW, MacDonald JM, eds: *Current veterinary dermatology: the science and art of therapy,* St Louis, 1993, Mosby.
61. Gilson SD, Withrow SJ, Wheeler SL et al: Pheochromocytoma in 50 dogs, *J Vet Intern Med* 8:228, 1994.
62. Rosenstein DS: Diagnostic imaging in canine pheochromocytoma, *Vet Radiol Ultrasound* 41:499, 2000.

63. Suter M, Lott-Stoltz G, Wild P: Generalized nodular dermatofibrosis in six Alsatians, *Vet Pathol* 20:632, 1983.
64. Jonasdottir TJ, Mellersh CS, Moe L et al: Genetic mapping of a naturally occurring hereditary renal cancer syndrome in dogs, *Proc Natl Acad Sci USA* 97:4132, 2000.
65. Marks SL, Farman CA, Peaston A: Nodular dermatofibrosis and renal cystadenomas in a golden retriever, *Vet Derm* 4(3):133, 1993.
66. Atlee BA, DeBoer DJ, Ihrke PJ et al: Nodular dermatofibrosis in German shepherd dogs as a marker for renal cystadenocarcinoma, *J Am Anim Hosp Assoc* 27:481, 1991.
67. Moe L, Lium B: Hereditary multifocal renal cystadenocarcinomas and nodular dermatofibrosis in 51 German shepherd dogs, *J Small Anim Pract* 38:498, 1997.
68. Gaafer SM, Greve J: Natural transmission of *Demodex canis* in dogs, *J Am Vet Med Assoc* 148:1043, 1966.
69. Sako S, Yamane O: Studies on the canine demodicosis. III. Examination of the oral-internal infection, intrauterine infection, and infection through respiratory tract, *Jpn J Parasitol* 11:499, 1962.
70. Medleau L, Willemse T: Efficacy of daily amitraz therapy for refractory generalized demodicosis in dogs: two independent studies, *J Am Anim Hosp Assoc* 31:246, 1995
71. Mueller RS, Bettenay SV: Milbemycin oxime in the treatment of canine demodicosis, *Aust Vet Pract* 25:122, 1995.
72. Miller WH, Scott DW, Cayatte SM et al: Clinical efficacy of increased dosages of milbemycin oxime for treatment of generalized demodicosis in adult dogs, *J Am Vet Med Assoc* 207:1581, 1995.
73. Miller WH, Scott DW, Wellington JR et al: Clinical efficacy of milbemycin oxime in the treatment of generalized demodicosis in adult dogs, *J Am Vet Med Assoc* 203:1426, 1993.
74. Tranquilli WJ, Paul AJ, Todd KS: Assessment of toxicosis induced by high-dose administration of milbemycin oxime in collies, *Am J Vet Res* 52:1170, 1991.
75. Paradis M: New approaches to the treatment of canine demodicosis, *Vet Clin North Am* 29:1425, 1999
76. Tapp T, Muse R, Rosenkrantz WS: Efficacy of alternate day oral ivermectin in the treatment of generalized demodicosis, *Proc Am Acad Dermat and Am Coll Vet Dermatol* 14:25, 1998.
77. Mueller RS, Bettenay SV: A proposed new therapeutic protocol for the treatment of canine mange with ivermectin, *J Am Anim Hosp Assoc* 35:77, 1999.
78. Morris DO, Beale KM: Feline demodicosis. In Bonagura JD, ed: *Kirk's current veterinary therapy XIII*, Philadelphia, 2000, WB Saunders.
79. Medleau L, Brown CA, Brown SA et al: Demodicosis in cats, *J Am Anim Hosp Assoc* 24:85, 1988.
80. Morris DO: Contagious demodicosis in three cats residing in a common household, *J Am Anim Hosp Assoc* 32:350, 1996.
81. Angarano DW: Metabolic epidermal necrosis. In Griffin CE, Kwochka KW, MacDonald JM, eds: *Current veterinary dermatology: the science and art of therapy*, St Louis, 1993, Mosby.
82. Nyland TG, Barthez PY, Ortega TM et al: Hepatic ultrasonographic and pathologic findings in dogs with canine superficial necrolytic dermatitis, *Vet Radiol Ultrasound* 3:200, 1996.
83. Pascal-Tenorio A, Olivry T, Gross TL et al: Paraneoplastic alopecia associated with internal malignancies in the cat, *Vet Dermatol* 8:47, 1997.
84. Brooks DG, Campbell KL, Dennis JS et al: Pancreatic paraneoplastic alopecia in three cats, *J Am Anim Hosp Assoc* 30:557, 1994.
85. Godfrey DR: A case of feline paraneoplastic alopecia with secondary *Malassezia*-associated dermatitis, *J Small Anim Pract* 39:394, 1998.
86. Scott DW, Yager JA, Johnston KM: Exfoliative dermatitis in association with thymoma in three cats, *Feline Pract* 23:8, 1995.

Suggested Reading

Caciolo PL, Nesbitt GH, Patnaik AK et al: Cutaneous lymphosarcoma in the cat: A report of nine cases, *J Am Anim Hosp Assoc* 20:491, 1984.

CHAPTER 15

Ear Diseases and Altered Hearing

STEVEN A. MELMAN

Ear diseases in older dogs and cats are frequently chronic in nature. Their treatment and development often result in diminished hearing capacity. Management of chronic ear diseases requires definitive diagnosis and control of the numerous underlying causes and perpetuating factors. Cleaning of the external ear canal and middle ear cavity, along with the use of oral antimicrobial agents, oral corticosteroids, topical antimicrobials, and topical corticosteroids, may be necessary for the treatment of ear diseases (Table 15-1). Otitis externa involves inflammation and infection of the outer ear when the tympanic membrane is present. Otitis media involves inflammation and infection of the middle ear, frequently in cases in which the tympanic membrane is ruptured. In many cases lifelong ear cleaning and drying agents may be required to prevent relapse of ear diseases.

DISEASES OF THE PINNA

Lesions of the pinna may be an extension of more generalized skin diseases and can be bacterial, fungal, parasitic, immune-mediated, or vascular (drug-induced) in origin.[1] Bacterial and yeast folliculitis of the pinna with focal areas of alopecia occur in dogs, and dermatophytosis of the pinna with focal alopecia and extensive crust formation can be found in cats. *Sarcoptes* mites in dogs and *Notoedres* mites in cats can cause parasitic pruritus and crusting of the margins of the pinna.

Trauma

Trauma to the pinna can occur at any age. A tear in the pinna is usually the result of a fight with another dog or cat. The resulting bleeding may be impressive, and the placement of several sutures is often curative. A small, fresh tear (up to 1 cm in length) can be sutured after cleaning and removal of some of the hair. The skin on the concave side of the pinna is apposed and sutured with interrupted sutures, starting at the edge of the pinna. The skin on the convex side is then apposed and sutured in the same way. The cartilage is not included in these sutures. Bleeding stops during suturing but a resistant artery may have to be ligated separately. In all cases, the wound should be considered contaminated, and a short period of systemic antimicrobial treatment is indicated. When the wound is not fresh and inflammation is apparent, the surgical correction is postponed and the inflammation is treated first. Surgical correction then begins with refreshening of the wound edges.

Aural Hematoma

Aural hematomas occur at all ages. The bleeding occurs between the cartilaginous layers of the pinna and usually results from trauma, such as shaking the head or scratching the ear as a result of hypersensitivity. Other causes include immune-mediated factors, clotting defects, and hormonal imbalances. Surgical intervention is necessary,

TABLE 15-1. DRUGS USED IN TREATMENT OF EAR DISEASES

DRUG	DOSAGE	ROUTE	FREQUENCY	CONDITIONS FOR USE
Prednisone/ prednisolone	0.5-1 mg/kg	Oral	Once daily	Canine antiinflammatory and antipruritic
	1-2 mg/kg	Oral	Once daily	Feline antiinflammatory and antipruritic
	1-2 mg/kg	Oral	Twice daily	Canine immunosuppressive
	2-4 mg/kg	Oral	Twice daily	Feline immunosuppressive
Dexamethasone	0.1 mg/kg	Oral	Twice daily or once daily	Idiopathic pinnal erythema
Etretinate	1 mg/kg or 10 mg per cat total dose	Oral	Once daily	Canine acquired pattern alopecia, canine ear margin seborrhea, canine and feline actinic dermatitis, lichenoid-psoriasiform dermatitis
Ivermectin	0.3 mg/kg	Oral	Once weekly	Sarcoptic mange, notoedric mange, canine and feline ear mites
	0.3 mg/kg	SC	Every 10-14 days	
Lime sulfur	2%	Dip	Once weekly	Sarcoptic mange, notoedric mange
Amitraz	0.025%	Dip	Once weekly	Sarcoptic mange, notoedric mange
Sulfasalazine	20-40 mg/kg	Oral	Three times daily	Idiopathic vasculitis
Fluocinolone 0.01%, DMSO 60%	2-12 drops, varies with size of ear canal	Topical	Twice daily initially, every 48-72 hours for maintenance	Canine antiinflammatory; moderate to severe allergic otitis, hyperplastic and proliferative otitis
Hydrocortisone 1%	2-12 drops, varies with size of ear canal	Topical	Twice daily initially, every 48-72 hours for maintenance	Canine antiinflammatory and astringent; moderate to severe allergic otitis, swimmer's otitis, ceruminous otitis
Hydrocortisone 0.5%, sulfur 2%, acetic acid 2.5%	2-12 drops, varies with size of ear canal	Topical	Twice daily initially, every 48-72 hours for maintenance	Canine antiinflammatory, astringent, and germicidal; allergic otitis, swimmer's otitis, ceruminous otitis
Lactic acid 2.5%, salicylic acid 0.1%, dioctyl sodium sulfosuccinate, propylene glycol, malic acid, benzoic acid	Fill ear canal	Topical	Every 48-72 hours or as needed	Ceruminolytic and drying agent, mild antibacterial activity, mild antifungal activity
Propylene glycol, malic acid, benzoic acid, salicylic acid	Fill ear canal	Topical	Every 48-72 hours or as needed	Ceruminolytic and drying agent, mild antibacterial activity, mild antifungal activity
Dioctyl sodium sulfosuccinate 6.5%, urea (carbamide) peroxide 6%	1-2 ml per ear canal	Topical	As needed	May be irritating to inflamed ear canal
Povidone-iodine 10%	Dilute 1:10 to 1:50 in water	Topical	As needed	Ear canal flushing
Polyhydroxidine iodine 0.5%	Dilute 1:1 to 1:5 in water	Topical	As needed	Ear canal flushing, weekly use for ear mites, twice daily for resistant *Pseudomonas* otitis
Acetic acid 5%	Dilute 1:1 to 1:3 in water	Topical	As needed	Ear canal flushing, may be irritating to inflamed ear canal on more concentrated solutions
Acetic acid 2%, boric acid 2%	Fill ear canal	Topical	Once daily for 7 days for *Malassezia,* then twice weekly	Ear canal flushing; *Malassezia* otitis, swimmer's otitis, antibacterial activity, antifungal activity
Neomycin 0.25%, triamcinolone 0.1%, thiabendazole 4%	2-12 drops, varies with size of ear canal	Topical	Twice daily	Bacterial, yeast, or allergic otitis, ear mite therapy
Neomycin 0.25%, triamcinolone 0.1%, nystatin 100,000 IU/ml	2-12 drops, varies with size of ear canal	Topical	Twice daily	Bacterial, yeast, or allergic otitis
Neomycin 1.75%, polymyxin B 5,000 IU/ml, penicillin G procaine 10,000 IU/ml	2-12 drops, varies with size of ear canal	Topical	Twice daily	Bacterial otitis

TABLE 15-1. DRUGS USED IN TREATMENT OF EAR DISEASES—cont'd

DRUG	DOSAGE	ROUTE	FREQUENCY	CONDITIONS FOR USE
Gentamicin 0.3%, betamethasone valerate 0.1%	2-12 drops, varies with size of ear canal	Topical	Twice daily	Bacterial otitis
Gentamicin 0.3%, betamethasone valerate 0.1%, clotrimazole 1%	2-12 drops, varies with size of ear canal	Topical	Twice daily	Bacterial otitis, refractory *Malassezia* otitis
Polymyxin B 10,000 IU/ml, hydrocortisone 0.5%	2-12 drops, varies with size of ear canal	Topical	Twice daily	Bacterial otitis
Pyrethrins 0.05%, squalene 25%	2-12 drops, varies with size of ear canal	Topical	Once daily	Ear mite otitis
Acetic acid 2%, aluminum acetate	Fill ear canal	Topical	Twice daily to every 48 hours	Astringent activity; swimmer's otitis
Silver sulfadiazine 1%	Dilute 1:1 with water	Topical	Twice daily for 2 weeks	*Pseudomonas* otitis, *Malassezia* otitis; use only in a clean ear canal
Tris-EDTA, +/– Baytril 5%	Add 6 ml large animal Baytril to 114 ml TrizEDTA; 0.5-1.5 ml/bid	Topical	Twice daily for 14 days	Resistant *Pseudomonas* otitis; may use alone or mix with Baytril to achieve 5% Baytril/TrizEDTA solution
TrizEDTA	Fill ear canal	Topical	Twice daily initially followed by 2-3 times weekly	*Pseudomonas* otitis and other bacterial otitis
Silver nitrate 5%	Use sparingly	Topical	As needed	Cauterization for ulcerative otitis externa
Miconazole 1%	2-12 drops, varies with size of ear canal	Topical	Once daily to twice daily	May use with or without a topical corticosteroid, can add 7.5 ml of dexamethasone phosphate (4 mg/ml) to 10 ml of 1% miconazole
Enrofloxacin	2-12 drops, varies with size of ear canal	Topical	Once daily	*Pseudomonas* otitis externa, other bacterial otitis
Enrofloxacin	2.5-5 mg/kg	Oral	Twice daily	*Pseudomonas* otitis externa, otitis media
Ketoconazole	5-10 mg/kg	Oral	Twice daily for 2-4 weeks, every other day for long-term maintenance	Refractory *Malassezia* otitis externa, *Malassezia* otitis media
Itraconazole	10 mg/kg	Oral	Once daily	Refractory *Malassezia* otitis externa
Cephalexin	10-20 mg/kg	Oral	Three times daily	Bacterial otitis externa, otitis media
	20-30 mg/kg	Oral	Twice daily	
Marbofloxacin		Oral	Once daily	Bacterial otitis externa, otitis media

DMSO, Dimethyl sulfoxide; *EDTA,* ethylenediaminetetraacetic acid; *SC,* subcutaneous administration; *Triz,* tromethamine.

because without treatment, the pinna will shrivel, and subsequent ossification of the cartilage will cause continuous irritation. In addition, shriveling of the pinna may cause obstruction of the external ear canal and thus induce chronic otitis externa. Surgery allows for removal of the blood clots and presses the layers of the pinna together long enough to effectuate reunion of the layers. A reliable surgical method consists of suturing through all layers of the pinna, placing sutures over the entire surface of the pinna.

Abscesses

In cats, a penetrating wound inflicted by the claw of another cat usually causes an abscess of the pinna. The skin over the abscess should be opened and the suppurative material removed by gentle compression, followed by flushing with copious amounts of sterile saline solution. A systemic antimicrobial agent should be administered for 10 to 14 days. In some older cats, both pinnae are shriveled because of multiple abscesses. The shriveled pinna can cause occlusion of the external ear canal, and continuous otitis externa may be the result. Ossification of the pinna usually causes continuous irritation to the cat, and amputation of the pinna results in remarkable relief.

Abscesses of the pinna are uncommon in the dog, but they are treated in the same way as in the cat. The healing of the pinna can be slow and painful, and hence an analgesic agent should be given in addition to antimicrobial therapy. In addition, in the dog a shriveled pinna can cause considerable irritation and chronic otitis externa. When complications in the external ear canal are also present, such as ossification of the cartilage or chronic proliferation of the skin, removal of the pinna and the ear canal in one procedure may be the preferred long-term solution.[2] This surgery may seem radical, but there is no reason to exclude older dogs from radical surgery when the alternative is continuous distress and pain.

Tumors of the Pinna

Tumors of the pinna occur at all ages in dogs and cats. Tumors in dogs may include squamous cell carcinomas, basal cell tumors, lymphomas, histiocytomas, mast cell tumors, sebaceous gland adenomas, fibromas, and hemangiopericytoma.[3] Squamous cell tumors are most commonly seen in white dogs and cats. Dog breeds most frequently affected by histiocytomas are retrievers and boxers; those most frequently affected by mast cell tumors are boxers and rottweilers; and those most frequently affected by sebaceous gland adenomas are cocker spaniels. Squamous cell tumors and histiocytomas can be removed by partial resection of the pinna. Amputation of the pinna may be necessary to prevent further extension of the tumor and potential metastasis. Mast cell tumors should be excised with a wide margin of surrounding tissue. The pinna and the external ear canal may have to be removed together.

Squamous cell carcinoma is the most common tumor affecting the pinna in the cat. Older white cats seem to be especially susceptible to the development of squamous cell carcinoma, but it does occur in any colored cat. Squamous cell carcinoma first appears as a nonhealing granulomatous inflammation at the edge of the pinna and is often misdiagnosed as an inflammatory lesion. As the squamous cell carcinoma grows, hemorrhage from the lesion at the edge of the pinna becomes a frequent nuisance. Cytologic examination of material collected by fine needle aspiration biopsy or histopathologic examination of surgical biopsy material will confirm the diagnosis. Unilateral or bilateral amputation of the pinna is an effective therapy, especially because metastasis seldom occurs in an early stage. Unilateral or bilateral pinna amputation will change the appearance of the animal considerably so the owner needs to be informed of such changes prior to surgery (Figure 15-1).

The surgical removal of the pinna in the cat and dog are similar procedures, but along the base of the dog's pinna on the convex side the skin is incised, and the individual arteries and veins are freed and ligated separately for effective hemorrhage control. After hemorrhage is controlled, the pinna is removed by cutting the cartilage and the skin on the concave side, and the skin edges are closed using standard suturing techniques.

DISEASES OF THE EXTERNAL AND MIDDLE EAR

Dogs and cats with recurrent otitis externa should always be evaluated for coexisting otitis media. Sedation or general anesthesia is often required for the clinician to properly evaluate the external ear canal and middle ear cavity. The optimal indicator of otitis media is a ruptured tympanum. In cases in which the tympanic membrane is intact, a myringotomy is required. Magnetic resonance imaging (MRI) or computer tomography (CT) may also be used to diagnose otitis media.[4] Sudden onset of peripheral vestibular syndrome or deafness may occur after any

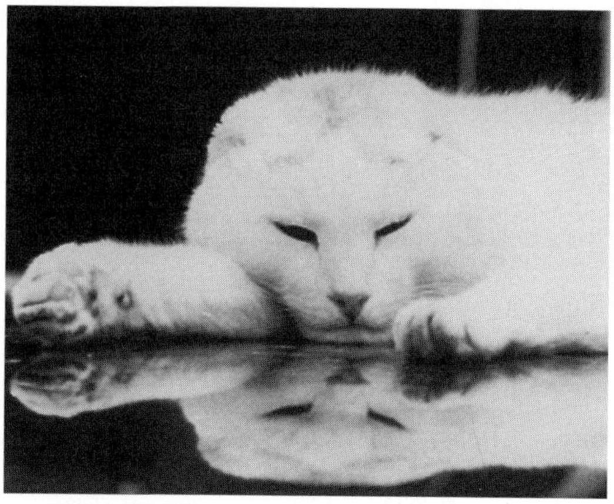

Figure 15-1. Bilateral pinna amputation changes the appearance of the cat considerably, but the cat lives in comfort.

otic flushing or dental cleaning procedure in older dogs and cats, especially when ototoxic drugs are used. Hearing return may take longer, if hearing returns at all, when ototoxic agents such as chlorhexidine are used, or hearing return may be more transient when alcohol is used.[5]

Ear Evaluation

The preferred method for flushing the external ear canal and middle ear cavity when the tympanic membrane is ruptured involves fiberoptic video–enhanced endoscopy.[4] This method ensures good visualization of the ear structures and safe flushing because the more delicate structures are located in the middle and dorsal areas of the middle ear cavity. Myringotomy allows the examiner to collect samples directly from the middle ear cavity and, therefore, is the practical method of diagnosing an otitis media when the tympanic membrane is intact in the presence of chronic ear problems. After the myringotomy, the middle ear cavity is flushed with about 200 to 300 ml of tepid sterile saline solution followed by a solution of tromethamine-ethylenediaminetetraacetic acid (Tris-EDTA)(TrizEDTA) then packed with 22 to 100 mg of fluoroquinolones (Baytril) and 2 to 6 mg of dexamethasone sodium phosphate. A serous, slightly sanguineous discharge may be observed for a few days after myringotomy. Postoperative analgesic agents can be used for at least 2 to 3 days. Insidious damage to the facial nerve can develop because of the existing otitis media or when cleaning, medicating, or performing diagnostic procedures in an ear with a ruptured tympanic membrane.

I do not perform standard culture and sensitivity testing unless there is a treatment failure. Some experts believe a primary indication for performing standard bacterial culture and sensitivity testing in dogs and cats is a diagnosis of severe proliferative otitis with bacterial rods, for which systemic antimicrobial therapy is indicated and management of otitis media is needed.[4] Cytologic examination in these cases usually shows numerous leukocytes in stained otic smears. Because multiple potentially pathogenic organisms may be cultured, it is important to combine the cytologic examination with bacterial culture results. The bacteria in the highest numbers may be identified, and this allows a more appropriate antimicrobial regimen to be chosen. Laboratories that report antimicrobial sensitivities with minimum inhibitory concentration information rather than the standard Kirby-Bauer susceptibility test allow for better determination of systemic antimicrobial dosages.[4] For example, *Pseudomonas* organisms may show intermediate or sensitive patterns to enrofloxacin by Kirby-Bauer susceptibility tests but be resistant on the minimum inhibitory concentration tests.

Otitis Externa

Otitis externa has both primary and secondary causes.[6] Primary causes of otitis externa in older dogs other than bacterial, fungal, and yeast infections are hypersensitivity such as atopic dermatitis, food allergy and contact hypersensitivity, and *Otodectes* infestation. Otitis externa may be the only presenting sign in atopic dogs. Often, dogs with diagnosed food allergy will show their allergic disease with only an otitis externa.

Food allergy should be the primary differential consideration in any older dog with an acute onset of otitis externa without previous history of otic disease. Flea allergy does not usually cause just an otitis externa, but instead causes total body skin disease. Prophylactic treatment for ear mites is essential to be certain that mites are not a component of otitis externa. Systemic therapy for ear mites is safer and easier with the use of selamectin or various ivermectin products.

Secondary causes of otitis externa include topical irritant reactions and *Pseudomonas* or *Malassezia* infection. Topical irritant reactions should be considered any time a case of otitis externa fails to respond or worsens with topical therapy. Therapeutic ingredients in ear medications such as propylene glycol (>10%) may induce inflammation in the previously damaged aural epidermis. Treatment of topical irritant reactions consists of discontinuation of topical therapies and limitation of topical products to normal saline solution or aqueous-based products. Systemic therapy for topical irritant reactions is preferred.

Most cases of *Pseudomonas* otitis externa are sensitive to polymyxin B, ticarcillin, or enrofloxacin. Polymyxin B is inactivated by purulent debris and must be applied only in clean external ear canals.

Malassezia otitis externa is best treated with a nonototoxic combination of 2% acetic and 2% boric acid (DermaPet Ear/Skin Cleanser; MalAcetic Otic) aqueous solution by flushing daily for 7 days. Signs including erythema, pain, and discharge as well as cytology were reversed in 17 dogs.[7] *Malassezia* otitis media occurs infrequently and is treated with systemic antifungal agents such as ketoconazole (10 mg/kg orally once daily) or itraconazole (10 mg/kg orally once daily).

Veterinarians previously have compounded enrofloxacin with a normal saline solution (4 ml of 22.7 mg/ml enrofloxacin with 12 ml of normal saline solution, acetic-boric acid cleanser, or Tris-EDTA (TrizEDTA). Topical enrofloxacin may be effective even when sensitivity testing indicates a resistance because of the increased concentration achieved when applied topically. Silver sulfadiazine (2%) solution is also effective against *Pseudomonas.* A formulation of enrofloxacin (5 mg/ml) combined with 1% silver sulfadiazine (Baytril Otic) is effective for bacterial and, to a much lesser extent, *Malassezia* otitis externa; it has not been proved to be safe or effective in cases in which there is a ruptured tympanum. Acetic acid (2%) is effective against *Pseudomonas* organisms after 1 minute of contact time. However, 2% acetic-2% boric acids are proven to be synergistic against *Pseudomonas.*[8]

EDTA has a direct bactericidal action against *Pseudomonas aeruginosa* by chelating metal ions important for the integrity of its cell wall, inactivating the efflux pump in gram-negative bacteria and inactivating enzymes secreted by *Pseudomonas* that would otherwise cause ulceration and tissue necrosis. Buffer solutions containing Tris are used to enhance the effects of EDTA on the *Pseudomonas aeruginosa* and other gram-negative organisms. The EDTA binds to metal ions, which compete with aminoglycosides for cell-wall receptors. Thus, the combination of aminoglycoside and Tris-EDTA is effective against bacteria causing an otitis externa or media infection, including *Staphylococcus intermedius, Proteus mirabilis, Escherichia coli,* and *Pseudomonas aeruginosa.* The Tris-EDTA buffer solution (TrizEDTA) is less effective at inhibiting gram-positive bacteria than gram-negative bacteria. The optimal pH for the activity of aminoglycosides and Tris-EDTA buffer solution is approximately 8[9]; many antimicrobial agents are enhanced at alkaline pH and have diminished efficacy at an acidic pH. The Tris-EDTA buffer solution is most effective as it approaches body temperature, at which point it has been demonstrated to irreversibly bind enzymes that would otherwise cause ulceration. Tris-EDTA is not considered to be ototoxic.

TrizEDTA buffer solutions are beneficial for long-term therapy for preventing the recurrence of *Pseudomonas* infection, as part of a regular ear-cleaning regimen, or as a presoak solution before the instillation of antimicrobial solutions into the external ear canal. Such solutions are typically applied two to three times a week as needed for preventive purposes.

Otitis Media

Most dogs with chronic otitis externa have concurrent otitis media that is frequently accompanied by an intact tympanic membrane.[10] Evidence of inflammation to the tissues surrounding the middle ear cavity, or even the inner ear, indicates that otitis media may be present. The entire tympanic membrane in most older dogs and cats is difficult to completely visualize by using the standard otoscopic evaluation procedure. Even with an intact tympanic membrane, various abnormalities of the middle ear cavity in dogs and cats may be visualized by using fiberoptic video-enhanced endoscopy.[4] The affected tympanic membrane is nontransparent and usually red or ruptured.[10] The discharge from the middle ear cavity may be mucopurulent in acute inflammation and drier and whiter in chronic inflammation. If the tympanic membrane is intact and otitis media is suspected, a myringotomy may be necessary to confirm the otitis media. The tympanic membrane should close within 4 weeks when middle ear disease is cured.

TUMORS OF THE EXTERNAL EAR CANAL

Tumors in the external ear canal more often occur in older cats than in older dogs. The tumors in the external ear canal of older dogs may include ceruminal gland adenomas, papillomas, ceruminal gland carcinomas, and squamous cell carcinomas.[3] The tumors in the external ear canal in older cats may include ceruminal gland adenomas, ceruminal gland carcinomas, sebaceous gland adenomas (Figure 15-2), papillomas, mast cell tumors, and rhabdomyosarcoma.[11] The unilateral or bilateral tumor can be diagnosed by otoscopic examination. Because each tumor damages the external ear canal and causes pain and continuous secondary inflammation, wide surgical excision or application of laser surgery is always indicated. Malignant tumors are especially threatening because they will eventually invade the tissues around the ear canal. Total ablation of the external ear canal is always indicated when a malignant tumor is confirmed and as long as the tumor is still confined within the cartilaginous wall.

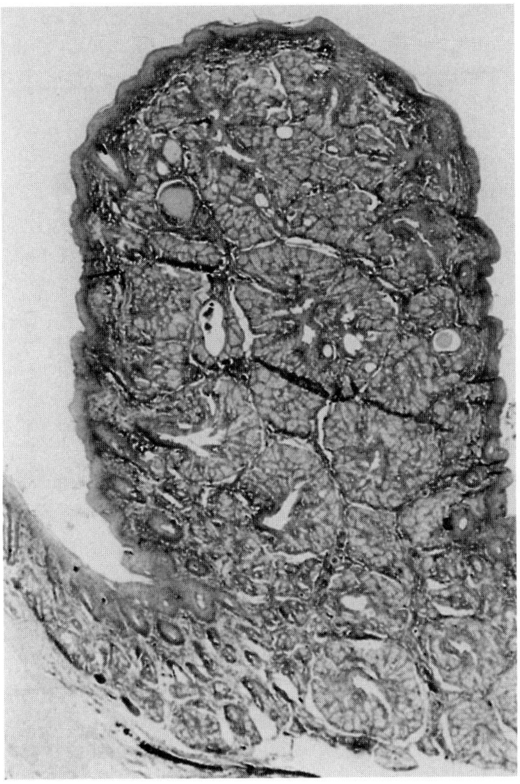

Figure 15-2. Sebaceous gland adenoma of the ear canal in a 10-year-old male European shorthair cat (H & E stain, × 36).

LOSS OF VESTIBULAR FUNCTION

The loss of vestibular function may be caused by middle ear disease, trauma, or ototoxicity in dogs and cats of all ages. Idiopathic vestibular disease commonly occurs in dogs, with an average age of onset of 12.5 years.[12] In cats with signs of peripheral vestibular dysfunction, the seemingly idiopathic vestibular syndrome is most often associated with middle ear disease.[13]

The case history of idiopathic vestibular disease in dogs is characterized by a peracute onset (within hours) of head tilt, incoordination, and nystagmus. The incoordination may be so severe that the dog cannot effectively rise and walk. Vomiting that is secondary to vertigo may be seen during the first 24 to 48 hours. The neurologic examination shows a head tilt, falling or rolling toward the head tilt, and horizontal to rotary nystagmus. Spontaneous nystagmus may be present, with the fast phase of the nystagmus occurring away from the head tilt. The type of nystagmus typically does not change. Generalized incoordination and a base wide stance are often present. No cranial nerve deficits will be noted, and no weakness or postural test deficit is present. If these signs are seen, then a brain stem lesion involving the central vestibular system is most likely. If the nystagmus type is vertical, a brain stem lesion is most likely to be present.

On the initial day of presentation, the incoordination and disorientation are often too severe to allow for adequate assessment of strength and postural test reactions. It may take 48 hours before any assessment can be used to help separate central vestibular disease from peripheral vestibular disease. Once vestibular signs have been localized to the peripheral vestibular system, the primary differential diagnoses are otitis interna and head trauma with resultant fracture of the petrous temporal bone. If facial nerve paralysis and Horner's syndrome are present on the same side of the head tilt, coexisting otitis media and interna are usually indicated.

Treatment involves supportive care because the peripheral vestibular problem will resolve on its own. The resolution timetable is usually consistent from case to case, and if the dog does not follow the timetable, there should be concern that the initial diagnosis was wrong. The nystagmus should disappear within 4 days, the dog should be able to rise and walk fairly well within 7 days, and the dog's gait should be normal by 3 weeks. A few dogs may have a residual head tilt or some incoordination after complete recovery when performing quick movements that require agility. Treatments that may be helpful during the first few days include fluid therapy for maintaining normal hydration, diazepam (5 to 15 mg three times daily) for sedation if disorientation is severe, meclizine (25 mg orally once daily) for vertigo, and diphenhydramine (4 to 8 mg/kg orally). These treatments are usually unnecessary after 72 to 96 hours after onset of peripheral vestibular signs.

PRIMARY MIDDLE EAR TUMORS

Primary middle ear tumors are uncommon in dogs and cats.[14,15] Tumors are suspected when the external ear canal is narrowed near the osseous external meatus and the otic discharge is hemorrhagic. Clinical signs include pain on the affected side and vestibular dysfunction. Survey radiographs may show densities in and around the tympanic bulla, but these findings do not differentiate between chronic inflammatory disease and tumor. CT is helpful for detection of lesions in the tympanic bulla and the petrosal bone. The destruction caused by the tumor at the time of diagnosis precludes any attempt at surgery.

SYSTEMIC ANTIMICROBIAL THERAPY

Systemic antimicrobial therapy is indicated for management of severe otitis externa or media, topical irritant reactions, poor response to topical otic therapy, and when severe proliferative otitis externa is present and the owner cannot administer regularly scheduled topical treatments. Antimicrobial agents that are known to penetrate into bone, concentrate within inflammatory cells, and have an excellent success in the treatment of otitis media should be selected and given at doses that are at the high end of the recommended dosage range. Antimicrobial and antifungal agents should be administered for at least 14 days after a complete clinical cure is obtained; often up to 6 to 12 weeks of therapy are necessary. Examples of systemic antimicrobial agents that are useful for the management of otitis media and proliferative otitis externa are clindamycin 7 to 10 mg/kg twice daily, sulfadimethoxine-ormetoprim 55 mg/kg for first day and 25 mg/kg once daily on subsequent days, enrofloxacin 5 to 20 mg/kg once daily, marbofloxin 2.5 to 5 mg/kg, and orbifloxacin 2.5 to 12.5 mg/kg once daily. In general, for *Pseudomonas aeruginosa* infections in dogs fluoroquinolones are needed at higher doses such as 10 to 20 mg/kg enrofloxacin once daily, 5 to 12.5 mg/kg orbifloxacin once daily, or 5 mg/kg marbofloxacin once daily.

INTRALESIONAL THERAPY

Stenosis of the vertical portion of the external ear canal occasionally may be nonresponsive to the administration of systemic corticosteroids. In these cases, intralesional triamcinolone acetonide (4 mg/ml) may be useful in widening the lumen of the vertical portion of the external ear canal. After effective cleaning of the external ear canal, multiple injections of triamcinolone acetonide at 0.1 ml per injection site are made as deep as possible into the proliferative tissue lining in a ringlike fashion around the external ear canal.

BACTERIAL OTITIS MEDIA PROTOCOL

Following is a protocol for the treatment of bacterial otitis media.

1. After choosing an antimicrobial agent through culture and sensitivity testing, start the agent systemically for at least 30 to 60 days. I currently prefer fluoroquinolones.
2. Clean with TrizEDTA twice daily. Do not refrigerate, as one mechanism of action is to reverse the activity of elastase enzymes, which occurs when the solution is at body temperature.
3. Instill topical antimicrobial agents (I currently prefer Baytril) in either a TrizEDTA "gemish" (a 5% Baytril injectable solution in TrizEDTA which can be attained by adding 600 mg large animal Baytril to 114 ml of TrizEDTA) or diluted with normal saline solution; for the first 3 weeks add 6 mg dexamethasone sodium phosphate per 15 ml of gemish).
4. For the first 14 days, I would use systemic prednisone at 1 to 2 mg/kg if otitis media has been diagnosed. The rationale is to decrease the inflammation, mucous secretion from the mucoperiosteum, pain, and viscosity of the exudate in the tympanic cavity.
5. If otitis media has been diagnosed, I would anesthetize the animal and with visualization flush the ear with TrizEDTA and directly instill Baytril and sodium dexamethasone phosphate into the tympanum. If the tympanum is present and otitis media is suspected, then I would do a myringotomy. The location of the myringotomy should be ventral. Maintenance therapy would include long-term biweekly TrizEDTA cleansing.

SURGICAL INTERVENTION FOR EAR DISEASES

In dogs with recurrent otitis, surgical intervention may be indicated. Such instances may include:

- Progressive otic changes, such as calcification, proliferation, and stenosis of the external ear canal, that result in permanent ear canal occlusion and are nonresponsive to intralesional therapy.
- Otitis media that fails to respond to myringotomy, ear canal flushing, and aggressive medical management.
- Inadequate response of the recurrent otitis to medical management because of poor owner compliance or the presence of resistant bacterial or fungal agents.

LOSS OF HEARING

Loss of hearing in older dogs and cats is well recognized. The cause of hearing loss may be related to a loss of spiral ganglion cells in the cochleas and secondary to hair cell loss.[16,17] Hearing in older dogs and cats may be tested most effectively by using brain stem auditory evoked responses.[18,19] The case histories provided by owners of older dogs and cats examined for hearing deficits usually suggest a progressive elevation of the hearing threshold rather than acute total hearing loss. However, hearing loss may be associated with existing otitis media, sudden onset immune-mediated otitis media or interna, or ototoxicity.

References

1. Roth L: Pathologic changes in otitis externa, *Vet Clin North Am* 18:755, 1988.
2. Venker-van Haagen AJ, Siemelink RJ, Smoorenburg GF: Auditory brain stem responses in the normal beagle, *Vet Q* 11:129, 1989.
3. Van der Gaag I: The pathology of external ear canal in dogs and cats, *Vet Q* 8:307, 1986.
4. Cole LK, Kwochka KW, Kowalski JJ et al: Microbial flora and antimicrobial sensitivity testing of isolated pathogens from the horizontal ear canal and middle ear of dogs with otitis media, *J Am Vet Med Assoc* 212:534, 1998.
5. Mansfield, S: Ototoxicity. In Gotthelf LN, ed: *Small animal ear diseases,* Philadelphia, 2001, WB Saunders.
6. Logas DB: Diseases of the ear canal, *Vet Clin North Am* 24:905, 1994.
7. Gotthelf LN, Young SE: New treatment of *Malassezia* otitis externa in dogs, *Vet Forum* 14:47, 1997.
8. Benson CE: Efficacy of acetic and boric acids against selected microbial flora seen in otitis externa, *Proc Am Acad Vet Derm,* 1999.
9. Wooley R: In-vitro effect of combinations of antimicrobial agents and tris-EDTA on *Pseudomonas, J Am Vet Med Assoc* 44:1521, 1983.
10. Little CJL, Lane JG, Gibbs C et al: Inflammatory middle ear disease of the dog: the pathology of otitis media, *Vet Rec* 128:293, 1991.
11. Rogers KS: Tumors of the ear canal, *Vet Clin North Am* 18:860, 1988.
12. Schunk KL, Averill DR: Peripheral vestibular syndrome in the dog: a review of 83 cases, *J Am Vet Med Assoc* 182:1354, 1983.
13. Burke EE, Moise NS, de Lahunta A et al: Review of idiopathic feline vestibular syndrome in 75 cats, *J Am Vet Med Assoc* 187:941, 1985.
14. Fiorito DA: Oral and peripheral vestibular signs in a cat with squamous cell carcinoma, *J Am Vet Med Assoc* 188:71, 1986.
15. Indrieri RJ, Taylor RF: Vestibular dysfunction caused by squamous cell carcinoma involving the middle ear and inner ear in two cats, *J Am Vet Med Assoc* 184:471, 1984.
16. Knowles K, Blauch B, Leipold H et al: Reduction of spiral ganglion neurons in the aged canine with hearing loss, *J Am Vet Med Assoc* 36:188, 1989.
17. Schuknecht HF, Igarashi M, Gacek RR: The pathological types of cochleo-saccular degeneration, *Acta Otolaryngol* 59:154, 1965.
18. Sims MH: Electrodiagnostic evaluation of auditory function, *Vet Clin North Am* 18:913, 1988.
19. Venker-van Haagen AJ: Disease and surgery of the ear. In Sherding RG, ed: *The cat: diseases and clinical management,* New York, 1989, Churchill Livingstone.

Suggested Readings

Cole LK, Kwochka KW, Podell M et al: Radiography, otoscopy, pneumotoscopy, impedance audiometry, and endoscopy for the diagnosis of otitis media in the dog, Proceedings of the Fourth World Congress of Veterinary Dermatology, San Francisco, Calif, 4:3, 2000.

Gotthelf LN: *Small animal ear diseases,* Philadelphia, 2001, WB Saunders.

Melman SA: New approach to pruritic otitis. In Gotthelf LN, ed: *Small animal ear diseases,* Philadelphia, 2001, WB Saunders.

CHAPTER 16

Ophthalmic Diseases and Their Management

JOHNNY D. HOSKINS

Older dogs and cats are often presented to a veterinary practice with an ocular problem. The examiner must obtain a history relating to the ocular problem and perform complete diagnostic testing for its diagnosis and treatment.

GENERAL OCULAR EXAMINATION

During the performance of the general ocular examination, several important points must be kept in mind. The Schirmer tear test and thorough eyelid examination should be the first procedures performed, and they should be performed before the application of any topical anesthetic agent or corneal stain.[1] The Schirmer tear test should measure both basal and reflex aqueous tear production for best diagnostic results.

Several types of corneal staining tests are used. One type is the dry fluorescein test strip that must be prewetted, with several fluorescein drops applied to the animal's corneal surface. The eyelids are then gently massaged, and the excess fluorescein stain is flushed away from the eye with sterile saline solution. Illumination of the globe will reveal fluorescein stain uptake if there is disruption to the epithelial layer. Another type of corneal staining makes use of a sterile ophthalmic solution that combines the disclosing action of fluorescein stain with the anesthetic action of proparacaine hydrochloride; one drop is applied to each eye, the excess is flushed with sterile saline solution, and the globe is illuminated. An additional type of corneal stain is rose bengal, which stains the dying corneal epithelial tissue that still adheres to the surface of the cornea. When illuminated with white light, rose bengal produces a bright pink color. The ocular diseases for which rose bengal staining may be diagnostic are feline herpesvirus infection and keratoconjunctivitis sicca.

Another important diagnostic procedure in older dogs and cats is measurement of the intraocular pressure (IOP). The normal IOP range is 15 to 30 mm Hg. There are several methods that can be used, but only two are of diagnostic quality for animals. Indentation tonometry involves use of the Schiotz tonometer and, if performed properly, can produce accurate readings. For the examiner to obtain a reading with the Schiotz tonometer, specific positioning is required that may be uncomfortable for the animal. Three readings are required to obtain an average IOP, and a species-specific conversion chart is used to determine actual IOP. The Tonopen method uses the technique of applanation tonometry and is considered the most practical and accurate method for determining IOP in animals. The examiner can place the animal's head in any position, only one reading is required, and no conversion is needed to determine the actual IOP measurement. Both the Schiotz and Tonopen tonometers must be cleaned before and after every use and should be calibrated before use.[2,3]

The examiner generally must rely on outside laboratory resources to confirm a cytologic, cultural, or histopathologic diagnosis. Most veterinary practices send out cytologic and tissue specimens for evaluation and will choose specific laboratories and pathologists based on their experience and preference. Pathologists who specialize in ocular diseases can better examine tissue for changes characteristic of disease; not all pathologists can perform this service well. Cytologic specimens can be sent to a laboratory for interpretation, bacterial and fungal culture, and sensitivity testing. Animals with chronic recurring ocular infections, corneal ulcers, keratomalacia, and refractory conjunctivitis are good candidates for cytologic evaluation. Owners should also be given the option of biopsy or fine-needle aspiration, once an ocular condition has been noticed. Biopsies should be performed for all enucleations, intraocular masses, and enlarging eyelid or scleral tumors.

OCULAR AND ORBITAL IMAGING TECHNIQUES

During the past 20 years, imaging of ocular and orbital structures has been improved by the development of ultrasonography, computed tomography (CT), and magnetic resonance imaging (MRI). Two-dimensional real-time ultrasonography of the eye and orbit is ideally suited for examination of opaque eyes and soft tissues of the retrobulbar space.[4-6] It can usually be performed in awake and unsedated animals and provides good imaging detail of soft tissues. Ultrasonograms may be acquired using an eyelid contact method, a corneal contact method, or a gel offset method. The eyelid contact and gel offset methods allow better delineation of the cornea and anterior chamber. The direct corneal method is used when posterior segment or retrobulbar disease is suspected. The ultrasonography may be performed with either sector scanners or linear array transducers, with 7.5-MHz or 10-MHz probes providing the best resolution. Imaging is useful in identifying intraocular lesions such as lens luxations, retinal detachments, hemorrhages, masses, and certain foreign bodies, especially in an eye with an opaque cornea or lens.

CT is a radiographic technique that involves serial transverse scanning of a particular organ or area of the body.[7,8] The differential imaging of tissues with CT scanning relies on x-ray attenuation or absorption characteristics of the tissues. The presence of retrobulbar fat, which absorbs x-rays to a lesser extent than water, provides excellent contrast differences between orbital soft tissues. Because of this natural contrast, the use of intravenous contrast agents is not usually required with orbital scans. CT scanning requires the animal to be anesthetized, exposes the animal to x-rays, is more complicated technologically than ultrasonography, and is expensive. It offers little advantage over ultrasonography when images of the globe and adnexa are desired but provides superior resolution of retrobulbar structures and the surrounding bony orbit. CT scanning is useful in animals for localizing intraocular and orbital foreign bodies, identifying and characterizing the invasiveness of orbital masses, and determining the presence of bony lysis or soft tissue mineralization.

MRI is based on the spinning behavior of atomic nuclei with odd numbers of protons when they are exposed to a magnetic field.[9] In MRI images, tissues with high signal intensity appear white, and tissues with low signal intensity appear black. Compared with CT scanning, MRI has the advantages of no exposure to ionizing radiation, direct multiplanar imaging, enhanced tissue characterization, and better imaging of the optic nerve, chiasm, and optic pathways. Disadvantages include the need for nonmetallic ventilation during inhalant anesthesia, long data acquisition time, increased tissue slice thickness with poorer spatial resolution, poor detection of bone, and certain image artifacts. MRI does provide precise, high-definition images of the eye, orbit, and optic pathway.[10-12] MRI images obtained in the oblique dorsal and oblique sagittal planes allow visualization of both the globe and retrobulbar structures within the same tissue slice section. MRI appears to provide precise localization and characterization of both intraocular and extraocular lesions, including retinal detachments, chorioretinal and iridal thickening, orbital cysts, orbital and optic pathway neoplasms, and extraocular muscle disorders.

Color Doppler ultrasonography and magnetic resonance angiography of the orbit have some clinical usefulness.[13,14] Color Doppler ultrasonography identifies the major vessels or vascular regions of the orbit and allows diseased orbits to be classified as hypovascularized, hypervascularized, or neovascularized. Magnetic resonance angiography circumvents intraarterial catheterization for contrast angiography by exploiting the different physical properties of moving protons versus stationary tissue.

Perhaps the most exciting development in advanced ocular imaging is that of ultrasound biomicroscopy. Ultrasound biomicroscopy uses high-frequency (60-MHz to 100-MHz) ultrasound waves to image the anterior segment of the eye. This imaging technique sacrifices penetration of the ultrasound waves in favor of extremely high resolution. Images of the cornea, anterior chamber, and iris have a high degree of resolution that mimics actual histopathologic sections.

Only those structures anterior to the lens can be imaged, however.

SENILE OCULAR CHANGES

Iris Atrophy

Iris atrophy is a common aging change in both dogs and cats and is the single most common cause of sluggish and incomplete pupillary light responses. Pupils may appear dissimilar in size and shape, with an irregular or threadlike edge to the pupillary margin. Affected areas appear as translucent patches or openings within the iris when light is reflected from the tapetal fundus. Occasionally, atrophy will cause large holes within the iris stroma, resembling multiple pupillary openings. Although iris atrophy may occur in any breed, toy and miniature poodles, miniature schnauzers, and Chihuahuas appear to have a higher incidence than other breeds. Vision is unaffected, but animals are sometimes sensitive to bright light. Sunglasses and sunglass holders (Sunpups, DogWorks, Inc., Ball Ground, Ga.) may be beneficial in the rare case of extreme photophobia.[15]

Lenticular Nuclear Sclerosis

Lenticular nuclear sclerosis generally begins in dogs and cats at 6 years of age.[15] The nucleus of the lens becomes increasingly dense as newer fibers laid down at the lens equator compress the central fibers. A concurrent decrease in soluble protein contributes to the loss of lens clarity. When the pupil is dilated, the nucleus appears homogeneously opalescent, with smooth boundaries separating it from the peripheral lens cortex (Figure 16-1). The tapetal reflection can be easily seen through the opacity, as can retinal detail. The increased translucency is more apparent when the eye is observed from the side. Nuclear sclerosis is unlikely to influence vision to a significant degree, although near and night vision may diminish slightly. If owners complain of vision loss in an animal with nuclear sclerosis in a "quiet" eye, the examiner should consider other causes of blindness, particularly retinal and optic nerve diseases.

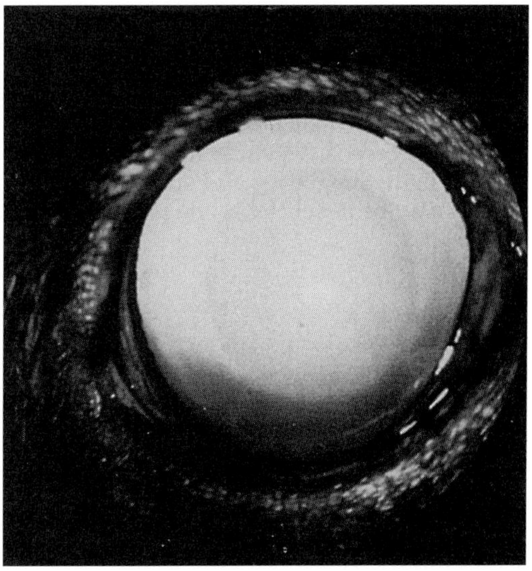

Figure 16-1. Senile nuclear sclerosis is characterized by a homogeneous grayness in the central lens. The tapetal reflection can be easily visualized, and the fundus can still be examined. Impact on vision is negligible. (From Glaze MB: Ophthalmic disease and its management, *Vet Clin North Am Small Anim Pract* 27:1505, 1997.)

Peripheral Cystoid Degeneration

Peripheral cystoid degeneration develops within the peripheral sensory retina near its junction with the posterior ciliary body.[15] The single or multiple, nonpigmented cystoid structures are most easily seen using indirect ophthalmoscopy in the maximally dilated eye. They are of no functional significance.

NEOPLASIA: EYE, ADNEXA, AND ORBIT

Orbital Neoplasia

Orbital neoplasia usually invades the orbital space by direct extension from the nasal cavities or sinuses as well as by hematogenous spread. Clinical signs of orbital neoplasia include unilateral exophthalmos, periorbital swelling or prominent third eyelid, exposure keratitis, deviated globe, dilated or eccentric pupil, chemosis, scleral injection, and possible vision loss (Figure 16-2).

Orbital neoplasias are osteosarcoma, lymphosarcoma, adenocarcinoma, and squamous cell carcinoma.[16,17] Osteosarcoma causes severe osteolytic and osteoproductive reactions in the orbit. Presenting signs of multicentric lymphosarcoma of older dogs and cats typically include exophthalmos, periorbital swelling (invasions of optic nerve and extraocular muscles), and possible globe collapse. Lymphosarcoma may cause globe indentation as a readily recognized finding in MRI studies. Squamous cell carcinomas arise from the eyelids, bulbar conjunctiva, orbit, and orbital

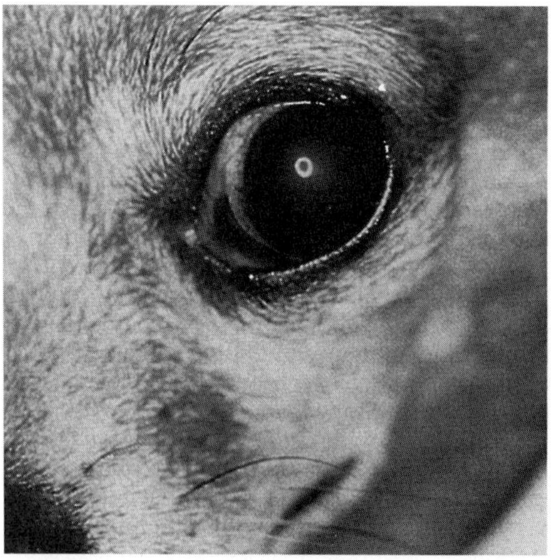

Figure 16-2. Moderate exophthalmos and lateral strabismus associated with a retrobulbar adenocarcinoma in a 14-year-old Chihuahua. (From Glaze MB: Ophthalmic disease and its management, *Vet Clin North Am Small Anim Pract* 27:1505, 1997.)

bones and are characterized by necrosis, hemorrhage, and generalized ulceration. Nests, cords, and columns of neoplastic squamous epithelial cells often invade with fingerlike projections beyond obvious tumor margins. Metastasis occurs to the regional lymph nodes, lungs, liver, and kidneys. Other orbital tumors include neurofibrosarcoma, rhabdomyosarcoma, melanoma, chondrosarcoma, chondroma rodens, reticulosis, meningioma, and hemangiosarcoma.

Surgery is the primary therapeutic option for most orbital neoplasms (Table 16-1). The invasive limit of many orbital neoplasms is poorly defined and, therefore, renders complete excision unlikely. Exenteration of the orbital contents is often the preferred treatment. Radiation and chemotherapy are additional treatment modalities to consider. Complications that commonly arise after surgery, radiation, and chemotherapy of orbital neoplasia include incomplete excision of the tumor, side effects induced by chemotherapy, and cosmetic alteration. Radiation therapy may induce a nonresponsive conjunctivitis, keratoconjunctivitis sicca, nasolacrimal duct stenosis, cataract formation, and retinal degeneration.

Eyelid Neoplasia

Eyelid neoplasia is primarily found in older dogs. [18,19] Sebaceous gland adenoma is the most common. Other epithelial or mesenchymal types of eyelid neoplasia are melanoma, papilloma, squamous cell carcinoma, basal cell tumor, trichoepithelioma, fibroma, fibrosarcoma, neurofibroma, hemangioma, hemangiosarcoma, mast cell tumor, cutaneous histiocytoma, and transmissible venereal tumor. Adenomas, adenocarcinomas, melanomas, papillomas, fibromas, and fibrosarcomas most often affect the canine eyelid. Malignant canine eyelid neoplasia is infiltrative and destructive but rarely metastasizes. Squamous cell carcinomas, papillomas, adenomas, adenocarcinomas, basal cell tumors, fibromas, fibrosarcomas, hemangiomas, hemangiosarcomas, and mast cell tumors most often affect the feline eyelid. Feline eyelid neoplasia is often locally invasive but rarely metastasizes. Several factors should be considered regarding eyelid neoplasia: most canine eyelid neoplasia is benign; most feline eyelid neoplasia is malignant; all eyelid tumors should be surgically removed and submitted for histopathologic examination; and early detection and removal bode best for complete excision and retention of eyelid function and appearance (see Table 16-1).

Although early excision of an eyelid tumor is the best means of eliminating potential irritation or enlargement, removal of small, asymptomatic or slow-growing canine eyelid masses is considered cosmetic because of the low incidence of malignancy.[15] Although many canine eyelid tumors may be conservatively observed, masses that develop near a nasolacrimal punctum, enlarge rapidly, or secondarily irritate the ocular surface should be removed. Feline eyelid masses should be completely and widely excised as soon as possible. Excised tissue should always be submitted for histopathologic examination.

For excision of a marginal eyelid neoplasm, a simple four-sided excision spares a greater proportion of the eyelid margin and provides a stable suture line when compared with the triangular wedge excision.[15] The extent of the defect should not exceed one fourth to one third the length of the eyelid, which is usually tolerated only in spaniels and hounds. A two-layer closure is recommended: simple continuous 6-0 absorbable sutures are placed in the tarsoconjunctiva, and simple interrupted 4-0 to 6-0 nonabsorbable sutures are used to reappose skin and muscle. A permanent lateral canthotomy may be used to provide relief when removal of tissue compromises the length of the palpebral fissure. More extensive tumors generally require rectangular or square "en bloc" excisions, followed by sliding skin grafts, as in the modified H-plasty. Care must be taken to ensure that the transposed tissue is lined by conjunctiva.

Ancillary treatments for eyelid neoplasms include cryotherapy, radiofrequency hyperthermia, brachytherapy, radiation therapy, and laser

TABLE 16-1. COMMON NEOPLASIA OF THE EYE, ADNEXA, AND ORBIT

HISTOPATHOLOGIC TYPE	TREATMENT	PROGNOSIS
Older Dogs		
EYELID MASS		
Meibomian gland adenoma	Surgical resection or cryosurgery	Excellent
Papilloma	Surgical resection or spontaneous remission	Excellent
Melanoma	Surgical resection	Guarded
LIMBAL MASS		
Melanoma	Monitor or surgical resection	Excellent
INTRAOCULAR MASS		
Lymphosarcoma	Chemotherapy	Guarded
Iris or ciliary body melanoma	Enucleation or exenteration	Good
Ciliary body adenoma	Enucleation or exenteration	Good
Older Cats		
EYELID MASS		
Squamous cell carcinoma	Surgical resection or cryosurgery	Good to excellent
CONJUNCTIVAL MASS		
Squamous cell carcinoma	Surgical resection or cryosurgery	Good to excellent
IRIS MASS		
Diffuse iris melanoma	Monitoring if small; enucleation if large	Guarded to good
INTRAOCULAR MASS		
Lymphosarcoma	Chemotherapy	Guarded
Iris or ciliary body melanoma	Enucleation or exenteration	Good
Sarcoma	Exenteration	Guarded to poor

resection.[15] In geriatric animals, cryotherapy may be used to manage small masses, using only local anesthesia. The eyelid site is clipped and cleansed with a topical antiseptic. Debulking prior to freezing provides adequate tissue for histopathologic examination. A chalazion clamp placed around the mass compromises blood flow and facilitates the rapid freeze and slow thaw essential for successful cryotherapy. Two freeze-thaw cycles are performed with either liquid nitrogen or nitrous oxide, targeting a minimum peripheral temperature of −25° C for most tumors and −30° C for squamous cell carcinoma. Mild discomfort occurs for approximately 12 hours following treatment. A tissue scab develops in a matter of days, then sloughs 10 to 20 days following the procedure. Secondary skin depigmentation usually resolves over a period of months, but whitening of the hair is permanent. Even in extensive lesions, cryotherapy characteristically causes minimal scarring or deformity.

Conjunctival and Third Eyelid Neoplasia

The diagnosis and treatment of conjunctival and third eyelid neoplasia—often benign in dogs and malignant in cats—are similar to those of eyelid neoplasia. Because of the close proximity to the globe, an incisional biopsy of a conjunctival or third eyelid mass may be used to diagnose and prognosticate. Complete excision may involve delicate adnexal and periocular structures with the need for adjunct therapy (see Table 16-1).

Canine Melanogenic Neoplasia

The melanoma is the most common intraocular tumor.[20] The primary melanogenic tumor in dogs is the anterior uveal melanoma. The canine melanogenic mass is usually localized in the anterior uveal tract with low metastatic potential, whereas the feline melanogenic mass is localized in the anterior uveal tract with high metastatic potential.[21] The clinical appearance of melanogenic neoplasia is heavily pigmented, tan to white, and associated with diffuse iris thickening. The melanogenic neoplasia causes an irregular pupil, blindness, and ocular pain. Glaucoma may occur secondary to the exfoliation or proliferation of cells within the uveal tract. Local infiltration and destruction occur as the neoplasm grows. Enucleation is usually required, although laser surgery may be used to selectively reduce intraocular masses. In addition, a sector iridectomy is possible for uveal mass excision (see Table 16-1).

Limbal and scleral melanocytic neoplasms (epibulbar melanoma) in dogs are usually benign. The epibulbar melanoma often arises in the superior temporal quadrant of the eye and is slower growing, less invasive, and well delineated in the sclera of older dogs. As the normal canine globe has melanocytes traversing the limbic sclera, conversion to abnormal growth occurs when the pigmented cells proliferate and invade the sclera, cornea, and conjunctiva. Surgical correction by full thickness corneal or scleral resection, laser reduction, or cryosurgery may be curative, because growth and extension of the neoplasm is slow.

Choroidal melanomas are infrequently seen in older dogs. Clinical signs include raised darkly pigmented areas of the fundus and domed thickening of the choroid with extension to the iris.

Feline Iris Melanoma

The diffuse iris melanoma is the most common intraocular tumor in cats. It begins on the anterior iris surface and progresses to diffuse darkening of the entire iris.[22,23] The cellular proliferation will eventually distort the iris and obstruct the iridocorneal angle, causing secondary glaucoma. The thickening and irregularity of the iris margin must be differentiated from normal local pigmentary changes of the feline iris. Early pigmentary changes should be monitored monthly. Early enucleation is still the safest treatment, and cats with secondary glaucoma, uveitis, and ocular pain should also have an enucleation performed. Metastatic disease to the liver and lungs is possible months to years after enucleation. The long-term prognosis for cats with intraocular malignant melanoma is guarded owing to the high metastatic rate. Adjunct chemotherapy may help to slow recurrence.

Ciliary Body Epithelial Neoplasia

Ciliary body neoplasia is identified as a visible mass in the anterior chamber.[24] Pigmentary changes are variable and depend on the cell layer involved, with possible occurrence of intraocular hemorrhage, pupillary blockade, neovascular angle closure, and secondary glaucoma. Ciliary body neoplasias, especially adenoma and adenocarcinoma, represent the second most common intraocular tumor in older dogs and cats. The origin of this neoplasm is the inner nonpigmented or outer pigmented layers of the ciliary body. Nonpigmented ciliary body tumors are more common as white-to-gray pupillary, anterior chamber or posterior chamber masses. Adenomas are usually retroiridal lesions, whereas adenocarcinomas are usually pink masses in the anterior chamber involving the iris root. Secondary uveitis, intraocular hemorrhage, glaucoma, and retinal detachment are possible. The diagnosis is confirmed by ocular ultrasonography or centesis of the mass. Although incisional or excisional biopsies are often heroic, exfoliation of neoplastic cells into the aqueous humor may offer a diagnosis by anterior chamber centesis (see Table 16-1). This occurs most commonly with medulloepithelioma and lymphosarcoma.

Feline Posttraumatic Sarcoma

Feline posttraumatic sarcoma is an aggressive intraocular tumor in cats.[25,26] The sarcomatous anaplastic spindle cells are thought to arise from disrupted lens epithelial cells and appear as a distinct mass between 1 to 10 years after the traumatic event. Affected cats seldom exhibit irritation or signs of pain. Clinical signs are nonspecific but usually involve the presence of an intraocular white-to-gray mass that may invade the anterior chamber and cause complete opacity to the cornea. The sarcoma usually invades circumferentially around the globe and involves the retina, optic nerve, and optic chiasm, and then progressive extension to the central nervous system occurs. The lens is generally destroyed. Retinal detachment and intraocular hemorrhage with secondary glaucoma may be present. Cats may be blind or have nonspecific neurologic disease. Local recurrence is common, and distant metastasis is possible. Cats can have widely disseminated disease to the spleen, liver, lung, kidney, lymph nodes, brain, heart, and adrenal glands. The preferred treatment is aggressive surgery with adjuvant radiation therapy; however, the long-term prognosis is poor.

Secondary Ocular Neoplasia

Although the eye is an unusual site for the occurrence of metastatic disease, lymphosarcoma, hemangiosarcoma, mammary gland carcinoma, and oral malignant melanoma are possibilities for metastasis with intraocular hemorrhage and glaucoma. Most metastatic lesions to the eye are lymphosarcomas, meningiomas, neurofibromas, hemangiosarcomas, rhabdomyosarcomas, or myeloproliferative disease of cats. Clinical signs associated with metastasis to the eye include anisocoria, unilateral glaucoma, scleral congestion, protruding third eyelid, corneal edema, intraocular hemorrhage, blindness, and an obvious mass.

Ocular Lymphosarcoma

Ocular lymphosarcoma warrants specific mention owing to its prominence in clinical veterinary oncology.[27] Dogs usually have bilateral involvement, whereas it is usually unilateral in cats. The neoplastic cells have most likely disseminated before ocular involvement. Clinical signs of ocular lymphosarcoma include intraocular hemorrhage, uveitis, secondary glaucoma, iritis, and corneal edema. Ocular lymphosarcoma may be diagnosed by cytologic examination of the aqueous humor, because neoplastic cells often exfoliate into the anterior chamber. Topical and systemic anti-inflammatory or glaucoma therapy is warranted during chemotherapy to control the associated uveitis and possible secondary glaucoma. Ocular lymphosarcoma is amenable to treatment with systemic chemotherapy, although relapses and incomplete control are expected. Thorough funduscopic examination of the animal with lymphosarcoma is always warranted, because the retina may exhibit pathologic changes that are consistent with systemic disease. Metastatic disease to the eye may cause severe retinal changes and includes retinal edema, retinal vessel attenuation or tortuosity, retinal hemorrhage, retinal detachment, and subretinal cellular infiltration.

KERATOCONJUNCTIVITIS SICCA

Older dogs, especially neutered females, are predisposed to keratoconjunctivitis sicca (KCS). Although senile atrophy of the lacrimal glands has been traditionally blamed for the lack of tear production in older dogs, chronic inflammation of the lacrimal glands caused by immune-mediated disease is the likely culprit.[15]

Clinical signs of KCS typically include sticky and mucopurulent discharge, conjunctival hyperemia, progressive corneal vascularization, and superficial pigmentation. Definitive diagnosis is made by the Schirmer tear test, with affected dogs measuring less than 10 mm of wetting per minute. Any breed may be affected; most commonly affected breeds include the cocker spaniel, English bulldog, schnauzer, West Highland white terrier, Yorkshire terrier, and beagle.

Topically applied cyclosporine has been shown to improve tear production and reduce corneal changes associated with the dry eye (KCS) condition.[15] This T-cell inhibitor is believed to counteract immune-mediated changes within the lacrimal gland, improving its function. Its efficacy in older dogs with KCS secondary to senile atrophy of the lacrimal glands should be minimal, but a therapeutic trial is nevertheless recommended in light of the current theory regarding pathogenesis in the geriatric dog. Twice-daily application of 0.2% cyclosporine ointment (Optimmune Ophthalmic Ointment) is recommended initially. Because response is seldom seen before 2 weeks, adjunct therapy should be considered until tear production increases. Some dogs may be maintained on a once-daily application, although indefinite therapy is indicated. Tear production can decrease precipitously if daily cyclosporine is not continued. Dogs that do not respond to cyclosporine ointment may respond to a 1% or 2% cyclosporine solution, which is available from compounding pharmacies. Of course, owners should be informed that the cyclosporine solution represents an extralabel drug application.

Conventional medical therapy may be used while one awaits initial response to cyclosporine ointment or in dogs that fail to respond to cyclosporine ointment after an adequate therapeutic trial period.[15] Medical therapy may combine acetylcysteine solution to break up the heavy mucus, an antibiotic-corticosteroid solution to control infection and inflammation, and artificial tears to supplement the tear volume. This mixture of ingredients can be formulated and refrigerated in a single solution: 10% acetylcysteine (5 ml) and triple antibiotic with 0.1% dexamethasone (10 ml) combined with as much as will suffice to make one ounce with artificial tears (Adsorbotear or Tears Naturale, Alcon Laboratories, Fort Worth, Tex.). Frequency of application is indicated by the severity of the dryness and accompanying changes. The chronic use of topical ophthalmic corticosteroid preparations can lead to iatrogenic hyperadrenocorticism; thus, intermittent application is preferred. An artificial tear ointment (Akwa Tears, Akorn, Buffalo Grove, Ill.) may be applied as needed for additional lubrication, especially at bedtime. Use of one to two drops of 2% pilocarpine twice daily in the food may also stimulate tear production. Parotid duct transposition may be considered in nonresponsive dogs.

OTHER IMMUNE-MEDIATED DISEASES

Allergic Blepharitis

Allergic blepharitis, the most common form of immune-mediated eyelid disease, occurs in association with generalized allergic dermatitis or as a localized eyelid disease.[28] The eyelids typically respond immunologically as the skin does. Causes of allergic blepharitis include vaccine reactions, insect stings, atopy, bacterial antigens, and exposure to contact allergens, including drugs. Severe acute-onset edema of the eyelids occurs when antigen-antibody complexes, toxins, or venom stimulates release of histamine and other vasoactive substances. Atopic blepharitis and conjunctivitis are mediated by IgE-mast cell interaction and are characterized by edematous, hyperemic, pruritic eyelids and conjunctiva. In chronic atopy, eyelid thickening and seborrhea may result from self-trauma secondary to marked pruritus. Skin or serologic testing to determine sensitivity to inhaled and ingested antigens may be useful in defining the allergen(s) and thereby limiting exposure. When a cause-effect sequence is apparent, the offending agent is removed and appropriate antiinflammatory therapy is initiated.

Chronic allergic blepharitis of dogs is initiated most commonly by bacterial infection. Clinically, the eyelids usually appear thickened, and the Meibomian glands are swollen and inflamed. With chronicity, nodular pyogranulomatous thickenings may be observed and are perpetuated by rupture of Meibomian gland follicles, with release of lipid secretions into periglandular connective tissues. Bilateral ulcerative blepharitis of the inferior medial canthus occurs in dogs and may be seen with chronic superficial keratitis (pannus) in German shepherds. Cytologic examination reveals lymphocytes and plasma cells, and the condition responds to topical corticosteroids.

Immune-mediated blepharitis occurs in dogs affected with lupus erythematosus and pemphigus foliaceous. Discoid lupus erythematosus commonly involves the planum nasale, but erosions, ulcers, and crusts may also affect the eyelids. Lesions of pemphigus foliaceous involve the face and head including the periocular area. Diagnosis is indicated by the presence of histopathologic changes in the deep epidermis and basement membrane.

Allergic Conjunctivitis

Allergic conjunctivitis results from localized reaction to antigen or as a manifestation of generalized hypersensitivity.[28] Allergic conjunctivitis is an immediate hypersensitivity involving binding of IgE and antigen with degranulation of mast cells and release of vasoactive amines causing vasodilation and chemosis. Spontaneous noninfectious necrotizing conjunctivitis in dogs appears to be unique to the Doberman pinscher and is presumed to be an immune-mediated disease. Systemic antiinflammatory and immunosuppressive therapies are needed to control these diseases.

Conjunctival lymphoid follicle formation is an immune response to a variety of surface antigens. These follicles are usually most noticeable on the anterior third eyelid conjunctiva. The third eyelids protrude, with diffuse fleshy thickenings on the anterior surfaces and leading edges, most notably in German shepherd dogs. Affected tissues often appear mottled and are sometimes described as "cobblestone" in appearance. Conjunctival scrapings and cytologic examination reveal plasmacytic and lymphocytic infiltrates. Topical corticosteroids afford reasonable control of this condition.

Chronic Superficial Keratitis

Chronic superficial keratitis (pannus) is a progressive corneal disease seen most frequently in the German shepherd dog.[28] Exposure to ultraviolet light appears to influence the disease progression. The disease affects both corneas usually beginning in the ventrolateral quadrant. As the disease progresses nasally the entire cornea may become involved, with increasing superficial vascularization, granulation, pigmentation, and scarring. Lesions may also be noted on the medial canthus and third eyelid. The infiltrative cell types support an immune-mediated pathogenesis and the dramatic response observed following topical corticosteroids.

Superficial Punctate Keratitis

Superficial punctate keratitis involves the corneal epithelium that results in small multifocal superficial opacities.[28] Lesions may be smooth or pitted and may or may not retain the fluorescein stain. Discomfort is associated with stain retention, indicating localized epithelial defects. Although superficial punctate keratitis may not always require treatment, topical corticosteroids will alleviate discomfort and result in healing of punctate ulcers. Because of a prompt response to topical antiinflammatory treatment, an immune-mediated cause is suspected.

Dachshund Keratitis

Multifocal corneal stromal ulcerations and chronic keratitis occur in dachshund dogs; this condition is termed *dachshund keratitis.*[28] Dachshund keratitis is an aggressive corneal disease and is not typically self-limiting; it is associated with diffuse inflammatory infiltration and marked corneal superficial vascularization. Dramatic response to topical corticosteroids suggests an immune-mediated disease. With topical treatment, multiple corneal ulcers usually epithelialize rapidly forming corneal facettes. In cases where large deep ulcers are present, conjunctival grafting may be needed. In chronic cases, progressive vascularization and pigmentation may result in severe opacities.

Feline Proliferative Keratitis

Progressive perilimbal keratitis of cats occurs as a unilateral or bilateral disease and is referred to as *feline proliferative* (or *eosinophilic) keratitis.*[28,29] Clusters of beige inflammatory cells accompany superficial corneal vascular infiltrates. Findings of eosinophils and mast cells on cytologic examination strongly suggest an immune-mediated pathogenesis. If left untreated the disease is progressive, with infiltration of the entire corneal surface resulting in reduced or lost vision. Feline proliferative keratitis can be managed effectively with oral megestrol acetate and local corticosteroid application. Following a favorable response, long-term maintenance therapy may be needed.

Scleritis and Episcleritis

Scleritis and episcleritis may occur as a nodular or diffuse inflammation of one or both eyes.[30] Scleritis involves the sclera proper, with potential for concurrent intraocular disease, whereas episcleritis affects the epibulbar connective tissues overlying the sclera. Either condition may involve adjacent cornea with stromal infiltration and edema. Although the onset of inflammation is usually insidious, the course is typically progressive. A breed predilection for the American cocker spaniel has been suggested. Diagnosis is made by signalment, appearance, elimination of other causes of "red eyes," and histopathology. The cellular response is typical of subacute nonseptic inflammation, such as numerous plasma cells and lymphocytes with occasional histiocytes.

Nodular Granulomatous Episclerokeratitis

Nodular granulomatous episclerokeratitis is a proliferative, presumably immune-related disease involving the ocular surface of dogs.[28] The disorder is also called *proliferative keratoconjunctivitis, nodular fasciitis, fibrous histiocytoma, inflammatory pseudotumor,* and *collie granuloma.* Lesions typically originate as localized proliferative vascularized growths on the scleral side of the lateral limbus. Lesions may be multifocal, involving one or both eyes. Medial limbus, third eyelid margin, and eyelids are less common sites. Large lesions may interfere with blinking, and progressive invasion of adjacent cornea may reduce vision. Lesions tend to be recurrent, even after surgical removal.

GLAUCOMA

Glaucoma is defined as an increase in IOP. The normal range of IOP is 15 to 30 mm Hg.[31] Primary glaucoma occurs when there is abnormal development of the iridocorneal angle. Secondary glaucoma occurs when a primary problem affects the drainage of aqueous humor out of the eye, such as in anterior lens luxation and uveitis. Secondary glaucoma will resolve once the source of the increased IOP is managed. Clinical signs of glaucoma include corneal edema, scleral injection, dilated pupil, blindness, and buphthalmos.

Chronic glaucoma is difficult for most owners to recognize in the older dog or cat. Animals adapt to a gradual increase in IOP and become tolerant of the ocular discomfort. This is the primary reason that IOP should be measured annually in older animals. Acute glaucoma is usually a cause for visits to the emergency clinic. Affected animals will not "act like themselves," prompting owners to find out the reason for the abnormal behavior. Glaucoma is not life threatening, but the animal is uncomfortable and in pain and, if the condition is not immediately managed, may experience visual impairment. Secondary glaucoma requires treatment or surgery to correct the underlying cause of the increase in IOP.

Medical treatment for canine glaucoma remains frustrating.[31,32] Medical treatment is not as effective in canine glaucoma because most cases of canine glaucoma involve narrow angle, closed angle, or secondary glaucoma rather than the open angle glaucoma that occurs in humans. Nevertheless, acute glaucoma should be treated medically to bring the IOP into the expected normal range in an attempt to preserve vision. Treatments with hyperosmotic agents, carbonic anhydrase inhibitors, antiinflammatory drugs, and miotics are used to decrease the rate of aqueous humor production, to increase the rate of outflow of aqueous humor, or both. Lifelong treatment is usually necessary in the medical management of canine and feline glaucoma. Animals with manageable glaucoma will also require periodic ophthalmic examination and monitoring of IOP for the remainder of their lives.

Surgery is still, unfortunately, the most effective therapy in canine glaucoma.[32] If medical management becomes less effective, or owners wish to decrease the amount and types of medication, the examiner may offer the owner surgical options, such as laser surgery, cyclocryotherapy, enucleation, globe evisceration, and chemical injection into the vitreal chamber. Chemical injection should be reserved for those animals with current medical conditions that exclude any surgical procedures and for owners who are not interested in cosmesis because phthisis bulbi and marked discoloration of the cornea will result from chemical injections.

Carbonic Anhydrase Inhibitors

Although carbonic anhydrase inhibitors have been used as systemic drugs for treatment of glaucoma for more than 40 years, a more recent shift in carbonic anhydrase inhibitor use has been from systemic to topical treatment to reduce systemic side effects.[32,33] These drugs decrease aqueous humor production by a mechanism separate from the diuretic effect on the kidneys. Use of topical or systemic carbonic anhydrase inhibitors with other antiglaucoma drugs can be more effective in the treatment of glaucoma than use of a single therapeutic agent alone. The topical commercially available drugs are dorzolamide (available as a 2% solution) and brinzolamide. These drugs have good corneal penetration and few systemic effects. Dorzolamide has been shown to decrease IOP in dogs and cats by 15% to 65%. A recent study in dogs showed that a three-times-a-day dosage decreased IOP by 24% and was more effective than a twice-a-day administration, although both lowered IOP significantly. Dorzolamide is also available as a combination drug with timolol. Systemic carbonic anhydrase inhibitors include acetazolamide, dichlorphenamide, ethoxzolamide, and methazolamide. Methazolamide is the most commonly used of these drugs at this time. It is, however, very expensive, and the cost of chronic treatment becomes a significant economic consideration for some owners. Cats are more susceptible to the side effects than are dogs.

Beta-Blockers

Although beta-blockers have been used in human medicine, their effectiveness in treatment of canine and feline glaucoma has not been established. Commercially available beta-blockers include timolol, levobunolol, metipranolol, and arteolol, and the 1-selective drug betaxolol. Timolol and metipranolol decrease IOP in normal dogs, and timolol decreases IOP in glaucomatous dogs.[32] Ocular side effects for timolol in dogs and cats include miosis and corneal epithelial toxicity. Systemic side effects include bradycardia.

Prostaglandin Analogues

One potentially useful product for glaucoma management is latanoprost 0.005% solution. The mechanism of action of this class of drugs is an increase in uveoscleral outflow of aqueous humor. Latanoprost has been shown to decrease IOP in normal dog eyes but as reported by Krohne did not decrease IOP in cats.[32] Both dogs and cats had miosis from once-a-day topical therapy. Mild conjunctival irritation was reported.

Cholinergic Drugs

The cholinergic drugs have been used for treatment of glaucoma for many years.[32] These drugs cause miosis and a decrease in IOP and are commonly used for acute and chronic glaucoma when miosis will not cause pupillary blockage. Commercially available direct-acting parasympathomimetic drugs used to treat acute glaucoma include pilocarpine solution (used four times a day) and gel (used once daily). The decrease in IOP, however, may decrease over time with pilocarpine use—that is, the eye may become refractory to the use of pilocarpine. Indirect-acting parasympathomimetic drugs are used for chronic glaucoma because they have a longer duration of action and may be administered twice daily. These include demecarium bromide and echothiophate iodide (Phospholine Iodide). Ocular side effects include topical irritation and a transient, minor breakdown in the blood-aqueous barrier. Miosis may cause pupillary blockage and, therefore, increase

IOP. Systemic side effects include salivation, lacrimation, vomiting, diarrhea, abdominal cramps, and cardiac problems. These topical agents should be avoided in animals that are being treated with flea products containing organophosphates, especially cats and small dogs.

Osmotic Diuretics

Osmotic diuretics have been used for many years to treat acute glaucoma.[32] They should not be used to treat chronic glaucoma; however, they can be administered intermittently for acute glaucoma flare-ups. Because their mechanism of action differs from that of the carbonic anhydrase inhibitors, the use of these drugs together is additive. They are effective for treating any type of glaucoma, unless the blood aqueous barrier is seriously disrupted. Commercially available and commonly used products include 20% mannitol, which is given intravenously, and 50% to 75% glycerin (glycerol), which is administered orally. Both drugs decrease IOP for approximately 8 to 10 hours. It is important to be aware that glycerin is metabolized to glucose and so should not be given to animals with diabetes mellitus.

CATARACTS

Senile cataracts are lens opacities that begin to develop in dogs and cats older than 6 years.[15] Their cause is generally unknown, although changes in composition and metabolism of the aging lens may contribute to cataract development or render the lens more susceptible to cataractogenic changes. Recurrent uveitis, chronic glaucoma, trauma, degenerative retinal disease, or diabetes mellitus may also produce cataracts in older animals. If cataracts are seen in the geriatric dog, they are no doubt of chronic duration. The most common cause of cataracts in the older cat is chronic uveitis. In either species, cataracts should be differentiated from senile nuclear sclerosis, a normal aging change produced by compression of central lens fibers.

Surgery has proved to be the only successful means of restoring sight.[15] Owing to the expense and potential risks of surgery as well as the ability of most visually impaired animals to adjust to their home environment, cataract extraction should be considered only for selected candidates. The preferred surgical candidates are those in good general health as determined by a comprehensive physical examination, including complete blood cell count, serum chemistry profile, and urinalysis. The eye should have no other abnormalities such as uveitis, keratoconjunctivitis sicca, or glaucoma. These stipulations often exclude most cats from consideration as preferred surgical candidates. Retinal function should be normal, as determined by electroretinography and ocular ultrasonography. The temperament of the dog or cat should also be considered, as well as the likelihood of owner compliance with postoperative management.

The preferred surgical procedure for cataract extraction is phacoemulsification, which fragments the lens nucleus by ultrasonic vibration and aspirates the particles through a small corneal incision.[15] Residual cortical material is also aspirated to minimize postoperative immunologic reaction to retained lens protein. Reported success rates are as high as 95% at 1 month following surgery, 86% at 2 years, and 71% at 4 years.[34] Intraocular lens implants have been designed for use in the dog and cat, but controversy still exists regarding their benefits to the animal. An animal without an implant usually functions well in its environment, despite its significant postoperative hyperopia. Although a successful intraocular lens implant provides the animal with more normal postoperative vision, intraocular lens implants have been associated with chronic, low-grade uveitis that may compromise ocular clarity and vision.

LENS-INDUCED UVEITIS

Geriatric dogs with long-standing cataracts may develop lens-induced uveitis, an inflammatory response of the uvea to lens protein. The most commonly affected breeds are the toy and miniature poodle and cocker spaniel. The interval between recognition of the cataract and diagnosis of the uveitis is typically 1 to 2 years.[35] Dogs with lens-induced uveitis usually show mature cataract, scleral injection, aqueous flare, decreased IOP, and poor response to topical mydriatic agents. Advanced chronic uveitis results in synechiae, keratic precipitates, hypopyon, and iris hyperpigmentation (Figure 16-3). Secondary glaucoma or phthisis bulbi may develop in the most severely or chronically inflamed eyes. Treatment is directed at control of inflammation through administration of topical 1% prednisolone acetate four to six times daily and 1% atropine sulfate ophthalmic solution until effective. Systemic prednisone may be needed in some dogs. Maintenance therapy may be necessary indefinitely to prevent recurrence. Cataract surgery following

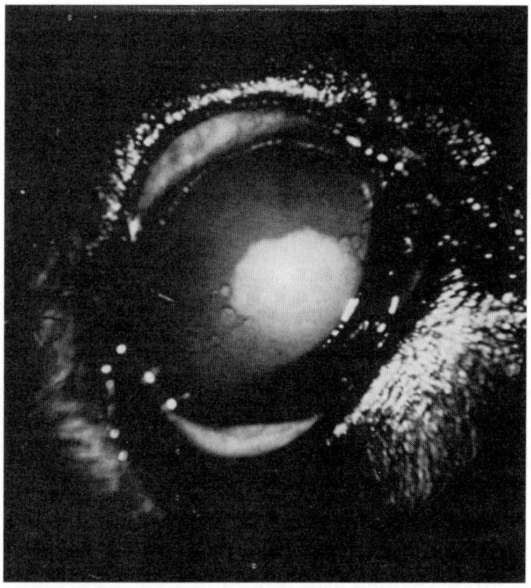

Figure 16-3. Chronic lens-induced uveitis accompanies a mature cataract in a 12-year-old mixed-breed dog. Uveal reaction to lens protein leads to corneal opacity, aqueous turbidity, keratic precipitates, posterior synechiae, and the threat of secondary glaucoma or phthisis bulbi. (From Glaze MB: Ophthalmic disease and its management, *Vet Clin North Am Small Anim Pract* 27:1505, 1997.)

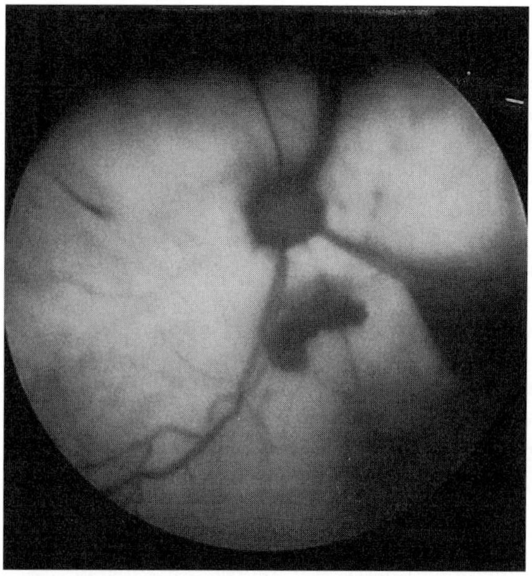

Figure 16-4. An 11-year-old domestic shorthair cat demonstrates the classical signs of acute hypertensive retinopathy, with retinal detachment and hemorrhage. (From Glaze MB: Ophthalmic disease and its management, *Vet Clin North Am Small Anim Pract* 27:1505, 1997.)

control of lens-induced uveitis is less successful than that in dogs without lens-induced uveitis.[35]

LENS LUXATION

Lens luxation may occur in older dogs and cats secondary to zonular weakness or rupture related to chronic lens-induced uveitis or capsular contracture of a mature cataract. Loss of lens support may also accompany age-related vitreous degeneration. Lens luxation occurs most often in miniature poodles older than 11 years of age.[36] The position of the lens and vitreous humor determines the accompanying clinical signs. Subluxated lenses may be relatively asymptomatic or may contribute to wide fluctuations in IOP, culminating in lesions typical of chronic glaucoma. Rarely will IOP increase beyond the 30- to 45-mm Hg range unless complete anterior luxation has occurred. In asymptomatic eyes, periodic evaluation of IOP is recommended. Medical therapy to reduce IOP is palliative but fails to correct the underlying cause. For that reason, intracapsular lens extraction and vitrectomy are recommended in eyes that have vision. Unfortunately, retinal detachment occurs in approximately 15% of animals postoperatively. Medical therapy is not generally recommended in blind eyes because of the unpredictability of the lens position, the expense of long-term therapy and repeated reevaluations, and the potential adverse side effects of systemic antiglaucoma agents. Preferable surgical options are removal of the intraocular contents followed by implantation of an intrascleral silicone prosthesis or enucleation.

RETINAL DISORDERS AND BLINDNESS

Acute-onset hypertension can result in unilateral or bilateral bullous retinal detachment (Figure 16-4). If the retinal detachment is bilateral, the cat or dog is often presented with an acute onset of blindness. Blood pressure elevation of a more chronic nature may result in retinal hemorrhages alone. In general, antihypertensive therapy is recommended if the indirect systolic pressure is greater than 170 mm Hg.[37] The return of vision is best if blood pressure control is reestablished within 2 to 3 days of the onset of blindness. Unfortunately, retinal reattachment in some cats does not always result in restoration of vision.

Geriatric miniature poodles appear predisposed to spontaneous bilateral retinal detachments resulting in irreversible blindness. The retina usually tears completely from its peripheral attachments and appears as a gray veil of tissue resting on the floor of the vitreous cavity. The tapetal region appears hyperreflective and avascular because the retina no longer overlies that portion of the fundus. It is unclear whether both eyes are affected simultaneously or whether the animal is presented only after the second eye is affected. The cause of the detachments is unknown. Surgical repair of giant retinal tears is possible, but experienced surgeons are few, and the likelihood for return to vision is guarded.[38]

Progressive retinal atrophy usually appears in young to middle-aged dogs, but owners may sometimes fail to recognize the slowly progressive loss of vision until the animal has reached the later stages of the disease.[15] Poodles and Labrador retrievers are most commonly presented with this history. Signs include progressive vision loss, first occurring in dim light and ultimately resulting in total blindness. Because of the late clinical presentation, owners may also complain of "green" or "yellow" eyes—caused by the reflection of the tapetum through the persistently dilated pupils. Other signs include retinal vessel attenuation and tapetal hyperreflectivity from the retinal thinning. Secondary cataract formation is common and may be incorrectly blamed for the vision loss. No treatment is available.

Sudden acquired retinal degeneration occurs most commonly in dogs 6 to 11 years of age.[39] Seventy percent are females, with the miniature schnauzer and the dachshund having breed predispositions. Affected dogs often present with a history of rapid vision loss occurring over 24 hours to 1 month. Polyuria or polydipsia, polyphagia, and hepatomegaly are often noted. Pupillary light responses are usually absent, but initial retinal appearance may be normal. The serum chemistry profiles show an increased alkaline phosphatase and alanine aminotransferase activities. Urine specific gravity is often below 1.025. Definitive diagnosis of sudden acquired retinal degeneration and differentiation from optic neuropathy is based on electroretinography. The affected dog will have an extinguished electroretinogram. The cause is unknown, and the blindness is irreversible.

BLINDNESS

Vision involves reception of an image on retinal sensors. In the retina, the image initiates a chemical reaction that converts the image into a neural impulse. That image travels via the second cranial nerve to the optic chiasm, optic tract, optic radiations, and finally to the visual cortex where it is processed. Damage to any portion of the visual pathway has the capacity to produce altered or impaired vision.[40] The examiner's ability to detect the visual deficits depends on the astuteness of the owner's observations of the animal, the ability to perform a thorough visual evaluation, and the mental status of the animal.

Localizing the site of the damage along the visual pathways is critical to making a tentative diagnosis, as many causes of visual impairment are relatively specific to certain locations. Additionally, diagnostic testing that is appropriate for visual loss from cerebral damage will not provide meaningful information in an animal with retinal damage. The keys to localizing visual damage are to determine whether the damage is unilateral or bilateral, whether the pupillary light reflexes are affected, and whether other parts of the neuraxis are also affected. It also important to remember that not all acute blindness is actually acute blindness. Owners may interpret vision loss as being acute in onset when the animal has adapted to its familiar environment; however, when the animal is placed in unfamiliar surroundings, such as when the owners move the furniture or take the animal on vacation with them, then the signs of blindness are apparent.

The following information is helpful in evaluating animals with presenting signs of blindness[40]

Asymmetric Visual Loss

- Determine if the visual loss is in a visual field or in one eye. Blindfolding one eye and then testing the visual field in the opposite eye may do this. If the visual loss is confined to one eye, it suggests that the lesion is cranial to the optic chiasm (toward the eye). If the visual loss involves both eyes, it suggests that the lesion is caudal to the optic chiasm (toward the brain).
- Determine if the pupils are normally responsive to light. If the visual loss is the result of damage to retinal function or the optic nerve, the pupillary light reflex (PLR) will be abnormal. In these animals, when the affected (abnormal) eye is illuminated, there will be a diminished or absent PLR in both the illuminated eye (direct PLR) and the opposite eye (consensual PLR). When the light illuminates the visual eye, there will be a normal PLR in both eyes. There may be no other signs of neurologic disease. The pupils may be symmetric, or the pupil in the blind eye may be minimally larger than the pupil in

the sighted eye (especially true in cats). In animals with glaucoma or certain other ophthalmic disorders, the PLR may be abnormal in the affected eye regardless of which eye is being illuminated. If the damage has occurred in the optic tracts, optic radiations, or cerebral cortex, there is usually a normal PLR. The visual loss is on the side opposite (contralateral) to the disease. The pupils are equal in size.

Bilateral Visual Loss

- If the damage is in the retina, optic nerve, or optic tract, there is complete blindness with pupils that are maximally dilated and do not respond to light. If the damage is confined to these locations, there are no other signs of neurologic disease. If the damage is systemic or diffuse, there may be other clinical signs seen. If the damage is in both optic radiations or the visual cortex, there is bilateral absence of vision; however, the pupils remain normal in size and still respond normally to light stimulation. The reason for this is that the visual and light reflex pathways separate at the lateral geniculate nucleus. Damage cranial to this causes both abnormal vision and an abnormal PLR. Focal damage caudal to this causes only a visual deficit or light reflex changes.

Acute blindness may occur with or without other systemic signs of illness (Figures 16-5 and 16-6). The cause may be primary damage to the ocular visual apparatus or the visual pathways in the central nervous system.[40] Generally, if the damage is to the ocular visual apparatus, the animal may accommodate to the visual loss. As long as the animal is in a familiar environment, it will show few signs of blindness. In animals with central blindness, especially if the damage is in the association areas of the cerebrum, the animal may be unaware of its blindness. Accommodation does not occur, because the animal is not aware of the visual loss. Such animals will continue to show signs of blindness, including behaviors that may possibly be injurious to themselves, because they have not developed the protective cautions of a blind animal. In some animals, depending on the location of damage and the cause, the blindness may be reversible if the disease process is treated promptly. In most animals the blindness will be permanent, even if the disease process is halted, because of irreversible damage to the visual system.

Most animals that have blindness of cerebral origin have damage to their cerebrum or diencephalon.[40] Most of these animals have other neurologic signs in addition to the blindness. The signs may include seizures, personality changes, abnormal mentation, circling, proprioceptive loss, sensory deficits, and deficiency of other cranial nerve functions. These signs may occur in any combination, and not all of these signs must be present in all cases of cerebral disease. The potential causes of cerebral diseases may include the following.[40]

Cerebral Diseases of Extracranial Origin

Cerebral diseases of extracranial origin (includes the metabolic and toxic encephalopathies) result from systemic metabolic and toxic processes that cause secondary cerebral signs. The predominant signs are personality changes, waxing and waning dementia, and seizures. The physical examination, not including the neurologic examination, is usually abnormal in these animals. The neurologic examination is frequently normal. The disease process is diagnosed on the basis of laboratory results of blood, urine, or body tissue testing, as well as by diagnostic imaging procedures. Examples include hepatoencephalopathy, lead poisoning, hypoglycemia, uremic encephalopathy, and hypothyroidism.

Cerebral Diseases of Intracranial Origin

Cerebral diseases of intracranial origin are neurologic disorders that result from central nervous system dysfunction. The predominant signs include seizures, visual loss, circling, weakness, personality changes, and other neural deficits. The physical examination in these animals is usually normal. The neurologic examination usually reveals abnormalities, even between seizures. The diagnosis in these cases requires specific neurologic testing, such as cerebrospinal fluid analysis, skull radiography, CT or MRI, and indirect blood pressure measurements. Examples include neoplasia, granulomatous meningoencephalitis, meningitis, lysosomal storage disorders, vascular disorders (systemic hypertension with retinal detachment or subretinal hemorrhage, severe anemia, thrombocytopenia, and hyperviscosity

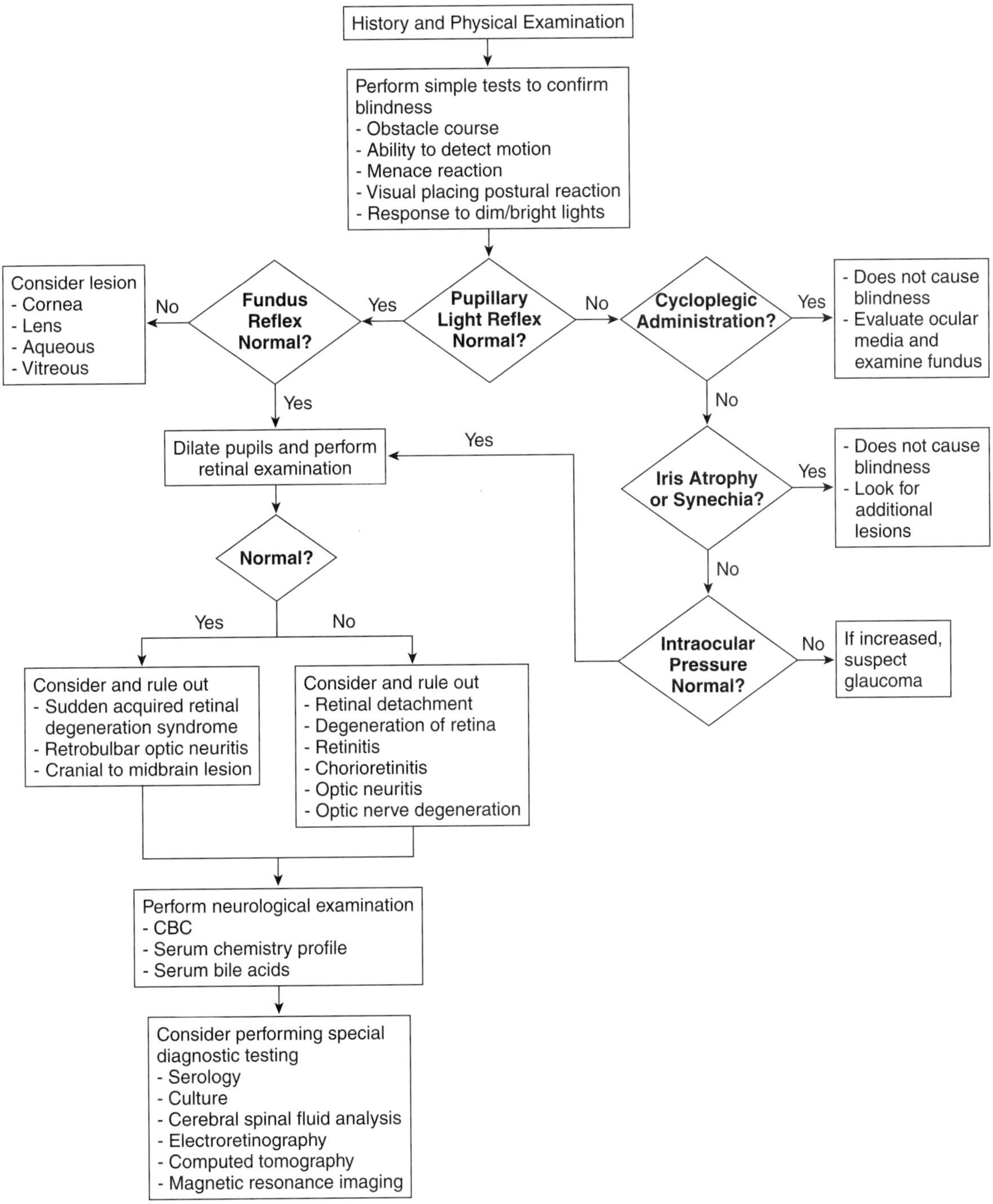

Figure 16-5. Decision tree for acute blindness.

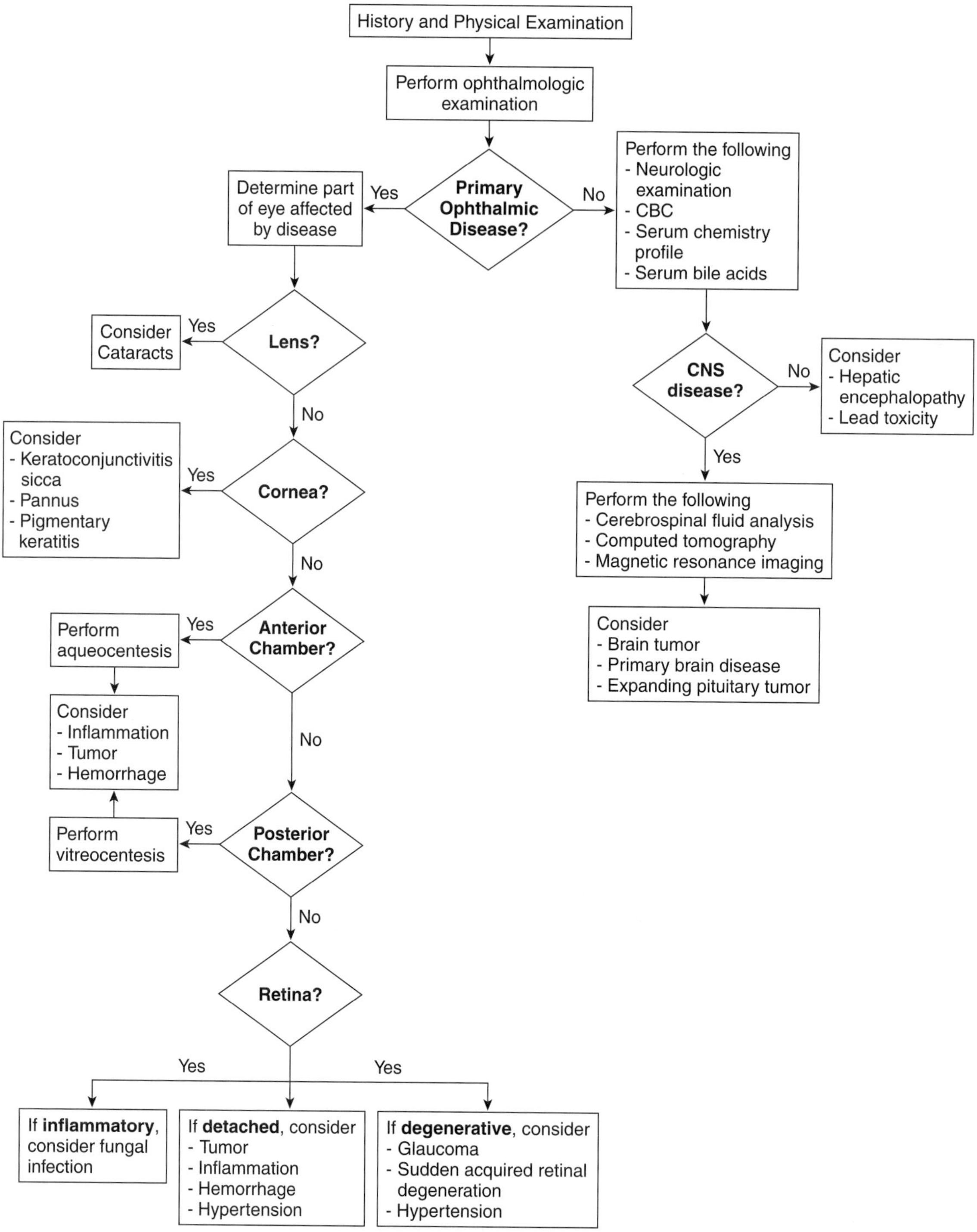

Figure 16-6. Decision tree for determining the cause of blindness.

syndromes), and trauma. In idiopathic epilepsy, seizures are the only clinical abnormality. Except during the seizure and the postictal period, the animal is normal. All laboratory test results are normal. Idiopathic epilepsy is a diagnosis of exclusion of other disease processes.

References

1. Hamor RE, Roberts SM, Severin GA et al: Schirmer tear test as a diagnostic tool for keratoconjunctivitis, *Am J Vet Res* 61:1422, 2000.
2. Peiffer RL: Glaucoma. In Morgan RV, ed: *Handbook of small animal practice,* ed 3, Philadelphia, 1997, WB Saunders.
3. Peiffer RL, Gelatt KN, Jessen CR et al: Calibration of the Schiotz tonometer for the canine eye, *Am J Vet Res* 38:1881, 1977.
4. Morgan RV: Ultrasonography of retrobulbar diseases of the dog and cat, *J Am Anim Hosp Assoc* 25:393, 1989.
5. Dziezyc J, Hager DA, Millichamp NJ: Two-dimensional real-time ocular ultrasonography in the diagnosis of ocular lesions in dogs, *J Am Anim Hosp Assoc* 23:501, 1987.
6. Hager DA, Dziezyc J, Millichamp NJ: Two-dimensional real-time ocular ultrasonography in the dog, *Vet Radiol* 28:60, 1987.
7. Calla CM, Kirschner SE, Baer KE et al: The use of computed tomography scan for the evaluation of orbital disease in cats and dogs, *Vet Comp Ophthalmol* 4:24, 1994.
8. LeCouteur RA, Fike JR, Scagliotti RH et al: Computed tomography of orbital tumors in the dog, *J Am Vet Med Assoc* 180:910, 1982.
9. Thomson CE, Kornegay JN, Burn RA et al: Magnetic resonance imaging—a general overview of principles and examples in veterinary neurodiagnosis, *Vet Radiol Ultrasound* 34:2, 1993.
10. Grahn BH, Stewart WA, Towner RA et al: Magnetic resonance imaging of the canine and feline eye, orbit, and optic nerves and its clinical application, *Can Vet J* 34:418, 1993.
11. Morgan RV, Daniel GB, Donnell RL: Magnetic resonance imaging of the normal eye and orbit of the dog and cat, *Vet Radiol Ultrasound* 35:102, 1994.
12. Morgan RV, Ring RD, Ward DA et al: Magnetic resonance imaging of ocular and orbital disease in 5 dogs and a cat, *Vet Radiol Ultrasound* 37:185, 1996.
13. Schmid Y: Color doppler investigation of the orbita in dogs, *Vet Radiol Ultrasound* 35:245, 1994.
14. Hamed LF, Silbiger J, Silbiger M et al: Magnetic resonance angiography of vascular lesions causing neuro-ophthalmic deficits, *Surv Ophthalmol* 37:425, 1993.
15. Glaze MB: Ophthalmic disease and its management, *Vet Clin North Am Small Anim Pract* 27:1505, 1997.
16. Gilger BC, McLaughlin SA, Whitley RD et al: Orbital neoplasms in cats: 21 cases (1974-1990), *J Am Vet Med Assoc* 201:1083, 1992.
17. Kern TJ: Orbital neoplasia in 23 dogs, *J Am Vet Med Assoc* 186:489, 1985.
18. Nasisse MP: Feline ophthalmology. In Gelatt KN, ed: *Veterinary ophthalmology,* ed 2, Philadelphia, 1991, Lea & Febiger.
19. Roberts SM, Severin GA, Lavach JD: Prevalence and treatment of palpebral neoplasms in the dog: 200 cases (1975-1983), *J Am Vet Med Assoc* 189:1355, 1986.
20. Wilcock BP, Peiffer RL: Morphology and behavior of primary ocular melanomas in 91 dogs, *Vet Pathol* 23:418, 1986.
21. Duncan DE, Peiffer RL: Morphology and prognostic indicators of anterior uveal melanoma in cats, *Prog Vet Comp Ophthalmol* 1:23, 1991.
22. Acland GM, McLean IW, Aguirre GD et al: Diffuse iris melanoma in cats, *J Am Vet Med Assoc* 176:52, 1980.
23. Dubielzig RR, Lindley DM: The transition from iris freckle to diffuse iris melanoma of cats: a histopathologic study, *Proc Am Coll Vet Ophthalmol* 24:56, 1993.
24. Peiffer RL: Ciliary body epithelial tumors in the dog and cat: a report of 13 cases, *J Small Anim Pract* 24:374, 1983.
25. Dubielzig RR, Everitt J, Shadduck JA et al: Clinical and morphologic features of post-traumatic ocular sarcomas in cats, *Vet Pathol* 27:62, 1990.
26. Barrett PM, Merideth RE, Alarcon FL: Central amaurosis induced by an intraocular, posttraumatic fibrosarcoma in a cat, *J Am Anim Hosp Assoc* 31:242, 1995.
27. Krohne SDG, Henderson NM, Richardson RC et al: Prevalence of ocular involvement in dogs with lymphosarcoma: prospective evaluation of 94 cases, *Vet Comp Ophthalmol* 4:127, 1994.
28. Moore CP: Immune-mediated ocular surface disease, *Proc Am Coll Vet Intern Med* 14:6, 1996.
29. Morgan RV, Abrams KL, Kern TJ: Feline eosinophilic keratitis: a retrospective study of 54 cases (1989-1994), *Vet Comp Ophthalmol* 6:131, 1996.
30. Murphy CJ: Disorders of the cornea and sclera. In Kirk RW, ed: *Current veterinary therapy XI,* Philadelphia, 1992, WB Saunders.
31. Miller PE: Glaucoma. In Bonagura JD, ed: *Kirk's current veterinary therapy XII,* Philadelphia, 1995, WB Saunders.
32. Krohne S: Antiglaucoma drugs, *Proc Am Coll Vet Intern Med* 18:29, 2000.
33. Brechue WF, Maren TH: A comparison between the effects of topical and systemic carbonic anhydrase inhibitors on aqueous humor secretion, *Exp Eye Res* 57:67, 1993.
34. Miller TR, Whitley RD, Meek LA et al: Phacofragmentation and aspiration for cataract extraction in dogs: 56 cases (1980-1984), *J Am Vet Med Assoc* 190:1577, 1987.
35. van der Woerdt A, Nasisse MP, Davidson MG: Lens-induced uveitis in dogs: 151 cases (1985-1990), *J Am Vet Med Assoc* 201:921, 1992.
36. Fischer CA: Geriatric ophthalmology, *Vet Clin North Am Small Anim Pract* 19:109, 1989.
37. Henik RA: Diagnosis and treatment of feline systemic hypertension, *Compend Contin Educ Pract Vet* 19:163, 1997.
38. Vainisi SJ, Packo KH: Management of giant retinal tears in dogs, *J Am Vet Med Assoc* 206:491, 1995.
39. van der Woerdt A, Nasisse MP, Davidson MG: Sudden acquired retinal degeneration in the dog: clinical and laboratory findings in 36 cases, *Prog Vet Comp Ophthalmol* 1:11, 1991.
40. Fenner WR: Mind blind: neurologic evaluation of the blind patient, *Proc Am Coll Vet Intern Med* 14:4, 1996.

Supplemental Reading

Regnier A: Antimicrobials, anti-inflammatory agents, and antiglaucoma drugs. In Gelatt KN, ed: *Veterinary ophthalmology,* Philadelphia, 2000, Lea & Febiger.

CHAPTER 17

The Endocrine and Metabolic Systems

CLAUD B. CHASTAIN

Endocrine and metabolic diseases in older dogs and cats are more commonly being recognized and treated. Old age has been defined as more than 12 years in cats, 11 years in small-sized dogs, 9-10 years in medium-sized dogs, and 7 years in giant breed dogs. The most common endocrine and metabolic diseases in dogs of these age groups are diabetes mellitus (especially hyperosmolar nonketotic), hyperadrenocorticism, insulinoma, and hyperlipidemia. In older cats, hyperthyroidism, diabetes mellitus, and hyperkalemia are the most common endocrine and metabolic diseases.

Aging, without concurrent disease, is associated with only a slight gradual decline in the functional reserve of endocrine organs. Because the functional reserve for endocrine organs is manyfold more than the resting level, no clinical change is generally evident except under severe stress.

Other important endocrine and metabolic diseases, for example, primary hypothyroidism, hypoparathyroidism, primary hypoadrenocorticism, hyperkalemia, hypocalcemia, hypolipidemia, and inborn errors of metabolism, have an average peak incidence during youth or middle age. These disorders are not discussed in this chapter.

PHYSICAL EXAMINATION

The presenting signs of geriatric endocrine and metabolic diseases are presented in Box 17-1. There are some physical findings of particular importance in the older dog or cat relating to possible endocrine or metabolic disease. For example, an older dog with sudden onset cataracts, polyuria-polydipsia, or weight loss without anorexia should be evaluated for diabetes mellitus. An older cat with weight loss and without anorexia should be evaluated for diabetes mellitus and hyperthyroidism, including palpation of the ventral neck for a thyroid nodule. The finding of calcinosis cutis in a dog is highly suggestive of hyperadrenocorticism. Superficial necrolytic dermatitis in dogs is usually associated with glucagonomas or severe liver disease.

DISORDERS OF DOGS

Endocrine Disorders

Primary Hyperparathyroidism

Cause. Primary hyperparathyroidism is generally caused by neoplasia of the parathyroid glands, which secrete excessive amounts of parathyroid hormone (PTH) and are unresponsive to the suppressive effects of hypercalcemia. Rarely, hyperplasia may cause primary hyperparathyroidism.[1] Affected parathyroid tissue may be found near or in the thyroid gland, the neck, the pericardial sac, or the cranial mediastinum.

Incidence. Affected dogs are usually older than 8 years. The incidence of primary hyperparathyroidism in dogs is rare, but undiagnosed cases may be common. One reason for the seemingly rare occurrence of the disorder is that clinical signs are slow developing and nonspecific. Most cases are recognized only after considerable alterations in the bones or after urinary calculi have occurred. Except for the rare carcinomas, parathyroid tumors are not palpable. There is no sex predisposition. However, Keeshonden dogs may be predisposed.

BOX 17-1 Presenting Signs of Geriatric-Onset Endocrine and Metabolic Diseases

Weight Loss and Weakness
Diabetes mellitus
Hyperthyroidism
Pheochromocytoma
Hypercalcemia of malignancy

Anorexia
Ketoacidotic diabetes mellitus
Primary hyperparathyroidism
Gastrinoma
Hypercalcemia of malignancy

Increased Appetite
Diabetes mellitus
Hyperthyroidism
Insulinoma

Obesity
Hyperadrenocorticism
Insulinoma

Mental Disturbances
Hyperthyroidism
Hypothalamic or pituitary tumors
Hyperadrenocorticism
Primary hyperparathyroidism

Pathologic Fractures
Primary hyperparathyroidism

Polyuria and Polydipsia
Diabetes insipidus
Diabetes mellitus
Primary hyperparathyroidism
Hyperadrenocorticism
Hyperthyroidism
Hypercalcemia of malignancy

Tetany, Muscle Spasms, and Muscle Cramps
Hyperadrenocorticism
Postsurgical hypoparathyroidism

Alopecia
Hyperadrenocorticism

Clinical Features. The clinical signs of primary hyperparathyroidism are produced by hypercalcemia, bone resorption, and calcium nephropathy resulting from the excessive secretion of PTH. The early signs are subtle and cause little concern with owners until anorexia or signs of renal failure are manifested. Effects and clinical signs resulting from hypercalcemia, excess PTH, and the uremic syndrome resulting from calcium nephropathy are listed in Box 17-2. Parathyroid gland adenomas or hyperplasia are rarely palpable. Calcium phosphate or oxalate uroliths may occur in affected dogs. Bony facial swelling (hyperostosis), loose teeth, and pliability of the mandible ("rubber jaw") are thought to result from demineralization, multiple infractions, hemorrhage, and replacement of bone by fibrous connective tissue and osteoid.

Laboratory Findings and Diagnosis. Persistent hypercalcemia is the best single diagnostic determinant of hyperparathyroidism. Rarely, serum calcium levels may be normal or intermittently elevated. Possible causes for hypercalcemia are listed in Box 17-3. The primary causes for serum calcium levels that exceed 15 mg/dl are malignancies, primary hyperparathyroidism, and hypervitaminosis D.

BOX 17-2 Clinical Signs of Primary Hyperparathyroidism and Their Causes

Excessive Parathyroid Hormone
Pathologic fractures
Facial hyperostosis
Loosening and loss of teeth
Painful mastication and malodorous breath
Bone pain, lameness, or neck pain

Hypercalcemia
Anorexia and vomiting
Constipation
Muscle weakness
Bradycardia and arrhythmias
Depression, coma, or seizures
Polyuria and polydipsia
Gastric ulcers

Uremic Syndrome
Depression and vomiting
Diarrhea
Oral ulcerations
Anemia
Dyspnea (compensation for metabolic acidosis)
Polyuria and polydipsia
Bleeding tendency (thrombocytopathy)
Immunosuppression

BOX 17-3 Differential Causes for Hypercalcemia

Primary hyperparathyroidism
Increased release of calcium from bone
- Nonparathyroid malignancies
- Acute immobilization
- Hyperthyroidism
- Septic osteomyelitis
- Hypervitaminosis A

Increased renal tubular reabsorption of calcium
- Thiazide diuretics
- Severe hypoadrenocorticism

Spurious laboratory results (hyperlipidemia)
Congenital renal diseases (decreased glomerular clearance and increased circulating complexed calcium)
Hypervitaminosis D
- Owner error in diet
- Calcitriol rodenticides
- Granulomatous disease (blastomycosis, schistosomiasis)

Repeated measurements (at least three) of serum calcium levels are recommended in dogs with clinical signs and history suggestive of primary hyperparathyroidism. Although compensatory changes in calcium regulation, calcitonin secretion, or concurrent diseases that cause hypoalbuminemia can cause normocalcemia in cases of primary hyperparathyroidism, these instances are rare. Early in the development of primary hyperparathyroidism, hypercalcemia often is accompanied by serum phosphorus levels below normal or in the low end of the normal range and by decreased plasma bicarbonate levels. As renal failure ensues, serum phosphorus concentrations become higher.

A radioimmunoassay for PTH and a determination of concurrent serum ionized calcium level may be considered. A two-site immunoradiometric assay for intact human PTH has been validated for the dog. A mid-molecule PTH assay is also validated for the dog. Normal ranges for PTH should be age adjusted; plasma PTH concentrations increase significantly with age in healthy dogs.[2] Plasma samples for PTH assay should be shipped overnight packed in ice.

Excessive calcium in the filtrate leads to impaired tubular reabsorption caused in part by decreased sodium reabsorption and decreased medullary tonicity. In addition, tubular calcification, tubular degeneration, and tubular necrosis can occur, especially if serum calcium levels exceed 15 mg/dl. Mineralization first becomes evident at the corticomedullary junction. The polyuria that results is not responsive to water deprivation or administration of antidiuretic hormone. All dogs with calcium phosphate or oxalate nephroliths or uroliths should be suspected of having primary hyperparathyroidism. Fractional clearance of calcium is variable and phosphorus is high (>12%), despite hypophosphatemia in the early stages.

Radiographic and Ultrasound Findings. Skeletal demineralization—osteopenia (osteomalacia)—can be seen radiographically in dogs with primary hyperparathyroidism; however, mineralization must be severely depleted before it becomes evident on routine radiographs. The earliest detectable changes usually are radiolucency of the laminae dura dentes of the teeth, the vertebral bodies, and the dorsal processes of the vertebrae. Eventually there is a general loss of bone density, but the overall site of the bones may increase with fibrous connective tissue and osteoid. Subperiosteal cortical resorption and bone cysts may be visualized radiographically in long bones. Multiple pathologic fractures are rare but may occur in advanced cases. Neurologic impairment may occur if a fracture compresses or severs the spinal cord. Subclinical demineralization may be made evident by a technetium pyrophosphate bone scan. Demineralization of the skeleton can be reduced or delayed if dietary intake of calcium is high.

In primary hyperparathyroidism, the incidence of soft-tissue metastatic mineralization outside the kidney is uncommon compared with secondary hyperparathyroidism or vitamin D intoxication. The risk of soft-tissue mineralization is decreased by hypophosphatemia and hyperchloremic metabolic acidosis in animals with early primary hyperparathyroidism.

When present, nephroliths and uroliths are seen easily in radiographs, because they are composed of calcium phosphate or oxalate. Renal calculi can also be detected by abdominal ultrasonography. Nephrocalcinosis is less distinct in radiographs, but it may appear as diffuse mild radiopacity of the kidneys. Chondrocalcinosis and periarticular calcification may be noted.

Nodules of the parathyroid glands that are 4 or more millimeters in diameter on high-resolution sonograms are parathyroid neoplasia.[3-5] Parathyroid gland scintigraphy with technetium 99m sestamibi has poor sensitivity and specificity in the dog.[6]

Management. Emergency treatment is necessary for severe hypercalcemia. Isotonic saline solution should be administered intravenously to rehydrate, dilute serum calcium, and cause diuresis. If hypercalcemia persists, furosemide should also be used.

Surgical removal of the parathyroid neoplasm is recommended for treatment of primary hyperparathyroidism. Ethanol injection and ultrasonographically guided radiofrequency heat ablation of parathyroid adenomas have been reported.[7,8] However, for most practice situations these techniques are more hazardous than parathyroidectomy.

Before surgery, the dog should be evaluated for the extent of functional renal impairment. Thoracic radiographs are also indicated to search for metastasis of parathyroid carcinomas or for cranial mediastinal ectopic parathyroid neoplasms. Exploratory surgery of the parathyroids should not be performed until all noninvasive diagnostic tests have been considered.

During surgery the parathyroid glands should be examined and their sizes compared. Enlarged glands should be removed, with the exception that if all are enlarged, then three glands should be removed and one cranial parathyroid gland should be left.

Transient but serious hypocalcemia may develop 12 to 96 hours after the operation because the source of excess PTH has been removed with uncompensated parathyroid tissue remaining and because of rapid calcium uptake by mineral-starved bone. Possible signs and effects of acute hypocalcemia are muscle fasciculations and tremors, nervousness and restlessness, tetanic convulsions, and death from laryngeal spasm. The risk of postparathyroidectomy hypocalcemia increases with the degree of presurgical hypercalcemia.

Because of the risk of postsurgical hypocalcemia, prophylactic postsurgical dihydrotachysterol (DHT) has been recommended. The recommended dosage is 0.02 mg/kg body weight per day for 3 days, then 0.01 mg/kg body weight per day for 1 week; the dosage is then reduced 25% to 50% per week, and the drug is discontinued in 2 months. By adjusting oral doses of calcium gluconate and vitamin D to maintain serum calcium levels between 7.5 and 9 mg/dl, the production of PTH from the remaining parathyroid tissue will normalize without the risk of acute hypocalcemia. If postoperative serum calcium levels are lower than 7.5 mg/dl, and no hypocalcemic signs are noted, oral calcium gluconate should be given in divided doses of 50 to 75 mg/kg of body weight per day.

Postoperative hypocalcemia with tetany or seizures is an emergency situation. An intravenous (IV) solution of 10% calcium gluconate should be slowly administered in a dose of 1 ml/kg body weight, up to a total of 10 ml. The heart rate and electrocardiogram (ECG) should be monitored for bradycardias and dysrhythmias. Prolonged administration as a slow drip with 5% dextrose may be continued. Hypomagnesemia (magnesium levels <0.41 mmol/L or 1 mEq/L) and hyperkalemia (potassium levels >5.5 mmol/L or mEq/L) potentiate the effects of hypocalcemia. Postoperative hyperkalemia is uncommon. When it occurs, hyperkalemia responds adequately to correction of hypocalcemia.

Serum magnesium levels should be monitored with serum calcium levels after parathyroid surgery. Hypomagnesemia may require correction by administration of 0.8 to 1 mmol/kg body weight of magnesium sulfate given intravenously over a 4-hour period.

The production of PTH by the remaining parathyroid tissue should normalize in 1 to 3 weeks. Dihydrotachysterol and oral calcium, in that order, can usually be tapered to discontinuation. Skeletal recovery after successful surgery should be nearly complete in 2 months. If serum calcium remains elevated after surgery, additional ectopic tissue in the neck or cranial mediastinum should be sought, or the diagnosis of primary hyperparathyroidism reevaluated.

Diabetes Mellitus

Cause. Diabetes mellitus results from an absolute or relative deficiency of insulin. Carbohydrate intolerance resulting from an insufficiency or deficiency of insulin is the hallmark of diabetes mellitus.

The most common cause in dogs is not known. Possible causes are genetic, pancreatic injury, beta-cell exhaustion from insulin antagonism, target tissue insensitivity, and insulin dyshormonogenesis. The most common known cause is pancreatitis. Approximately one third of diabetic dogs have acute or chronic pancreatitis lesions, and nearly half of those examined have active mononuclear islet infiltration.

There are three types of diabetes mellitus: insulin-dependent diabetes, non–insulin-dependent diabetes, and diabetes that is secondary to other conditions such as estrus, hyperadrenocorticism, acromegaly, and glucagonomas, or drugs such as progestogens and glucocorticoids. Non–insulin-dependent diabetes mellitus is rare in dogs.

Incidence. Diabetes mellitus most frequently occurs in small breeds, especially the dachshund (standard, miniature, longhaired, and wirehaired) and poodle (toy, miniature, and standard), but all breeds are affected. A familial tendency for insulin-dependent diabetes mellitus has been reported in the Samoyed.[9] German shepherd dogs, cocker spaniels, collies, and boxers are at significantly decreased risk. The age of onset is usually 8 to 9 years. Affected intact and neutered female dogs outnumber affected male dogs by twofold to fourfold. The onset of diabetes may be more common in dogs during winter months.

Clinical Features. The clinical signs of diabetes mellitus depend on the type of insulin insufficiency, the degree of insulin insufficiency, and the conditions preceding the onset of insulin insufficiency. Clinical forms of diabetes are categorized as nonketotic, ketoacidotic, and nonketotic hyperosmolar.

Approximately 25% to 50% of dogs with diabetes are seen for examination in a nonketotic state. Dogs with uncomplicated diabetes mellitus are usually afebrile and are mentally alert. They also have nocturia, polyuria, and polydipsia with mild dehydration and are losing weight although the appetite is excessive. Clinical signs have a known duration of about 1 week to 1 month before presentation.

Polyuria, nocturia, and compensatory polydipsia with mild dehydration are the most frequent presenting signs. Most dogs are obese but have recently been losing weight because of the uninhibited gluconeogenesis. Hepatomegaly may be palpable in 10% to 20%. Diabetic dogs are at higher risk than normal for systemic hypertension.[10] Bacterial and yeast dermatitis and otitis are also more common in diabetic dogs.[11]

Diabetic dogs are uniquely susceptible to cataracts (Figure 17-1).[12] Increased aldose reductase in the lens reduces excessive glucose to sorbitol and fructose. Increased intralenticular sorbitol and fructose cause the lens to draw in water, causing cataracts in the anterior and especially the posterior cortex. Cataracts are found at presentation in about half of all dogs with canine diabetes. In many cases, stellate cataracts are the major presenting complaint. The development typically occurs over a period of a few days to 2 weeks. If diabetes has been present for several years, there can be microaneurysms, exudates, and small hemorrhages in the retina.

Ketoacidosis is present in most dogs that initially are presented with diabetes mellitus. It represents the uncompensated stage of the body's attempts to buffer the ketoacids formed as an alternate energy source during severe or prolonged insulin deficiency (Figure 17-2). Dogs with ketoacidosis have a greater deficiency of endogenous insulin production.[13] All the clinical signs of ketoacidotic diabetes mellitus may be

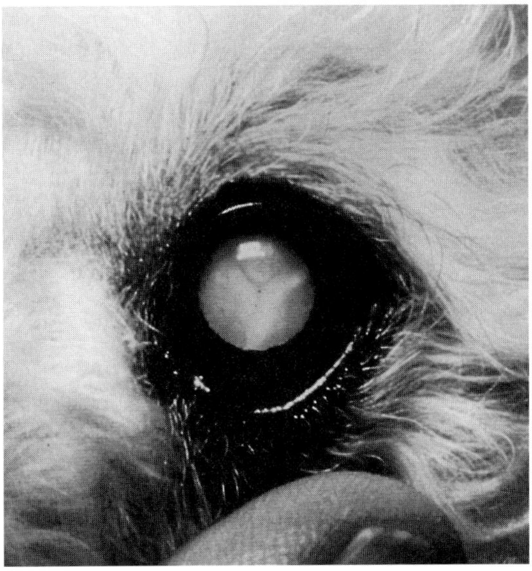

Figure 17-1. Diabetic cataract in a poodle. (From Chastain CB, Ganjam VK: *Clinical endocrinology of companion animals*, Philadelphia, 1986, Lea & Febiger.)

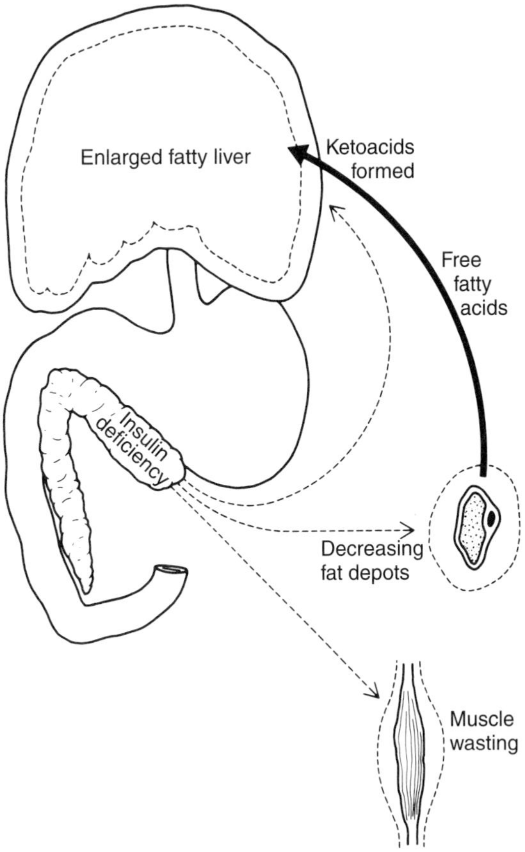

Figure 17-2. The general effects of diabetes mellitus. (From Chastain CB, Ganjam VK: *Clinical endocrinology of companion animals*, Philadelphia, 1986, Lea & Febiger.)

explained by the greater insulin deficiency, longer duration of deficiency, metabolic derangements caused by the acidosis, and serum hyperosmolarity resulting from hyperglycemia. Common initiating factors that cause diabetic dogs to produce more ketones than they can buffer and excrete include infections, acute pancreatitis, administration of diabetogenic drugs, spontaneous hyperadrenocorticism, dehydration, and anorexia.

Compensatory respiratory efforts occur in the form of labored expirations—Kussmaul's breathing—to expire carbon dioxide and correct the metabolic acidosis. In addition to a history consistent with having had previous uncomplicated diabetes mellitus, affected dogs may be febrile, have moderate to severe dehydration, be anorectic and mentally depressed, be vomiting or have diarrhea, and have oliguria or anuria.

Nonketotic hyperosmolar syndrome is a diabetic condition most common in older dogs. Cardiac or renal disease impairs the body's ability to retain water and excrete sodium, which leads to nonketotic hyperosmolar coma in affected animals with diabetes. Renal excretion should prevent blood glucose from exceeding 500 mg/dl if the glomerular filtration rate is normal. The blood glucose level exceeds 600 mg/dl, serum sodium is often more than 145 mmol/L (mg/dl), and the plasma osmolality exceeds 340 mOsm. Each time blood glucose level increases by 100 mg/dl, the plasma osmolality increases 5.6 mOsm/kg. Ketonemia is not present.

In dogs with nonketotic hyperosmolar diabetic coma, stupor or coma is caused by the plasma's hyperosmolality. Central nervous system dysfunction is not likely to occur until the serum osmolality exceeds 340 mOsm/L. This is when blood glucose levels approach 800 mg/dl.

Laboratory Findings and Diagnosis. Overt diabetes mellitus may be diagnosed if repeated fasting blood glucose values exceed 140 mg/dl or if fasting or postprandial blood glucose values exceed 200 mg/dl. Occasionally, fasting blood glucose values may only periodically or transiently be in excess of 140 mg/dl, which may be caused by a mild to moderate impairment in dogs that have glucose tolerance or a stress-related hyperglycemia.

Common abnormal laboratory findings in dogs with nonketotic diabetes mellitus, ketoacidotic diabetes mellitus, and nonketotic hyperosmolar syndrome vary. In general, the only laboratory abnormalities in uncomplicated diabetes mellitus are hyperglycemia and glucosuria. In ketoacidosis, a low blood pH, ketonemia, hypokalemia, hypophosphatemia, and hyperosmolality in addition to hyperglycemia and glucosuria are common. Ketonemia is the result of free fatty acid mobilization. Nonketotic hyperosmolar diabetes is characterized by extreme hyperglycemia (>500 mg/dl), hyperosmolality, azotemia, and no ketonemia or ketonuria.

Mobilization of peripheral fat and the development of hepatic lipidosis are at least partially responsible for a tendency for elevated serum enzymes (alanine transaminase and alkaline phosphatase) from the liver. Uninhibited hormone sensitive lipase is also responsible for serum elevations of cholesterol and triglyceride. Diabetic dogs are predisposed to hepatic abscess, which could contribute to increased hepatic enzyme activities.[14]

Some serum electrolyte concentrations tend to decrease with increasing blood glucose levels. Serum sodium and potassium levels are lowered by the osmotic diuretic action of glucosuria and ketonuria when organic anions cannot be adequately provided by hydrogen or ammonium ions. The production of metabolic acidosis by ketoacids and by lactic acid depresses serum pH and bicarbonate. Approximately one-fourth to one-half of female canine diabetics have bacterial cystitis at initial presentation, but there is a low incidence of expected clinical signs. All diabetic dogs, with or without clinical signs of lower urinary infection, should have urine cultures performed.[15] Rarely, proliferation of gas-forming bacteria (*Escherichia coli, Aerobacter aerogenes,* or *Clostridium* species) or yeast may cause emphysematous cystitis or cholecystitis.

Management. The initial goals of therapy are to normalize the hyperglycemia, fluid balance, electrolyte balance, and plasma osmolality as carefully as possible.

After the diagnosis of diabetes mellitus is established, dogs should be characterized in stages as having uncomplicated, ketoacidotic, or nonketotic hyperosmolar syndrome. Dogs that are alert, with little or no dehydration and little or no ketonuria, and that are also willing and able to eat without vomiting, can be treated as having uncomplicated diabetes.

Treatment of uncomplicated diabetes mellitus with insulin may begin with the subcutaneous (SC) administration of an intermediate-acting insulin, NPH or insulin zinc suspension (Humulin L and Humulin N), at 0.5 U/kg of body weight 30 minutes before a morning meal and before an evening meal. Although diabetes in some dogs may be controlled by once-daily injections, the majority of dogs require twice-daily injections for effectiveness and reduction of the risk of insulin shock (iatrogenic hypoglycemia).[16] Currently avail-

BOX 17-4 Types of Insulin

Short-Acting (up to 8 hours)
Insulin injection USP (Humulin R)

Intermediate-Acting (up to 24 hours)
Isophane insulin suspension USP (NPH; Humulin N)
Insulin zinc suspension USP (Humulin L)

Long-Acting (possibly more than 24 hours)
Extended insulin zinc insulin suspension USP (Humulin U)
Protamine zinc insulin USP (PZI VET)

able insulins are listed in Box 17-4. Recombinant human insulin is the most commercially available.

The response to intermediate-acting insulin should be evaluated 8 to 12 hours after the injection, and the insulin dose should be appropriately modified in 1- to 2-U increments to attain a blood glucose value between 100 and 150 mg/dl in the morning and evening. If the insulin dose is 10 U or less, a dilution of 9:1 diluent/insulin should be used to facilitate accurate dosing and SC absorption. Normal saline may be used as a diluent if used within 24 hours. Otherwise, an insulin diluent formulated for the proper pH and buffer should be used if storage for more than 24 hours is desired.

Urinary glucose concentrations should not be used to monitor response to treatment. The concentration of urinary glucose does not correlate well with concentrations of plasma glucose. The concentration of urinary glucose varies with differences in the individual dog's urinary glucose thresholds, volume output, and renal concentrating ability.

Exercise and caloric intake should remain as static as possible. It is best to determine caloric requirements based on ideal body weight rather than on the present body weight. Reduction in excess body fat is beneficial because obesity reduces insulin receptors and receptor binding of insulin and causes a defect in post–insulin receptor events. Most 10- to 15-kg house dogs are estimated to require 40 to 60 kcal/kg of body weight per day. Canned dog food can be estimated to contain approximately 500 to 600 kcal/lb. The total daily diet should be evenly divided into morning and evening meals when twice-per-day insulin injections are required. Dietary chromium is needed for normal insulin action.[17] However, supplements of chromium to typical commercial balanced dog diets are probably of no benefit.[18]

Increasing the fiber in diets to more than 15% of dry matter and increasing the complexed carbohydrates in the diet are possibly beneficial for the control of diabetes mellitus. Serum fructosamine concentrations (indicator of mean blood glucose concentrations for a couple of weeks) are lower in dogs on high-fiber diets than those on low-fiber diets.[19] Glycemic control and quality of life has been reported to improve if additional fiber is added to a standard diet.[20] However, others have not found improved glucose tolerance with added dietary fiber, but fat absorption can be reduced, leading to adverse effect on the skin and haircoat.[21]

Soluble fiber reduces the postprandial rise in blood glucose and may improve glycemic control in diabetic dogs. Soluble fiber absorbs water, slows gastric emptying time, and reduces the rate of intestinal absorption of glucose. Soluble fiber may be poorly tolerated, causing difficulty in swallowing, poor haircoat, and soft feces. Insoluble fiber may also be beneficial and be better tolerated, although it can cause constipation. Some commercial high-fiber diets are Prescription Diets (Hills Pet Products) Canine r/d, w/d, and g/d; Science Diet Canine Maintenance Light (Hills Pet Products); and Purina Fit & Trim. Added fiber must be mixed into the food and not given separately to be of value. High-fiber diets should not be given to cachectic diabetic dogs.

The most frequent causes of death during treatment for diabetic ketoacidosis are cerebral edema caused by a rapid decline in blood glucose concentration or by the injudicious use of hypotonic fluids; hypokalemia caused by the administration of insulin and bicarbonate plus fluid dilution and fluid-induced diuresis; and iatrogenic hypoglycemia or insulin shock.

Successful treatment of diabetic ketoacidosis depends on an accurate assessment of the dog's initial status, frequent reassessment of the dog's change in status during treatment, and appropriate therapeutic modifications during treatment. An active, mentally alert dog that will eat and does not vomit does not have ketoacidosis to a degree sufficient to require intensive care.

Frequent monitoring of the initial response to insulin is essential for the successful management of diabetic ketoacidosis. The blood glucose level is generally determined each hour until it is less than 250 mg/dl. This can be done in a little over 1 minute with a few drops of whole blood using glucose oxidase–impregnated strips and a reflectance colorimeter such as Accu-Chek Test Strips

(Roche Diagnostics, Basel, Switzerland) and Accu-Chek II meters (Roche Diagnostics).

Assessment of serum osmolality also should be included in the initial evaluation of depressed diabetic dogs. The serum of diabetic dogs can become severely hyperosmolar with or without ketoacidosis. If the dog is clinically ill, as shown by such signs as depression, anorexia, weakness, and vomiting, serum hyperosmolality is possible. Tonicity or "effective osmolality" can be calculated in diabetics by the following formula:

$$\text{mOsm/L} = 2\,(\text{Na}) + \frac{\text{Glucose}}{20}$$

Normal plasma effective osmolality in the dog is about 280 to 310 mOsm/L. Serum osmolality above 340 mOsm/L can be dangerous.

Indwelling urethral catheterization is inadvisable unless the dog is comatose, markedly azotemic, or apparently oliguric or anuric because of the risk of bacteremia and ascending urinary infections. Nonspecific host-defense mechanisms are impaired in diabetics. Even using a closed system with urinary catheterization for a few days will result in the development of urinary infections in half or more of diabetic dogs. Prophylactic antibiotics used while the catheter is in place does not reduce the risk of infection, but does increase the risk of antibiotic resistance with the infections.

Hypotension is particularly likely if hyperosmolality is present, because the resulting cellular dehydration of the myocardium weakens myocardial strength of contraction. Proper administration of fluids should improve cardiac output, decrease serum osmolality, reduce hyperglycemia, reduce ketonemia, buffer ketoacids, maintain urinary excretion, and correct electrolyte imbalances.

The IV route of administration should be used in all cases of clinically significant ketoacidosis. In most cases, a rate of IV administration of 20 to 40 ml/kg of body weight per hour is adequate until rehydration is complete, and then a slower rate is used to maintain urinary output. The rate of the IV administration of fluids should not exceed 90 ml/kg of body weight per hour. Slower rates are especially advisable if insufficiencies of cardiac or renal function are present.

The selection of fluids is based on the dog's serum osmolality and blood pH. Lactated Ringer's solution, half-strength normal saline solution (0.45% NaCl), and 5% dextrose solution are the most useful fluids in the treatment of diabetic ketoacidosis. Lactated Ringer's solution can be used whenever the blood pH and serum osmolality are near normal. At half-strength, saline solution reduces serum hyperosmolality caused by profound hyperglycemia and dilutes the hyperosmolality of administered bicarbonate. Dextrose (5%) solution is reserved for whenever the administration of fluid and insulin lowers plasma glucose concentrations to less than 250 mg/dl. Normal saline may aggravate acidosis and should be avoided.

The need for fluid additives, such as potassium phosphate and sodium bicarbonate, is determined by the blood pH and serum potassium concentration. Bicarbonate should be administered when serum bicarbonate (or total CO_2) levels are less than 50% of normal (<12 mEq/L) or when the blood pH is <7.1. Total bicarbonate deficit is calculated as follows: bicarbonate deficit × kg body weight × 0.4. One half the calculated deficit should be given over 4 to 6 hours, then the blood gases should be reevaluated.

Insulin facilitates the intracellular entry of phosphate as well as potassium. Resulting hypophosphatemia (<1 mg/dl) decreases the transfer of oxygen from hemoglobin to the tissues. Phosphate is also required for the cellular energy source, adenosine triphosphate. Phosphate is the major intracellular anion. Severe hypophosphatemia can cause hemolytic anemia, seizures, an altered mental state, cardiomyopathy, and skeletal muscle weakness. Hypophosphatemia in diabetics is associated with hypokalemia and ketonemia. Most have acute pancreatitis and have been given SC insulin.

Total body potassium is always decreased in untreated diabetics. In severe cases, serum potassium is less than normal. Normal concentrations of serum potassium are about 3.5 to 5.5 mmol/L. The initial replacement dose is 0.01 to 0.03 mmol/kg of body weight per hour. A combination of 2 parts potassium chloride and 2 parts potassium phosphate should be administered if serum phosphorus is low. Twenty mmol/L of potassium is placed in 5% dextrose or sterile saline solution. The administration of potassium should never exceed 0.5 mmol/kg of body weight per hour. Urine potassium levels, as well as serum potassium levels, can be monitored to verify adequate supplementation.

IV low-dose administration of short-acting insulin (Humulin R) is the preferred insulin treatment if the dog is severely hypotensive or hypothermic and if adequate supervision is available to prevent malpositioning of catheters and to assure a regular rate of administration.[22] Recommended IV low-dose therapy is 0.1 U/kg of body weight, followed by a dose of 0.1 U/kg of body weight per hour of short-acting insulin diluted in replacement fluids, such as lactated Ringer's solution, and administered by slow drip.

Low-dose, intramuscular administration of short-acting insulin permits more accurate measurement of administered insulin and requires a minimum of equipment and supervision compared with IV administration. If the dog is adequately hydrated and has normal cardiovascular function, intramuscular crystalline insulin is effective in 30 minutes and lasts 81% longer than intravenously administered insulin.

The initial intramuscular dose is 2 U of short-acting insulin, administered in the thigh muscles for small dogs weighing less than 10 kg. Very small dogs under 3 kg should be treated initially with only 1 U of short-acting insulin followed by 1 U each hour. For dogs weighing more than 10 kg, the initial dose is 0.25 U/kg of body weight. Treatment continues each hour thereafter until blood glucose levels are less than 250 mg/dl: for small dogs, 1 U is administered; for dogs weighing more than 10 kg, 0.1 U/kg of body weight is administered. Syringes measuring 1 U (Lo-Dose Insulin Syringes, Becton Dickinson, Franklin Lakes, NJ) and a fresh dilution of short-acting insulin in sterile saline solution should be used.

After the blood glucose level has been reduced to a concentration ranging between 150 and 250 mg/dl, the administration of intramuscular administered insulin is discontinued. The mean time required to reduce the blood glucose level to this range is about 4 hours. Fluids are then changed to 5% dextrose solution with potassium phosphate added to prevent dilutional hypokalemia and hypophosphatemia. If the blood glucose is less than 150 mg/dl, a solution of 5% dextrose with 20 mmol/L of potassium phosphate and potassium chloride (50:50) is administered. Insulin is not given. If the blood glucose ranges between 150 and 250 mg/dl, the IV administration of 5% dextrose with potassium phosphate and potassium chloride is given, and 0.5 U/kg of body weight of short-acting insulin is administered SC every 6 to 8 hours. Doses are then changed by 1 to 2 U to maintain blood glucose concentrations between 100 and 200 mg/dl at 4 hours after the last injection. When the dog is able to eat without vomiting, fluids and regular administration of insulin can be discontinued. Maintenance therapy with intermediate-acting insulin can then begin in a conventional manner.

Nonketotic hyperosmolar coma should also be treated with short-acting insulin. Because the coma is due to hyperosmolality, the reduction in hyperglycemia should be gradual to minimize the risk for iatrogenic cerebral edema. Low-dose insulin administration is appropriate and preferred for the treatment of nonketotic hyperosmolar coma, as well as diabetic ketoacidosis. Once diabetic dogs with ketoacidosis or nonketotic hyperosmolar coma are stabilized and willing to eat, and capable of doing so without vomiting, they can be treated as uncomplicated diabetics.

Possible responses to insulin are illustrated in Figure 17-3. Type A reactions may be caused by the Somogyi effect, an exaggerated response to insulin-induced hypoglycemia, or by a transient effect of intermediate-acting insulin. Transient effects are presumably due to excessive insulinase activity, called the *dawn phenomenon.* Transient

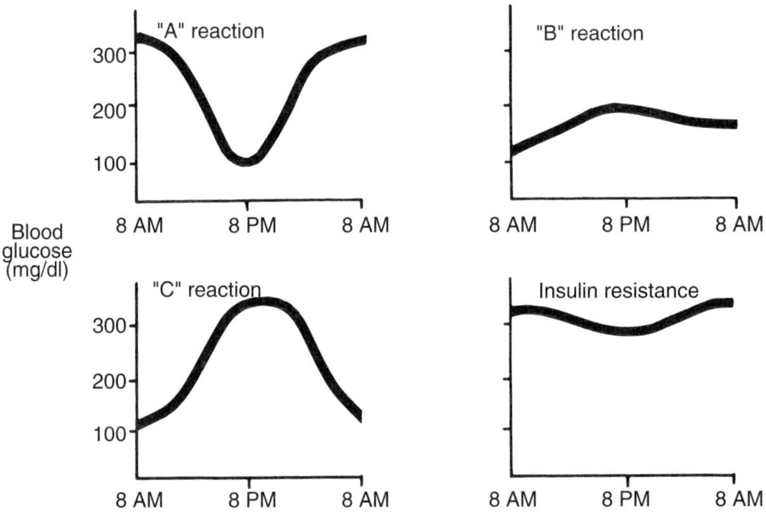

Figure 17-3. Possible responses to a single administration of intermediate- or long-acting insulin. (From Chastain CB, Ganjam VK: *Clinical endocrinology of companion animals,* Philadelphia, 1986, Lea & Febiger.)

insulin activity is more common than is the Somogyi effect. Type B reaction is the desired response.

Insulin resistance is arbitrarily defined as the failure to reduce blood glucose to normal levels with the administration of less than 2.2 U/kg of body weight per injection (not per day). Insulin resistance may be caused by decreased receptor affinity for insulin, the induction or administration of insulin-antagonistic hormones, insulin-antagonistic endocrinopathies, inactivation of insulin at the site of injection, antiinsulin antibodies, or postreceptor defects in the action of insulin.

Antibodies against administered older type insulins have been detected in dogs. However, their significance in impeding insulin action is now considered low because of the current purity of insulin preparations.

Insulin resistance may be corrected by successful management of the concurrent infectious disease, pancreatitis, obesity, pregnancy, estrus, uremia, or insulin-antagonistic endocrinopathy or by the discontinuation of the administration of insulin-antagonistic drugs. Hormones antagonistic to insulin actions are epinephrine, glucagon, growth hormone, glucocorticoids, progesterone, and thyroid hormones. Sexually intact females should be spayed.

In the case of type A reactions caused by the Somogyi effect, reducing the insulin dose will correct the hypoglycemic episodes and subsequent early morning hyperglycemia. Somogyi reactions do not seem to be common in dogs. Type A reactions resulting from the transient effect of intermediate acting insulin are quite common in diabetic dogs. One solution to this problem may be the use of a long-acting insulin, extended insulin zinc insulin suspension Humulin U (Lilly). After a long-acting insulin injection (with the same number of units as had previously been given with the intermediate-acting insulin), measurements of blood glucose should be made every 2 to 4 hours to assess the timing and quantity of its effects.

The first recheck examination should be scheduled for 2 weeks after the initial discharge. All recommended subsequent rechecks should take place every 3 months, provided the dog is well regulated by the treatment. The owner should keep a log of the parameters (Box 17-5) to be reviewed by the veterinarian at times of apparent poor control and at routine reexaminations. Diabetic dogs should be examined by a veterinarian if abnormalities are detected during home monitoring for 2 or more days in a row or whenever ketones are detected in the urine. Review of the owner's log of observations, findings from the physical examination of the animal, and monitoring of body weight changes are sufficient to assess glycemic control.[23] However, ambitious owners may check their diabetic dog's blood glucose at home if they have been instructed in the proper use of a lancet and finger vacuum (Microlet Vaculance, Bayer Diagnostics, Tarrytown, NY) to collect blood and a portable reflectance colorimeter.[24,25]

BOX 17-5 Home Assessments of Diabetic Control

Daily
Attitude
Appetite
Physical activity
Water consumption
Urinary continence

Weekly
Body weight

As Necessary
Urine ketones and glucose

Diabetic dogs should be physically reexamined, their home-monitoring log reviewed, and blood examinations repeated every 3 months. Glycohemoglobin is the result of a slow nonenzymatic combination of glucose with certain types of hemoglobin throughout the life of a red blood cell (120 days in the dog).[26] Glycohemoglobin levels parallel the mean blood glucose level over the preceding 8 to 12 weeks. Normal blood glycohemoglobin concentration in dogs is less than 6%. It is elevated only by persistent hyperglycemia.[27] Serum fructosamine is a glycosylation product of serum proteins, particularly albumin.[28] Normal serum fructosamine concentration in dogs is less than 3.5%. Its value reflects the state of glycemic control over the preceding 2 weeks. Hypoproteinemia can lower serum fructosamine concentration without a change in mean blood glucose concentration.[29,30] Recommended components of an outpatient recheck examination are listed in Box 17-6.

Elective surgeries should be postponed until the dog is well managed for at least 1 to 2 weeks. Hypoglycemia is more likely if full maintenance doses of insulin are given on the day of surgery.[31] A safer approach is to administer twice the normal morning maintenance dose, administer 5% dextrose as a slow IV drip during induction and surgery, and monitor the blood glucose to

BOX 17-6 Routine Outpatient Assessments Of Diabetic Control

Review of owner's observations and home records
Body weight and routine physical examination
Urinalysis and urine culture (collection by cystocentesis)
Blood and serum examinations
- Hemogram
- Blood glucose
- Serum urea nitrogen
- Cholesterol
- Triglycerides
- Serum alanine aminotransaminase
- Serum alkaline phosphatase
- Glycohemoglobin or serum fructosamine

administer short-acting insulin intravenously, if necessary for marked hyperglycemia.

Beta-Cell Tumors (Insulinoma)

Cause. Most islet tumors in dog are multihormone producing. Insulin is most frequently produced in enough excess to cause a disease, hypoglycemia. Insulinomas are beta-cell tumors of the pancreatic islets that predominately produce an excess of insulin (Figure 17-4). Even though about 40% of canine insulinomas appear histologically benign, clinically malignant tumors of the islets outnumber benign tumors by more than four to one in dogs.

The incidence of insulinomas is about equal in both pancreatic limbs. Multiple pancreatic masses are present in 10% to 20% of cases, and nearly half have grossly visible metastasis at the time of surgery.

Incidence. The average age of an affected dog is 9 years (range, 3 to 12 years). Breeds larger than 25 kg in body weight have the greatest incidence. There is no predisposition for either sex. German shepherd dogs, Irish setters, golden retrievers, collies, standard poodles, boxers, and fox terriers are considered predisposed for insulinomas.

Clinical Features. The presenting signs are either those resulting from a deficient supply of glucose to the brain (neuroglucopenia) or release of catecholamines (adrenergic response). Abdominal enlargement and signs of encroachment on surrounding organs such as icterus or abdominal pain are not manifestations of insulinomas.

When the amount of glucose available to the brain is decreased, the use of oxygen by the brain is also decreased. The clinical signs of neuroglucopenia are the same as those of hypoxia.

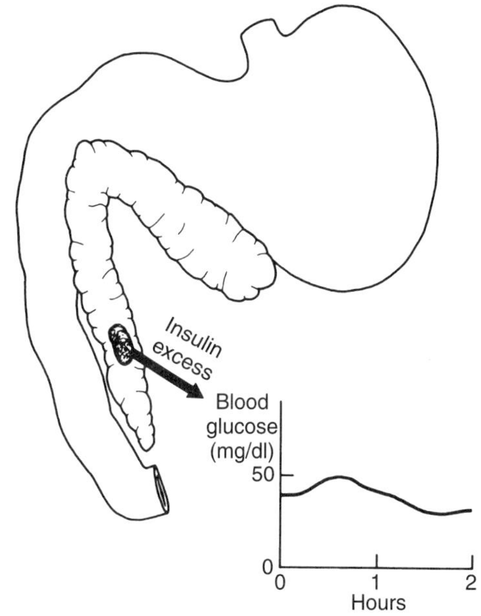

Figure 17-4. The effect of excessive insulin secretion by an insulinoma. (From Chastain CB, Ganjam VK: *Clinical endocrinology of companion animals,* Philadelphia, 1986, Lea & Febiger.)

Presenting clinical signs and owner complaints are seizures, weakness and incoordination, depression, change in behavior, polyphagia, and syncope. Half of insulinoma cases are presented with seizures. Unequivocal signs are usually not noticed until blood glucose levels are less than 40 mg/dl. Signs may develop during fasting, exercise, periods of excitement, or eating a meal. Mild weight gain may occur from hypoglycemia because of the inhibition of the hypothalamic satiety center and unchecked activity of the feeding center in the hypothalamus. Degenerative or immune-mediated peripheral polyneuropathy characterized by proprioceptive deficits and depressed reflexes may occur.[32]

The degree of hypoglycemia does not always correlate with clinical signs of the neural dysfunction. The brain is able to adapt to low glucose, particularly in periods of rest. The rate of fall of blood glucose and the degree of neural adaptation are important factors governing the clinical signs produced.

Laboratory Findings and Diagnosis. Postprandial or fasting hypoglycemia less than 50 mg/dl is the hallmark of insulinomas in older dogs with muscle weakness, personality changes, and episodic seizures. Insulinoma is the most common cause for hypoglycemia in dogs over 5 years of age, but other causes can include abdominal smooth muscle tumors.[33,34] Hypoglycemia may occur during fasting or in the postprandial period.

Abnormal routine laboratory findings other than hypoglycemia are uncommon. Mild hypokalemia occurs in about 20% of cases. Liver metastasis from insulinomas usually does not result in elevated serum liver enzyme levels. Because insulin inhibits the production of ketones, the finding of ketonemia or ketonuria with hypoglycemia eliminates the diagnosis of insulinoma.

Taking four random blood samples during a day of fasting is generally sufficient to detect a period of hypoglycemia in a dog with an insulinoma.[35] Once fasting hypoglycemia is noted, a fasting immunoreactive insulin (IRI) assay should be done. Shipments of serum to reference laboratories require packing with ice owing to degradation of insulin in unfrozen serum. The measurement of blood glucose levels should be determined with blood samples drawn at the same time as serum for IRI determination. Serum fructosamine concentrations may be below normal limits in a dog that has had frequent periods of hypoglycemia in the prior 2 weeks.[36]

Normal fasting serum IRI levels in dogs are less than 30 μU/ml. The glucose/insulin ratio is generally sufficient for a diagnosis. Ratios of <2.5 mg/μU are diagnostic. The amended insulin/glucose ratio has fewer false negative but more false positive results. The tolbutamide, glucagon, L-leucine, ethanol, and glucose tolerance tests are potentially serious, even lethal, hazards of induced hypoglycemia. Their clinical indications are restricted to cases that have equivocal insulin/glucose ratios. Even then, their diagnostic accuracy can be questionable.

Radiographic Findings. Computed tomography (CT) or selective arterial angiography has been successfully used to show pancreatic tumors larger than 2 cm. However, many tumors are smaller than 2 cm, and radiographic proof of the tumor is generally unnecessary for diagnosis or management. Less than half are large enough to be detected by ultrasonography. An insulinoma has been detected in dogs using scintigraphy with selenomethionine 75 or Indium In-111 pentetreotide.[37]

Management. Excision of insulinomas should be attempted whenever possible. Insulinomas are nearly always grossly evident at surgery.

Insulinomas in dogs are slow-growing malignant tumors with few exceptions. Two thirds appear histologically malignant. Of insulinomas, 45% have metastasis to the liver and regional lymph nodes that is evident at laparotomy. Virtually all tumors eventually recur after excision, but excision of the primary tumor can eliminate clinical signs in most cases for as long as 3 years. Mean survival after surgery is 1 year. Survival times are shorter without surgery.

Recommended presurgical, surgical, and postsurgical care is listed in Box 17-7. If the insulinoma has been sufficiently excised, the blood glucose should rise to normal levels within 2 hours. Postsurgical complications include persistent seizures from cerebral laminar necrosis, diabetes mellitus, and trauma-induced pancreatitis. Diabetes occurs in 20% to 25% of animals treated surgically. In most, the hyperglycemia is mild and transient, lasting only 3 to 5 days. Treatment for hyperglycemia is not necessary unless the fasting blood glucose level exceeds 250 mg/dl or is above 140 mg more than 1 week after surgery.

If surgical treatment is not possible or not successful, or if hypoglycemic episodes recur after surgery, medical therapy is indicated. Medical therapy alone for insulinomas is less desirable than surgical excision. Medical management should not be recommended to owners as an alternative to surgery, only as a supplement.

Initial medical management for hypoglycemia from insulinomas should include giving small, frequent (three or more) meals high in protein, complex carbohydrates, and fat, plus prednisolone in a dose of 0.5 mg/kg of body weight per day in divided doses. Should dietary management and prednisolone be inadequate, diazoxide (Proglycem), 10 mg/kg of body weight per day in divided doses, may be tried. It is an effective adjunctive treatment in about 70% of cases.

BOX 17-7 Recommended Surgical Care for Islet Cell Tumors

Before Surgery

Feed several small, high-protein meals per day.
Give no food by mouth for 8 hours before surgery.
Give 5% to 10% dextrose IV at a slow constant rate for several hours before surgery.
Monitor serum potassium and blood glucose every 8 hours until time of surgery.

During Surgery

Infuse 10% dextrose IV.
Monitor blood glucose levels every 30 minutes.

After Surgery

Measure blood glucose every 8 hours.
Administer 5% to 10% dextrose IV as necessary for hypoglycemia.
Give no food or water by mouth for 3 days.
Monitor serum potassium, urea nitrogen, lipase, and amylase at least once a day for 3 days.
After 3 days, begin feeding small frequent meals.

Diazoxide is a benzothiadiazide derivative that has hyperglycemic effects. It inhibits insulin secretion and promotes gluconeogenesis and glycogenolysis. The dosage may be increased to 40 mg/kg/day in divided doses, if necessary. Its hyperglycemic actions include the inhibition of insulin secretion, enhancement of epinephrine-induced glycolysis, decreased peripheral use of glucose, and increased mobilization of glycerol and free fatty acids. Common adverse effects are vomiting and anorexia. Chlorothiazide, given in twice-daily doses of 20 to 40 mg/kg of body weight, should be used with diazoxide to reduce sodium retention and potentiate the hyperglycemic effects.

Hyperadrenocorticism

Cause. Spontaneous hyperadrenocorticism may have its origin in the pituitary gland or the adrenal cortex. Pituitary-dependent causes represent about 80% of the total spontaneous causes in dogs. Reports on the incidence of pituitary neoplasms associated with pituitary-dependent hyperadrenocorticism (PDH) in dogs vary widely (from 15% to 85%). Adrenocorticotropic hormone (ACTH)–producing pituitary tumors may or may not compress the remaining adenohypophysis and the area dorsal to the hypophysis, the hypothalamus. In dogs, two thirds of these tumors are situated in the pars distalis; the remaining tumors are found in the pars intermedia. Generally, pituitary tumor growth rate is slow. PDH in dogs is not caused by continuous hyperstimulation of pituitary corticotrophs by corticotropin-releasing hormone.

Small, 3- to 10-mm tumors constituting the presurgical undetectable group are usually referred to as *pituitary microadenomas.* When immunocytochemical stains for ACTH are used, more than 80% of dogs with PDH are proved to have pituitary adenomas. Approximately one fourth of dogs with pituitary tumors causing PDH have macrotumors; about half of these have neurologic signs.

The remaining 10% to 20% of spontaneous cases of hyperadrenocorticism in dogs are caused by unilateral or bilateral adrenocortical neoplasms. Adrenocortical adenomas are well-circumscribed tumors that do not metastasize and are not locally invasive. Adrenocortical carcinomas by the time of diagnosis are large, hemorrhagic, and necrotic. Carcinomas, especially of the right adrenal, frequently invade the caudal vena cava and metastasize to the liver, lungs, kidney, or regional lymph nodes. The occurrence of adrenocortical adenomas and carcinomas in dogs is nearly equal.

Some adrenal tumors predominately or exclusively produce an excess of mineralocorticoids: aldosterone or desoxycorticosterone.[38,39] These may be referred to as *aldosteronomas.*

Incidence. Hyperadrenocorticism occurs more frequently in dogs than in any other domestic species. There is no sex predilection for PDH. There is a threefold greater incidence of adrenocortical tumors in female dogs. Boston terriers, dachshunds, boxers, miniature poodles, and toy poodles are the breeds most frequently affected by spontaneous hyperadrenocorticism. Brachycephalic breeds have a higher incidence of ACTH-producing pituitary tumors than do other breeds. A familial tendency for PDH has been reported in Dandie Dinmont terriers.[40]

Adrenocortical neoplasms most frequently occur in large-breed dogs. Adrenal tumors occur on either side with equal incidence. Ages affected range from 3 to 15 years; most dogs are 7 to 9 years old when hyperadrenocorticism occurs.

Clinical Features. Most of the clinical signs of hyperadrenocorticism in dogs are caused by excessive levels of cortisol and corticosterone, but in about 30% of the female dogs, clitoral hypertrophy is noted. This effect is caused by excessive levels of adrenocortical sex hormones.[41] Possible clinical signs, in order of their reported occurrence, are listed in Box 17-8.

Most dogs with hyperadrenocorticism develop a triad of polyuria-polydipsia, pendulous abdomen, and bilateral alopecia (Figure 17-5). Polyuria-polydipsia is defined as the intake of water in excess of 100 ml/kg/day and production of urine in excess of 50 ml/kg/day.

Alopecia most often first affects the caudal and lateral aspects of the hind legs and then the trunk.

BOX 17-8 Possible Clinical Signs of Hyperadrenocorticism in Dogs in Decreasing Order of Occurrence

Polyuria and polydipsia
Pendulous abdomen
Bilateral alopecia
Hepatomegaly
Polyphagia
Muscular weakness and atrophy
Lethargy
Persistent anestrus or atrophied testes
Hyperpigmentation of the skin
Calcinosis cutis
Heat intolerance
Hypertrophy of the clitoris
Neurologic deficits

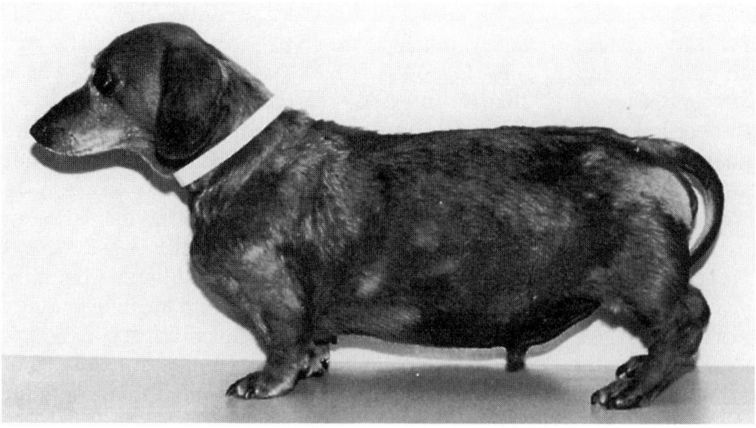

Figure 17-5. Most dogs with hyperadrenocorticism exhibit pendulous abdomen, bilateral alopecia, and polyuria and polydipsia. (From Chastain CB, Ganjam VK: *Clinical endocrinology of companion animals,* Philadelphia, 1986, Lea & Febiger.)

The head and distal extremities are little affected, if at all. Skin changes are manifested as thin, wrinkly, inelastic skin with excessive surface scaling and small papules or comedones caused by follicular hyperkeratosis. Comedones are most prominent on the ventral abdomen. Protein catabolism causing atrophic collagen also frequently leads to easy bruising, either spontaneously or after a vein is punctured for blood samples.

Calcinosis cutis is a cutaneous change that occurs in about 25% of dogs with hyperadrenocorticism. The development of calcinosis cutis is thought to result from the calcium-attracting alteration of collagen's ionic charge.

All skeletal muscles are affected by the catabolic action of excessive glucocorticoids. Besides the development of a pendulous abdomen, affected animals may assume a straight- or stiff-legged stance caused by muscular weakness. Myotonia or pseudomyotonia in dogs with hyperadrenocorticism results in extensor rigidity of the proximal appendicular muscles. Rigidity usually begins in one hind leg, then progresses to the other hind leg, and finally affects the front legs. The gait is stiff, especially after the animal has rested or has been exposed to cold.

Nearly one in three sexually intact dogs with hyperadrenocorticism has persistent anestrus or atrophied testes. Perianal adenomas in a neutered dog can indicate excessive adrenal androgens associated with hyperadrenocorticism.

Intolerance to heat is noted in some dogs with hyperadrenocorticism. Heat intolerance may lead to respiratory distress. In addition to heat intolerance, congestive heart failure and impaired diaphragmatic movements resulting from obesity and hepatomegaly are common causes of respiratory distress in cases of hyperadrenocorticism.

Sudden development of respiratory distress, right-sided heart failure, or sudden death may be the result of pulmonary thromboemboli.[42] Thrombosis risks are increased by thrombocytosis, hypertensive and catabolic endothelial vascular damage, increased production of clotting factors, recumbency, and urinary losses of antithrombin III caused by glomerulonephrosis.[43] Sudden weakness and anemia in older dogs can be caused by rupture of an adrenocortical carcinoma.[44]

Excessive levels of glucocorticoids can produce behavioral changes, psychoses, depression, and mania. Some neurologic clinical abnormalities are more likely the result of an enlarging pituitary tumor or, possibly, metastasis from an adrenocortical carcinoma. These signs include seizures, somnolence, aimless wandering, blindness, head pressing, anisocoria, and Horner's syndrome.

Hypertension and proteinuria are often manifestations of hyperadrenocorticism.[45] Intravascular volume is expanded and plasma renin substrate is elevated, which leads to higher blood pressure. Hypertension increases the risks of thrombosis, intrarenal hypertension with glomerulopathy, and left-side heart failure. Hypertension can be a prominent feature of aldosteronomas, mineralocorticoid-producing adrenal tumors. Aldosteronomas also cause hypokalemia, metabolic alkalosis, and hyporeninemia.[38,39]

Certain types of hyperadrenocorticism can be easily missed. Hyperadrenocorticism caused by adrenal carcinomas can develop rapidly, precluding development of "classic" clinical signs.

Laboratory Findings and Diagnosis. The most consistent routine hematologic and serum findings with hyperadrenocorticism are relative and absolute lymphopenia (less than $1000/mm^3$) and marked increased levels of serum alkaline phosphatase (SAP).

In addition to lymphopenia, common hematologic findings include neutrophilia, eosinopenia ($<100/mm^3$), and monocytosis. Occasionally, polycythemia, hypersegmented neutrophils, and increased platelets are seen.

Abnormalities other than increased levels of SAP found in most serum analyses include increases in alanine transaminase (ALT), cholesterol, and glucose. Serum phosphorus levels may be decreased. With the exception of SAP, the increase in serum enzymes is usually mild to moderate. The increase in SAP, which is more than four times the upper normal limit and can be greater than 3000 IU/L, generally exceeds all other abnormalities seen in the serum analyses. The origin of the increased SAP is the liver, which responds to excessive levels of glucocorticoids by inducing enzyme production from biliary epithelium. Corticosteroid-induced alkaline phosphatase levels can be determined. Corticosteroid-induced alkaline phosphatase isoenzyme in the diagnosis of canine hyperadrenocorticism has low specificity (many false positive results) but high sensitivity (95%). Elevated corticosteroid-induced alkaline phosphatase also occurs with diabetes mellitus, primary liver diseases, acute pancreatitis, chronic heart failure, and neoplasia. However, the absence of corticosteroid-induced alkaline phosphatase activity in a dog virtually rules out the presence of hyperadrenocorticism associated with hypercortisolemia.[46,47]

Serum glucose is usually in the high normal range, but the response to glucose tolerance tests is abnormal in about two thirds to three fourths of affected cases. Fasting serum insulin levels are abnormally elevated in more than three fourths of dogs with hyperadrenocorticism. Approximately 10% to 20% of dogs with hyperadrenocorticism, especially miniature poodles, develop overt diabetes mellitus caused by insulin antagonism and pancreatic islet exhaustion. A decrease in the number of insulin receptors may be a primary event to insulin resistance, or it may be a downregulation secondary to hyperinsulinemia from other causes.

Well-regulated diabetic dogs have normal plasma cortisol levels and dynamic responses to stimulation and suppression. Some unregulated diabetic dogs do not. There should be a history of hyperadrenocorticism signs before the development of diabetes mellitus. This history aids in differentiating stress-induced hypercortisolemia caused by unregulated diabetes mellitus from hyperadrenocorticism.

Serum electrolyte levels (sodium, potassium, calcium, and phosphorus) are usually normal. Hypokalemia with hyperadrenocorticism is suggestive of a mineralocorticoid-producing adrenal tumor. Arterial blood gas changes if thromboembolism occurs. The changes often include a low PO_2 (<70 mm Hg) and a low PCO_2 (<30 mm Hg).

Urinalysis often shows hyposthenuria caused by diuresis. Urine specific gravity is frequently less than 1.012 unless water is being withheld. The urine should be routinely cultured because the incidence of urinary infections is about 50% in cases of hyperadrenocorticism; pyuria is inconsistently present because of the antiinflammatory and urine-dilutional effects of excessive glucocorticoids. Proteinuria from glomerulopathy occurs in more than 60% of dogs with hyperadrenocorticism.

Baseline levels of serum thyroxine (T_4) have been reported to be secondarily decreased in approximately 70% of dogs with hyperadrenocorticism. Thyroid hormone serum levels become normal in most dogs after the hyperadrenocorticism is controlled.

The baseline plasma cortisol value is rarely, if ever, diagnostically useful by itself. Over half the dogs with hyperadrenocorticism have baseline plasma cortisol values within ranges considered normal. The ability to suppress plasma cortisol levels to a significant extent with a low dose of dexamethasone usually rules out hyperadrenocorticism. The inability to suppress the plasma cortisol with the low-dose administration of dexamethasone (0.01 mg/kg IV) may result from hyperadrenocorticism of either pituitary or adrenal origin, from some drugs, and from some nonadrenocortical illnesses. Plasma cortisol samples should be taken at baseline, then 4 and 8 hours later. Normal dogs suppress and maintain their plasma cortisol levels to <1.5 μg/dl. If the level achieved is less than 50% of the baseline at 4 hours and higher later, PDH is probable.

Exaggerated responses to the exogenous stimulation of ACTH are seen in most dogs (>80%) with bilateral adrenocortical hyperplasia, more than half of those dogs with adrenocortical neoplasms, and in some dogs with nonadrenocortical illnesses. However, it is more specific for the diagnosis of hyperadrenocorticism than the low-dose dexamethasone test.[48] Dogs with adrenocortical carcinomas have exaggerated plasma cortisol values more often and to a greater degree than dogs with adrenocortical adenomas. Dogs should be given at least 5 μg/kg of cosyntropin (Cortrosyn) IV, with samples taken at baseline and 1 hour later. Cosyntropin can be reconstituted and frozen in one-dose aliquots in plastic syringes for at least 6 months without loss of efficacy.[49]

Normal dogs elevate their plasma cortisol levels up to 20 μg/dl.

Another useful screening test is the urine corticoid/creatinine (C/Cr) ratio.[50] Of urine corticoids, 70% are free cortisol. However, other steroids may be detected. Urinary C/Cr ratio is more accurate and more sensitive than the low-dose IV dexamethasone suppression test, particularly if urine samples are collected at the dog's home to reduce the risk of stress-induced changes.[51] Normal values vary among laboratories. Two morning urine samples are preferred. If results are normal, this test rules out hyperadrenocorticism. If results are abnormally high, additional tests such as the ACTH stimulation test are needed to confirm the diagnosis and differentiate the cause.

Some cases of hyperadrenocorticism do not produce excesses of cortisol. If clinical signs are consistent with the diagnosis but plasma cortisol levels are within normal limits, 17-hydroxyprogesterone and possibly adrenal sex hormone plasma concentrations should be determined.[41,52-54]

Once the diagnosis of hyperadrenocorticism is determined, a high-dose dexamethasone suppression test (0.1 mg/kg IV) should be done to determine the cause and to facilitate rendering a prognosis. Suppression is reduction from baseline levels by 50% or more. All adrenal tumor-dependent hyperadrenocorticism (ATDH) cases do not suppress, but 10% to 30% of PDH cases also do not suppress. Those PDH cases that do not suppress are more likely to be macrotumors, >1 cm in diameter, or located in the pars intermedia.

A high-dose dexamethasone suppression test can also be done on an outpatient basis by the owner, who gives three doses of 0.1 mg of dexamethasone/kg per dose at 8-hour intervals before a urine sample is taken for C/Cr-ratio determination. In most animals with PDH the ratio is suppressed to <50% of the mean resting ratio. If the ratio is not suppressed, an endogenous ACTH test is indicated to differentiate PDH from ATDH with more certainty.

Endogenous ACTH levels fluctuate in bursts throughout the day. Random plasma ACTH samples can be very helpful in differentiating the cause of hyperadrenocorticism in selected cases that cannot be classified otherwise. Plasma ACTH collection and transport require special handling—that is, the use of glass tubes is avoided, centrifugation is performed promptly, and transport occurs overnight, with samples packed in ice. Normal dogs have endogenous ACTH levels of 10 to 70 pg/ml. High or normal plasma ACTH levels (40 to 500 pg/ml) with concurrently elevated plasma cortisol levels are suggestive of PDH. The magnitude of the endogenous ACTH level above normal often correlates with the size of pituitary tumors producing the excessive ACTH. Low plasma ACTH levels (less than 20 pg/ml) with concurrently elevated plasma cortisol levels are suggestive of ATDH (Box 17-9 and Table 17-1).

BOX 17-9 Testing Protocol for Hyperadrenocorticism in Dogs

Obtain urine for corticoid/creatinine ratio.
If urine corticoid/creatinine ratio is abnormally high, perform the following:
- ACTH stimulation test
- Low-dose dexamethasone suppression test
- Radiographic imaging of abdomen

If either ACTH stimulation or low-dose dexamethasone suppression test is abnormal and abdominal radiographs are normal, perform abdominal ultrasonography and high-dose dexamethasone suppression test.
If pituitary-dependent hyperadrenocorticism is suspected, assay endogenous ACTH levels and, if possible, perform CT scan on pituitary.

ACTH, Adrenocorticotropic hormone; *CT,* computed tomography.

Radiographic and Other Imaging Findings. The most consistent radiographic finding of hyperadrenocorticism is hepatomegaly. Other possible findings include soft-tissue mineralization (skin, adrenals, bronchi, branches of the abdominal aorta, kidney, gastric mucosa, and liver capsule), mild osteoporosis, and an enlarged adrenal silhouette (Figure 17-6). With pulmonary thromboembolism, thoracic radiographs may reveal pleural effusion, blunting of pulmonary arteries, and decreased vascularity of affected lung lobes.

No one evaluation method is reliable for the detection of adrenal tumors. Multiple testing (endogenous ACTH, abdominal radiographs, and abdominal ultrasound) are needed.[55] The thorax and abdomen should be radiographed to search for adrenal tumors and metastasis. Ultrasonography is also helpful in detecting about two thirds of adrenal tumors. Ultrasonography can also determine the presence of vena cava compression or invasion; in addition, it is excellent for screening for liver metastasis. Tumors as small as 1.2 cm can be detected with ultrasonography, but it is not reliable in differentiating benign from malignant adrenocortical tumors.[56] Routine radiography

TABLE 17-1. INTERPRETATION OF BASELINE PLASMA CORTISOL, URINE CORTICOID/CREATININE RATIO, ACTH STIMULATION, LOW-DOSE DEXAMETHASONE SUPPRESSION (LDDS), HIGH-DOSE DEXAMETHASONE (HDDS) SUPPRESSION, AND ENDOGENOUS ACTH TEST RESULTS

	NORMAL	PDH	ATDH
Urine corticoid (nmol/L)/creatinine (mmol/L) ratio	8-24	High	High
Baseline plasma cortisol (μg/dl)	<1-4	Normal to high	Normal to high
Plasma cortisol after LDDS (μg/dl)	<1.5	>1.5	>1.5
Plasma cortisol after ACTH (μg/dl)	<20	High	Normal to high
Plasma cortisol after HDDS (μg/dl)	<50% of baseline	<50% of baseline	>50% of baseline
Endogenous plasma ACTH (pg/ml)	10-70	>40	<20

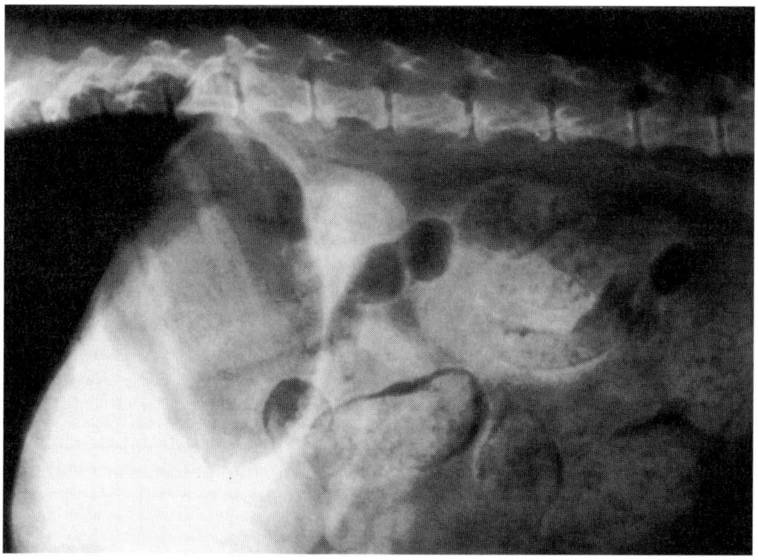

Figure 17-6. A radiograph of enlarged mineralized adrenal tumor in a dog with hyperadrenocorticism.

cannot detect adrenal tumors of 2 cm or less unless they have mineralized. Because of its location dorsal to the liver, the right adrenal is more difficult to assess by radiography or ultrasonography than is the left adrenal.

Approximately 50% of adrenocortical neoplasms are visible on routine abdominal radiographs. Thirty percent to 40% are mineralized. Bilateral adrenal tumors occur in 7%. Ultrasonography is more sensitive than abdominal radiography for detection of adrenal tumors, but false positive results may be more likely, too. Carcinomas are more likely to be detected by either method. Vena cava invasion usually is caused by carcinomas on the right side. Special imaging examinations of the adrenals include nephrotomography, ultrasonography, magnetic resonance imaging (MRI), and CT scans.

MRI or CT scans are ideal to search for the presence of pituitary tumors. MRI is capable of revealing tumors as small as 4 mm in diameter. Cisternography combined with linear tomography has also been useful in detecting pituitary enlargement. The severity of neurologic clinical signs does not correlate well with the size of pituitary tumors causing hyperadrenocorticism.

The incidence of calcium-containing uroliths is higher in dogs with hyperadrenocorticism. These are detectable by routine radiography.[57]

Management. The treatment of hyperadrenocorticism can be done by pharmacologic control, surgical correction, or a combination. For treatment of PDH, the most economic and safest form of treatment is the pharmacologic approach with mitotane. For radiographically demonstrable adrenocortical tumors (enlarged carcinomas), surgical excision should be attempted, and if necessary, pharmacologic control of metastasis used.

Adrenocortical hyperplasia is usually treated with mitotane (o,p′DDD; Lysodren). The exact mechanism of action is unknown, but mitotane seems to block the stimulation of steroidogenesis by ACTH, to hasten the catabolism of cortisol, and to block extraadrenal cortisol effects. The recommended dose for adrenal hyperplasia in the dog is 50 mg/kg every day until a satisfactory response is noted. A response should be evident within 10 days of treatment, or a reevaluation for adrenocortical tumors should be done.[58] An alternative initial treatment consists of administration of mitotane for 5 to 14 days with glucocorticoid replacement. An ACTH stimulation test is always necessary before mitotane administration to serve as a baseline for evaluation of subsequent effectiveness of treatment. Post-ACTH plasma cortisol levels are below 5 μg/dl after sufficient mitotane treatment. Urine C/Cr ratio is inferior to ACTH stimulation for monitoring mitotane treatment.[59-61]

For maintenance, a weekly administration of 50 mg/kg of body weight is required indefinitely, because the zona arcuata or zona intermedia will regenerate the hyperplastic zona fasciculata and zona reticularis if not continually suppressed. Dogs with adrenocortical tumors that are not surgical candidates may respond to mitotane at higher than usual dosage or for longer initial daily treatments, or both, than for PDH.[58,62] Mitotane is best absorbed with food.

The toxic effects of mitotane are primarily dose dependent. At the recommended dosage for adrenocortical hyperplasia, few toxic effects occur. About 25% of dogs treated show mild adverse effects. The most frequent adverse effects are temporary anorexia, weakness, and dizziness for 2 to 12 hours. Pretreatment with low-dose prednisolone may preclude such adverse effects in affected dogs. Hair grown in areas of previous alopecia may be darker and longer than the dog's previous haircoat.

Decreasing plasma cortisol levels may allow the pituitary growth to proceed without inhibition. Signs of an enlarging pituitary macrotumor become more likely while adrenocortical function is being suppressed. These signs include disorientation, anorexia, wandering, restlessness, staring, ataxia, head pressing, circling, or seizures. Less commonly, abnormal body temperature, aggressive behavior, or blindness may occur.

If persistent clinical signs of glucocorticoid deficiency such as vomiting, diarrhea, marked depression, or total anorexia develop, replacement glucocorticoid therapy should be initiated. When necessary, the dose of 0.22 mg/kg/day of prednisone or prednisolone will replace baseline glucocorticoid effects of normal cortisol levels. Addison's disease occurs in about 5% of treated cases. It should be suspected if there is poor response to glucocorticoid replacement alone. In such cases, serum sodium and potassium levels should be reassessed.

The reexamination of treated dogs is recommended 6 weeks after dismissal from the hospital and every 3 to 6 months thereafter. Approximately one half of dogs with PDH develop partial resistance to treatment with mitotane because of a compensatory increase in the secretion of ACTH resulting from lowered levels of plasma cortisol. This is because of increased ACTH secretion, accelerated elimination of mitotane, or decreased intestinal absorption associated with the decrease in intestinal fat absorption caused by reduced cortisol secretion.

An alternative medical treatment to mitotane is ketoconazole (Nizoral). Ketoconazole inhibits cortisol synthesis by inhibiting P450 enzymes. The dosage required exceeds the dose required for antifungal effects. It may be used to prepare dogs for surgery or when mitotane cannot be tolerated. Presurgical therapy should begin 4 to 8 weeks before the surgery. The dose is 10 to 15 mg/kg twice per day on an indefinite basis. Potential adverse effects include anorexia, vomiting, and lightening of the haircoat. Treatment failures for long-term maintenance are at least 50%. The cause is unknown, although poor gastrointestinal absorption is suspected. Endogenous ACTH secretion or stimulation of pituitary tumor growth is not believed to increase secondarily to ketoconazole therapy. Mitotane should not be used concurrently with ketoconazole.

Aminoglutethimide, another steroidogenesis inhibitor, is not consistently effective, and mild to moderate adverse effects are common.[63] Selegiline (L-Deprenyl; Anipryl) is a monoamine oxidase-B inhibitor approved for the treatment of PDH, but it is not effective by itself.[64] Trilostane (not currently available in the United States) is a safe and effective inhibitor of steroidogenesis.[65,66]

Surgical procedures such as adrenalectomy or hypophysectomy are possible means of correcting hyperadrenocorticism. Both procedures require the skill of an experienced surgeon and are expensive compared with drug therapy. Bilateral adrenalectomy should not be performed on diabetic patients because loss of medullary epinephrine allows hypoglycemia to be more severe. The long-term prognosis for dogs having adrenalectomy is good if they survive more than 2 weeks after surgery.[67]

Pituitary macroadenomas and macroadenocarcinomas have been successfully managed with external beam, photon radiotherapy. The dose used is 40 Gy in 10 equal doses over 22 days. Tumor size decreases approximately 50% every 6 months. Neural and ocular complications are common with radiation exposure to the head. Although radiotherapy can reduce the size of macroadenomas, it may not control hyperadrenocorticism.[68]

The treatment of hyperadrenocorticism concurrent with insulin-dependent diabetes mellitus requires insulin therapy until the blood glucose has been near normal limits for at least 1 week. Treatment with mitotane is then begun, and the previous insulin dosage is reduced 50% to reduce the risk of hypoglycemia caused by decreasing concentrations of plasma cortisol while still inhibiting ketogenesis and ketoacidosis. After a satisfactory response to mitotane is attained, the insulin dosage is readjusted to produce more desirable blood glucose levels.

If polyuria and polydipsia do not correct after plasma cortisol levels are normal, central diabetes insipidus from a pituitary, especially pars intermedia, tumor should be suspected. Mitotane therapy removes the negative feedback on the pituitary, and ACTH secretion increases. In some cases, successful suppression of cortisol excess may augment pituitary tumor enlargement from lack of negative feedback.

There is a 50% chance that dogs with PDH will live more than 2 years if they are treated with mitotane. Death is usually from bacterial complications, congestive heart failure, or pulmonary thromboembolism.

Pheochromocytoma

Cause. Pheochromocytomas are usually slow-growing, well-encapsulated, red-brown tumors of the adrenal medulla or sympathetic paraganglia. They constitute about 1.5% of canine tumors. One-third to two-thirds are incidental findings at necropsy. Half, based on evidence of metastasis, are malignant.[69,70] Their histologic appearance may, however, appear misleadingly benign. Canine pheochromocytomas can secrete excessive amounts of catecholamines.

About half of pheochromocytomas occur concurrently with other endocrine neoplasia.[69,70] These occurrences are classified as multiple endocrine neoplasia (MEN) syndromes. MEN type IIA, which has been reported in dogs, is the concurrent presence of pheochromocytoma, medullary carcinoma of the thyroid gland, and parathyroid gland hyperplasia. Pheochromocytoma has also occurred with pituitary and adrenocortical adenomas in one dog and with a thyroid follicular cell adenoma and islet cell carcinoma in another.

Incidence. The true incidence of excess catecholamine-secreting pheochromocytomas in dogs is not currently known because the clinical signs of excessive catecholamines are vague and secretion may be intermittent. In addition, routine screening of peripheral arterial blood pressure on annual physical examinations and measurements of urinary catecholamine metabolites, the basis of diagnosis of excessive catecholamine secretion by pheochromocytomas in humans, are not performed on dogs.

There is no predisposition for sex or breed. The incidence, based on canine necropsies, is about 0.5% of all dogs examined postmortem. Pheochromocytomas in dogs may be associated with tumors of the carotid body and aortic body, which are nonchromophobe paraganglia. Extraadrenal pheochromocytomas can occur anywhere along the sympathetic ganglia from the cervical region to the pelvis.

Clinical Features. Pheochromocytomas can cause clinical signs by compression or invasion of surrounding structures, especially the caudal vena cava, or by secretion of excessive catecholamines. Some dogs may be presented with signs of spinal cord compression caused by extension of the tumor into the vertebral canal.[71] Clinical signs vary, depending on whether an excess of epinephrine or norepinephrine is predominant. More common possible clinical signs and their causes are listed in Box 17-10. The ability to secrete excessive catecholamines is not related to tumor size, but most tumors with invasiveness will cause cardiovascular collapse or arrhythmias. Other clinical signs can include palpable abdominal mass, ascites, flushing of mucous membranes, fever, constipation, paresthesias, and various neurologic abnormalities caused by hypertension or cerebral hemorrhage. Secretion of catecholamines from pheochromocytomas may be caused by palpation of the tumor, beta-adrenergic blockers, induction of anesthesia, exercise, eating, and exposure to cold temperatures.

Dogs with pheochromocytomas apparently secreting excessive levels of catecholamines indicate that the clinical signs and postmortem lesions such as cardiomyopathy, arteriolar sclerosis, and tunica media hyperplasia of arterioles are consistent with an excess of norepinephrine. Nearly all the clinical signs caused by pheochromocytomas secreting excessive levels of norepinephrine are the result of persistent or intermittent hypertension. A combination of the hypertension and tissue damage by malignancy can cause acute spontaneous hemorrhage into the retroperitoneal space.[72]

BOX 17-10 Possible Clinical Signs Caused by Adrenal Medullary Pheochromocytomas

Compression of Surrounding Structures
Enlarged caudal superficial abdominal veins
Edema of the caudal extremities
Weakness of the hind legs

Secretion of Excessive Catecholamines
Excessive Epinephrine
Hypotension
Noncardiac pulmonary edema
Ventricular arrhythmias

Predominant Norepinephrine-secreting
Tachycardia and tachyarrhythmias
Congestive heart failure
Excessive panting
Weakness and trembling
Epistaxis
Seizures
Retinal hemorrhage
Head pressing
Weight loss

Laboratory Findings and Diagnosis. Clinical laboratory findings associated persistently or intermittently with pheochromocytomas secreting excessive amounts of catecholamines include hyperglycemia, polycythemia, and hypertriglyceridemia. Packed cell volumes may be increased as a result of decreased plasma volume or of hemorrhage. Urinalysis may show proteinuria and hematuria.

Determination of the urinary excretion of catecholamines and their metabolites is the standard screening test for the presence of pheochromocytomas secreting excessive amounts of catecholamines in humans. Frequently, a definitive diagnosis can be made without further tests. Unfortunately, the diagnostic value of this test has not been evaluated in dogs with pheochromocytomas.

The diagnosis in dogs can be based on routine abdominal radiography, pneumoperitoneal radiography, angiography, CT scan, or ultrasonography. The sensitivity of transabdominal ultrasonography in detecting pheochromocytomas is an enlargement of >2 cm, and for a CT scan, it is >0.5 to 1 cm. Either CT scan or ultrasonography may detect invasion or compression of the vena cava (Figure 17-7).

Blood pressure response tests to phentolamine, histamine, tyramine, or glucagon are risky and should be reserved for normotensive dogs with equivocal abdominal imaging results.

Radiographic Findings. Radiographic examinations of the abdomen may show an enlarged adrenal shadow in about one third of the cases. The left adrenal is more easily seen. The right adrenal is normally covered by the liver. Adrenal calcification is more suggestive of adrenocortical carcinoma than pheochromocytoma.[70] Appreciation of the adrenal enlargement may require ultrasonography, scintigraphy, tomography, retroperitoneal pneumography, IV pyelography, contrast venography of the caudal vena cava, or selective angiography. Nonselective vena caval venography can show a tumor thrombus in about 50% of the cases. Selective angiography is the most dangerous

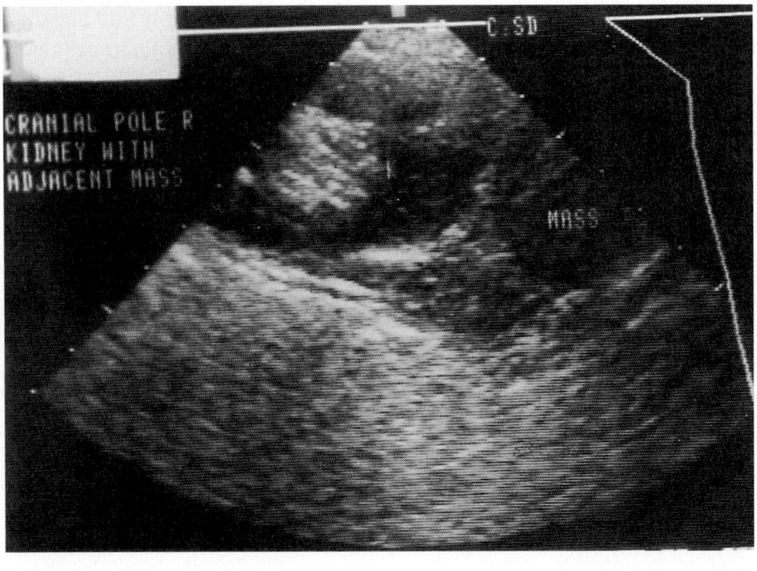

Figure 17-7. An abdominal sonogram showing an enlarged adrenal gland from a pheochromocytoma in a dog.

procedure because of the risk of vascular rupture. Scintigraphy may be performed using ^{123}I-labeled metaiodobenzylguanidine.[73] If available, CT scans of the abdomen are particularly useful.

Management. Excision is the only satisfactory treatment for pheochromocytomas. If tachycardia or tachyarrhythmias are present before surgery, the nonselective β-blocker propranolol hydrochloride (Inderal) may be given in an oral dose of 0.15 to 0.5 mg/kg three times daily, but after the administration of an oral α_1- and α_2-blocker phenoxybenzamine hydrochloride (Dibenzyline) has begun. Phenoxybenzamine in an oral, twice daily dose of 0.2 to 1.5 mg/kg should be begun 10 to 14 days before surgery to stabilize blood pressure. Otherwise, vasoconstriction and severe hypertension may result from unopposed α-adrenergic effects. Prazosin (Minipress) has a shorter duration of activity, is a selective α_1-blocker, and may be preferable to phenoxybenzamine.

Preoperative administration of atropine or phenothiazines should be avoided to reduce risks of tachycardia or sudden hypotension. Equipment for measuring the ECG and blood pressure should be connected to the dog before induction. Induction should be with narcotics or thiobarbiturate combined with glycopyrrolate. Anesthesia should be done with enflurane and nitrous oxide. Halothane can induce arrhythmias and should be avoided. Phentolamine, an α-blocker for IV use, can be used in a dose of 0.02 to 0.1 mg/kg during surgery to lower blood pressure while manipulating the tumor. Propranolol can be given intravenously in a dose of 0.3 to 1 mg/kg, or lidocaine without epinephrine can be administered intravenously, as necessary, during the surgery to control tachycardia or tachyarrhythmias. Immediately after the adrenalectomy, the rate of fluid administration should be increased. If blood pressure cannot be maintained, norepinephrine (Levophed) should be given carefully in an IV dose. Adrenocortical steroids should not be replaced or supplemented unless both adrenals must be removed.

Metabolic Disorders

Hypercalcemia of Malignancy

Cause. Hypercalcemia of malignancy (HCM) is more common than primary hyperparathyroidism. Hypercalcemia in adult dogs is defined as >12 mg/dl. HCM is the most common paraneoplastic disorder of the dog. In comparison with primary hyperparathyroidism, HCM is usually characterized by a more rapid onset of weight loss, lack of overt bone demineralization, and hypercalcemia of greater magnitude.

Hypercalcemia is caused by malignancies by one of at least three mechanisms: a humoral substance, osteoclast-activating factor by cells within the bone marrow, or bone destruction from solid tumor bone metastasis.

Most cases of lymphosarcoma in dogs associated with hypercalcemia seem to cause hypercalcemia by producing PTH-related peptide (PTHrP) or a lymphokine, osteoclast activity factor, or both. PTHrP is a peptide with a molecular weight of 16,000 daltons and contains eight of the first 13 amino acids of PTH. Although its plasma level is elevated with lymphosarcomas associated with hypercalcemia, the level is not in a linear relationship with the degree of hypercalcemia. Therefore, other factors may be involved in mediating hypercalcemia caused by lymphosarcoma. In some cases, 1, 25-dihydroxyvitamin D may contribute to hypercalcemia of malignancy associated with lymphosarcoma.[74]

Multicentric and thymic (cranial mediastinal) forms of lymphosarcoma are most commonly associated with hypercalcemia. About 10% of dogs with multicentric lymphosarcoma and half of dogs with thymic forms develop hypercalcemia. Over 80% of dogs with hypercalcemia from lymphosarcoma have a cranial mediastinal mass. Most of these have bone marrow involvement.

The term *pseudohyperparathyroidism* has been used to describe any hypercalcemia resulting from malignancy not caused by metastasis to bone. About 50% to 80% of malignancies causing hypercalcemia in people are associated with PTHrP. PTHrP has also been demonstrated in apocrine gland adenocarcinoma (AGAC) of the anal sacs in dogs.[75] The degree of hypercalcemia caused by AGAC is in a linear relationship with the PTHrP produced. Other malignancies often causing HCM are multiple myeloma, malignant melanoma, and a variety of carcinomas.[76]

Incidence. Hypercalcemia resulting from malignancy is most frequently associated with lymphosarcoma in dogs. Lymphosarcoma constitutes about 4.5% of all canine neoplasia, and 10% to 40% of dogs with lymphosarcoma develop hypercalcemia. Canine breeds considered at a greater-than-expected risk for lymphosarcoma include the boxer, basset hound, Saint Bernard, Scottish terrier, and various hunting breeds. The second most common cause of hypercalcemia in dogs is AGAC of the anal sacs. Lymphosarcoma primarily affects middle-aged dogs. AGAC of the anal sacs usually affects dogs older than 10 years.

More than 90% of dogs affected with AGAC of the anal sacs are female dogs, with an average age of 10 years. It is the most common malignant perineal tumor in older female dogs. German shepherd dogs may have a higher than expected incidence of AGACs of the anal sacs. About 80% of AGACs are unilateral, and despite the relative lack of anaplastic appearances, more than 90% have metastasized to the iliac or sublumbar lymph nodes by the time of diagnosis. This tumor usually, but not invariably, causes hypercalcemia. It is often occult, not being discovered until a digital examination of the anus and rectum is done. About 60% of affected dogs have a perineal mass or dyschezia.

Clinical Features. Many of the clinical signs of HCM are attributable to hypercalcemia and are identical to those seen in animals with primary hyperparathyroidism (Box 17-11). Clinical signs are often not evident until the serum calcium concentration exceeds 14 mg/dl. Additional clinical signs may be produced by the nonparathyroid tumor itself, including such signs as enlarged lymph nodes, perianal tumors, mammary tumors, cough from lung metastasis, and others. The osteomalacia seen in subjects with primary hyperparathyroidism is not evident radiographically in subjects with humoral mediated HCM.

Signs of AGAC of the anal sacs include tenesmus, constipation, ribbon stools, perineal swelling, polyuria-polydipsia, pelvic limb edema, and cough. AGAC of the anal sacs metastasizes early. Most cases, but not all, have hypercalcemia and hypophosphatemia until renal failure occurs.

Laboratory Findings and Diagnosis. The clinical diagnosis of HCM is based on correction of the elevated serum calcium levels after the removal, destruction, or suppression of the nonparathyroid neoplasm suspected to be producing hypercalcemia-promoting substances. A minimal data base necessary for arrival at a tentative diagnosis of HCM requires a thorough and accurate history. Physical examination should include palpation of the skeleton, all superficial lymph nodes, anal sacs, deep abdominal structures, and an ophthalmologic examination. Other causes of hypercalcemia include hypervitaminosis D, primary hypoadrenocorticism, end-stage renal failure, granulomatous diseases (blastomycosis, schistosomiasis), and primary or metastatic bone neoplasia.[77]

BOX 17-11 Possible Clinical Signs of Hypercalcemia of Malignancy

Polyuria and polydipsia
Vomiting
Constipation
Weight loss
Anemia
Weakness and depression

Elevated serum alkaline phosphatase levels occur more often, and to a greater magnitude, in animals with HCM than in animals with primary hyperparathyroidism.

Calcium nephropathy is present in most cases of HCM. Urinalysis usually shows isosthenuria or hyposthenuria, no casts, and an occasional red or white blood cell in the sediment. Crystals of calcium phosphate or oxalate may be found. Retention of blood urea nitrogen, creatinine, organic acids, and other metabolic waste products depends on the severity of renal failure at the time of examination. Mineralization of soft tissue outside the kidneys is rare in animals with HCM.

Malignancies causing hypercalcemia are occult in nearly half the cases. Recommended laboratory data useful for detection of occult nonparathyroid malignancies and differentiation of HCM from primary hyperparathyroidism include a complete hemogram, serum chemistries (urea nitrogen, alanine transaminase, alkaline phosphatase, creatinine, total protein, albumin, calcium, phosphorus, and magnesium), urinalysis, thoracic and abdominal radiographs, bone marrow biopsy, and an aspirate biopsy of the lymph nodes. A low serum phosphorus level with hypercalcemia is suggestive of excessive PTH or PTHrP production.

Radiographic Findings. Radiologic examination of the bones for subperiosteal resorption should include the dental arcade and metacarpals-phalanges. Radiographs of the thorax and abdomen are also recommended to search for nonparathyroid malignancies and skeletal demineralization typical of primary hyperparathyroidism. Thyroid or bone radioisotope scans may be useful in selected cases.

AGAC of the anal sacs has metastasis in more than 50% of cases. Metastasis is usually recognized by radiographic enlargement of the iliac lymph nodes.

Management. Ideally, the nonparathyroid tumor responsible for HCM should be excised or totally destroyed by radiation or immunotherapy. Within 2 days of excision, the hypercalcemia should be resolved. The degree of functional renal disability should be determined before any form of therapy is undertaken. Pathologic changes in the kidneys caused by calcium may not be reversible.

Hypercalcemic crisis resulting from serum calcium levels in excess of 14 mg/dl occurs more often with HCM than with primary hyperparathyroidism. Clinical signs of hypercalcemic crisis can include constipation, muscle tremors, and mental depression. Serum calcium levels that exceed 18 mg/dl can result in renal failure and shock, rapidly leading to death.

It is advisable to attempt to reduce the serum calcium levels with an IV solution of sterile isotonic saline solution with added potassium chloride, 10 mmol/L, and furosemide, 1 mg/kg of body weight, every 2 hours. In addition to the dilutional effects of an IV saline solution, sodium loading with saline solution and treatment with furosemide inhibit calcium's reabsorption in the renal tubules. Thiazide diuretics can aggravate hypercalcemia and should be avoided.

Other means of reducing hypercalcemia can be considered after conservative attempts with the IV administration of saline solution, furosemide, and glucocorticoids have failed. Etidronate disodium (Didronel IV), a diphosphonate that inhibits osteoclastic activity, should be tried if conservative therapy has been unsuccessful. The dosage is 7.5 mg/kg diluted in at least 250 ml of saline. It is given IV over a minimum of 2 hours each day for 3 consecutive days. Other treatments for refractory hypercalcemia include calcitonin and gallium nitrate.

Calcitonin (Calcimar), 4 U/kg, given IV or SC, is effective, but it has a short duration and is expensive. Gallium nitrate (Ganite) inhibits bone resorption, but is nephrotoxic to the tubules. It, too, is very expensive.

Plicamycin (Mithracin) is an antibiotic anticancer agent that decreases DNA-directed RNA synthesis and decreases osteoclastic activity. However, because of significant toxicities in dogs with malignancies, it should be considered only for cases that are unresponsive to other treatments for hypercalcemia.[78]

Excision is the preferred treatment for AGAC of the anal sacs. AGAC of the anal sacs should not be confused with the more common perianal gland adenomas in older male dogs. One half of excised AGAC of the anal sacs recur. The mean survival after excision is 1 year. Response to chemotherapy is generally disappointing, but treatment with cisplatin or carboplatin may be more effective than treatment with most chemotherapeutic drugs.[79]

DISORDERS OF CATS

Endocrine Disorders

Cause. Hyperthyroidism in cats is usually caused by a solitary adenoma or multinodular adenomatous hyperplasia. Thyroid carcinomas (mixed compact and follicular carcinomas, and occasionally follicular and papillary carcinomas) are rare in cats, constituting 2% of all hyperthyroid cases.

The inciting cause for thyroid adenomas in cats is unknown. Hyperthyroidism in cats is not caused by autoantibodies to thyroid-stimulating hormone (TSH) receptors or other thyroid-stimulating factors in serum, as is typically the case in humans.[80] It is not analogous to Graves' disease in people. Potential causes of hyperthyroidism in cats are controversial. There is no evidence of a genetic predisposition, but there is precedence in humans for dietary factors being involved in the growth of thyroid adenomas. Risk surveys of cats have shown that cats that eat canned cat food are at two to three times the risk, and those that use cat litter are at three times the risk (perhaps because they are indoor cats), of the general population of cats to develop hyperthyroidism.[81] Cats that eat canned fish or liver- and giblet-flavored food have a significantly increased risk for hyperthyroidism.[82] Iodine content of commercial foods varies widely.[83] Serum free T_4 is suppressed in cats by excessive iodine in commercial diets but not by adding potassium iodate to a standard diet.[84,85] Persistently suppressed T_4 levels could lead to persistent overstimulation of the growth of thyroid glands by TSH and, in theory, could induce adenomatous changes.

Incidence. Hyperthyroidism is the most commonly diagnosed endocrinopathy in the cat. It is estimated to affect one in 300 cats. Older cats (6 to 20 years old) are most often affected. There is no predisposition with regard to breed or sex for adenomas or adenomatous hyperplasia of the thyroid. Thyroid carcinomas most commonly occur in castrated males. Both thyroid lobes are involved in about 70% of adenoma or adenomatous hyperplasia cases; 30% are unilateral. Thyroid lobes that are bilaterally affected are usually asymmetrically enlarged.

Clinical Features. Clinical signs are caused by an increased metabolic rate and increased sensitivity to catecholamines. Most thyroid tumors (90%) are palpable near the larynx. The most frequently recognized clinical signs are weight loss with a good appetite. Other common signs are listed in Box 17-12. Less common clinical signs include anorexia, apathy, mild fever, polypnea and dyspnea, irritability when handled, muscle weakness and tremors, congestive heart failure, unkempt hair coat, hair loss, and increased nail growth (Figure 17-8). In about 10% of affected cats, severe depression, anorexia, and weakness occur. This "apathetic hyperthyroidism" is usually

BOX 17-12 Common Clinical Signs of Hyperthyroidism in Cats in Decreasing Order of Occurrence

- Weight loss
- Polyphagia
- Hyperactivity
- Tachycardia
- Polyuria and polydipsia
- Vomiting
- Cardiac murmur
- Diarrhea and increased fecal volume

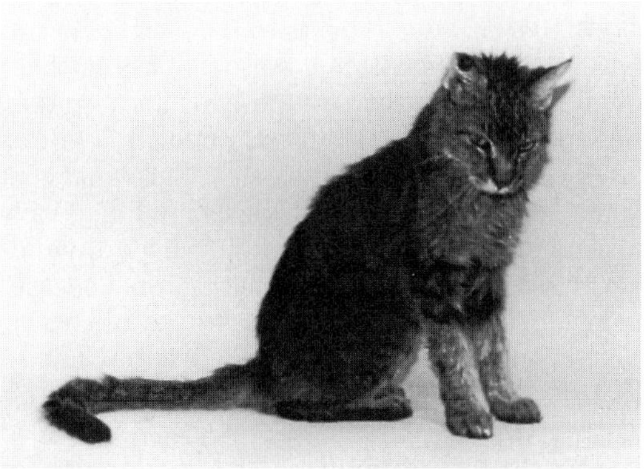

Figure 17-8. A hyperthyroid cat presented because of weight loss despite a good appetite.

associated with cardiac arrhythmias or congestive heart failure. Many of the classical signs of hyperthyroidism are less common or milder than in the past because of earlier detection today.[86,87]

Cardiac complications can be life threatening. More than 80% of thyrotoxic cats have cardiomegaly, and 10% to 15% have congestive heart failure. Some have pulmonary edema and pleural effusion. Two thirds have sinus tachycardia (heart rates exceeding 240 beats per minute) and tachyarrhythmias. One third have increased QRS voltages in lead II exceeding 0.9 mv. Many have second-degree atrioventricular blocks and left anterior fascicular blocks. Echocardiograms usually reveal hypertrophy of the left ventricular caudal wall, enlarged left atrial diameter, and hypertrophy of the interventricular septum. Hypertension occurs in 87% of cats with hyperthyroidism. However, hypertensive vascular accidents, such as retinal hemorrhage, are not common.[88] Hypertrophic cardiomyopathy will resolve after therapy. The left ventricular caudal wall and the interventricular septal wall thickness decreases after therapy, if the animal is hypertrophic from hyperthyroidism. Changes in the ECG revert to normal in at least 80% of cats in which serum T_4 and T_3 levels are successfully lowered. If the cardiomyopathy is congestive, it is not reversible. All cases of feline cardiomyopathy should be screened by measuring serum T_4 levels to rule out or substantiate hyperthyroidism as a cause.

Laboratory Findings and Diagnosis. Laboratory findings associated with feline hyperthyroidism include a stress leukogram, mild to moderate erythrocytosis, macrocytosis, increased serum inorganic phosphorus, increased fecal fat, hyperbilirubinemia, and elevated serum hepatic enzymes. Hypercalcemia may occur if a carcinoma is present. Increased serum enzymes of hepatic origin occur in more than one half the affected cats. These serum enzymes include alkaline phosphatase, lactic dehydrogenase, aspartate transaminase, and alanine transaminase. All older cats with weight loss and elevated serum liver enzymes should be screened for hyperthyroidism by measurement of serum T_4 levels. Hyperthyroid cats may be predisposed to developing hypokalemia.[89] Serum fructosamine concentration is lowered in hyperthyroidism, which causes difficulty in interpreting fructosamine concentration in cats with concurrent hyperthyroidism and diabetes mellitus.[90]

The definitive diagnosis of feline hyperthyroidism is usually based on elevated serum T_4 levels (above 4 μg/dl). Cats with early or mild hyperthyroidism combined with a severe nonthyroidal illness may have baseline serum T_4 levels within high normal range.[91] In such cases, the serum T_4 level should be rechecked in 1 to 2 weeks. If both T_4 levels are normal but hyperthyroidism is suspected, serum free T_4 concentration measured by equilibrium dialysis may be diagnostic.[92] In rare cases in which T_4 and free T_4 concentrations are within normal ranges but the affected animal is still suspected to have hyperthyroidism, a T_3 suppression test or a thyrotropin-releasing hormone (TRH) stimulation test can be performed.

A T_3 suppression test is done by giving 25 μg of T_3 (Cytomel) orally, three times per day until seven doses have been administered. Two to 4 hours after the last dose of T_3, serum T_4 and T_3 samples should be taken. Cats with hyperthyroidism have an unsuppressed serum T_4 of >1.5 μg/dl and <50% drop from baseline T_4 levels. The serum T_3 level should be normal to elevated to verify the last dose was administered and absorbed.

A TRH stimulation test can be performed by administering 0.1 mg/kg of protirelin (Thyrel) IV.

Normal cats double their baseline serum T_4 level by 4 hours after the injection. Hyperthyroid cats show no significant change after TRH stimulation. Hypersalivation and vomiting are common adverse effects.[93] TRH stimulation test results may be unreliable in hyperthyroid cats with nonthyroidal illnesses.[94]

Radiographic and Other Diagnostic Imaging Findings. Thyroid scans (1 mCi sodium pertechnetate IV) can detect aberrant "hot" thyroid nodules or metastasis (Figure 17-9). Thyroid images that are darker than the salivary glands are diagnostic for hyperthyroidism. Thyroid–salivary gland scintigraphic image ratio is a good predictor of thyroid metabolic status.[95] Scans also indicate whether involvement is unilateral or bilateral. Scans of carcinomas often reveal multiple nodular lesions in the neck, thoracic inlet, and cranial mediastinum. When unilateral hyperthyroid neoplasia exists, the contralateral lobe should not be evident on a thyroid scan. If serum T_4 or T_3 levels are persistently high, any thyroid tissue visible on thyroid scans should be excised if surgery is planned. Recent treatment with methimazole and withdrawal for diagnostic examinations increases the uptake of pertechnetate or radioactive iodine (^{131}I) in otherwise normal atrophied thyroid lobes.[96] Methimazole should not be used for 3 weeks before thyroid scans or radioiodine therapy.

High-resolution ultrasonography is helpful in diagnosis of thyroid nodules but not as helpful as scintigraphy in the diagnosis of hyperthyroidism or possible metastasis.[97]

Management. Treatment of hyperthyroidism can be accomplished with antithyroid drugs, radioactive iodine, and surgery. If surgery is planned, the hypermetabolism and hypersensitivity to catecholamines should first be medically controlled. Methimazole is preferred to suppress thyroid hypersecretion.

Hyperthyroidism increases renal blood flow and glomerular filtration rate. Many older cats with hyperthyroidism have masked renal failure that has been stabilized by increased glomerular filtration rate produced by hyperthyroidism.[98-101] When these cats are effectively treated for hyperthyroidism, the concurrent renal failure may become clinically significant. Evaluations of renal function should be done before the animals are treated for hyperthyroidism. If any indication of impaired renal function is found, methimazole should be used as a reversible trial for control of hyperthyroidism. If a euthyroid state can be achieved without the development of serious renal failure, more permanent means of treatment (radioiodine or thyroidectomy) can be considered.

Treatment with methimazole is begun orally with a dose of 5 mg every 8 hours and continued for 2 weeks before the thyroidectomy. Because methimazole primarily blocks organification in the thyroid, stored hormone continues to be released and must be allowed to dissipate before surgery. Serum T_4 levels begin to drop within 24 to 48 hours of treatment, but it should be confirmed that serum T_4 levels are less than 4 μg/dl before surgery is done. If there is little decline in serum T_4 levels after 2 weeks' treatment, methimazole can be increased to a dose of 20 to 30 mg/day. Methimazole is also available for transdermal administration in an organogel and applied to the

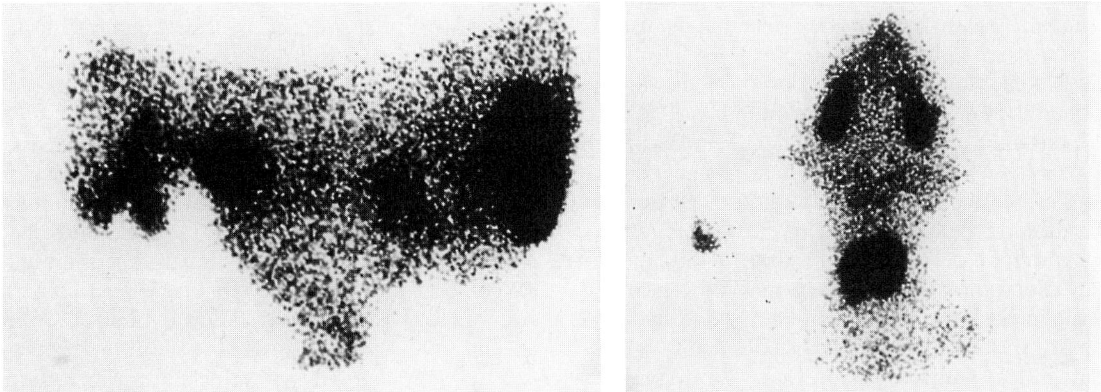

Figure 17-9. A, A lateral view of a thyroid scan with pertechnetate in a cat with bilateral multinodular adenomatous hyperplasia. **B,** A ventrodorsal view of a thyroid scan with pertechnetate in a cat with bilateral multinodular adenomatous hyperplasia.

inside surface of the pinna of the ear. Propranolol for 10 days followed by potassium iodate for 10 days may be considered as an alternative to presurgical treatment with methimazole.[102]

Propranolol should be considered if tachyarrhythmias or other excessive adrenergic effects are present. The initial dosage of propranolol should be 2.5 to 5 mg three times per day for at least 2 days before the thyroidectomy is done. Propranolol should not be used if congestive heart failure is evident.

Because of the risks of the surgical procedure and those inherent in doing surgery on debilitated aged cats, thyroidectomies should be done by an experienced surgeon. Presurgical thyroid scans are recommended because bilateral involvement may not be grossly evident based on intraoperative appearance. If an external parathyroid is evident, a modified extracapsular technique has been recommended as superior to intracapsular (subcapsular) thyroidectomy. The subcapsular method is best for preservation of a parathyroid, but postsurgical relapse of hyperthyroidism is a greater risk. Staged bilateral thyroidectomy has the fewest postoperative complications but is expensive and requires two periods of anesthesia. Overall, surgically related mortality rate is 5% to 10%.

The use of atropine and halothane should be avoided because of their adverse effect on tachyarrhythmias. A cardiac monitor should be used throughout the procedure. If a unilateral thyroidectomy is done, the cranial parathyroid should be spared in case a relapse necessitates later removal of the remaining thyroid. If a bilateral thyroidectomy is done, at least one cranial parathyroid should be preserved.

After the surgery, serum calcium levels should be monitored for signs of hypocalcemia for at least 3 days. Parathyroid function may be temporarily or permanently impaired by postsurgical trauma. Treatment for hypocalcemia is usually unnecessary in half the cases, or more. However, treatment should be considered if the serum calcium levels have fallen below 7 mg/dl. Severe hypocalcemia should be treated with an IV dose of 10% calcium gluconate (1 to 3 ml) followed by 6 to 8 ml in 100 ml of saline solution twice per day. In addition, 0.03 mg/kg/day of dihydrotachysterol is given for 3 days, followed by 0.01 to 0.02 mg/kg/day. Persistent hypocalcemia may be controlled with an oral dose of 0.02 mg/kg/day of dihydrotachysterol and 750 mg/kg/day of calcium gluconate. Most animals can be weaned off, because accessory parathyroid tissue occurs in more than 60% of cats. Also, serum calcium can normalize through a PTH-independent mechanism.

After a unilateral thyroidectomy, serum T_4 levels should be monitored. Because the remaining thyroid will have been suppressed, serum T_4 levels will be low and may remain so for 2 to 3 months, but replacement therapy with thyroid hormone should not be administered unless marked lethargy occurs or low serum T_4 levels persist more than 3 months. Other possible postsurgical problems include Horner's syndrome or laryngeal paralysis. The recurrence rate following thyroidectomy may be 5% to 10% within 3 years after surgery.

Therapy with ^{131}I can be safer than a thyroidectomy in many cats.[103] Anesthetics are not necessary, and no hypoparathyroidism results. Therapy with ^{131}I is also a valuable salvage procedure when subtotal thyroidectomy is not curative. The disadvantages of ^{131}I therapy are the need for postadministration isolation, the cost of treatment, and the necessity for specialists to administer the treatment and monitor the posttreatment isolation.

If a methimazole trial suggests ^{131}I treatment will probably not precipitate renal failure, recent treatment with and withdrawal from methimazole may increase the risk of ^{131}I destruction to healthy thyroid tissue. Antithyroid drug therapy should be discontinued at least 3 weeks prior to ^{131}I treatment to reduce the risk of TSH-stimulated growth of healthy tissue during the recovery from methimazole. Carcinomas are treated with three to 10 times the usual dose of ^{131}I, 20 to 30 mCi. Or instead, cobalt 60 may be used at 48 Gy in 12 fractions of four each given three times per week.

An SC dose of 4 to 5 mCi of ^{131}I is administered to destroy the hyperactive nodules. Improvement should be noticeable within 1 to 2 weeks. Over half of treated animals have normal serum T_4 levels in 4 days; three fourths have normal levels in 8 days. Relapses occur in less than 10% of cases. Most relapses occur within 9 months of the initial treatment. Reevaluation of serum T_4 for hyperthyroidism in cats should be done 6 months and 12 months after treatment.[104,105]

If thyroidectomy or therapy with radioactive iodine is not possible or is undesirable, indefinite therapy using methimazole may be tried. Percutaneous ethanol ablation of thyroid nodules has been successful in selected unilateral cases, but the efficacy and safety for most hyperthyroid cats are less than with methimazole treatment.[106-108]

The maintenance dose for methimazole is 2.5 to 20 mg/day. Adverse effects occur in 10% to 20% of animals in the first month. These include anorexia, vomiting, lethargy, self-induced excoriation of face and neck, bleeding, and icterus. Ten percent to 20% have eosinophilia, lymphocytosis, and a slight leukopenia. Three percent to 4% have agranulocytosis and thrombocytopenia. One in five are antinuclear antibody (ANA)–positive (two after 6 months of treatment), but no lupus syndrome occurs. Initially 10 to 15 mg/day should be given and the serum T_4 and hemogram routinely monitored every 3 to 6 months. Hyperthyroid levels return in 2 days after cessation. Methimazole's effects last longer than the duration in the plasma because it is concentrated in the thyroid.

Diabetes Mellitus

Cause. As in dogs, the most common cause of diabetes mellitus in cats is unknown. However, the incidence of islet cell amyloidosis is higher in diabetic cats than in nondiabetic cats. An insulin-related protein, possibly from proinsulin or preproinsulin, is involved in the formation of feline islet amyloid. Selective islet cell amyloidosis may contribute to the loss of ability to secrete insulin in normal amounts.[109] Controversy exists on whether immune-mediated islet cell destruction may cause some cases of diabetes mellitus in cats.[110,111] Megestrol acetate or other progestogens can precipitate diabetes mellitus in predisposed cats by antagonizing the action of insulin.

Pituitary tumors causing hyperadrenocorticism or acromegaly should be investigated in cases of insulin resistance and failure to lose weight as expected.[112,113] However, insulin-like growth factor I cannot be used to diagnose acromegaly in diabetics. Insulin-like growth factor I concentrations are increased in diabetics with or without acromegaly.[114]

Incidence. Feline diabetes mellitus is most common in castrated male cats. The incidence in male cats is 1.5 times higher than in female cats. Most of the affected cats are neutered. Three fourths of diabetic cats are older than 7 years. One in 400 to 500 cats at risk develops diabetes, and the risk increases with obesity.[115] The occurrence in cats may be more common in spring and summer.

Clinical Features. The clinical signs of diabetes in cats are similar to those in dogs. Exceptions are that cats develop diabetes more slowly and go through periods of transient diabetes for months before having persistent hyperglycemia.[116] Cats also do not develop clinically significant diabetic cataracts as compared with diabetic dogs. Diabetic cats are more likely than dogs to develop a peripheral polyneuropathy. This is characterized by a plantigrade stance, depressed patella reflexes, apparent paresthesias, and weakness. It may be first recognized by owners as cat litter that sticks to the plantar surface of the metatarsals because of glucosuria stickiness and plantigrade stance from peripheral neuropathy.

Laboratory Findings and Diagnosis. Persistent fasting hyperglycemia (>140 mg/dl) is the hallmark of diabetes mellitus. Stress from struggling during an examination or during blood collection is common in cats. Gentle restraint is important for meaningful assessment of blood glucose concentrations.[117] A single IV glucose tolerance test is too variable to be reliable for diagnostic assessment.[118] The renal threshold for glucose in cats (about 290 mg/dl) is much higher than in dogs (about 180 mg/dl). At presentation for initial diagnosis, more than one third of diabetic cats will be in ketoacidosis.[119] The number of Heinz bodies directly correlates with β-hydroxybutyrate concentrations from ketoacidosis.[120]

Management. The management of diabetes in cats is similar to that in dogs, except that 20% to 50% of diabetic cats do not require insulin. They have non–insulin-dependent diabetes mellitus (NIDDM). These cats do not have ketonuria or anorexia. The degree of hyperglycemia is mild. NIDDM in affected cats may be controlled with avoidance of stress and hypoglycemic drugs.

High fiber diets are possibly beneficial in overweight diabetic cats.[121] Prescription Diet Feline w/d or r/d and Science Diet Feline Maintenance Light are high-fiber, low-caloric density diets for cats. Soft-moist foods are not recommended because they contain corn syrup and propylene glycol, which will rapidly raise the blood glucose level. Obesity should be corrected and then prevented from recurring. Older diabetic cats usually require 60 to 70 kcal/kg of ideal body weight. However, high-fiber diets should not be used if the cat is cachectic.

Dietary chromium is needed for normal insulin action.[17] However, supplementation of typical commercial balanced cat diets with chromium is probably of no benefit.[122]

If high-fiber diets and calorie control are not effective in normalizing blood glucose levels within 1 week, hypoglycemic drugs should be tried. Glipizide (Glucotrol) has been reported effective in some animals that have not had ketonemia or ketonuria. The recommended dosage of glipizide is 5 mg two to three times per day with food. Possible adverse effects are vomiting, hypoglycemia, blood dyscrasias, and hepatopathy. Islet cell amyloidosis is progressive. Therefore, the beneficial response to glipizide may not be permanent.

Response to glipizide therapy should be evaluated for 1 month. If during the trial course of therapy the clinical signs become worse, ketoacidosis occurs, the blood glucose exceeds 300 mg/dl, or the owners are dissatisfied, glipizide therapy should be discontinued.

Insulin therapy is necessary if ketonuria, anorexia, or a failed response to diet and hypoglycemic drugs has occurred. Maintenance insulin therapy usually requires twice-per-day SC injections of an intermediate-acting or long-acting insulin. Although several preparations are effective in many cases, protamine zinc insulin (PZI VET) is the most popular preparation. Initial dosage is 1 U per injection for an average-sized cat.[123]

At least one fourth of poorly regulated diabetic cats do not absorb long-acting insulins well enough to control their diabetes. Intermediate-acting insulins are more reliable. A dilution of 100 U/ml of insulin 1:9 with the proper insulin diluent (Lilly) to make 10 U/ml is recommended to facilitate accurate measurement and reliable SC absorption. It is best to use 0.5 ml syringes with 27-gauge needles. The use of morning urine glucose samples for regulation of diabetes is not helpful in detecting overdosage or underdosage of insulin. Obese diabetic cats are at increased risk of hypoglycemia from insulin overdosage without typical clinical signs of low blood glucose.[124]

Home monitoring of blood glucose concentrations by ambitious owners may be achieved by marginal ear vein blood drop collection and a portable reflectance colorimeter.[125] Glycohemoglobin or fructosamine can be used to assess average blood glucose during the weeks preceding an examination in a veterinary clinic.[126-128]

Metabolic Disorders

Hypokalemia

Cause. Hypokalemia in the cat is defined as a serum potassium level of 3.6 mmol/L. Low serum levels may occur with increased, normal, or subnormal total body potassium concentration. Approximately 98% of the body's exchangeable potassium is intracellular. It is the most important intracellular cation in the body, with an intracellular concentration of approximately 150 mmol/L. Maintenance of the higher intracellular potassium concentration is a function of the cell membrane sodium-potassium pump.

Hypokalemia is due primarily to either potassium loss or to redistribution (intracellular shift), although anorexia can aggravate hypokalemia by preventing the intake necessary to compensate for potassium losses. Shifts to the inside of cells are due to acute metabolic alkalosis, insulin, anabolic steroids, or stimulation of adrenergic receptors (Box 17-13). Acute alkalosis may be caused by overtreatment with excessive bicarbonate therapy or by overventilating during anesthesia.

BOX 17-13 Causes of Hypokalemia

Poor Dietary Intake
Anorexia
Inability to eat
Excessive use of potassium-free fluid therapy

Increased Loss of Potassium
Gastrointestinal Loss
Vomiting
Diarrhea

Renal Loss
Diuretics
Renal tubular acidosis
Chronic renal failure
Administration of urinary acidifiers
Hyperaldosteronism

Intracellular Shift
Insulin therapy
Anabolic steroid administration
Mineralocorticoid administration

Specific causes of potassium loss are vomiting, diarrhea, and urinary losses. Potassium is lost with the intestinal contents in diarrhea. With vomiting, the primary cause of hypokalemia is potassium loss in the urine secondary to compensation for gastric hydrogen ion losses. Urinary losses can also be from diuretic therapy with potassium wasting drugs, diuresis with potassium-deficient fluid therapy, mineralocorticoid excess, and renal tubular acidosis. Chronic acidosis as occurs with chronic renal failure or the oral administration of acidifiers can cause potassium depletion.

Incidence. Polyuric renal failure has been found to be the most important cause of hypokalemia in cats. Affected cats were fed diets with marginal potassium content and acidifiers. The incidence of severe hypokalemia in cats has declined in recent years because of the increased concentrations of potassium that have been added to some commercial feline diets.

Clinical Features. Severe depletion of potassium can cause muscular weakness, stiff gait, apparent muscle pain, ileus, arrhythmias, and primary polyuria. Weakness is often of acute onset and associated with apparent pain. Persistent ventroflexion of the neck is a characteristic finding in cats. Hypermetria and a wide-based stance is also common.

Laboratory Findings and Diagnosis. Serum potassium concentrations of <3.6 mmol/L are diagnostic for hypokalemia. Serum potassium levels of <3 mmol/L indicate severe hypokalemia. A hemogram, serum biochemistry profile, blood pH measurement, and a complete urinalysis are indicated. The serum bicarbonate level is often elevated. Serum creatine kinase activity can be elevated with severe hypokalemia because of resulting rhabdomyolysis. Pseudohypokalemia can be caused by extreme serum elevations of glucose, proteins, lipids, or urea nitrogen.

The history should be evaluated for recent vomiting, diarrhea, use of potassium wasting diuretics, and insulin or anabolic steroid therapy. Metabolic alkalosis with hypokalemia is usually due to vomiting of gastric acid or administration of diuretics.

Low fractional excretion of potassium as calculated below suggests nonrenal potassium losses:

$$\frac{\text{Urine K}}{\text{Serum K}} \times \frac{\text{Serum creatinine}}{\text{Urine creatinine}} \times 100$$

Fractional excretion of potassium in excess of 4% suggests an inappropriate renal loss. Chronic hypokalemia can cause tubular nephropathy and impair urine concentrating ability of the kidneys.

Management. The long-term successful management of hypokalemia depends on finding and correcting the cause. It is impractical to measure total body potassium for clinical purposes. Repeated measurement of serum potassium concentration during therapy with appropriate adjustments of fluid rates is the only means of safely administering potassium.

Immediate therapy is necessary for severe and acute hypokalemia. Oral potassium should be given whenever possible. An estimated beginning oral dose of potassium gluconate (Tumil-K) is 1 mmol/kg twice per day. The dosage should be adjusted based on serum potassium concentrations.

Potassium can be given SC if diluted in isotonic fluids such as lactated Ringer's solution at up to 30 mmol potassium chloride per liter of lactated Ringer's solution. Potassium given IV should never exceed the rate of 0.5 mmol/kg/hour. An estimated daily potassium requirement for moderate to severe hypokalemia is 4 to 8 mmol/kg. Chloride, as in physiologic saline or potassium chloride, is necessary if metabolic alkalosis is present with hypokalemia. Dextrose infusions should be avoided as they stimulate insulin release and an intracellular shift of potassium. IV solutions of >40 mmol/L may cause phlebitis.

References

1. DeVries SE, Feldman EC, Nelson RW et al: Primary parathyroid gland hyperplasia in dogs: six cases (1982-1991), *J Am Vet Med Assoc* 202:1132, 1993.
2. Aguilera-Tejero E, Lopez I, Estepa JC et al: Mineral metabolism in healthy geriatric dogs, *Res Vet Sci* 64:191, 1998.
3. Feldman EC, Wisner ER, Nelson RW et al: Comparison of results of hormonal analysis of samples obtained from selected venous sites versus cervical ultrasonography for localizing parathyroid masses in dogs, *J Am Vet Med Assoc* 211:54, 1997.
4. Wisner ER, Nyland TG, Feldman EC et al: Ultrasonographic evaluation of the parathyroid glands in hypercalcemic dogs, *Vet Radiol Ultrasound* 34:108, 1993.
5. Wisner ER, Penninck D, Biller DS: High resolution parathyroid sonography, *Vet Radiol Ultrasound* 38:462, 1997.
6. Matwichuk CL, Taylor SM, Daniel GB et al: Double-phase parathyroid scintigraphy in dogs using Technetium-99M-Sestamibi, *Vet Radiol Ultrasound* 41:461, 2000.
7. Long CD, Goldstein RE, Hornof WJ et al: Percutaneous ultrasound-guided chemical parathyroid ablation for treatment of primary hyperparathyroidism in dogs, *J Am Vet Med Assoc* 215:217, 1999.
8. Pollard RE, Long CD, Nelson RW et al: Percutaneous ultrasonographically guided radiofrequency heat ablation for treatment of primary hyperparathyroidism in dogs, *J Am Vet Med Assoc* 218:1106, 2001.
9. Kimmel SE, Ward CR, Henthorn PS et al: Familial insulin-dependent diabetes mellitus in Samoyed dogs, *J Am Anim Hosp Assoc* 38:235, 2002.
10. Struble Al, Feldman EC, Nelson RW et al: Systemic hypertension and proteinuria in dogs with diabetes mellitus, *J Am Vet Med Assoc* 213:822, 1998.
11. Peikes H, Morris DO, Hess RS: Dermatologic disorders in dogs with diabetes mellitus: 45 cases (1986-2000), *J Am Vet Med Assoc* 219:203, 2001.
12. Beam S, Correa MT, Davidson MG: A retrospective-cohort study on the development of cataracts in dogs with diabetes mellitus: 200 cases, *Vet Ophthalmol* 2:169, 1999.
13. Parsons SE, Drobatz KJ, Lamb SV et al: Endogenous serum insulin concentration in dogs with diabetic ketoacidosis, *J Vet Emerg Crit Care* 12:147, 2002.
14. Grooters AM, Sherding RG, Biller DS et al: Hepatic abscesses associated with diabetes mellitus in two dogs, *J Vet Intern Med* 8:203, 1994.
15. Forrester SD, Troy GC, Dalton MN et al: Retrospective evaluation of urinary tract infection in 42 dogs with hyperadrenocorticism or diabetes mellitus or both, *J Vet Intern Med* 13:557, 1999.
16. Hess RS, Ward CR: Effect of insulin dosage on glycemic response in dogs with diabetes mellitus: 221 cases (1993-1998), *J Am Vet Med Assoc* 216:217, 2000.
17. Appleton DJ, Rand JS, Sunvold GD et al: Dietary chromium tripicolinate supplementation reduces

glucose concentrations and improves glucose tolerance in normal-weight cats, *J Feline Med Surg* 4:13, 2002.

18. Schachter S, Nelson RW, Kirk CA: Oral chromium picolinate and control of glycemia in insulin-treated diabetic dogs, *J Vet Intern Med* 15:379, 2001.
19. Kimmel SE, Michel KE, Hess RS et al: Effects of insoluble and soluble dietary fiber on glycemic control in dogs with naturally occurring insulin-dependent diabetes mellitus, *J Am Vet Med Assoc* 216:1076, 2000.
20. Graham PA, Maskell IE, Rawlings JM et al: Influence of a high fibre diet on glycaemic control and quality of life in dogs with diabetes mellitus, *J Small Anim Pract* 43:67, 2002.
21. Hoenig M, Laflamme D, Klaser DA et al: Glucose tolerance and lipid profiles in dogs fed different fiber diets, *Vet Ther* 2:160, 2001.
22. Macintire DK: Treatment of diabetic ketoacidosis in dogs by continuous low-dose intravenous infusion of insulin, *J Am Vet Med Assoc* 202:1266, 1993.
23. Briggs CE, Nelson RW, Feldman EC et al: Reliability of history and physical examination findings for assessing control of glycemia in dogs with diabetes mellitus: 53 cases (1995-1998), *J Am Vet Med Assoc* 217:48, 2000.
24. Wess G, Reusch C: Evaluation of five portable blood glucose meters for use in dogs, *J Am Vet Med Assoc* 216:203, 2000.
25. Casella M, Wess G, Reusch CE: Measurement of capillary blood glucose concentrations by pet owners: a new tool in the management of diabetes mellitus, *J Am Anim Hosp Assoc* 38:239, 2002.
26. Elliott DA, Nelson RW, Feldman EC et al: Glycosylated hemoglobin concentrations in the blood of healthy dogs and dogs with naturally developing diabetes mellitus, pancreatic B-cell neoplasia, hyperadrenocorticism, and anemia, *J Am Vet Med Assoc* 211:723, 1997.
27. Marca MC, Loste A, Unzueta A et al: Blood glycated hemoglobin evaluation in sick dogs, *Can J Vet Res* 64:141, 2000.
28. Thoresen SI, Lorenzen FH: Treatment of diabetes mellitus in dogs using isophane insulin penfills and the use of serum fructosamine assays to diagnose and monitor the disease, *Acta Vet Scand* 38:137, 1997.
29. Loste A, Marca MC: Study of the effect of total serum protein and albumin concentrations on canine fructosamine concentration, *Can J Vet Res* 63:138, 1999.
30. Reusch CE, Haberer B: Evaluation of fructosamine in dogs and cats with hypo- or hyperproteinaemia, azotaemia, hyperlipidaemia and hyperbilirubinaemia, *Vet Rec* 148:370, 2001.
31. Kronen PWM, Moon-Massat PF, Ludders JW et al: Comparison of two insulin protocols for diabetic dogs undergoing cataract surgery, *Vet Anaesth Analg* 28:146, 2001.
32. Van Ham L, Braund KG, Roels S et al: Treatment of a dog with an insulinoma-related peripheral polyneuropathy with corticosteroids, *Vet Rec* 141:98, 1997.
33. Beaudry D, Knapp DW, Montgomery T et al: Hypoglycemia in four dogs with smooth muscle tumors, *J Vet Intern Med* 9:415, 1995.
34. Bagley RS, Levy JK, Malarkey DE: Hypoglycemia associated with intra-abdominal leiomyoma and leiomyosarcoma in six dogs, *J Am Vet Med Assoc* 208:69, 1996.
35. Siliart B, Stambouli F: Laboratory diagnosis of insulinoma in the dog: a retrospective study and a new diagnostic procedure, *J Small Anim Pract* 37:367, 1996.
36. Thoresen SI, Aleksandersen M, Lonaaas L et al: Pancreatic insulin-secreting carcinoma in a dog: fructosamine for determining persistent hypoglycaemia, *J Small Anim Pract* 36:282, 1995.
37. Lester NV, Newell SM, Hill RC et al: Scintigraphic diagnosis of insulinoma in a dog, *Vet Radiol Ultrasound* 40:174, 1999.
38. Reine NJ, Hohenhaus AE, Peterson ME et al: Deoxycorticosterone-secreting adrenocortical carcinoma in a dog, *J Vet Intern Med* 13:386, 1999.
39. Rijnberk A, Kooistra HS, van Vonderen et al: Aldosteronoma in a dog with polyuria as the leading symptom, *Domest Anim Endocrinol* 20:227, 2001.
40. Scholten-Sloof BE, Knol BW, Rijnberk A et al: Pituitary-dependent hyperadrenocorticism in a family of Dandie Dinmont terriers, *J Endocrinol* 135:535, 1992.
41. Frank LA, Schmeitzel LP, Oliver JW: Steroidogenic response of adrenal tissues after administration of ACTH to dogs with hypercortisolemia, *J Am Vet Med Assoc* 218:214, 2001.
42. Berry CR, Hawkins EC, Hurley KJ et al: Frequency of pulmonary mineralization and hypoxemia in 21 dogs with pituitary-dependent hyperadrenocorticism, *J Vet Intern Med* 14:151, 2000.
43. Jacoby RC, Owings JT, Ortega T et al: Biochemical basis for the hypercoagulable state seen in Cushing syndrome, *Arch Surg* 136:1003, 2001.
44. Whittemore JC, Preston CA, Kyles AE et al: Nontraumatic rupture of an adrenal gland tumor causing intra-abdominal or retroperitoneal hemorrhage in four dogs, *J Am Vet Med Assoc* 219:329, 2001.
45. Ortega TM, Feldman EC, Nelson RW et al: Systemic arterial blood pressure and urine protein/creatinine ratio in dogs with hyperadrenocorticism, *J Am Vet Med Assoc* 209:1724, 1996.
46. Jensen AL, Poulsen JSD: Preliminary experience with the diagnostic value of the canine corticosteroid-induced alkaline phosphatase isoenzyme in hypercorticism and diabetes mellitus, *J Am Vet Med Assoc* 39:342, 1992.
47. Solter PF, Hoffman WE, Hungerford LL et al: Assessment of corticosteroid-induced alkaline phosphatase isoenzyme as a screening test for hyperadrenocorticism in dogs, *J Am Vet Med Assoc* 203:534, 1993.
48. Van Liew CH, Greco DS, Mowafak DS: Comparison of results of adrenocorticotropic hormone stimulation and low-dose dexamethasone suppression tests with necropsy findings in dogs: 81 cases (1985-1995), *J Am Vet Med Assoc* 211:322, 1997.
49. Frank LA, Oliver JW: Comparison of serum cortisol concentrations in clinically normal dogs after administration of freshly reconstituted versus reconstituted and stored frozen cosyntropin, *J Am Vet Med Assoc* 212:1569, 1998.
50. Kolevska J, Svoboda M: Immunoreactive cortisol measurement in canine urine and its validity in hyperadrenocorticism diagnosis, *Acta Vet Brno* 69:217, 2000.
51. van Vonderen IK, Kooistra HS, Rijnberk A: Influence of veterinary care on the urinary corticoid:creatinine ratio in dogs, *J Vet Intern Med* 12:431, 1998.
52. Norman EJ, Thompson H, Mooney CT: Dynamic adrenal function testing in eight dogs with hyperadrenocorticism associated with adrenocortical neoplasia, *Vet Rec* 144:551, 1999.

53. Syme HM, Scott-Moncrieff C, Treadwell NG et al: Hyperadrenocorticism associated with excessive sex hormone production by an adrenocortical tumor in two dogs, *J Am Vet Med Assoc* 219:1725, 2001.
54. Ristic JME, Ramsey IK, Heath FM et al: The use of 17-hydroxyprogesterone in the diagnosis of canine hyperadrenocorticism, *J Vet Intern Med* 16:433, 2002.
55. Gould SM, Baines EA, Mannion PA et al: Use of endogenous ACTH concentration and adrenal ultrasonography to distinguish the cause of canine hyperadrenocorticism, *J Small Anim Pract* 42:113, 2001.
56. Besso JG, Penninck D, Biller DS et al: Retrospective ultrasonographic evaluation of adrenal lesions in 26 dogs, *Vet Radiol Ultrasound* 38:448, 1997.
57. Hess RS, Kass PH, Ward CR. Association between hyperadrenocorticism and development of calcium-containing uroliths in dogs with urolithiasi, *J Am Vet Med Assoc* 212:1889, 1998.
58. Behrend EN, Kemppainen RJ, Clark TP et al: Treatment of hyperadrenocorticism in dogs: a survey of internists and dermatologists, *J Am Vet Med Assoc* 215:938, 1999.
59. Angles JM, Feldman EC, Nelson RW et al: Use of urine cortisol:creatinine ratio versus adrenocorticotropic hormone stimulation testing for monitoring mitotane treatment of pituitary-dependent hyperadrenocorticism in dogs, *J Am Vet Med Assoc* 211:1002, 1997.
60. Guptill L, Scott-Moncrieff JC, Bottoms G et al: Use of the urine cortisol:creatinine ratio to monitor treatment response in dogs with pituitary-dependent hyperadrenocorticism, *J Am Vet Med Assoc* 210:1158, 1997.
61. Randolph JF, Toomey J, Center SA et al: Use of the urine cortisol-to-creatinine ratio for monitoring dogs with pituitary-dependent hyperadrenocorticism during induction treatment with mitotane (o,p′-DDD), *Am J Vet Res* 59:258, 1998.
62. Kintzer PP, Peterson ME: Mitotane treatment of 32 dogs with cortisol-secreting adrenocortical neoplasms, *J Am Vet Med Assoc* 205:54, 1994.
63. Perez Alenza MD, Guerrero B, Melian C et al: Use of aminoglutethimide in the treatment of pituitary-dependent hyperadrenocorticism in the dog, *J Small Anim Pract* 43:104, 2002.
64. Reusch CE, Steffen T, Hoerauf A: The efficacy of L-deprenyl in dogs with pituitary-dependent hyperadrenocorticism, *J Vet Intern Med* 13:291, 1999.
65. Neiger R, Ramsey I, O'Connor J et al: Trilostane treatment of 78 dogs with pituitary-dependent hyperadrenocorticism, *Vet Rec* 150:799, 2002.
66. Ruckstuhl NS, Nett CS, Reusch CE: Results of clinical examinations, laboratory tests, and ultrasonography in dogs with pituitary-dependent hyperadrenocorticism treated with trilostane, *Am J Vet Res* 63:506, 2002.
67. Anderson CR, Birchard SJ, Powers BE et al: Surgical treatment of adrenocortical tumors: 21 cases (1990-1996), *J Am Anim Hosp Assoc* 37:93, 2001.
68. Goossens MMC, Feldman EC, Theon AP et al: Efficacy of cobalt 60 radiotherapy in dogs with pituitary-dependent hyperadrenocorticism, *J Am Vet Med Assoc* 212:374, 1998.
69. Gilson SD, Withrow SJ, Wheeler SL et al: Pheochromocytoma in 50 dogs, *J Vet Intern Med* 8:228, 1994.
70. Barthez PY, Marks SL, Woo J et al: Pheochromocytoma in dogs: 61 cases (1984-1995), *J Vet Intern Med* 11:272, 1997.
71. Platt SR, Sheppard BJ, Graham J et al: Pheochromocytoma in the vertebral canal of two dogs, *J Am Anim Hosp Assoc* 34:365, 1998.
72. Williams JE, Hackner SG: Pheochromocytoma presenting as acute retroperitoneal hemorrhage in a dog, *J Vet Emerg Crit Care* 11:221, 2001.
73. Berry CR, Wright KN, Breitschwerdt EB et al: Use of 123-Iodine metaiodobenzylguanidine scintigraphy for the diagnosis of a pheochromocytoma in a dog, *Vet Radiol Ultrasound* 34:52, 1993.
74. Rosol TJ, Nagode LA, Couto CG et al: Parathyroid hormone (PTH)–related protein, PTH, and 1,25-dihydroxyvitamin D in dogs with cancer-associated hypercalcemia, *Endocrinology* 131:1157, 1992.
75. Grone A, Weckmann MT, Blomme EAG et al: Dependence of humoral hypercalcemia of malignancy on parathyroid hormone-related protein expression in the canine anal sac apocrine gland adenocarcinoma (CAC-8) nude mouse model, *Vet Pathol* 35:344, 1998.
76. Pressler BM, Rotstein DS, Law JM et al: Hypercalcemia and high parathyroid hormone-related protein concentration associated with malignant melanoma in a dog, *J Am Vet Med Assoc* 221:263, 2002.
77. Fradkin JM, Braniecki AM, Craig TM et al: Elevated parathyroid hormone-related protein and hypercalcemia in two dogs with schistosomiasis, *J Am Anim Hosp Assoc* 37:349, 2001.
78. Rosol TJ, Chew DJ, Hammer AS et al: Effect of mithramycin on hypercalcemia in dogs, *J Am Anim Hosp Assoc* 30:244, 1994.
79. Bennett PF, DeNicola DB, Bonney P et al: Canine anal sac adenocarcinomas: clinical presentation and response to therapy, *J Vet Intern Med* 16:100, 2002.
80. Nguyen LQ, Arseven OK, Gerber H et al: Cloning of the cat TSH receptor and evidence against an autoimmune etiology of feline hyperthyroidism, *Endocrinology* 143:395, 2002.
81. Kass PH, Peterson ME, Levy J et al: Evaluation of environmental, nutritional, and host factors in cats with hyperthyroidism, *J Vet Intern Med* 13:323, 1999.
82. Martin KM, Rossing MA, Ryland LM et al: Evaluation of dietary and environmental risk factors for hyperthyroidism in cats, *J Am Vet Med Assoc* 217:853, 2000.
83. Johnson LA, Ford HC, Tarttelin ME et al: Iodine content of commercially prepared cat foods, *N Z Vet J* 40:18, 1992.
84. Tarttelin MF, Johnson LA, Cooke RR et al: Serum free thyroxine levels respond inversely to changes in levels of dietary iodine in the domestic cat, *N Z Vet J* 40:66, 1992.
85. Kyle AHM, Tarttelin MF, Cooke RR et al: Serum free thyroxine levels in cats maintained on diets relatively high or low in iodine, *N Z Vet J* 42:101, 1994.
86. Broussard JD, Peterson ME, Fox PR: Changes in clinical and laboratory findings in cats with hyperthyroidism from 1983 to 1993, *J Am Vet Med Assoc* 206:302, 1995.
87. Bucknell DG: Feline hyperthyroidism: spectrum of clinical presentations and response to carbimazole therapy, *Aust Vet J* 78:462, 2000.
88. van der Woerdt A, Peterson ME: Prevalence of ocular abnormalities in cats with hyperthyroidism, *J Vet Intern Med* 14:202, 2000.
89. Nemzek JA, Kruger JM, Walshaw R et al: Acute onset of hypokalemia and muscular weakness in four hyperthyroid cats, *J Am Vet Med Assoc* 205:65, 1994.
90. Reusch CE, Tomsa K: Serum fructosamine

concentration in cats with overt hyperthyroidism, *J Am Vet Med Assoc* 215:1297, 1999.
91. McLoughlin MA, DiBartola SP, Birchard SJ et al: Influence of systemic nonthyroidal illness on serum concentration of thyroxine in hyperthyroid cats, *J Am Anim Hosp Assoc* 29:227, 1993.
92. Peterson ME, Melian C, Nichols R: Measurement of serum concentrations of free thyroxine, total thyroxine, and total triiodothyronine in cats with hyperthyroidism and cats with nonthyroidal disease, *J Am Vet Med Assoc* 218:529, 2001.
93. Peterson ME, Broussard JD, Gamble DA: Use of the thyrotropin releasing hormone stimulation test to diagnose mild hyperthyroidism in cats, *J Vet Intern Med* 8:279, 1994.
94. Tomsa K, Glaus TM, Kacl GM et al: Thyrotropin-releasing hormone stimulation test to assess thyroid function in severely sick cats, *J Vet Intern Med* 15:89, 2001.
95. Daniel GB, Sharp DS, Nieckarz JA et al: Quantitative thyroid scintigraphy as a predictor of serum thyroxin concentration in normal and hyperthyroid cats, *Vet Radiol Ultrasound* 43:374, 2002.
96. Nieckarz JA, Daniel GB: The effect of methimazole on thyroid uptake of pertechnetate and radioiodine in normal cats, *Vet Radiol Ultrasound* 42:448, 2001.
97. Wisner ER, Theon AP, Nyland TG et al: Ultrasonographic examination of the thyroid gland of hyperthyroid cats: comparison to 99mTcO4-scintigraphy, *Vet Radiol Ultrasound* 35:53, 1994.
98. Graves TK, Olivier NB, Nachreiner RF et al: Changes in renal function associated with treatment of hyperthyroidism in cats, *Am J Vet Res* 55:1745, 1994.
99. DiBartola SP, Broome MR, Stein BS et al: Effect of treatment of hyperthyroidism on renal function in cats, *J Am Vet Med Assoc* 208:875, 1996.
100. Adams WH, Daniel GB, Legendre AM: Investigation of the effects of hyperthyroidism on renal function in the cat, *Can J Vet Res* 61:53, 1997.
101. Becker TJ, Graves TK, Kruger JM et al: Effects of methimazole on renal function in cats with hyperthyroidism, *J Am Anim Hosp Assoc* 36:215, 2000.
102. Foster DJ, Thoday KL: Use of propranolol and potassium iodate in the presurgical management of hyperthyroid cats, *J Small Anim Pract* 40:307, 1999.
103. Slater MR, Geller S, Rogers K: Long-term health and predictors of survival for hyperthyroid cats treated with iodine 131, *J Vet Intern Med* 15:47, 2001.
104. Theon AP, Van Vechten MK, Feldman E: Prospective randomized comparison of intravenous versus subcutaneous administration of radioiodine for treatment of hyperthyroidism in cats, *Am J Vet Res* 55:1734, 1994.
105. Peterson ME, Becker DV: Radioiodine treatment of 524 cats with hyperthyroidism, *J Am Vet Med Assoc* 207:1422, 1995.
106. Walker MC, Schaer M: Percutaneous ethanol treatment of hyperthyroidism in a cat, *Feline Pract* 26:10, 1998.
107. Goldstein RE, Long C, Swift NC et al: Percutaneous ethanol injection for treatment of unilateral hyperplastic thyroid nodules in cats, *J Am Vet Med Assoc* 218:1298, 2001.
108. Wells AL, Long CD, Hornof WJ et al: Use of percutaneous ethanol injection for treatment of bilateral hyperplastic thyroid nodules in cats, *J Am Vet Med Assoc* 218:1293, 2001.
109. Lutz TA, Rand JS: Plasma amylin and insulin concentrations in normoglycemic and hyperglycemic cats, *Can Vet J* 37:27, 1996.
110. Hall DG, Kelley LC, Gray ML et al: Lymphocytic inflammation of pancreatic islets in a diabetic cat, *J Vet Diagn Invest* 9:98, 1997.
111. Hoenig M, Reusch C, Peterson ME: Beta cell and insulin antibodies in treated and untreated diabetic cats, *Vet Immunol Immunopathol* 77:93, 2000.
112. Elliott DA, Feldman EC, Koblik PD et al: Prevalence of pituitary tumors among diabetic cats with insulin resistance, *J Am Vet Med Assoc* 216:1765, 2000.
113. Norman EJ, Mooney CT: Diagnosis and management of diabetes mellitus in five cats with somatotrophic abnormalities, *J Feline Med Surg* 2:183, 2000.
114. Lewitt MS, Hazel SJ, Church DB et al: Regulation of insulin-like growth factor-binding protein-3 ternary complex in feline diabetes mellitus, *J Endocrinol* 166:21, 2000.
115. Appleton DJ, Rans JS, Sunvold GD: Insulin sensitivity decreases with obesity, and lean cats with low insulin sensitivity are at greatest risk of glucose intolerance with weight gain, *J Feline Med Surg* 3:211, 2001.
116. Nelson RW, Griffey SM, Feldman EC et al: Transient clinical diabetes mellitus in cats: 10 cases (1989-1991), *J Vet Intern Med* 13:28, 1999.
117. Rand JS, Kinnaird E, Baglioni A et al: Acute stress hyperglycemia in cats is associated with struggling and increased concentrations of lactate and norepinephrine, *J Vet Intern Med* 16:123, 2002.
118. Sparkes AH, Adams DT, Cripps PJ et al: Inter- and intraindividual variability of the response to intravenous glucose tolerance testing in cats, *Am J Vet Res* 57:1294, 1996.
119. Crenshaw KL, Peterson ME: Pretreatment clinical and laboratory evaluation of cats with diabetes mellitus: 104 cases (1992-1994), *J Am Vet Med Assoc* 209:943, 1996.
120. Christopher MM, Broussard JD, Peterson ME: Heinz body formation associated with ketoacidosis in diabetic cats, *J Vet Intern Med* 9:24, 1995.
121. Nelson RW, Scott-Moncrieff JC, Feldman EC et al: Effect of dietary insoluble fiber on control of glycemia in cats with naturally acquired diabetes mellitus, *J Am Vet Med Assoc* 216:1082, 2000.
122. Cohn LA, Dodam JR, McCaw DL et al: Effects of chromium supplementation on glucose tolerance in obese and nonobese cats, *Am J Vet Res* 60:1360, 1999.
123. Nelson RW, Lynn RC, Wagner-Mann CC et al: Efficacy of protamine zinc insulin for treatment of diabetes mellitus in cats, *J Am Vet Med Assoc* 218:38, 2001.
124. Whitley NT, Drobatz KJ, Panciera DL: Insulin overdose in dogs and cats: 28 cases. (1986-1993), *J Am Vet Med Assoc* 211:326, 1997.
125. Thompson MD, Taylor SM, Adams VJ et al: Comparison of glucose concentrations in blood samples obtained with a marginal ear vein nick technique versus from a peripheral vein in healthy cats and cats with diabetes mellitus, *J Am Vet Med Assoc* 221:389, 2002.
126. Crenshaw KL, Peterson ME, Heeb LA et al: Serum fructosamine concentration as an index of glycemia in cats with diabetes mellitus and stress hyperglycemia, *J Vet Intern Med* 10:360, 1996.
127. Thoresen SI, Bredal WP: Clinical usefulness of fructosamine measurements in diagnosing and monitoring feline diabetes mellitus, *J Small Anim Pract* 37:64, 1996.
128. Elliot DA, Nelson RW, Feldman EC et al: Glycosylated hemoglobin concentration for assessment of glycemic control in diabetic cats, *J Vet Intern Med* 11:161, 1997.

CHAPTER 18

Spleen and Lymph Nodes

JOHNNY D. HOSKINS

THE SPLEEN

The spleen is an important organ for many pathologic processes because it is located between the portal and systemic circulatory systems. The spleen may be affected with primary disease that may be the reason a dog or cat is ill. The spleen can also be secondarily affected by a systemic disease and act as a sentinel organ for an underlying disease process.

Splenic Storage Function

The spleen in dogs and cats has a large capacity to store blood and may contain 10% to 20% of the total blood volume.[1-3] This blood storage capacity is related to the abundance of venous sinuses in the spleen. For example, the blood volume in awake nonsplenectomized cats is approximately 26 ml/lb (56 ml/kg) of body weight, whereas that of splenectomized cats is approximately 20 ml/lb (44 ml/kg).[3] The reservoir function of the spleen serves to release erythrocytes into the circulation during strenuous exercise and also to retain a mass of erythrocytes that are readily available in case of acute blood loss or hemolysis. An appreciable decrease in the packed cell volume after hemorrhage may not occur for several hours because this mass of erythrocytes has contributed to the blood volume by splenic contraction.

SPLENOMEGALY

Splenomegaly may be a focal or generalized enlargement of the spleen (Box 18-1). Focal enlargement of the spleen may be caused by neoplasia or by a nonneoplastic condition. Generalized enlargement of the spleen may be caused by inflammatory or infectious conditions, lymphoreticular hyperplasia, congestion, and infiltrative disease.

Focal splenic tumors may include hemangioma, hemangiosarcomas, fibrosarcoma, leiomyosarcoma, leiomyoma, myelolipoma, and lymphoma; nonneoplastic conditions may include hematoma, abscess, nodular hyperplasia, infarction, and cyst formation following traumatic-induced hematoma. Inflammatory splenomegaly (splenitis) usually results from the effects of an infectious agent. Inflammatory splenomegaly can be suppurative, necrotizing, eosinophilic, lymphoplasmacytic, or granulomatous or pyogranulomatous splenitis.[4]

Suppurative splenitis is generally associated with penetrating wounds to the abdomen, migrating foreign bodies, hematogenous dissemination of bacterial infection from endocarditis or pyogenic sepsis, secondary to splenic torsion, and protozoal infections, such as toxoplasmosis. Necrotizing splenitis may be caused by gas-forming anaerobes or *Salmonella* species and is often seen in cases of splenic torsion or neoplasia. Eosinophilic infiltrates in the spleen can be seen with hypereosinophilic syndrome of cats and eosinophilic gastroenteritis of dogs. Lymphoplasmacytic splenitis is usually associated with infectious conditions, such as infectious canine hepatitis, ehrlichiosis, pyometra, brucellosis, and hemobartonellosis. Granulomatous or pyogranulomatous splenitis occurs secondarily to blastomycosis, sporotrichosis, mycobacteriosis, and feline infectious peritonitis.

BOX 18-1 Causes of Splenomegaly

Generalized Splenomegaly

Inflammatory

Suppurative
- Bacterial emboli
- Foreign bodies
- Splenic torsion toxoplasmosis

Eosinophilic
- Hypereosinophilic syndrome (cat)
- Eosinophilic gastroenteritis (dog)

Granulomatous
- Systemic mycoses
- Mycobacterial infections
- Brucellosis

Pyogranulomatous
- Systemic mycoses

Focal Splenomegaly

Neoplastic Lesions

Hemangioma
Hemangiosarcoma
Fibrosarcoma
Leiomyosarcoma
Leiomyoma
Myelolipoma
Lymphoma

Nonneoplastic Lesions

Hematomas
Abscess
Nodular hyperplasia
Infarction
Cysts (resolution of hematoma)

Noninflammatory, Nonneoplastic

Chronic antigenic stimulation
- Chronic bacterial infections
  - Endocarditis
  - Diskospondylitis
  - Brucellosis
- Immune-mediated diseases
  - Systemic lupus erythematosus
  - Immune-mediated hemolytic anemia
  - Immune-mediated thrombocytopenia
- Congestion
  - Tranquilizers and barbiturates
  - Congestive heart failure
  - Splenic torsion
- Extramedullary hematopoiesis
  - Pyometra
- Immune-mediated hemolytic anemia
  - Chronic anemia of any cause
  - Immune-mediated thrombocytopenia
- Amyloidosis

Neoplastic (Infiltrative)

Leukemia
Mastocytoma
Lymphoma
Myeloma
Malignant histiocytosis (dogs)

Nodular hyperplastic splenomegaly is a spleen that reacts to blood-borne antigens or erythrocytic destruction, with resultant hyperplasia of its mononuclear and lymphoid components. This form of splenomegaly is common in dogs with bacterial endocarditis, chronic bacteremic disorders such as diskospondylitis and brucellosis, systemic lupus erythematosus, and hemolytic disorders resulting in erythrocytic destruction. Congestive splenomegaly develops when the venous drainage from the spleen is impaired or obstructed. Administration of most tranquilizers and barbiturates will immediately cause smooth muscle relaxation in the splenic capsule and a congestive splenomegaly. Right-sided heart failure and portal hypertension may also lead to congestive splenomegaly. Splenic torsion is another example of congestive splenomegaly.

Torsion of the spleen is often associated with the gastric dilatation-volvulus syndrome in dogs and manifests as sudden-onset acute abdominal pain and distention, depression, anorexia, and vomiting.[5] Infiltrative splenomegaly with neoplastic cells is one of the more common causes of generalized splenic enlargement in dogs and cats. Neoplastic cellular infiltration into the spleen may be seen in cases of acute and chronic leukemia, systemic mastocytosis, malignant lymphoma, multiple myeloma, and malignant histiocytosis. Splenomegaly from metastatic dissemination of nonhematologic neoplasms occurs infrequently in dogs and cats.

Nonneoplastic causes of infiltrative splenomegaly are less common than neoplastic causes. Splenic extramedullary hematopoiesis may result in splenomegaly and is more common in dogs than in cats. Extramedullary hematopoiesis can be seen in conditions such as pyometra, immune-mediated hemolytic anemia, immune-mediated thrombocytopenia, chronic anemia, infectious disease, malignancy, amyloidosis, hypereosinophilic syndrome, and systemic lupus erythematosus.

Clinical Approach to Splenomegaly

The clinical signs and historical aspects of dogs and cats with splenomegaly are often vague and nonspecific and may result from the underlying disease rather than be due to the splenic enlargement. History may reveal anorexia, weight loss, weakness, abdominal enlargement, vomiting, or polyuria-polydipsia. The cause of the polyuria-polydipsia is unclear, but it may be caused by psychogenic polydipsia that results from abdominal pain or distention of the capsular stretch receptors of the spleen.[4] Splenectomy in these animals usually results in prompt resolution of the polyuria and polydipsia.

Physical examination of animals with splenic disorders may be normal or may reveal various abnormalities. Pallor of the mucous membranes and signs of bleeding (e.g., petechiae or ecchymoses) may be seen. The spleen may be palpable, but all palpable spleens are not abnormal (especially in German shepherds) and not all enlarged spleens are palpable.[4] The spleen is usually located in the cranial abdominal quadrant, although in some breeds, such as miniature schnauzers, cocker spaniels, Irish setters, greyhounds, and German shepherds, it may also be located in the ventral midabdomen.[6] Peripheral lymph nodes should be examined for size since many diseases that cause splenomegaly may also cause lymphadenopathy. In most cats with splenomegaly, the splenic surface will be smooth; in dogs, an enlarged spleen can be either smooth or irregular (i.e., "lumpy-bumpy"). Localized splenic masses are common in the dog but not in the cat. Finally, associated hepatomegaly may be present, depending on the underlying cause of the splenomegaly (e.g., posthepatic portal hypertension).

Diagnostic Evaluation

The complete blood count including buffy coat smears, serum chemistry profile, urinalysis, fine-needle aspiration of the spleen, bone marrow aspiration, ultrasonography, thoracic and abdominal radiography, and exploratory laparotomy may be performed during the clinical evaluation process. These tests are not listed in order of preference; they should be selected based on the individual case. In addition, tests to assess for the existence of feline leukemia virus infection, feline immunodeficiency virus infection, feline infectious peritonitis, bartonellosis, and toxoplasmosis should be performed in all cats with splenomegaly.

The spleen can exert a marked influence on the hemogram. Two patterns of hematologic changes are recognized in the dog and cat with splenomegaly: hypersplenism and hyposplenism.[2] Hypersplenism occurs as a result of increased reticuloendothelial activity and is uncommon; hyposplenism is more common and results in changes similar to those seen in the splenectomized animal. In hypersplenism, the changes are those of cytopenias. In hyposplenism, changes may include thrombocytosis, presence of nucleated red blood cells and nuclear red blood cell remnants, presence of acanthocytes and fragments, and reticulocytosis.

Extramedullary hematopoiesis in the spleen may effect a change in the complete blood count that is referred to as the *leukoerythroblastic effect.* In this situation, there is loss of normal inhibitory influences on the bone marrow because inhibitory influences are not operative at extramedullary sites (e.g., the spleen). Because the spleen retains its fetal hematopoietic potential during adult life, the extramedullary hematopoiesis may cause significant increases in nucleated red blood cells and immature white blood cells that result in a substantial left shift of the white blood cells, which at first glance may appear to represent an underlying infectious cause. In a study of 100 dogs with splenomegaly, schistocytosis was seen in 23% of the dogs with neoplastic disease, whereas it was seen in only 3% of the dogs with nonneoplastic disease.[7] In the same study, the authors found that dogs with anemia, increased numbers of nucleated red blood cells, and abnormal red blood cell morphology or splenic rupture had a greater chance of having splenic neoplasia.

Abnormalities in serum chemistry profile and urinalysis are uncommon. These tests seldom provide a definitive diagnosis, but they may give supportive evidence of an underlying disease process. For example, hypercalcemia and hyperglobulinemia may be associated with neoplastic disease (e.g., lymphosarcoma, multiple myeloma), and hemoglobinemia, hemoglobinuria, hyperbilirubinemia, bilirubinuria, and elevated serum alkaline phosphatase are common findings in dogs with splenic torsion.

Fine-needle aspiration of an enlarged spleen is a safe and reliable method for evaluation of animals with splenomegaly.[8] The procedure can be performed with the animal in right lateral or dorsal recumbency using manual restraint or mild sedation. A handheld 12-ml disposable plastic syringe or an aspiration gun using a 20-ml plastic syringe can be used to obtain an aspiration biopsy specimen from the spleen. A 25- or 23-gauge 1- to 1½-inch needle can be used. The area to be aspirated is identified by palpation or ultrasonography, and the overlying abdominal wall is clipped and surgically prepared. The spleen is then localized by palpation or ultrasonography, and the needle is quickly advanced into the spleen. After suction is applied one time without moving the needle, the needle and syringe are quickly removed. The normal splenic cytology consists primarily of small lymphocytes with an occasional neutrophil and large lymphocyte. The fine-needle aspiration may reveal a definitive diagnosis such as hematopoietic neoplasia or an infectious disease (identification of organisms), but can also be beneficial in the categorization of generalized splenomegaly. Fine-needle aspiration is less effective in establishing a diagnosis in localized splenomegaly than in generalized splenomegaly.

Abdominal radiography may differentiate between diffuse and localized splenomegaly and may also provide evidence for a definitive diagnosis. For example, dogs with splenic torsion usually have massive splenomegaly with distinct edges and markedly increased density.[4] In addition, dogs with splenic torsion may have decreased visceral abdominal detail because of abdominal effusion or because the dorsal extremity or body of the spleen may not be observed in its normal position (caudal and to the left of the stomach).[9] Hepatomegaly along with diffuse splenomegaly may indicate that congestive splenomegaly secondary to right-sided heart disease or infiltrative splenomegaly affecting the liver and spleen (e.g., lymphosarcoma, hematopoietic neoplasia, or amyloidosis) is present. Evaluation of thoracic radiographs to assess for metastatic disease is of paramount importance in dogs and cats with splenic disease (especially those with focal splenomegaly).

Abdominal ultrasonography may define the underlying disease by a noninvasive means. Diffuse enlargement with normal splenic parenchyma is seen in acute (sepsis, toxemia) or passive congestion (chronic liver disease, right-sided heart failure), vascular compromise, and diffuse cellular infiltration. Reduced echogenicity can be seen with torsion of the spleen, splenic vein thrombosis, and lymphoma or leukemia. Focal hypoechoic regions in the spleen can be another pattern visualized secondary to lymphoma or infarction.[10] Ultrasonography of splenic hemangiosarcoma has variable echo patterns (anechoic to hyperechoic).[11] Hematomas (<5 cm) are usually hypoechoic to anechoic, whereas large ones (>6 cm) contain a mixture of anechoic, hypoechoic, hyperechoic, and isoechoic material.[12] Dogs with splenic torsion have severely enlarged spleens, with diffuse anechoic areas separated by small linear echoes.[13] Splenic congestion from splenic torsion is suggested by the presence of enlarged splenic veins at the hilus and within splenic parenchyma. Splenic ultrasonography in dogs with lymphosarcoma has most consistently had a focal to diffuse hypoechoic pattern.[14,15] The multifocal hypoechoic foci have been described as having a "Swiss-cheese" appearance. Ultrasonographic evaluation of the right atrium for masses should be performed in dogs with suspected splenic hemangiosarcoma. If right atrial masses are found to exist in conjunction with splenic ultrasound abnormalities, the likelihood is higher that the animal has hemangiosarcoma versus a more benign disease such as hematoma or hemangioma of the spleen. Hepatic ultrasonography may also be useful in determining whether metastatic disease exists in association with a splenic mass. If multiple nodules are visualized in the liver by ultrasound evaluation, and there is a splenic mass, a greater likelihood exists that the hepatic nodules represent metastatic disease. If only one or two hepatic nodules are present, nodular regeneration of the liver should be considered.

If a diagnosis cannot be obtained by the previously mentioned diagnostic procedures, or if the animal has suffered significant blood loss from the spleen, exploratory laparotomy may be indicated. Splenectomy may cause pronounced leukocytosis after splenectomy, decrease in the packed cell volume and increase in platelet numbers, increased numbers of nucleated red blood cells and Howell-Jolly bodies, altered immune defenses, and decreased body iron for a short period of time, and affected animals may be more prone to parasitic infections of the red blood cells (e.g., *Hemobartonella* and *Babesia* species). One additional concern should be given consideration when planning exploratory laparotomy: the association between cardiac arrhythmias and mass lesions of the canine spleen. A recent report described 106 dogs with splenic masses (which were composed of hemangiosarcomas, hematomas, and leiomyosarcomas), and 35% (37 of 106) had ventricular arrhythmias.[16] All dogs with diagnosed or suspected mass lesions of the spleen should be evaluated prior to anesthesia for cardiac arrhythmias with an electrocardiogram or simultaneous cardiac auscultation and pulse palpation for the detection of pulse deficit. Inhalation anesthesia is recommended if arrhythmias are present or as a method to prevent or minimize their occurrence. Continuous cardiac monitoring is recommended during the surgical procedure, and postoperative monitoring is indicated in the form of lead II electrocardiogram recordings and careful examination for pulse deficits daily for at least 3 days.

THE LYMPH NODES

One of the most common clinical abnormalities seen in veterinary practice is lymph node enlargement (Box 18-2). The peripheral lymph nodes are frequently evaluated because of their accessibility; however, radiographic and ultrasonographic evaluation of the thorax or abdomen can reveal masses that represent enlarged visceral lymph nodes. Evaluation of changes in lymph nodes usually involves fine-needle aspiration or core biopsy of the affected tissue. If aspiration cytology is not conclusive, an excisional biopsy is preferable to a core biopsy. Histopathologic evaluation of lymph node architecture is often crucial for a diagnosis of lymphoma, especially in the case of lymphocytic lymphoma. With metastatic lesions or inflammation caused by fungal agents, a core biopsy may miss the affected area and, hence, the diagnosis. Markedly enlarged lymph nodes often have a necrotic center resulting either from an inflammatory process causing abscess or from a neoplastic process that has outgrown its blood supply, causing ischemic necrosis. If possible, the smaller lymph nodes should be evaluated in a patient with generalized or regional lymphadenopathy. If a solitary node is markedly enlarged, the center of the lymph node should be avoided during sampling.

Lymph nodes consist of a capsule, subcapsular sinus, cortex, paracortex, postcapillary venules, medullary cords, and medullary sinuses. The primary function of the lymph node is directing the immune response toward antigens that filter into the lymph node from peripheral tissue. Antigens are processed by the dendritic reticular cells (macrophages that are most likely of bone marrow origin) and are presented to the lymphocytes, which make up most of the lymph node cell population. Fine-needle aspiration cytology of a normal lymph node demonstrates primarily small lymphocytes (more than 90%); smaller numbers of intermediate lymphocytes and lymphoblasts can be found, as well. An occasional plasma cell, neutrophil, mast cell, or eosinophil may be present. If a large amount of blood contamination is evident in the aspirate, peripheral blood leu-

BOX 18-2 Disorders Affecting the Lymph Nodes and Lymphatic Vessels

Lymph Node Hypoplasia

Advanced age
FeLV
Malnutrition
Hyperadrenocorticism
- Drugs
- Corticosteroids
- Antineoplastic agents
- Radiation therapy

Lymph Node Hyperplasia +/− Inflammation

Infectious agents
- Bacterial *(Mycobacteria, Streptococcus)*
- Viral (FeLV, FIV)
- Fungal *(Blastomyces, Cryptococcus)*
- Rickettsial *(Ehrlichia, Neorickettsia helminthoeca)*
- Parasitic *(Leishmania, Toxoplasma)*
- Algal *(Prototheca)*

Immune-mediated diseases
Chronic dermatopathies (usually eosinophilic)
Vaccine-associated
Feline lymphadenopathies
- Plexiform vascularization of lymph nodes
- FeLV/FIV-associated
- Eosinophilic granulomas complex
- Hypereosinophilic syndrome

Lymphangitis

Infectious agents
- Bacterial
- Fungal

Neoplasia (metastatic)
Trauma

Neoplasia

Lymphoma
Hematopoietic neoplasia
Metastatic neoplasia
- Melanoma
- Squamous cell carcinoma
- Perirectal adenocarcinoma
- Mammary adenocarcinoma
- Prostatic adenocarcinoma
- Osteosarcoma
- Mast cell tumors

FeLV, Feline leukemia virus; *FIV,* feline immunodeficiency virus.

kocytes such as neutrophils and eosinophils may occur in higher numbers. The cell population of a lymph node changes significantly with various causes of lymphadenopathy. Both neoplastic and nonneoplastic disorders can be recognized with aspirate cytology.

Nonneoplastic causes of lymphadenopathy can be divided into two categories: hyperplasia or inflammation. Lymphoid hyperplasia is characterized by increased numbers of intermediate lymphocytes, lymphoblasts, and plasma cells. With marked hyperplasia, Mott cells—plasma cells containing Russell bodies (distinct, empty appearing vesicles that represent dilated endoplasmic reticuli)—are often present. Lymphoid hyperplasia can be the result of systemic or localized antigenic stimulation. Generalized lymphoid hyperplasia can be seen with widespread dermatologic diseases (eosinophilic inflammation as well as hyperplasia may be evident in such cases) or canine ehrlichiosis or as an idiopathic syndrome in cats that may be associated with feline immunodeficiency virus, feline leukemia virus, or argyrophilic bacteria.[17,18] Localized lymphadenopathy is seen in lymph node draining sites of local inflammation, including inflammation associated with neoplasia. Because of the high incidence of dental disease in older dogs, the submandibular lymph nodes and tonsils are often mildly enlarged as a result of lymphoid hyperplasia.

Inflammatory lymphadenopathy, or lymphadenitis, is usually accompanied by some degree of lymphoid hyperplasia and is characterized by an increase in reactive lymphoid cells. The predominant cytologic change in lymphadenitis is increased numbers of neutrophils, eosinophils, or macrophages or of a mixed population of inflammatory cells. Suppurative or neutrophilic lymphadenitis is commonly seen with bacterial infection, whereas a granulomatous or pyogranulomatous lymphadenitis is most often seen with fungal diseases such as blastomycosis, coccidioidomycosis, or sporotrichosis. Mycobacterial infections, however, are associated with granulomatous rather than suppurative inflammation, as is brucellosis. Cryptococcosis is unique in that the host may not produce any inflammatory reaction to the organism. Lymph nodes may become completely effaced with the organism and appear soft and gelatinous. A mixed inflammatory response characterized by increases in neutrophils, macrophages, eosinophils, plasma cells, and mast cells is often seen with dermatopathies. Eosinophils may predominate in cases of flea allergy dermatitis or other causes of cutaneous hypersensitivity and the hypereosinophilic syndrome seen in cats. It is important to remember that mast cells and eosinophils are often increased in these disorders, and such increases should not be considered indicative of metastatic mast cell neoplasia.

Neoplastic diseases can cause either generalized or localized lymphadenopathy. Mast cell tumor, squamous cell carcinoma, melanoma, mammary gland adenocarcinoma, and perianal gland adenocarcinoma have a propensity for spread to regional lymph nodes via the lymphatic vessels. Osteosarcoma may metastasize to or infiltrate regional lymph nodes. The presence of neoplastic cells in a lymph node can elicit an immune response and result in lymphoid hyperplasia. Metastatic neoplasia, particularly squamous cell carcinoma, can also be accompanied by neutrophilic inflammation. In the case of squamous cell carcinoma, the keratin produced by the neoplastic squamous cells elicits a profound neutrophilic inflammatory response.

The primary differential diagnosis for generalized lymphadenopathy in the geriatric dog is lymphoma. Lymphoma is the most common hemolymphatic neoplasm in dogs, and the incidence of lymphoma increases with age. The diagnosis of lymphoma is often made cytologically but may require histopathologic confirmation in cases of lymphocytic or intermediate cell lymphoma. Quality cytologic preparations are necessary for diagnosis, and intact cells must be present for evaluation. Many enlarged lymph nodes, regardless of whether they are neoplastic, have necrotic centers. Aspiration into the necrotic center will result in a nondiagnostic sample consisting of necrotic debris and broken cells. Neoplastic lymphocytes have a tendency to be fragile, and gentle handing of the aspirated material is required to provide intact cells for evaluation. With an adequate sample, diagnosis of lymphoblastic lymphoma can be quite straightforward; cytology will demonstrate a homogenous population of large, deeply basophilic lymphoblasts with prominent nucleoli. However, lymphocytic lymphoma, follicular lymphoma, and lymphoma of mixed cell type can be difficult to distinguish from atypical benign hyperplasia. It is very important to obtain diagnostic samples before anticancer therapy is initiated because the character of the neoplastic cells can change significantly in response to the anticancer drugs used.[19] Once a diagnosis of lymphoma is made, clinical staging for prognosis includes a complete blood count, bone marrow biopsy, and serum chemistry profile. Several bone marrow samples obtained from different sites may be necessary to rule out bone marrow involvement. Even with a thorough evaluation, only 60% of cases with metastasis to bone marrow will be identified.[19] A core biopsy using a Jamshidi needle increases the chances of finding the neoplasm in the bone marrow.

Several studies of prognostic correlations of clinical findings (clinical stage, hypercalcemia, age, and body weight) have suggested that dogs with liver or spleen involvement have a poor prognosis and increased risk of organ failure as a result of tumor lysis syndrome (i.e., therapy-induced tumor necrosis).[20] Dogs with high-grade disease (lymphoblastic or immunoblastic) appear to have better survival times as well as better response to anticancer therapy.[21]

Unlike canine lymphoma, feline lymphoma has a bimodal age distribution that reflects the feline leukemia virus–associated lymphomas of young cats (average age at diagnosis, 3 years) and the non–virus-associated lymphomas of older cats (average age at diagnosis, 7 years). The alimentary form is more common in geriatric cats (average age at diagnosis, 8 years).[22] Prognosis in the cat is significantly affected by clinical stage, with complete remission occurring in 90% of cases in stages I and II and in 50% of cases in stages III, IV, and V. Additional negative prognostic indicators in the cat are presence of leukemia, anemia, neutropenia, feline leukemia virus infection, and sepsis. Several idiopathic lymphadenopathies have been reported, but all cases were in cats younger than 2 years of age. Plexiform vascularization of lymph nodes is a benign solitary lymphadenopathy that can affect geriatric cats.

Multiple myeloma is an uncommon neoplasm of lymphoid origin. It is seen most often in the dog, occurring in an estimated 3.6% of primary and secondary bone marrow neoplasms.[23] Multiple myeloma is characterized by proliferation of malignant plasma cells along with production of a monoclonal gammopathy of IgG or IgA isotype. Clinical findings in dogs include lameness associated with pathologic fractures and punctate osteolytic lesions, hemorrhage caused by decreased platelet function, polyuria-polydipsia, and retinal hemorrhage resulting from hyperviscosity. Clinicopathologic findings seen with multiple myeloma include nonregenerative anemia, leukopenia, and thrombocytopenia. The hematologic changes are often associated with plasma cell infiltration of the bone marrow. It is important to remember that other causes of bone marrow plasmacytosis should not be confused with multiple myeloma. Ehrlichiosis is associated with a significant infiltration of the bone marrow by plasma cells and can also be associated with a monoclonal gammopathy. Plasma cell proliferation may also be present in the lymph nodes and spleen of any animal demonstrating chronic antigenic stimulation.

The hemorrhagic diathesis associated with multiple myeloma can have several causes. Hyperviscosity alone will increase bleeding times, as the paraproteins present in the serum are thought to interfere with the coagulation cascade. In addition, paraproteins interfere with platelet adhesion and aggregation.[24] Serum chemical profile abnormalities often indicate renal dysfunction. Renal disease associated with multiple myeloma may be due to concurrent hypercalcemia or glomerular damage associated with filtration of myeloma proteins.

References

1. Barton CL: The spleen: pathophysiology of disease. In Bojrab MJ, ed: *Pathophysiology in small animal surgery,* Philadelphia, 1981, Lea & Febiger.
2. Couto CG: Lymphadenopathy and splenomegaly. In Couto CG and Nelson RW, eds: *Essentials of small animal internal medicine,* St Louis, 1992, Mosby.
3. Breznock EM, Strack D: Blood volume of nonsplenectomized and splenectomized cats before and after hemorrhage, *Am J Vet Res* 43:1811, 1982.
4. Couto CG: Splenomegaly: a diagnostic approach, *Proc Am Coll Vet Intern Med Forum* 7:194, 1989.
5. Stead AC, Frankland AL, Borthwick R: Splenic torsion in dogs, *J Small Anim Pract* 24:549, 1983.
6. Couto CG: A diagnostic approach to splenomegaly in cats and dogs, *Vet Med* March:220, 1990.
7. Johnson KA, Powers BE, Withrow SJ et al: Splenomegaly in dogs predictors of neoplasia and survival after splenectomy, *J Vet Intern Med* 3:160, 1989.
8. O'Keefe DA, Couto CG: Fine-needle aspiration of the spleen as an aid in the diagnosis of splenomegaly, *J Vet Intern Med* 1:102, 1987.
9. Stickle RL: Radiographic signs of isolated splenic torsion in dogs: eight cases (1980-1987), *J Am Vet Med Assoc* 194:103, 1989.
10. Nyland TG, Hager D: Sonography of the liver, gallbladder, and spleen, *Vet Clin North Am Small Anim Pract* 15:1123, 1985.
11. Wrigley RH, Park RD, Konde LJ et al: Ultrasonographic features of splenic hemangiosarcoma in dogs: 18 cases (1980-1986), *J Am Vet Med Assoc* 192:1113, 1988.
12. Wrigley RH, Konde LJ, Park RD et al: Clinical features and diagnosis of splenic hematomas in dogs: 10 cases (1980-1987), *J Am Anim Hosp Assoc* 25:371, 1989.
13. Konde LJ, Wrigley RH, Lebel JL et al: Sonographic and radiographic changes associated with splenic torsion in the dog, *Vet Radiol* 30:41, 1989.
14. Lamb CR, Hartzband LE, Tidwell AS et al: Ultrasonographic findings in hepatic and splenic lymphosarcoma in dogs and cats, *Vet Radiol* 32:117, 1991.
15. Wrigley RH, Konde LJ, Park RD et al: Ultrasonographic features of splenic lymphosarcoma in dogs: 12 cases (1980-1986), *J Am Vet Med Assoc* 193:1565, 1988.

16. Knapp DW, Aronsohn MG, Harpster NK: Cardiac arrhythmias associated with mass lesions of the canine spleen, *J Am Anim Hosp Assoc* 29:122, 1993.
17. Kirkpatrick CE, Moore FM, Patnaik AK et al: Argyrophilic intracellular bacteria in some cats with idiopathic peripheral lymphadenopathy, *J Comp Pathol* 101:341, 1989.
18. Mooney S, Patnaik AK, Hayes AA et al: Generalized lymphadenopathy resembling lymphoma in cats: six cases (1972-1976), *J Am Vet Med Assoc* 190:897, 1987.
19. Carter RF, Valli VEO: Advances in the cytologic diagnosis of canine lymphoma, *Semin Vet Med Surg (Small Anim)* 3:167, 1988.
20. MacEwen EG, Hayes AA, Matus RE: Evaluation of some prognostic factors for advanced multicentric lymphosarcoma in the dog: 147 cases (1978-1981), *J Am Vet Med Assoc* 190:564, 1987.
21. Greenlee PG, Filippa DA, Quimby FW et al: Lymphomas in dogs: a morphologic, immunologic, and clinical study, *Cancer* 66:480, 1990.
22. Hardy WD: Hematopoietic tumors of cats, *J Am Anim Hosp Assoc* 17:921, 1981.
23. Matus RE, Leifer CE, MacEwen EG et al: Prognostic factors for multiple myeloma in the dog, *J Am Vet Med Assoc* 188:1288, 1986.
24. Shepard V, Dodds-Laffin W, Laffin R: Gamma A myeloma in a dog with defective hemostasis, *J Am Vet Med Assoc* 160:1121, 1972.

CHAPTER 19

The Urinary System

JOHNNY D. HOSKINS

Chronic renal failure (CRF) of older dogs and cats is defined as primary renal failure that has prevailed for a lengthy period, usually months to years. Other urinary disorders other than CRF that may concurrently be seen in middle-aged or geriatric dogs and cats include nephrolithiasis, urinary incontinence, urinary bladder tumors, pyelonephritis, amyloidosis, and perirenal pseudocysts. Diagnosis of these urinary disorders separate from the existing CRF can be a challenge because the signs of these related diseases are often insidious, nonspecific, and atypical in older dogs and cats.

CHRONIC RENAL FAILURE

Kidneys of geriatric dogs and cats are smaller in weight and size, which is reflected in decreased glomerular numbers, decreased tubular size and weight, and increased mesangium and fibrosis.[1] These changes in morphology are associated with decreased renal blood flow, glomerular filtration, urinary concentration ability, and ability to maintain sodium, water, and acid-base homeostasis. Decreased concentrations of renin, aldosterone, and activated vitamin D may also occur.

Clinical History

Polydipsia and polyuria, and sometimes nocturia, are among the earliest clinical signs of CRF. Cat owners, probably as a result of the cat's voiding habits, recognize these signs less often. Dehydration results if water intake fails to keep up with urinary water losses. Gastrointestinal complications are usually the clinical signs of uremia.[2] Anorexia may be manifested at first as a selective appetite. The dog or cat refuses its regular food but will eat a more palatable pet food (canned food); later this food is also refused, and the animal will eat only "table food." The inappetence may progress to complete refusal of all food. Weight loss may result from a combination of inadequate caloric intake, the catabolic effects of uremia, and intestinal malabsorption secondary to uremic gastroenteritis.

Vomiting results from the effects of uremic toxins on the medullary chemoreceptor trigger zone and from uremic gastroenteritis. Vomiting may not occur until the advanced stages of CRF. The severity of vomiting usually varies with the degree of azotemia. Hematemesis may occur if there is ulcerative uremic gastritis. Uremic stomatitis may be observed in the dog with severe uremia. Ulcerations may be located on the buccal mucosa and tongue, and necrosis and sloughing of the anterior portion of the tongue may occur. Diarrhea, frequently hemorrhagic, may occur with severe uremia because of uremic enterocolitis. Constipation may occur and is common in cats.

Neurologic abnormalities associated with uremia may include dullness, lethargy, tremors, altered gait, myoclonus, seizures, stupor, and coma. Many of the neurologic signs associated with CRF may be due to the effects of uremia or secondary hyperparathyroidism. Cats with hypokalemic polymyopathy may exhibit cervical ventroflexion, difficulty walking, inability to jump up onto resting areas, and generalized muscle weakness.[3,4] Cardiac arrhythmias may occur as a result of the hypokalemia or underlying cardiac disease.

Arterial hypertension is a common complication of CRF in older dogs and cats, occurring in 60% of cats and 50% of dogs.[5-7] CRF with associated hypertension should always be considered whenever dogs or cats experience sudden blindness and hyphema.

Physical Findings

Some dogs and cats with early CRF demonstrate no physical abnormalities. The body condition of symptomatic dogs and cats may be poor, with muscle wasting and a poor haircoat.[2,8,9] Renomegaly may be present and may be associated with hydronephrosis, renal tumors, pyelonephritis, and amyloidosis. In one CRF study, small and irregular kidneys were palpable in 25% and large kidneys in 25% of the cats studied.[8] Chronic renal diseases associated with large kidneys in older cats include renal lymphosarcoma, polycystic renal disease, perirenal pseudocyst, and feline infectious peritonitis.[8] Additional physical abnormalities include oral ulceration, pale mucous membranes, and retinal lesions. Ocular abnormalities may include reduced pupillary light reflexes, papilledema, retinal arterial tortuosity, retinal hemorrhage, retinal detachment, hyphema, anterior uveitis, and glaucoma.[5-7] A systolic murmur may result from underlying cardiac disease or from CRF, if there is severe anemia. Subcutaneous edema and hydrothorax may be observed in dogs and cats with nephrotic syndrome.

Laboratory Findings

In older dogs and cats with CRF, laboratory evaluation typically shows increased blood urea nitrogen and serum creatinine, hyperphosphatemia, metabolic acidosis, and nonregenerative anemia. The urine specific gravity is usually in the isosthenuric range (1.007 to 1.015). Some cats with CRF can have a urine specific gravity greater than 1.025.[8,10] Other abnormalities may include hypokalemia, hypercholesterolemia, hypercalcemia or hypocalcemia, hyperamylasemia, and proteinuria. Survey abdominal radiography most often reveals reduced renal size with irregular renal contours, renal mineralization, and possible evidence of skeletal osteopenia. Renal ultrasonography may reveal increased cortical echogenicity, renal mineralization, renoliths, and reduced renal size.

In addition to the evaluation of CRF and its vague history and physical findings, older dogs and cats should undergo thorough evaluation for the presence of coexisting diseases. Other diseases to consider include diabetes mellitus, hepatic disease, hyperadrenocorticism, cardiac disease, inflammatory bowel disease, chronic pancreatitis, and neoplastic disease. Hyperthyroidism should always be considered in cats older than 7 years.

Management

Specific therapy for CRF consists of treatment developed to slow the progression of renal lesions by influencing the disease responsible for the renal lesions. Examples include the administration of antimicrobial agents for treatment of bacterial pyelonephritis; correction of hypercalcemia that is causing hypercalcemic nephropathy; removal of tumors or uroliths responsible for obstructive uropathy; administration of antifungal drugs for treatment of fungal infections; and correction of abnormal renal perfusion that has caused ischemic renal lesions.[2]

General guidelines for the medical management of older dogs and cats diagnosed with CRF are presented in Boxes 19-1 and 19-2. The medical management is intended to maximize residual renal function, slow the progression of renal failure, and alleviate the signs of uremia; these effects are achieved by correcting fluid, electrolyte, acid-base, endocrine, and nutritional status. Those animals that have uncompensated CRF and are unable to eat or accept oral medications because of severe uremia will require intensive fluid therapy before any conservative therapy is attempted (Box 19-3). These animals usually require initial treatment with intravenous fluids for at least 24 to 72 hours.[11] In addition, symptomatic treatment of gastrointestinal signs (nausea, anorexia, vomiting, hematemesis, diarrhea, and oral ulcerations) is with an H_2-receptor blocker (cimetidine, ranitidine, or famotidine) to reduce gastric hydrochloric acid production. Sucralfate may be administered as a gastrointestinal protectant. Animals that are vomiting may be treated with antiemetics such as metoclopramide. Renal function is evaluated after prerenal azotemia is corrected. The ultimate disposition and long-term management of the animal is then outlined for the owner.

Dietary therapy remains the cornerstone of long-term management of the animal with

BOX 19-1 Guidelines for Long-Term Management of Older Dogs Diagnosed with Chronic Renal Failure

Dietary Therapy

- Dietary therapy remains the cornerstone of medical management of dogs with chronic renal failure.
- Commercially prepared renal diets provide the best nutritional support if the dog will eat the diet.
- Homemade or commercially prepared kidney diets may be modified with flavoring agents to provide favorable odors and enhance palatability.

Fluid Therapy as Needed

- Oral fluids are often preferable if frequent vomiting is not a problem.

Antimicrobial Therapy

- Therapy is based on urine culture and sensitivity test results, if possible.
- Active chronic pyelonephritis should be treated for at least 6 to 8 weeks or until urine culture results are negative.
- Reculture after antimicrobial therapy has been discontinued for 1 week.
- Reculture 1 to 2 months later and every 3 to 6 months thereafter.
- Routinely performed urinalysis in older dogs may not be accurate enough to detect a mild to moderate urinary tract infection.

Intestinal Phosphorus-Binding Agents

- Before intestinal phosphorus-binding agents are used, restricted phosphorus diets should be fed in an attempt to normalize serum phosphorus concentration.
- When feeding restricted phosphorus diets, do not normalize the serum phosphorus concentration and then start administering the intestinal phosphorus-binding agents.
- It is preferable to use oral sucralfate or aluminum hydroxide at 10 to 30 mg/kg twice a day; capsules are better than suspension; always give them with restricted phosphorus diets.

Control of Vomiting and Nausea

- Administer oral famotidine at 0.5 mg/kg once or twice daily.
- Administer oral or subcutaneous metoclopramide at 0.2 to 0.4 mg/kg every 6 to 8 hours.
- Administer drugs 30 minutes before forced feeding.

Bone Marrow Stimulation

- Administer recombinant human erythropoietin (r-HuEPO) and use daily iron supplementation with ferrous sulfate at oral dosage of 100 to 300 mg per day.
- r-HuEPO is indicated if PCV < 21% and clinical signs from the nonregenerative anemia exist. An initial dose of 50 to 100 units/kg is given subcutaneously three times weekly until PCV of 37% to 45% for dogs is achieved. The r-HuEPO dosage is then reduced to twice weekly as the dog's PCV approaches the desired PCV, and then once weekly to prevent polycythemia. Maintenance dosage is usually one to two times weekly to maintain PCV within the target reference range.
- Treatment with r-HuEPO is withheld if PCV exceeds the desired target reference range. During maintenance, dosage adjustments are made every 3 to 4 weeks because of lag phase between desired PCV and r-HuEPO response.
- Failure to respond to adequate r-HuEPO therapy includes the presence of iron deficiency, external blood loss, hemolytic process, concurrent diseases, and development of anti–r-HuEPO antibodies.
- PCV should be monitored weekly until PCV is established in target reference range for at least 4 weeks. The PCV is then checked bimonthly or monthly.
- r-HuEPO injections are discontinued if polycythemia, fever, anorexia, joint pain, cellulitis at the injection site, or cutaneous or mucosal ulceration occurs.
- r-HuEPO should be withheld until hypertension, iron deficiency, and polycythemia are corrected.
- Severe erythroid hypoplasia is consistent with serum antibody production that usually occurs within 4 to 16 weeks of initiating r-HuEPO therapy. Incidence is about 20% to 30% of treated animals. The PCV will return to the pretreatment low PCV value. Antibodies will decrease over a variable period after discontinuation of the r-HuEPO therapy.
- Dogs that respond well to r-HuEPO therapy will have the nonregenerative anemia corrected and will have an improved quality of life.

Control of Hypertension with Daily Administration of Antihypertensive Drugs and Restricted Sodium Diets

- Monitor the control of blood pressure every 6 months.

Administration of Anabolic Steroids if Weight Loss Is Occurring

- Anabolic steroids increase vigor and appetite in dogs almost immediately.
- Dogs need to be eating for anabolic steroids to be helpful.
- Anabolic steroids cause an increase in erythrocyte production in the bone marrow beginning about 100 days after initiation of therapy.
- Give stanozolol at 1 to 2 mg/kg intramuscularly every 4 to 6 weeks.

Psychosocial Care

- Manage most dogs at home if at all possible.
- Stress should be minimized for the affected dog by avoiding high environmental temperature, changes in residence, unnecessary travel, introduction of new pets, and hospitalization.

PCV, Packed cell volume.

BOX 19-2 Guidelines for Long-Term Management of Older Cats Diagnosed with Chronic Renal Failure

Dietary Therapy

- Dietary therapy remains the cornerstone of medical management of cats with chronic renal failure.
- Because nutritional support serves as the foundation for the long-term management of cats with chronic renal failure, strategies must be designed to minimize inappetence.
- Feeding methods may incorporate orogastric tube feeding or esophagostomy tube feeding.
- Commercially prepared renal diets provide the best nutritional support if the cat will eat the diet. Diet changes should be made gradually over a period of 2 to 4 weeks. If possible, commercially prepared renal diets should be chosen that resemble the cat's preferred diet with respect to texture and flavor.
- Foods may be warmed to enhance palatability. Dry foods may be moistened with water. Fresh and aromatic food is more likely to be desirable.
- Homemade or commercially prepared kidney diets may be modified with flavoring agents to provide favorable odors and enhance palatability. However, commercially prepared kidney diets are best fed unaltered.

Fluid Therapy

- Oral fluids are often preferable if frequent vomiting is not a problem.
- Administer intravenous or subcutaneous fluids supplemented with potassium chloride at 60 to 90 ml/lb per day.
- Subcutaneous fluids can be administered by owner or veterinary technician and should be given at a rate of about 150 ml one to three times per week.
- The addition of 1 ml B-complex vitamins per 250 ml of fluid solution may be desirable.

Antimicrobial Therapy

- Therapy should be based on urine culture and sensitivity test results, if possible.
- Active chronic pyelonephritis should be treated for at least 6 to 8 weeks or until urine culture results are negative.
- Reculture after antimicrobial therapy has been discontinued for 1 week.
- Reculture 1 to 2 months later and then every 3 to 6 months.

Intestinal Phosphorus-Binding Agents

- Before intestinal phosphorus-binding agents are used, a restricted phosphorus diet should first be fed in an attempt to normalize serum phosphorus concentration.
- When feeding restricted phosphorus diets, do not normalize the serum phosphorus concentration and then start administering the oral intestinal phosphorus-binding agents.
- Use of oral sucralfate or aluminum hydroxide at 10 to 30 mg/kg twice a day (usually 75 mg twice a day) may be preferred; capsules are better than suspension; always give them with restricted phosphorus diets.

Control of Vomiting and Nausea

- Administer oral famotidine at 0.5 mg/kg once or twice daily.
- Administer oral or subcutaneous metoclopramide at 0.2 to 0.4 mg/kg every 6 to 8 hours.
- Administer drugs 30 minutes before forced feeding.
- Use both drugs if the appetite is still poor.

Oral Potassium Supplementation

- Give potassium gluconate at 2 to 3 mEq per day.

Bone Marrow Stimulation

- Administer recombinant human erythropoietin (r-HuEPO), and use daily iron supplementation with ferrous sulfate at oral dosage of 50 to 100 mg/day for cats. Some cats do not tolerate the oral iron supplementation; in these cases administer iron dextran at 50 mg intramuscularly every 3 to 4 weeks.
- r-HuEPO is indicated if PCV <19% and clinical signs from the nonregenerative anemia exist. Administer an initial dose of 50 to 100 units/kg subcutaneously 3 times weekly until a PCV of 30% to 40% for cats is achieved. The r-HuEPO dosage is then reduced to twice weekly as the cat's PCV approaches the desired level and then once weekly to prevent polycythemia. Maintenance dose is usually given one to two times weekly to maintain PCV within the target reference range.
- Treatment with r-HuEPO is withheld if PCV exceeds the desired target reference range. During maintenance, dosage adjustments are made every three to four weeks because of lag phase between desired PCV and r-HuEPO response.
- Failure to respond to adequate r-HuEPO therapy may result from the presence of iron deficiency, external blood loss, hemolytic process, concurrent diseases, and development of anti–r-HuEPO antibodies.
- PCV should be monitored weekly until PCV is established in target reference range for at least 4 weeks. The PCV is then checked bimonthly or monthly.
- r-HuEPO injections are discontinued if polycythemia, fever, anorexia, joint pain, cellulitis at the injection site, or cutaneous or mucosal ulceration occurs.

PCV, Packed cell volume.

Box 19-2 Guidelines for Long-Term Management of Older Cats Diagnosed with Chronic Renal Failure—cont'd

- r-HuEPO should be withheld until hypertension, iron deficiency, and polycythemia are corrected.
- Severe erythroid hypoplasia is consistent with serum antibody production that usually occurs within 4 to 16 weeks of initiating r-HuEPO therapy. Incidence is about 20% to 30% of treated animals. The PCV will return to the pretreatment low PCV value. Antibodies will decrease over a variable period after discontinuation of the r-HuEPO therapy.
- Cats that respond well to r-HuEPO therapy will have corrected nonregenerative anemia and will have an improved quality of life.

Control of Hypertension with Daily Administration of Antihypertensive Drugs and Restricted Sodium Diets

- Monitor the control of blood pressure every 3 to 6 months.

Anabolic Steroids

- Administration of anabolic steroids increases vigor and appetite in cats almost immediately.
- Cats need to be eating for anabolic steroids to be helpful.
- Anabolic steroids cause an increase in erythrocyte production in the bone marrow beginning about 100 days after initiation of therapy.
- Give stanozolol at 1 to 2 mg/kg intramuscularly every 4 weeks.

Psychosocial Care

- Most cats should be managed at home if at all possible.
- Stress should be minimized for the affected cat by avoiding high environmental temperature, changes in residence, unnecessary travel, introduction of new pets, and hospitalization.

BOX 19-3 Guidelines for Intensive Diuresis Therapy for Dogs and Cats in Uremic Crisis

- Rehydrate with a balanced electrolyte solution in 4 to 6 hours.
- Evaluate the cardiac stasis of the animal after initial rehydration for potential signs of left-sided heart failure. Do not proceed further with intensive diuresis if any signs of left-sided heart failure are noted at any time during the intensive diuresis process.
- Weigh the animal after rehydration.
- Place and secure an indwelling urinary catheter in the urinary bladder to enable monitoring of urinary output.
- Intravenously administer a fluid load equal to 3% to 5% of the animal's body weight.
- Administer a diuretic such as furosemide intravenously or subcutaneously at a routine diuretic dosage.
- Administer two or three cycles of fluid load followed by diuretic administration every 24 hours.
- Fluid input and urine output should be approximately equal.
- Reevaluate serum chemistry profile every 24 hours while the animal is being diuresed.
- Serum potassium concentrations should be maintained at a level greater than 3 mEq/L.
- When blood urea nitrogen and serum creatinine concentrations are stable, stop the diuretic administration, slowly reduce intravenous fluids, and start feeding the animal.

compensated CRF. The goals of nutritional therapy are (1) to reduce or ameliorate the clinical signs of uremia by reducing the production of proteinaceous waste products; (2) to minimize the electrolyte, vitamin, and mineral disturbances associated with excessive consumption of protein and certain minerals; (3) to provide daily protein, calorie, and mineral requirements; and (4) to slow the progression of the CRF. It is currently recommended that dogs with mild to moderate CRF be fed a diet that contains at least 13% gross energy as protein.[2] It is also recommended that euhydrated dogs with serum creatinine concentration less than 4.5 mg/dl be maintained on 2 to 2.2 g of high biologic quality dietary protein per kilogram of body weight per day. Euhydrated dogs with serum creatinine concentrations greater than 4.5 mg/dl should be fed approximately 1.3 g of protein per kilogram of body weight per day. Cats have a dietary protein requirement that is substantially higher than that of dogs.[12] Cats with CRF should be fed a diet that provides at least 21% of gross energy as protein.[2] There are a number of commercially prepared dietary products available for feeding dogs and cats with varying degrees of CRF that achieve the above requirements when fed in quantities sufficient to maintain caloric requirements. The owner can also formulate homemade diets, such as those recommended in Box 19-4. These diets can then be tailored to suit an animal's palate.

Reducing phosphorus retention and hyperphosphatemia is a major medical goal in animals

BOX 19-4 Some Homemade Diets Formulated for Management of Chronic Renal Failure

Restricted Protein and Phosphorus Diet for Dogs

0.25 lb (115 g) ground beef (regular)
1 large egg (50 g) (hard cooked)
2 cups (350 g) cooked rice (without salt)
3 slices (75 g) white bread (crumbled)
1 t (5 g) calcium carbonate
Balanced supplement that will fulfill the AAFCO requirements for all vitamins and trace minerals for dogs.
Braise the meat, retaining the fat. Combine all ingredients and mix well. This mixture is somewhat dry. The palatability can be improved by adding some water (not milk). Yield: 1.25 lb (595 g).

Nutrient Contents

Protein:	20.00% (dry matter)
Phosphorus:	0.29% (dry matter)
Sodium:	0.26% (dry matter)

Restricted Protein and Phosphorus Diet for Cats

0.25 lb (115 g) liver
2 large eggs (100 g) (hard cooked)
2 cups (350 g) cooked rice (without added salt)
1 T (15 g) vegetable oil
1 t (5 g) calcium carbonate
Balanced supplement that fulfills the AAFCO feline requirements for all vitamins and trace minerals.
Dice and braise the liver, retaining the fat. Combine all ingredients and mix well. This mixture is somewhat dry, and the palatability may be improved by adding some water (not milk). Yield 1.25 lb (585 g).

Nutrient Contents

Protein:	24.30% (dry matter)
Phosphorus:	0.47% (dry matter)
Sodium:	0.17% (dry matter)
Potassium:	0.33% (dry matter)

AAFCO, Association of American Feed Control Officials.
From Lewis LD, Morris ML, Hand MS: *Small animal clinical nutrition III*, Topeka, Kan, 1987, Mark Morris Associates.

with CRF; it may reduce renal secondary hyperparathyroidism, renal osteodystrophy, soft-tissue calcification, and progression of renal failure.[2] An attempt should first be made to normalize serum phosphorus concentration by means of dietary therapy. As CRF progresses, dietary phosphorus restriction alone will fail to prevent hyperphosphatemia. Intestinal phosphate-binding agents can then be administered if hyperphosphatemia occurs despite dietary phosphorus restriction. Intestinal phosphate-binding agents that are aluminum based (aluminum carbonate, aluminum hydroxide, and aluminum oxide) or calcium based (calcium acetate, calcium citrate, and calcium carbonate) compounds are available over the counter from most pharmacies in liquid, tablet, and capsule forms. Sucralfate, a complex polyaluminum hydroxide salt of sulfate, may also be effective as an intestinal phosphate binder. The calcium-based products do pose a potential risk of causing hypercalcemia; calcium acetate is the most effective calcium-based phosphorus-binding agent and has the lowest risk of causing hypercalcemia.[2]

Phosphorus-binding agents should be given with each meal to enhance the effectiveness of the phosphorus-binding activity. They may be mixed with the food or given 15 to 30 minutes before each meal. These agents must be given with a phosphorus-restricted diet, and capsules or tablets are preferable. The dosage of phosphate-binding agents should be adjusted according to the serum phosphorus concentration. Serial monitoring of serum calcium and phosphorus concentrations at 14-day intervals should permit assessment of the adequacy of therapy.[2]

Oral alkalinization therapy is recommended when the serum bicarbonate decreases to or below 17 mEq/L.[2] Sodium bicarbonate and potassium citrate (most useful in cats) are the most commonly used alkalinizing agents for treatment of metabolic acidosis. Tablets may be crushed and given with food or administered in the form of a solution.[3,4] The alkalinizing agent should be administered in small divided doses throughout the day to minimize fluctuations in blood pH and to normalize serum bicarbonate concentration within the expected normal reference range. The serum bicarbonate should be assessed 14 days after initiating therapy.

Oral potassium replacement therapy is always indicated for cats with CRF, even in the absence of clinical signs of hypokalemia.[3] Potassium gluconate is the preferred form and may be administered orally in the form of a powder, tablets, a gel, or an elixir. In cats, oral potassium is usually given at a dose of 2 to 6 mEq per day, depending on the size of the cat and the severity of the hypokalemia. The dosage should then be adjusted based on clinical response. Long-term potassium supplementation at 2 to 3 mEq/day is recommended for all cats with CRF, irrespective of the measured serum potassium concentration.

Arterial hypertension should be confirmed by recording increased arterial blood pressures measured during three separate determinations by indirect Doppler ultrasonography or oscillometry. Hypertension exists when systolic blood pressures exceed 184 mm Hg in dogs and 165 mm Hg in cats; when diastolic blood pressures exceed 130 mm Hg in dogs and 124 mm Hg in cats; and when the mean arterial pressure exceeds 152 mm Hg in dogs and 139 mm Hg in cats.[2] Immediate medical therapy should be initiated in animals with obvious signs associated with hypertensive disease (ocular hemorrhage, hypertensive retinopathy, and retinal detachment) and coexistent elevations in measured arterial pressures.

Dietary sodium and protein restriction are the basis of nonpharmacologic control of hypertension.[6] Sodium intake should be reduced slowly over a period of 1 to 2 weeks to allow the animal to adapt to sodium restriction. Canine and feline diets formulated for CRF are both sodium and protein restricted. Unfortunately, dietary therapy alone is rarely effective in controlling hypertension.[13] This necessitates the administration of antihypertensive drugs, such as angiotensin-converting enzyme (ACE) inhibitors, calcium-channel blockers, adrenergic receptor antagonists, arteriolar vasodilators, and diuretics. ACE inhibitors are the preferred therapy for treatment of systemic hypertension for dogs; enalapril, benazepril, and lisinopril are the initial ACE inhibitors of choice.[13] Amlodipine, a calcium-channel blocker, is the current drug of choice for hypertension in cats.[13,14] Blood pressures often decrease within 12 to 48 hours of administration of these drugs.[13] Serial measurements of blood pressure and frequent monitoring of serum concentrations of creatinine, blood urea nitrogen, and electrolytes are important when these drugs are used.

The administration of low doses of vitamin D (calcitriol or 1,25 dihydroxyvitamin D) in combination with effective control of serum phosphorus concentrations reduces the degree of secondary renal hyperparathyroidism and its associated skeletal abnormalities in dogs with CRF.[15,16] Calcitriol is the most active form of vitamin D and is formed in the kidney by 1α-hydroxylation of 25-hydroxycholecalciferol. Renal 1α-hydroxylase activity and formation of calcitriol are stimulated by parathormone. Calcitriol normally regulates parathormone synthesis by feedback inhibition. Calcitriol deficiency develops early in the course of CRF as a result of the inhibitory effects of phosphate retention on 1α-hydroxylase activities in renal tubular cells. This is temporarily restored at the expense of a persistent increase in parathormone concentration. With progression of CRF, loss of viable renal tubular cells limits calcitriol synthetic capacity, and calcitriol concentrations remain low. Calcitriol deficiency causes skeletal resistance to parathormone action and raises the set point for calcium-induced suppression of parathormone release. These activities limit the skeletal release of calcium and allow hyperparathyroidism to persist regardless of whether serum ionized calcium concentrations are normal or increased.

Calcitriol supplementation at an oral dose of 2.5 to 3.5 ng/kg daily is initiated early in CRF (when serum creatinine is greater than 2 mg/dl, or 170 μmol/L).[16] At this stage of CRF, hyperparathyroidism is not established and low doses of calcitriol will prevent its development. It is suggested that a baseline serum parathormone concentration be determined before initiating calcitriol therapy to document the magnitude of hyperparathyroidism; serial measurements of serum parathormone concentration are performed to document the effectiveness of the combination of phosphorus restriction and the calcitriol treatment. Serum parathormone concentration should be measured 8 weeks after initiating calcitriol therapy to determine if a dosage increase is needed. The short half-life (4 to 6 hours) and short duration of action (4 days) allows adjustment in dosage to alleviate hypercalcemia, if present. Serum phosphorus concentrations should be decreased, if necessary, to 6 mg/dl (1.9 mmol/L) prior to initiation of calcitriol therapy. Phosphorus restriction and normalization of serum concentration of phosphorus are important to allow calcitriol therapy to effectively lower serum parathormone concentration.[16]

Animals with advanced hyperparathyroidism and serum parathormone concentrations in excess of 10 times normal may require twice-weekly pulse administration of calcitriol (20 ng/kg orally twice a week).[16] This allows the administration of higher doses and serum concentrations of calcitriol without causing hypercalcemia that would occur with daily administration of calcitriol. Serum calcium concentration is measured 1 and 2 days after the third dose of calcitriol to monitor for hypercalcemia, and the calcitriol dose is adjusted downward if hypercalcemia is detected. Serum parathormone concentration is measured 1 month after initiation of pulse therapy, and if it is not significantly suppressed, calcitriol dosage is adjusted upward by 5 ng/kg. Serum calcium concentration is again measured 1 and 2 days after the third dose of calcitriol to monitor for hypercalcemia. Pulse administration can then be replaced by daily administration (2.5 to 3.5 ng/kg daily) once the serum concentration of parathormone is normalized and maintained for 2 to 3 months.

A progressive, nonregenerative anemia is a characteristic finding in older dogs and cats with moderate to advanced CRF. The magnitude and the progression of the anemia correlate with the degree of CRF and worsen as renal function declines further. Erythropoietin deficiency has been identified as the primary cause of the nonregenerative anemia in animals with CRF.[17,18] Several strategies for the management of the nonregenerative anemia should be considered. Unnecessary blood loss can be prevented by reducing, if possible, the quantity of blood collected for diagnostic tests and monitoring purposes from animals with a small body size (cats and small dogs). Chronic low-grade gastrointestinal blood loss may contribute to the severe anemia in animals with CRF. Therapeutic trials with H_2-receptor antagonists may be necessary for chronic gastrointestinal blood loss to be reduced. Indicators of a positive response to H_2-receptor antagonist administration include improvements in hematocrit and appetite.[2]

A transfusion of whole blood or packed red cells may be necessary for the severely anemic CRF animal that needs rapid correction of their anemia. Compatible blood products, as determined by cross-matching or blood-typing procedures, should be used, even for the first transfusion. Repeated transfusions may be needed for long-term maintenance of the animal's hematocrit.[2] A posttransfusion target hematocrit should be in the low end of the normal reference range to minimize the complications of an abrupt increase in blood volume and viscosity, such as circulatory overload, hypertension, and seizures.[2]

Recombinant human erythropoietin produces a rapid and effective erythroid response in dogs and cats with naturally occurring CRF.[17,19] Significant increases in red blood cell count, hematocrit, and hemoglobin concentration can be found within the first month of initiating recombinant human erythropoietin therapy and may be sustained indefinitely.[19] In addition to the positive effects on hematopoiesis for dogs and cats with CRF, there are positive effects such as improved energy, increased appetite and alertness, and weight gain noted in most treated animals. Hypokalemia frequently observed in uremic cats resolves with recombinant human erythropoietin administration and is probably due to increased dietary intake of potassium.[19]

The most common problem associated with recombinant human erythropoietin administration in dogs and cats is the development of recombinant human erythropoietin antibodies, as indicated by the progressive decline in hematocrit, red blood cell count, and hemoglobin concentration. It is estimated that about 25% of treated animals develop anti–recombinant human erythropoietin antibodies.[19] These antibody titers decline after recombinant human erythropoietin therapy is stopped, and pretreatment levels of erythropoietin will be attained, reversing the suppressed erythropoiesis. Other side effects of recombinant human erythropoietin therapy include seizures, systemic hypertension, and iron depletion. Allergic reactions, including mucocutaneous or cutaneous drug reactions, fever, and arthralgia, have also been observed in dogs and cats early in the course of recombinant human erythropoietin therapy. Most adverse reactions resolve within a few days, and some adverse reactions do not return when recombinant human erythropoietin therapy is reinitiated.

Erythropoietin replacement is indicated for dogs and cats that are symptomatic for the nonregenerative anemia of CRF.[2,19] Erythropoietin-replacement is usually beneficial in animals with moderate to severe anemia (hematocrit <21% in dogs and hematocrit <19% in cats). The recommended initial dose of recombinant human erythropoietin is 50 to 100 U/kg of body weight subcutaneously three times a week (for instance, on Monday, Wednesday, and Friday) until the ideal target hematocrit of 37% to 45% for dogs and 30% to 40% for cats is attained. As the ideal target hematocrit range is approached, the recombinant human erythropoietin administration interval is decreased to twice a week. A lower initial dose (50 U/kg three times a week) is prescribed if a slower erythropoietic response is desired. If the ideal target hematocrit range is not attained within 8 to 12 weeks, then the initial amount of recombinant human erythropoietin administered per time may be increased by 25 U/kg in a stepwise manner. The amount of recombinant human erythropoietin administered to maintain the hematocrit within the desired target reference range varies by individual animal and must be established empirically by monitoring the animal's response. In general, a dose of 50 to 100 U/kg once or twice a week is usually sufficient. Temporary cessation of recombinant human erythropoietin treatment may be required if the animal's hematocrit exceeds the desired target reference range.

All animals receiving recombinant human erythropoietin therapy should be provided oral or parenteral iron supplementation to prevent iron depletion and facilitate the erythropoietic response. Oral supplementation with iron sulfate is preferred, and its starting dose is 50 to 100 mg per day for cats and 100 to 300 mg per day for dogs.[6] Some cats do not tolerate the oral iron supplementation; in these cases, administer iron dextran at 50 mg intramuscularly every 3 to 4 weeks.

Because commercial diets formulated to contain reduced quantities of protein, phosphorus, sodium, and acid metabolites are the cornerstone of managing compensated CRF, anorexia may pose a major therapeutic challenge.[2] Many animals with CRF, primarily older cats, refuse to eat some or all commercial diets. To avoid this food aversion, commercial diets formulated for long-term management of CRF should not be fed until the underlying causes of nausea, anorexia, and vomiting are resolved.[2] Dietary changes should always be made gradually, over a period of 1 to 2 weeks. If possible, commercial diets should be chosen that resemble preferred diets with respect to texture and flavor. Foods may be warmed to enhance palatability. Dry foods may be moistened with water. Fresh and aromatic food is more likely to be desirable. Homemade or commercial diets may be modified with flavoring agents to provide favorable odors and enhance palatability. A flavoring agent, such as clam juice, bouillon, gravy, animal fat, butter, garlic, or dehydrated cottage cheese, may be used to enhance the palatability of the commercial diet.

Cats that refuse protein-restricted diets should be allowed to eat as much protein as the uremia will allow. Some cats refuse protein-restricted diets entirely and eat only commercial cat food, chicken liver, chicken breast, all-meat baby food, fish, or shrimp. A general observation is that a cat or dog with CRF and uremia is more likely to die sooner if it eats nothing than if it is allowed to eat whatever it wants. Force feeding, tube feeding, or placing an esophagostomy tube or percutaneous gastrostomy tube may provide nutritional support to sustain the animal in the hope that it will eventually begin eating voluntarily.[20]

Pharmacologic appetite stimulants are usually only marginally successful in animals with CRF.[2] Benzodiazepines, such as oxazepam and diazepam, may be effective in some animals.[21] Diazepam may be given orally or intravenously but is most effective when given intravenously. In sick cats, the appetite-stimulating properties of benzodiazepines seem to wane in a few days and are generally unsatisfactory for long-term maintenance of the cat's appetite.[21]

Nausea, vomiting, and anorexia caused by uremic gastropathy may be treated with H_2-receptor antagonists such as cimetidine, ranitidine, or famotidine. Sucralfate may be used instead of an H_2-receptor antagonist. Because sucralfate may interfere with the absorption of many other drugs, the other drugs should be given 30 minutes prior to the administration of sucralfate. Antiemetic drugs such as metoclopramide may also be used alternatively or to supplement H_2-receptor antagonists and sucralfate.

Other key factors should also be considered in the management of CRF. Avoiding high environmental temperature, change of residence, unnecessary travel, introduction of a new pet, and hospitalization should minimize stress in animals with CRF. The veterinarian should avoid prescribing any nephrotoxic drugs or drugs that require renal excretion in animals with CRF. Dosage regimens should be adjusted to compensate for decreased renal function if circumstances dictate that drugs that require renal excretion must be administered.

NEPHROLITHIASIS

Renoliths of older dogs and cats account for less than 3% of all uroliths analyzed.[22] During a 12-year period, 17,610 uroliths from dogs have been analyzed by quantitative methods.[22] Of these, 226 (1.3%) were renoliths. Renoliths occurred more commonly in females (55%) than in males (45%). Sixty-eight percent (154 of 226) affected only the kidneys, and 32% (72 of 226) affected the kidneys and other portions of the urinary tract. The predominant mineral composition of the renoliths was calcium oxalate (39%), struvite (34%), ammonium urate (8%), mixed (8%), calcium phosphate (4%), compound (4%), matrix (2%), silica (<1%), and xanthine (<1%).

During an 11-year period, 284 uroliths of renal origin in dogs were analyzed.[23] These renoliths represented about 4% of all uroliths submitted from female dogs and 2% of uroliths submitted from male dogs. Fifty-nine percent (166 of 284) of the specimens were from female dogs and 31% (88 of 284) were from male dogs. Renoliths were present in the kidney(s) alone in male dogs at least 50% of the time and in female dogs at least 75% of the time. Most of the renoliths were composed of mixtures of mineral (41% in males and 55% in females) or of two or more mineralogically different layers (50% in males and 60% in females). The predominant mineral composition was struvite (38% of specimens in males and 58% of specimens in females). Other minerals included urate (33% in males and 12% in females), calcium oxalate (33% in males and 35% in females), calcium phosphate (32% in males and 38% in females), and silica (9% in males and 5% in females).

During a 12-year period, 3,989 uroliths from cats were analyzed by quantitative methods.[22] Of these, 113 (2.8%) were renoliths. Eight-four percent (95 of 113) affected only the kidneys, and 15.9% (18 of 113) affected the kidneys and other portions of the urinary tract. The predominant mineral composition of the renoliths was calcium oxalate (43%), matrix (25%), calcium phosphate (15%), mixed (11%), struvite (5%), and compound (1%). Renoliths occurred more commonly in males (63%) than in females (32%).

During an 11-year period, 62 renoliths from cats were analyzed.[22] These renoliths represented about 5% of all uroliths submitted from cats. Of the specimens, 55% (34 of 62) were from female cats, and 45% (28 of 62) were from male cats. About 15% of cats of both genders with renoliths also had uroliths in the urinary bladder. The mineral composition was similar for both genders. Of the renoliths, 73% were at least partially composed of calcium oxalate, 34% contained calcium phosphate, 6% contained struvite, and 1% contained urate. Eighteen percent of the renoliths were composed of mixtures of two or more mineral substances. Renoliths containing a single mineral layer constituted 71% of the specimens. Nineteen percent contained two distinct mineralogic layers, and 10% were composed of three or more different mineralogic layers.

Physical Findings

The history and clinical signs of older dogs and cats with renoliths depend on the presence or absence of infection and the degree of renal pelvic obstruction and hydronephrosis.[22] Most animals are asymptomatic when obstruction and infection are absent, and the renoliths are fortuitously seen on survey abdominal radiographs. Some animals may have intermittent or persistent hematuria or have recurrent urinary tract infection. Obstruction of one renal pelvis without infection is unlikely to cause noticeable clinical signs if the other kidney is functioning normally. Unilateral renal pelvic obstruction in the presence of infection may produce acute pyelonephritis, septicemia, and severe illness. Bilateral renal calculi often reduce renal function to such a degree that CRF and signs of uremia develop.

Laboratory Findings

There is considerable variability in laboratory findings in older dogs and cats with nephrolithiasis.[22,24,25] The findings depend on presence or absence of infection, degree of renal dysfunction, and amount of physical injury to adjacent tissues. Some animals will not have any abnormalities, whereas others will show hematuria and proteinuria. Some animals with nephrolithiasis will have abnormalities consistent with CRF or urinary tract infection. Survey abdominal radiography often shows obvious radiodense renoliths. Small renoliths may not be seen, and radiolucent renoliths cannot be seen. For these reasons, excretory urography is a more accurate method for the diagnosis of nephrolithiasis and ureterolithiasis than is survey abdominal radiography. Renal ultrasonography may be used for the detection of small renoliths, radiolucent renoliths, and obstructive disease. In addition, renal ultrasonography may be useful when renal dysfunction exists and is causing difficulty in evaluating the excretory urography. Whatever imaging techniques are used, renoliths should be differentiated from other radiodense structures and conditions that may resemble renoliths, including mineralization of the renal parenchyma, radiodense intestinal ingesta, calcified lymph nodes, osseous metaplasia of the transitional epithelium, choleliths, and radiodense medications in the intestinal tract.[22]

Management

The options for management of nephrolithiasis include medical dissolution, surgical removal, and disintegration by lithotripsy[22] (Box 19-5). The choice of treatment will depend on the animal's health status, the veterinarian's expertise, and the availability of lithotripsy. Simple diagnosis of renoliths is never an indication for surgical removal of the renoliths. Animals with renoliths and/or ureteroliths that are identified as causing an outflow obstruction and functional impairment of the affected kidney should be managed surgically or, if possible, with percutaneous nephropyelonephrostomy.[22]

Surgical removal of renoliths should be considered under several clinical scenarios. These include cases in which there is risk of further

BOX 19-5 Fact Sheet for Canine and Feline Nephrolithiasis

- Renoliths may cause potential complications such as obstruction of the renal pelvis or ureter, may predispose an animal to pyelonephritis, and may result in compressive injury of renal parenchyma leading to renal failure.
- Renoliths may be "inactive" because of lack of any complications. Inactive renoliths may not require removal but should be monitored periodically. Inactive renoliths should be monitored by urinalysis, urine culture, and abdominal radiography.
- Indications for renolith removal include obstruction, recurrent urinary tract infection accompanied by reduction in renal function, progressive renolith enlargement, and the presence of renoliths in a solitary functional kidney.
- Canine renoliths are usually composed of calcium oxalate and struvite. Breeds most commonly affected include Shih Tzu, Lhasa apso, miniature schnauzer, Yorkshire terrier, miniature poodle, bichon frise, and cocker spaniel.
- Feline renoliths are usually composed of calcium oxalate. Breeds most commonly affected include domestic shorthair and domestic longhair.
- Radiodense renoliths are diagnosed by survey abdominal radiography. Ultrasonography or excretory urography may confirm the presence, size, and number of renoliths and ureteroliths regardless of radiographic density. In cats, mineralization of the renal pelvis or diverticula should be differentiated from renoliths.
- Definitive identification of renolith type requires quantitative analysis of renolith or renolith fragments.
- Urinalysis may reveal hematuria, crystalluria, and proteinuria. Pyuria and bacteriuria may be noted in animals with concomitant urinary tract infection. Urine culture should be done on samples obtained by cystocentesis from all animals with renoliths.
- Evidence of inflammation revealed on the leukogram occurs with concurrent pyelonephritis and ureteral obstruction. Azotemia occurs if bilateral renal disease or obstruction is present. Hypercalcemia may be seen with calcium oxalate or calcium phosphate renoliths. Hyperadrenocorticism may be associated with calcium oxalate uroliths or urinary tract infection and with secondary struvite renoliths.
- Treatment includes surgery, monitoring of inactive renoliths, medical dissolution, and extracorporeal shock wave lithotripsy. Calcium oxalate renoliths, the most common urolith type, are not amenable to medical dissolution. Ureteroliths or obstructing renoliths are not amenable to medical dissolution.
- Nephrolithotomy may result in 27% to 52% reduction in glomerular filtration rate 3 weeks after surgery and 22% to 34% reduction in glomerular filtration rate 6 weeks after surgery.
- Renoliths recur frequently after surgical removal. Because nephrolithotomy results in reduced renal function, repeated nephrolithotomies for recurrent renoliths will result in progressive loss of renal function and quickly contribute to chronic renal failure.
- Medical dissolution for struvite renoliths includes calculolytic diet and appropriate antimicrobial agents if urinary tract infection is present. The animal should not be in renal failure and should not have evidence of obstructive disease.
- Medical dissolution of canine urate renoliths can be attempted using a protein-restricted, alkalinizing diet and administering allopurinol (15 mg/kg administered orally twice a day) and supplemental potassium citrate (Urocit-K) as needed to maintain a urine pH of approximately 7.

deterioration of renal function during the time required for medical dissolution and those in which obstructive disease is present. Surgery is also appropriate when renoliths are composed of calcium oxalate and when effective dissolution protocols have not yet been developed. Male animals with uroliths in multiple sites that require abdominal surgery and cystotomy to correct lower urinary tract obstruction are also potential candidates for removal of renoliths.

Surgical procedures that may be appropriate for removal of renoliths in animals include nephrolithotomy, pyelolithotomy, and nephrectomy.[22] Nephrectomy is always the last resort and should be reserved for those cases complicated by severe pyelonephritis or hydronephrosis and when the contralateral kidney is functional. The option of pyelolithotomy versus nephrolithotomy can be made at surgery. Pyelolithotomy is more desirable than nephrolithotomy because it does not require occlusion of renal blood supply and creation of a surgical incision in the kidney parenchyma. However, pyelolithotomy is feasible only when the renolith is located within a dilated portion of the ureter or the extrarenal portion of the renal pelvis. When the renolith is surrounded by kidney parenchyma, nephrolithotomy is required for renolith removal. Bilateral nephrolithiasis requires that the veterinarian choose between simultaneous procedures and staged unilateral procedures. Surgery on both kidneys can be performed at the same time if there is adequate urine-concentrating ability and absence of azotemia. When renal dysfunction is present, surgery should be performed on only one kidney initially. The choice of which kidney to treat first will require the veterinarian's judgment. The veterinarian should try and choose the kidney most likely to sustain the animal's renal function. Renal function should be assessed after the animal has recovered from surgery. Because nephrolithotomy produces additional renal dysfunction, staged procedures should be separated by several weeks in those animals with renal dysfunction (Osborne et al, 1995).[26]

Conservative medical management may be considered for struvite, cystine, or urate renoliths (see Box 19-5). Feeding of a calculolytic, acidifying diet (Hill's Prescription Diet Canine s/d) and antimicrobial treatment for coexisting urinary tract infection may produce dissolution of struvite uroliths.[22] One study reported that the average time for dissolution of bacterial-induced struvite renoliths in six dogs was 184 ± 99 days.[22] Cystine renolith dissolution may be achieved by feeding a restricted-protein diet (Hill's Prescription Diet Canine u/d) and administration of *N*-(2-mercaptopropionyl)-glycine (2-MPG).[22] Urate calculi may be dissolved with the administration of allopurinol and by feeding a low-purine diet (Hill's Prescription Diet Canine u/d).[22] Medical protocols for the dissolution of calcium oxalate uroliths have not been established.[22] However, dietary modification may prevent increases in the size and number of nonobstructing renoliths. The size and number of nonobstructing calcium oxalate renoliths did not increase in six dogs fed a restricted-protein, low-sodium, alkalinizing diet (Hill's Prescription Diet Canine u/d) for 5 to 8 months.[22]

Extracorporeal shock wave lithotripsy has been used in dogs with ureterolithiasis and nephrolithiasis.[27-29] The technique appears to be a safe and effective means of treating nephrolithiasis and ureterolithiasis in dogs. In addition, extracorporeal shock wave lithotripsy causes less parenchymal damage and renal dysfunction than nephrolithotomy.[28] Routine use of this method of management is unlikely because of the limited availability of shock-wave lithotriptor units as well as the actual expense involved.[29]

URINARY INCONTINENCE

The most common causes of acquired urinary incontinence in older dogs and cats are urethral incompetence, urinary tract infection, and polyuria-polydipsia.[30–32] Urethral incompetence (commonly referred to as *hormone-responsive incontinence*) often occurs in spayed female dogs and cats and infrequently in intact female and neutered and intact male dogs and cats. Urinary tract infection usually causes urge incontinence. Polyuria can be produced by a number of pathologic abnormalities and medications. Eliminating or ameliorating the increased urinary output may resolve or substantially decrease urinary incontinence. Behavioral problems or debilitating diseases may also cause urinary incontinence. Older dogs may become more dependent on their owners; these animals may urinate when they get excited while greeting their owners. Affected dogs may have to be retrained to empty their urinary bladders more frequently or to not become excited in stressful situations. Debilitated animals may have to be trained to void on newspapers or may require help to go outside for elimination.[30]

Determination of the causes of acquired urinary incontinence requires careful evaluation of information obtained from the history, physical examination, and laboratory and diagnostic imaging tests (Table 19-1). The history should include detailed information about the nature of the urinary incontinence. Urethral incompetence is most often seen when the dog or cat is relaxing or asleep. The physical examination should include a neurologic examination; abdominal palpation to evaluate the urinary bladder for distention, tenderness, and irregularities; inspection and palpation of the external genitalia; and digital rectal examination of the prostate gland, urethra, and adjacent structures in dogs. The physical examination should also include evaluation of the urine stream and the behavior of the dog or cat while it urinates. For assessment of urethral tone, the dog or cat should be interrupted while it is urinating so that its ability to stop urinating midstream can be evaluated. Residual urine volume should be measured after voiding is completed to determine if the dog or cat can completely empty the urinary bladder. Residual urine volumes should not be greater than 0.2 to 0.4 ml/kg.[31] Urinalysis and urine culture should be performed routinely to determine whether a urinary tract infection has developed. Other tests that may be included are complete blood cell count, serum chemistry profile, and abdominal radiography and ultrasonography.

Therapy should be directed at the specific cause of the acquired urinary incontinence. If a specific cause cannot be identified, nonspecific treatment of the urinary incontinence should be used (Table 19-2). Medications are available that

TABLE 19-1. ACQUIRED DISORDERS OF ABNORMAL VOIDING OF URINE IN OLDER DOGS AND CATS

DISORDER	CHARACTERISTICS OF URINARY BLADDER AND VOIDING PATTERN
Acquired Disorders with Increased Residual Volumes in the Urinary Bladder after Complete Voiding of Urine	
Urinary bladder dysfunction (hypocontractility) caused by acute or chronic overdistention of urinary bladder	Distended urinary bladder, intermittent overflow incontinence; absent or incomplete voiding
Urethral Dysfunction (Increased Outlet Resistance)	
Physical obstruction	Distended urinary bladder; dysuria with little or no urine voided; intermittent overflow incontinence if partial obstruction
Functional urethral obstruction	Same as physical obstruction
Detrusor-urethral dyssynergia	Distended urinary bladder, dysuric or interrupted voiding pattern
Acquired Disorders with Normal Residual Volumes in the Urinary Bladder after Complete Voiding of Urine	
Urinary bladder dysfunction (hypercontractility) from urinary tract infection, neoplastic infiltration or mass, or idiopathic causes	Small urinary bladder; intermittent urine leakage; animal may leak urine when active; possible urinary tract infection (urge incontinence) or feline leukemia virus infection
Urethral dysfunction (hypotonicity)	Small urinary bladder; voiding pattern normal; intermittent urinary incontinence, often when animal is recumbent
Hormone responsive incontinence	Small urinary bladder; voiding pattern normal; intermittent urinary incontinence, often when animal is recumbent
Prostatic disease	Small urinary bladder; voiding pattern normal if not obstructed; intermittent urinary incontinence, often when animal is recumbent

TABLE 19-2. MEDICATION USED IN THE MANAGEMENT OF URINARY INCONTINENCE

MEDICATION AND ITS TYPE OF ACTIVITY	RECOMMENDED DOSAGE BY SPECIES
Increase Urethral Resistance	
Stilbestrol	0.04-1 mg PO once a day for 7 days (about 0.2 mg/kg), followed by 0.1-1 mg PO every 7 days (dog)
Testosterone propionate	2.2 mg/kg SC or IM every 2-3 days (dog) 5-10 mg IM as needed (cat)
Testosterone cypionate	2.2 mg/kg IM every 30 days (dog)
Phenylpropanolamine	1.5 mg/kg PO three times a day (dog and cat)
Ephedrine	1.2 mg/kg PO three times a day (dog) 2-4 mg/kg PO two or three times a day (cat)
Decrease Urethral Resistance	
Phenoxybenzamine	0.25 mg/kg PO two times a day (dog and cat)
Diazepam	0.2 mg/kg PO three times a day (dog) 2.5-5 mg PO three times a day (cat)
Aminopromazine	2.2 mg/kg PO two times a day (dog and cat)
Acepromazine	1.1-2.2 mg/kg PO
Dantrolene	0.5-1 mg/kg PO three times a day (dog) 0.5-1 mg/kg PO two times a day (cat)
Nicergoline	1-5 mg PO three times a day (dog and cat)
Increase Urinary Bladder Contractility:	
Bethanechol	5-25 mg PO three times a day (dog) 1.25-7.5 mg PO three times a day (cat)
Decrease Urinary Bladder Contractility	
Propantheline	7.5-30 mg PO three times a day (dog) 5-7.5 mg PO three times a day (cat)
Oxybutynin	1.25-5 mg PO two to three times a day (dog) 0.5-1.25 mg PO two times a day (cat)
Imipramine	5-15 mg PO two times a day (dog) 2.5-5 mg PO two times a day (cat)

IM, Intramuscular administration; *PO*, oral administration; *SC*, subcutaneous administration.

can increase or decrease urinary bladder contraction or urethral contraction.[32] For these medications to be used appropriately, it is important to localize the problem to the urinary bladder or urethra and to determine if the problem is one of excessive contraction or relaxation.

URINARY BLADDER TUMORS

Urinary bladder tumors are the most common neoplasm of the urinary tract in older dogs and cats[33,34] (Box 19-6). Urinary bladder neoplasia occurs more frequently in female dogs than in male dogs.[35] Scottish terriers, Shetland sheepdogs, beagles, collies, cocker spaniels, springer spaniels, dachshunds, boxers, Labrador retrievers, West Highland white terriers, and cairn terriers are the breeds most commonly affected by urinary bladder tumors.[34,35] Transitional cell carcinomas, the most common urinary bladder tumor of older dogs and cats, may occur as a papillary projection into the urinary bladder lumen or infiltrate into the wall. Squamous cell carcinomas, adenocarcinomas, and other types of uncommon neoplasias may also occur.

A urinary bladder tumor should be suspected in any older dog or cat with persistent hematuria, pollakiuria, dysuria, or urinary incontinence that is not responsive to antimicrobial agents or other routine therapy. Urinary bladder masses can be identified by double-contrast cystography, urinary

BOX 19-6 Fact Sheet for Urinary Bladder Tumors in Dogs and Cats

- Urinary bladder neoplasia occurs more frequently in middle-aged to older female dogs and cats than in male dogs and cats.
- Scottish terrier, Shetland sheepdog, beagle, collie, cocker spaniel, springer spaniel, dachshund, boxer, Labrador retriever, West Highland white terrier, and cairn terrier are the breeds most commonly affected. No specific cat breed is overrepresented.
- Transitional cell carcinoma is the most common urinary bladder tumor of older dogs and cats and may occur as a papillary projection into the urinary bladder lumen and may infiltrate into the urinary bladder wall. Other, infrequently occurring tumors include squamous cell carcinoma, leiomyoma, leiomyosarcoma, rhabdomyosarcoma (seen primarily in young dogs), lymphosarcoma, and transmissible venereal tumor.
- Urinary bladder tumors should be suspected in older dogs and cats with persistent hematuria, pollakiuria, dysuria, or urinary incontinence that is not responsive to traditional antimicrobial or other routine therapy.
- The trigone region is the most common site for urinary bladder tumors, but tumors may originate from the urethra and prostate gland.
- Metastasis may occur to regional lymph nodes, lungs, and bone (especially the ribs). Up to 37% of dogs have metastatic disease at the time of initial examination.
- Urinary bladder masses may be identified by double contrast cystography, urinary bladder ultrasonography, or cystoscopy.
- Definitive diagnosis is based on biopsy of soft tissue mass(es) within the urinary bladder. Biopsies may be obtained by cystoscopy, laparoscopy, cystotomy, or urinary catheter aspirate biopsy.
- Urinalysis may reveal epithelial cells with multiple criteria of malignancy such as anisocytosis, anisokaryosis, increased nuclear to cytoplasmic ratio, and deeply staining cytoplasm. Caution should be used against over-interpreting cytologic findings if inflammation is also evident during urine sediment evaluation.
- Poorly differentiated urinary bladder tumors with distant metastasis have the worst prognosis.
- Successful treatment of urinary bladder tumors is primarily dependent on early diagnosis. Up to 50% of the urinary bladder can be resected with minimal loss of urinary bladder function.
- Symptomatic therapy usually includes treatment of secondary urinary tract infection and urolithiasis. In those animals with profuse bleeding to the point of declining PCV values, surgical resection or chemical cauterization of the urinary bladder lining may be needed. Intravesicular instillation of 10 to 20 ml of 1% formalin solution for 20 minutes followed by thorough rinsing with sterile saline solution may be used to cauterize the urinary bladder lining.
- Chemotherapy with mitoxantrone (dosed at 5.5 mg/m^2 and given intravenously at 3-week intervals) and piroxicam is the preferred way to treat urinary bladder neoplasia. This therapy should be continued as long as no adverse side effects are noted. The hemogram should be monitored before each mitoxantrone treatment and one week after its administration for myelosuppression. Piroxicam (0.3 mg/kg orally once a day with food for affected dogs; those dogs with compromised liver and/or kidney function or cats use the initial dosage to 0.15 mg/kg orally once a day with food) administration will minimize animal discomfort and somewhat decrease the size of the urinary bladder mass(es). Owners should watch for signs of gastrointestinal upset such as inappetence, vomiting, diarrhea, and change in color of stools passed when administering piroxicam. In addition, the hemogram and renal function should be monitored.

bladder ultrasonography, or cystoscopy. Detection of urinary bladder masses by any of these diagnostic means may include masses that represent resolving blood clots, organized granulomas, or neoplasia. If a urinary bladder mass is a non-neoplastic lesion such as resolving blood clots, the mass should resolve within 4 to 6 weeks of diagnosis; if it does not, one needs to reevaluate the urinary bladder for another cause. Definitive diagnosis of urinary bladder neoplasia is based on histopathologic evaluation of a urinary bladder tissue sample, which may be obtained via cystoscopy, laparoscopy, cystotomy, or urinary catheter biopsy technique. Cytologic evaluation of urine sediment or needle aspiration biopsies of the urinary bladder mass may also provide definitive evidence of neoplasia.[36]

Successful treatment of urinary bladder tumors is primarily dependent on early diagnosis. Unfortunately, however, most urinary bladder tumors are identified at an advanced stage, and therapy for affected animals is often aimed at relieving urinary discomfort, maintaining urinary continence, and preventing hydronephrosis and hydroureter. Curative treatment is rarely attainable. Surgically accessible tumors may be removed along with a wide zone of healthy tissue. Widespread tumors or tumors involving the neck region of the urinary bladder may be debulked. Total cystectomy with urinary diversion may be attempted but has been unrewarding with regard to long-term survival and quality of life. Nonsurgical therapy may include radiation and chemotherapy. Symptomatic therapy includes treatment of secondary urinary tract infection and urolithiasis and chemical cauterization of the urinary bladder lining to minimize profuse bleeding. Methenamine mandelate (10 mg/kg orally every 6 hours) or intravesicular instillation of a 1% formalin solution may be used to cauterize the urinary bladder mucosa.[36,37]

Chemotherapy with mitoxantrone (5.5 mg/m^2 given intravenously at 3-week intervals) and piroxicam is the preferred way to treat urinary bladder neoplasia. This therapy is continued for as long as no adverse side effects are noted. The hemogram should be monitored before each mitoxantrone treatment and 1 week after its administration for myelosuppression. Piroxicam, a nonsteroidal antiinflammatory drug, has also become popular in the clinical management of most urinary bladder tumors, because it seems to minimize animal discomfort and has some short-term antineoplastic activity. If a urinary bladder mass is a neoplastic lesion such as transitional cell carcinoma, and no evidence of metastatic disease exists, the prognosis with well-tolerated chemotherapy is good for survival beyond 9 months. If a urinary bladder mass is a neoplastic lesion such as transitional cell carcinoma, and evidence of metastatic disease in regional lymph nodes or lungs exists, the prognosis for survival beyond 3 months is poor, even with well-tolerated chemotherapy.

GLOMERULONEPHRITIS

Glomerulonephritis is common in older dogs and cats.[38,39] Most glomerulonephritides in older dogs and cats are caused by the presence of immune complexes in the glomerular capillary walls. Immune complexes accumulate in the glomerulus secondary to either deposition of preformed circulating complexes or by in situ immune complex formation. One of the earliest functional defects in glomerulonephritis is the loss of excessive plasma proteins into the urine. Clinical consequences of this continuous proteinuria observed in the affected animal are sodium retention, edema or ascites, hypercholesterolemia, hypertension, hypercoagulability, muscle wasting, and weight loss. Glomerular leakage of plasma proteins also allows protein to accumulate within the glomerular tuft, which results in mesangial cell proliferation and increased mesangial matrix production. With time, irreversible glomerular damage occurs in the form of glomerulosclerosis. Once the glomerulus is irreversibly damaged, the entire associated nephron becomes nonfunctional and is replaced by fibrous scar tissue.

Definite diagnosis of glomerulonephritis and related proteinuria is confirmed by measuring the urine protein-to-creatinine ratio and performing renal biopsies for histopathologic examination.[40] To determine the urine protein-to-creatinine ratio, the protein and creatinine concentrations are measured in a 10-ml urine sample collected from the animal's natural urine voiding or by cystocentesis and sent to a local reference laboratory for evaluation. Then, the measured urine protein concentration is divided by the measured urine creatinine concentration to derive the urine protein-to-creatinine ratio for the urine sample evaluated. The dog's or cat's normal urine protein-to-creatinine ratio is less than 1. If the urine protein-to-creatinine ratio is equal to or greater than 3, then medical management for the proteinuria is recommended. The urine protein-to-creatinine ratio in older dogs and cats should be screened in the following circumstances: 1) the serum albumin concentration is below or at least in the lower end of the expected normal reference value range; 2) renal-origin azotemia is present; 3) one is monitoring the medical response of an animal that is being treated for proteinuria; and 4) the screening is a component of the animal's annual or biannual wellness examination.

Specific therapy for glomerulonephritis should be directed at identifying and treating the primary underlying disease causing the chronic antigenic stimulation. Unfortunately, however, this is often not possible. An increasing amount of scientific evidence indicates that ACE inhibitors reduce protein excretion in human beings and animals with proteinuria. In dogs with unilateral nephrectomies, experimentally induced diabetes mellitus, or idiopathic glomerulonephritis, administration of an ACE inhibitor has been reported to reduce glomerular transcapillary hydraulic pressure and glomerular cell hypertrophy as well as the proteinuria.[41,42] In another study, ACE inhibitor treatment of Samoyed dogs with X-linked hereditary nephritis decreased proteinuria, improved renal excretory function, decreased glomerular basement membrane splitting, and prolonged survival when compared with control dogs.[43] It is, therefore, currently recommended that older dogs and cats with proteinuria and a urine protein-to-creatinine ratio equal to or greater than 3 be managed daily with an ACE inhibitor. The question is then what should be the recommended dose of the ACE inhibitor administered daily to these older dogs or cats with proteinuria? Currently, I prefer to start with an ACE inhibitor such as enalapril, benazepril, or lisinopril at one-half of the dose normally used for the management of canine or feline heart disease and to feed a commercially prepared senior diet (and not necessarily a restricted protein diet) that the animal will eat. Thereafter, the medicated dog or cat is monitored monthly for improvement in the urine protein-to-creatinine ratio and for any other medical problems. After 2 months of ACE inhibitor administration with no improvement in the urine protein-to-creatinine ratio, I then increase the daily dose of the ACE inhibitor to that used for canine or feline heart disease. In general, clinical results have shown that older dogs and cats can be effectively managed, at least on a short-term basis, for proteinuria with ACE inhibitors and have an improved quality of life.

AMYLOIDOSIS

Renal amyloidosis is characterized by extracellular deposition of amyloid in glomerular capillary walls, glomerular mesangium, and medullary interstitium.[44] Renal amyloidosis is usually observed in older unrelated dogs; however, familial renal amyloidosis occurs in Abyssinian, Oriental shorthair, and Siamese cats, and in beagle and Chinese Shar-Pei dogs.[45-48] The condition is usually recognized when clinical signs and laboratory abnormalities consistent with CRF and uremia occur. Affected Chinese Shar-Pei dogs may have a history of intermittent pyrexia or swelling of the tibiotarsal joints (so-called "swollen hock disease"). Unlike older animals with nonfamilial renal amyloidosis, severe proteinuria is an inconsistent clinical feature of familial renal amyloidosis in Abyssinian cats and Chinese Shar-Pei dogs. This disparity most likely reflects differences in the intrarenal location of amyloid deposits. The medullary interstitium is the primary site of amyloid deposition in these breeds. Diagnosis of renal amyloidosis is based on breed, clinical signs and laboratory findings consistent with CRF, and demonstration of renal amyloid deposits by light microscopy. No therapy is capable of slowing or eliminating renal amyloid deposition. Because renal amyloidosis often results in progressive nephron destruction and deterioration of renal function, symptomatic and supportive therapy may be of benefit.

PYELONEPHRITIS

Pyelonephritis is the consequence of ascending bacterial urinary tract infections.[49] Acquired abnormalities of the urinary tract that may compromise host defenses are important predisposing factors in the pathogenesis of pyelonephritis. Urinary stasis or obstruction, urolithiasis, and neoplasia are potentially important predisposing factors in older animals. Bacterial infections of the kidney may be acute or chronic, focal, or disseminated.[44] Animals with advanced chronic generalized pyelonephritis typically have small, scarred kidneys.

Clinical findings associated with pyelonephritis depend on the degree of renal involvement and the duration of infection.[49] Acute generalized pyelonephritis may be associated with varying degrees of pyrexia, lethargy, anorexia, vomiting, renal pain, leukocytosis, bacteriuria, pyuria, and casts. Finding white blood cell casts with bacteriuria is strongly suggestive of bacterial pyelonephritis. Manifestations of chronic generalized pyelonephritis are often subtle, but may include polyuria, polydipsia, isosthenuria, recurrent asymptomatic bacteriuria, or recurrent urethrocystitis.

If generalized involvement of both kidneys occurs, clinical signs and laboratory findings associated with renal failure may be present. A diagnosis of pyelonephritis is based on history, physical examination, and results of laboratory evaluations (complete blood count, serum chemistry profile, urinalysis, quantitative urine culture), and radiographic or ultrasonographic studies. Treatment of bacterial pyelonephritis consists of antimicrobial therapy and the elimination of predisposing factors. Because eradication of bacteria from the kidney may be difficult, antimicrobial therapy is usually continued for 6 to 8 weeks. In uremic animals, supportive therapy for renal failure should be provided.

PERIRENAL CYSTS (PSEUDOCYSTS)

Perirenal cyst is an uncommonly recognized disorder characterized by progressive abdominal enlargement owing to accumulation of fluid in a cyst-like structure surrounding one or both kidneys.[50] By definition, a cyst is a filled sac lined by an epithelium. The renal capsule is a mesenchymally derived connective tissue cover and, therefore, devoid of an epithelial lining. Consequently, the collection of fluid between the kidney and its capsule is best described as a pseudocyst. There is no definitive way to know how long a perirenal pseudocyst has been present.

Perirenal pseudocyst can be differentiated from hydronephrosis, polycystic kidneys, and neoplasia by ultrasonography or intravenous urography, which usually reveals a normal- to small-sized kidney encased in a fluid-filled sac.[50] Unilateral or bilateral entrapment of fluid within the renal capsule in cats can be a transudate, urine, or blood. The question that then arises is what is the type of fluid contained within this perirenal pseudocyst now? Is the cystic fluid leaked urine from a disrupted renal pelvis or proximal ureter, or is it a transudate (low protein content and low cellularity)? Accumulated urine is ruled out by doing an ultrasound-guided aspiration of the perirenal pseudocyst. The aspirated fluid is then evaluated for creatinine and potassium concentrations, and their concentrations are compared with the serum creatinine and potassium concentrations. If the aspirated fluid creatinine and potassium concentrations are higher than the respective serum concentrations, the aspirated fluid is accumulated urine—that is, urine has leaked into the renal capsule from the pelvic region of the kidney. If this is the case, exploratory laparotomy should be performed with the idea that the kidney and associated ureter should be removed. If the aspirated fluid is a transudate, then the perirenal pseudocyst can be aspirated under ultrasound guidance, as needed. If the perirenal pseudocyst refills quickly, then exploratory laparotomy can be performed to permanently open the renal capsule so that the accumulating perirenal fluid can easily escape into the abdominal cavity and subsequently be absorbed into circulation.

Accumulation of blood in perirenal pseudocysts can result from trauma, surgery, neoplastic erosion of blood vessels, rupture of aneurysms, or coagulopathies. After hematoma formation, clot retraction, and lysis, a clear or light yellow fluid may remain between the kidney and its capsule. Of these three fluid types, blood accumulates least commonly.

Affected cats may or may not be azotemic.[50] Repeated complete blood counts and serum chemistry profile monitoring and medical management of the CRF is recommended after the initial diagnosis. The short-term prognosis is usually favorable after transudative fluid removal from a perirenal pseudocyst via repeated ultrasound-guided aspirations or permanent capsulectomy in cats that have no evidence of renal dysfunction or only mild degrees of renal dysfunction. The long-term prognosis for cats with perirenal pseudocysts is not known, because acquired perirenal pseudocysts have not yet been determined to be in some way associated with underlying lesions in the renal parenchyma that may be progressive.

RECURRENT URINARY TRACT INFECTIONS

Recurrent urinary tract infections in dogs and cats are especially common. The way I generally manage recurrent urinary tract infections in dogs of all ages is as follows. First, I diagnose and manage any underlying cause of the problem. In older dogs, endocrine diseases such as hyperadrenocorticism, advanced dental disease, and urinary bladder neoplasia are likely primary causes. Then, I administer appropriate antimicrobial therapy to the affected dog until the urine cultures are negative. This usually requires standard antimicrobial therapy for at least 4 to 6 weeks. Thereafter, the dog receives a single standard dose of the appropriate antimicrobial agent each evening after complete voiding of the urinary bladder for the night, usually around 10 PM or 11 PM.

If the antimicrobial agent is administered each

evening, it should concentrate in the collecting urine during the night for an immediate antimicrobial effect and should help maintain a delayed antimicrobial effect that is known to occur with many antimicrobial agents in the urinary tract. This means that the antimicrobial agent will be incorporated into the surface epithelial cells of the urinary tract and maintain a bacteriostatic effect for an extended period, which will vary depending on which antimicrobial agent is used.

How long one should continue to administer the daily evening dose of an antimicrobial agent for recurrent urinary tract infection in older dogs and cats is unknown. It may be for months to years depending somewhat on the medical history and active clinical problems of the affected animal. I suspect that some recurrent urinary tract infections are related to impaired immune regulation in the urinary tract, and in such cases the animals may require antimicrobial therapy for life.

References

1. Cowgill LD, Spangler WL: Renal insufficiency in geriatric dogs, *Vet Clin North Am* 11:727, 1981.
2. Polzin DJ, Osborne CA, Jacob F et al: Chronic renal failure. In Ettinger SJ, Feldman EC, eds: *Textbook of veterinary internal medicine,* ed 5, Philadelphia, 2000, WB Saunders.
3. Dow S, Fettman M: Renal disease in cats: the potassium connection. In Kirk RW, Bonagura JD, eds: *Current veterinary therapy XI,* Philadelphia, 1992, WB Saunders.
4. Rubin SI: Diagnosis and management of chronic renal failure in geriatric cats, *Compend Contin Educ Pract Vet* 11:1065, 1989.
5. Morgan RV: Systemic hypertension in four cats: ocular and medical findings, *J Am Anim Hosp Assoc* 22:615, 1986.
6. Cowgill LD: Medical management of the anemia of chronic renal failure. In Osborne CA, Finco DR, eds: *Canine and feline nephrology and urology,* Baltimore, 1995, Williams & Wilkins.
7. Kobayashi DL, Peterson ME, Graves TK et al: Hypertension in cats with chronic renal failure or hyperthyroidism, *J Vet Intern Med* 4:58, 1990.
8. DiBartola SP, Rutgers HC, Zack PM et al: Clinicopathologic findings associated with chronic renal disease in cats: 74 cases (1973-1984), *J Am Vet Med Assoc* 190:1196, 1987.
9. Krawiec DR, Gelberg HB: Chronic renal disease in cats. In Kirk RW, ed: *Current veterinary therapy X: small animal practice,* Philadelphia. 1989, WB Saunders.
10. Ross LA, Finco DR: Relationship of selected clinical renal function tests to glomerular filtration rate and renal blood flow in cats, *Am J Vet Res* 42:1704, 1981.
11. Rubin SI, Outerbridge CA: Examining the links among potassium, diet, and renal disease in the cat, *Vet Previews* 2:14, 1995.
12. Rogers QR, Morris JG, Freedland RA: Lack of hepatic enzymatic adaptation to low and high levels of dietary protein in the adult cat, *Enzyme* 22:348, 1977.
13. Bartges JW, Willis AM, Polzin DJ: Hypertension and renal disease, *Vet Clin North Am Small Anim Pract* 26:1331, 1996.
14. Snyder PS: Evaluation of the antihypertensive agent amlodipine besylate in normotensive cats and a cat with systemic hypertension, *J Vet Intern Med* 8:147, 1994 (abstract).
15. Nagode LA, Chew DJ, Podell M: Benefits of calcitriol therapy and serum phosphorus control in dogs and cats with chronic renal failure, *Vet Clin North Am Small Anim Pract* 26:1293, 1996.
16. Nagode LA, Chew DJ, Steinmeyer CL et al: Renal secondary hyperparathyroidism: toxic aspects, mechanisms of development, and control by oral calcitriol treatment. In Proceedings of the 11th Annual Forum of the American College of Veterinary Internal Medicine, San Diego, Calif., 1993.
17. Cowgill L, Kallet A: Systemic hypertension. In Kirk RW, ed: *Current veterinary therapy IX,* Philadelphia, 1986, WB Saunders.
18. Esbach J: The anemia of chronic renal failure: pathophysiology and effects of recombinant erythropoietin, *Kidney Int* 35:134, 1989.
19. Cowgill LD: Application of recombinant human erythropoietin (r-HuEPO) in dogs and cats. In Kirk RW, ed: *Current veterinary therapy XI: small animal practice,* Philadelphia, 1992, WB Saunders.
20. Elliot DA, Riel DL, Rogers QR: Complications and outcomes associated with use of gastrostomy tubes for nutritional management of dogs with renal failure: 56 cases (1994-1999), *J Am Vet Med Assoc* 217:1337, 2000.
21. Macy DW, Ralston SL: Cause and control of decreased appetite. In Kirk RW, ed: *Current veterinary therapy X: small animal practice,* Philadelphia, 1989, WB Saunders.
22. Osborne CA, Lulich JP, Polzin DJ et al: Canine and feline nephrolithiasis: causes and cure. In Proceedings of the 11th Annual Forum of the American College of Veterinary Internal Medicine, San Diego, Calif., 1993.
23. Ling GV: Nephrolithiasis: prevalence of mineral type. In Kirk RW, Bonagura JD, eds: *Current veterinary therapy XII: small animal practice,* Philadelphia, 1995, WB Saunders.
24. Carter WO, Hawkins EC, Morrison WB: Feline nephrolithiasis: Eight cases (1984 through 1989), *J Am Anim Hosp Assoc*, 29:247, 1993.
25. Dieringer TM, Lees GE: Nephroliths: approach to therapy. In Kirk RW, ed: *Current veterinary therapy XI: small animal practice,* Philadelphia, 1992, WB Saunders.
26. Osborne CA, Unger LK, Lulich JP: Canine and feline nephroliths. In Kirk RW, Bonagura JD, eds: *Current veterinary therapy XII: small animal practice,* Philadelphia, 1995, WB Saunders.
27. Bailey G, Burk RL: Dry extracorporeal shock wave lithotripsy for treatment of ureterolithiasis and nephrolithiasis in a dog, *J Am Vet Med Assoc* 207:592, 1995.
28. Block G, Adams LG, Widmer WR et al: Use of extracorporeal shock wave lithotripsy for treatment of nephrolithiasis and ureterolithiasis in five dogs, *J Am Vet Med Assoc* 208:531, 1996.
29. Senior DF: Lithotripsy in companion animals. In Kirk RW, Bonagura JD, eds: *Current veterinary therapy XII: small animal practice,* Philadelphia, 1995, WB Saunders.
30. Krawiec DR: Urinary incontinence in dogs and cats, *Mod Vet Pract* 69:17, 1988.

31. Moreau PM: Neurogenic disorders of micturition in the dog and cat, *Compend Contin Educ Pract Vet* 4:12, 1982.
32. Krawiec DR: Diagnosis and treatment of acquired canine urinary incontinence, *Comp Anim Pract* 1:12, 1989.
33. Burnie AG, Weaver AD: Urinary bladder neoplasia in the dog: a review of seventy cases, *J Small Anim Pract* 24:129, 1983.
34. Osborne CA, Low DG, Perman V et al: Neoplasms of the canine and feline urinary bladder: Incidence, etiologic factors, occurrence and pathologic features, *Am J Vet Res* 29:2041, 1968.
35. Hayes HM: Canine bladder cancer: epidemiologic features, *Am J Epidemiol* 104:673, 1976.
36. Crow SE, Klausner JS: Management of transitional cell carcinomas of the urinary bladder. In Kirk RW, ed: *Current veterinary therapy VIII,* Philadelphia, 1983, WB Saunders.
37. Macy DW: Chemotherapeutic agents available for cancer treatment. In Kirk RW, ed: *Current veterinary therapy IX,* Philadelphia, 1986, WB Saunders.
38. DiBartola SP, Chew DJ: Glomerular disease in the dog and cat. In Kirk RW, ed: *Current veterinary therapy IX,* Philadelphia, 1986, WB Saunders.
39. Grauer GF, Frisbie DD, Snyder PS et al: Treatment of membranoproliferative glomerulonephritis and nephrotic syndrome in a dog with a thromboxane synthetase inhibitor, *J Vet Intern Med* 6:77, 1992.
40. Cook AK, Cowgill LD: Clinical and pathologic features of protein-losing glomerular disease in the dog: a review of 137 cases, *J Am Anim Hosp Assoc* 32:313, 1996.
41. Brown SA, Walton CL, Crawford P et al: Long-term effects of antihypertensive regimens on renal hemodynamics and proteinuria, *Kidney Int* 43:1210, 1993.
42. Grauer GF, Greco DS, Getzy DM et al: Effects of enalapril in dogs with glomerulopathy, *J Vet Intern Med* 13:250, 1999.
43. Grodecki KM, Gains MJ, Baumal R et al: Treatment of X-lined hereditary nephritis in Samoyed dogs with angiotensin converting enzyme (ACE) inhibitor, *J Comp Pathol* 117:209, 1997.
44. Maxie MG, Prescott JF: The urinary system. In Jubb KVF, Kennedy PC, Palmer N, eds: *Pathology of domestic animals,* vol 2, ed 4, New York, 1991, Academic Press.
45. Bowles MH, Mosier DA: Renal amyloidosis in a family of beagles, *J Am Vet Med Assoc* 201:569, 1992.
46. Chew DJ, DiBartola SP, Boyce JT et al: Renal amyloidosis in related Abyssinian cats, *J Am Vet Med Assoc* 181:139, 1982.
47. DiBartola SP, Tarr MJ, Webb DM et al: Familial renal amyloidosis in Chinese Shar Pei dogs, *J Am Vet Med Assoc* 197:483, 1990.
48. Zuber RM: Systemic amyloidosis in Oriental and Siamese cats, *Aust Vet Pract* 23:66, 1993.
49. Crowell WA, Neuwirth L, Mahaffey MB: Pyelonephritis. In Osborne CA, Finco DR, eds: *Canine and feline nephrology and urology,* Baltimore, 1995, Williams & Wilkins.
50. Lulich JP, Osborne CA, Polzin DJ: Cystic diseases of the kidney. In Osborne CA, Finco DR, eds: *Canine and feline nephrology and urology,* Baltimore, 1995, Williams & Wilkins.

Supplemental Reading

Lewis LD, Morris ML, Hand MS: *Small animal clinical nutrition III,* Topeka, Kan, 1987, Mark Morris Associates.

CHAPTER 20

The Prostate Gland

JOHNNY D. HOSKINS

Prostatic disease is common in the older dog but rarely occurs in the older cat. The canine prostatic diseases include benign prostatic hyperplasia (BPH), parenchymal and paraprostatic cysts, calculi, acute and chronic infectious prostatitis, abscess, squamous metaplasia, and neoplasia.[1] Prostatic disease occurs in both intact and neutered dogs, with an increased incidence of infectious and inflammatory disorders in intact males. The incidence of canine prostatic disease increases with advancing age for several reasons. As a dog ages, the prostate gland increases in size and develops an increased sensitivity to testosterone. Prostatic secretions, thought to have antibacterial properties, decline after 4 years of age. Communication with the urinary and reproductive tracts permits transfer of genitourinary pathogens into the parenchyma of the prostate gland. Neoplastic transformation occurs with increased frequency in older dogs, and early neutering does not appear to be protective against prostatic neoplasia.[2]

Diagnosis of canine prostatic disease is based on the case history, clinical signs (fecal tenesmus, dysuria, urethral discharge, systemic illness), and results of selected diagnostic tests (rectal or transabdominal palpation of the prostate gland, cytologic evaluation of urethral discharge, cytologic, bacterial, and fungal evaluation of ejaculated or aspirated prostatic fluid, ultrasonography and radiography of the prostate gland and surrounding structures, and prostatic gland aspiration or biopsy).

BENIGN PROSTATIC HYPERPLASIA

Although the definitive cause and pathogenesis of BPH are not known, it is clear that hormonal factors are involved.[3,4] BPH is associated with an altered androgen-to-estrogen ratio and requires the presence of functioning testes.[3] With advancing age, there is a modest decrease in serum androgen concentration but an accumulation of dihydrotestosterone within the prostate gland.[5] This increase in dihydrotestosterone may alter the growth and function of the prostate gland in BPH. In addition, an absolute or relative increase in estrogen concentration may also enhance the hyperplastic process.

Dogs with BPH are bright, alert, and nonfebrile (Figure 20-1). Clinical signs usually include constipation and tenesmus or a mild hemorrhagic urethral discharge. The incidence of clinical signs referable to the urinary tract (stranguria, dysuria, incontinence) varies from occasional to frequent.[6] Prostatic palpation often reveals a symmetrically enlarged, nonpainful gland of normal consistency, but occasionally an irregular, cobblestone-like surface may be felt. Radiographically, the prostate gland often appears enlarged, especially on the lateral radiographic view. Ultrasonographically, symmetric enlargement with a homogeneous echogenicity is observed, but in some cases small cavitary lesions are present that indicate cyst formation (Figure 20-2). Ejaculates and prostatic massages are normal to hemorrhagic. Definitive diagnosis can be made

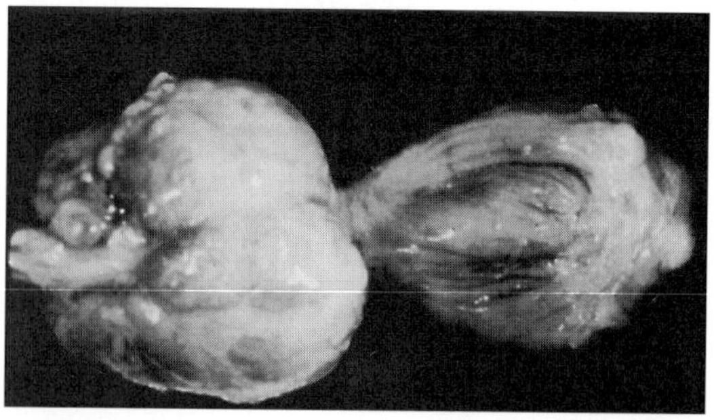

Figure 20-1. Benign prostatic hyperplasia in a dog. The circumscribed mass to the left is the enlarged prostate gland; the urinary bladder is to the right.

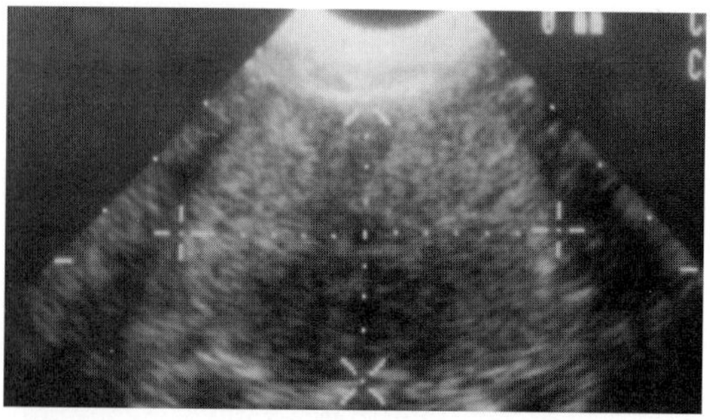

Figure 20-2. Cross-sectional ultrasonogram of an aged dog with benign prostatic hyperplasia. The prostate gland measures 5.4 × 3 cm in cross-sectional diameter and is uniformly hyperechoic and symmetric and contains no cavitations or mineralization. (Courtesy of Beth Partington, DVM, Louisiana State University, Baton Rouge, La.)

only by biopsy, but this is seldom necessary, as a presumptive diagnosis can usually be made on the basis of the case history, physical examination findings, and laboratory findings.

Treatment for BPH is directed at reducing the size of the prostate gland and eliminating clinical signs related to the benign hyperplasia. This is best accomplished by castration. Castration will cause the prostate gland to decrease in size over a 2- to 3-month period with few complications. Synthetic estrogens used in small doses and over short periods of time will cause atrophy of the prostate gland, but extended use may cause squamous metaplasia and enlargement of the prostate gland. Squamous metaplasia leads to secretory stasis, which may cause prostatic cyst or abscess formation.[7] In addition, severe bone marrow depression with pancytopenia may also result from prolonged use of estrogens or as an idiosyncratic reaction.[8] Diethylstilbestrol given orally at 0.5 to 1 mg daily for 5 days or every few days for 3 weeks has been recommended.[7]

Use of 5-Alpha-Reductase Inhibitors

The definitive treatment for most canine prostatic diseases is castration. However, if a dog is used for breeding purposes and castration is not an acceptable option, medical treatment with 5-alpha-reductase inhibitors is indicated.[9] Dogs medicated with 5-alpha-reductase inhibitors experience a significant decrease in prostatic size within 6 weeks, but the prostate gland will return to the previous enlarged size when the medication is withdrawn. Inhibiting 5-alpha-reductase blocks the conversion of testosterone to dihydrotestosterone within the prostate gland, protecting the prostate gland from the effects of androgens. The 5-alpha-reductase inhibitors do not affect semen quality, so the dog can still be used for breeding. Finasteride (Proscar) is a 5-alpha-reductase inhibitor approved for use in men. The dose used in dogs is 5 mg/kg given orally once daily for 6 to 8 weeks.[9,10] Treatment may be repeated as needed over time.

INFECTIOUS PROSTATITIS

Ascending infection from *Escherichia coli*, *Staphylococcus* species, or *Streptococcus* species most commonly causes bacterial prostatitis in older dogs. These bacteria ascend the urethra and progress through the ductal system into the parenchyma of the prostate gland.[7,11] Acute bacterial prostatitis may be initiated by any condition that alters the normal secretion of the prostatic gland, such as cystic hyperplasia and squamous metaplasia, or by an increase in bacterial numbers in the prostatic urethra, such as occurs with a lower urinary tract infection, urolithiasis, neoplasia, and trauma. Dogs with acute prostatitis may present with fever, anorexia, lethargy, urethral discharge, and painful prostate glands on rectal palpation. Inflammatory leukograms with or without a left shift are often seen. Urinalysis may reveal pyuria, hematuria, and bacteriuria. Prostatic fluid is often difficult to obtain from dogs that are in pain. Vigorous prostatic massage may be contraindicated because of the risk of inducing a bacteremia. Because the blood-prostatic barrier is disrupted in acute bacterial prostatitis, most antimicrobial agents will be distributed into the parenchyma of the prostate gland. Parenteral administration of an antimicrobial agent initially is recommended, followed by 3 to 4 weeks of oral antimicrobial therapy. The dog should be reevaluated 7 to 10 days after antimicrobial therapy is discontinued.

Chronic prostatic infections may be present without causing any signs of prostatic disease. Symptomatic dogs are presented for treatment of recurrent urinary tract infections but are not usually systemically ill.[12,13] Chronic infection alone will not cause changes in the size or symmetry of the prostate gland unless an abscess has formed or cystic disease has occurred. Rectal or transabdominal palpation of the prostate gland does not cause pain. The hemogram is usually normal. Urinalysis reveals pyuria, hematuria, and bacteriuria. Prostatic fluid usually contains inflammatory cells, and bacterial cultures may grow a single organism at >100,000 organisms per milliliter. No specific radiographic changes occur with chronic bacterial prostatitis, but ultrasonography may reveal echogenic parenchymal foci or diffusely increased echogenicity (Figure 20-3).[14]

In cases of chronic bacterial infections, bacteria may persist within the prostate gland in spite of antimicrobial therapy. Treatment of chronic bacterial prostatitis should be based on the bacterial isolation and sensitivity testing. In general, chloramphenicol, erythromycin, trimethoprim, ciprofloxacin, enrofloxacin, and carbenicillin are able to cross the prostatic epithelium and concentrate within prostatic fluid.[15] Antimicrobial agents such as ampicillin, cephalosporins, oxytetracycline, and the aminoglycosides are unable to readily cross the prostatic epithelium and concentrate within prostatic fluid. If gram-negative organisms are cultured, trimethoprim-sulfonamide, chloramphenicol, enrofloxacin, or ciprofloxacin should be used. If gram-positive organisms are cultured, clindamycin, erythromycin, chloramphenicol, or trimethoprim-sulfonamide may be used. Antimicrobial therapy should be continued for at least 4 to 6 weeks. If urine culture was positive, urine and prostatic fluid should be cultured at 4 to 7 days and again at 30 days after the completion of antimicrobial therapy. If the prostatic infection still persists, a 3-month course of antimicrobial agents should be administered. In addition to antimicrobial therapy, castration is recommended.[16]

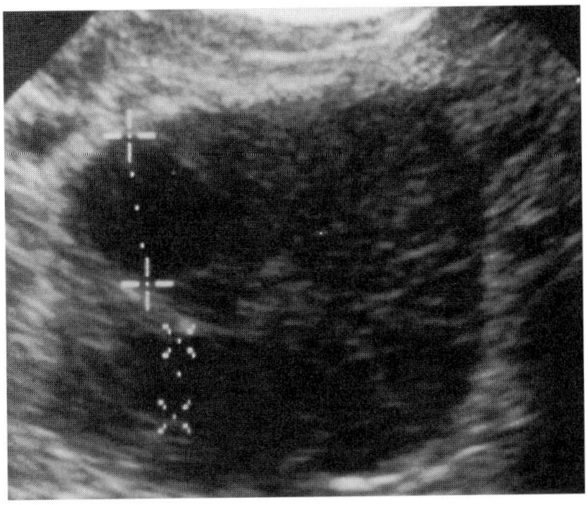

Figure 20-3. Cross-sectional ultrasonogram of a 5-year-old male dachshund with cavitating bacterial prostatitis. The prostate gland is enlarged, hypoechoic, and irregularly marginated and contains two anechoic circular cavitations identified with *t* and *x* measurement cursors. Ultrasound-guided fine-needle aspiration of the cavitations for cytology and bacterial culture confirmed the diagnosis. (Courtesy of Beth Partington, DVM, Louisiana State University, Baton Rouge, La.)

PROSTATIC ABSCESSES

Prostatic abscesses occur when large pockets of purulent material accumulate as a result of a bacterial infection of the prostate gland. Clinical signs such as tenesmus, dysuria, stranguria, and constant or intermittent urethral discharge may occur secondarily to prostatic enlargement.[9] In addition, the dog may be systemically ill from endotoxemia or peritonitis. Rectal examination findings vary depending on the size and location of the abscesses. Asymmetry of the prostate gland may be palpated. A neutrophilic leukocytosis with or without a left shift is usually present. Prostatic fluid may contain large numbers of bacteria, white blood cells, and, occasionally, red blood cells. On survey radiographs, prostatomegaly may be seen, and ultrasonographic findings include hypoechoic to anechoic areas within the prostatic parenchyma (see Figure 20-3). Most prostatic abscesses should be treated aggressively by either marsupialization of the prostate gland or placement of surgical drains. Alternatively, a prostatectomy may be performed. Associated with these procedures is a high incidence of complications including urinary incontinence, chronically draining stomas, septic shock, and death.[17,18] Castration is recommended as adjunctive therapy. Antimicrobial agents should be administered to dogs with abscessed prostate glands, as would be done for chronic infectious prostatitis.

SQUAMOUS METAPLASIA

Squamous metaplasia of the prostatic parenchyma may occur secondarily to endogenous or exogenous hyperestrogenism. Squamous metaplasia predisposes the prostate gland to cystic disease and infectious prostatitis. Identification and removal of the source of estrogen is recommended. Estrogen-producing Sertoli cell tumors are the most common cause of squamous metaplasia in older dogs.

PROSTATIC CYSTS

Prostatic cysts typically are multiple small cysts associated with benign hyperplasia, prostatic retention cysts, paraprostatic cysts, or cysts associated with squamous metaplasia. Except for the multiple small prostatic cysts associated with benign hyperplasia, the incidence of prostatic cysts in older dogs is low, ranging from approximately 2.6% to 5.3%.[19] Dogs with prostatic cysts often exhibit dysuria and tenesmus related to increased prostatic size. Large prostatic cysts place excessive pressure on the urinary bladder wall and may displace the neck of the urinary bladder cranially. A urethral discharge may occur if the prostatic cyst communicates with the urethra.[7,9] Small prostatic cysts may be palpated rectally as asymmetrically enlarged prostate glands. Soft, fluctuant areas are sometimes noted in the affected lobe. Large discrete prostatic cysts are usually palpated in the caudal abdomen and occasionally in the perineal area.[19] If the prostatic cyst becomes large enough, abdominal distention may be present. Aspirated cystic fluid will vary in color but is often light yellow with varying degrees of cloudiness.[7,19] Bacterial culture of the aspirated fluid is usually negative for bacterial growth. Large prostatic cysts appear radiographically as soft-tissue dense masses similar to the urinary bladder in the caudal-ventral region of the abdomen. Contrast cystography will outline the contour of the urinary bladder, and occasionally reflux of contrast material into the prostatic cyst will occur. Small prostatic cysts on ultrasonography appear as hypoechoic to anechoic foci located within the prostatic parenchyma or outside its capsule. Ultrasound-guided fine-needle aspirate of a prostatic cyst may yield fluid for cytologic examination and bacterial culture. The treatment for large prostatic cysts is resection and marsupialization.[17,19] However, these cysts must be large enough to reach the ventral abdominal wall for this surgical technique to be performed. Concurrent castration is recommended to reduce the size of the prostate gland and eliminate any effects an altered androgen-estrogen balance may be having on the disease process. Complications of surgery include infections or injury to the urinary bladder or ureters. Drainage and surgical resection alone are occasionally possible with some prostatic cysts. The treatment for small intraprostatic cysts is castration.

PROSTATIC NEOPLASIA

Both intact and neutered older dogs are at risk for primary neoplasia of the prostate gland. The most commonly reported neoplasm in dogs is adenocarcinoma, followed by transitional cell carcinoma (Figures 20-4 and 20-5). The primary site of metastasis of prostatic adenocarcinoma is the iliac lymph nodes, followed in decreasing order by the lungs, urinary bladder, mesentery, rectum, and bone.[20] Metastatic bone lesions can

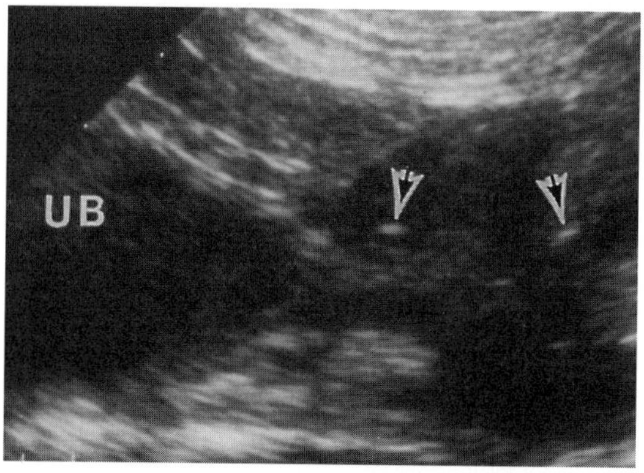

Figure 20-4. Longitudinal prostatic ultrasonographic examination of a 9-year-old castrated Airedale terrier with prostatic transitional cell carcinoma. The prostate gland is slightly enlarged, irregularly marginated, and complexly echogenic and contains several small mineralizations *(arrowheads)*. *UB,* Urinary bladder. (Courtesy of Beth Partington, DVM, Louisiana State University, Baton Rouge, La.)

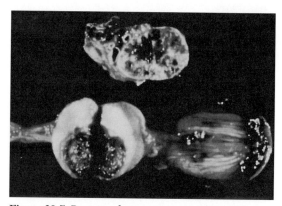

Figure 20-5. Prostatic adenocarcinoma in a dog. The prostate gland has been incised to expose the neoplasm; the urinary bladder is to the right of the prostate gland. Metastasis to a regional lymph node is included above.

be proliferative or lytic, and the most frequent sites include the pelvis, lumbar vertebrae, and femur. Presenting history is similar to other prostatic diseases; however, about 70% of older dogs with lameness or ambulatory difficulties have prostatic neoplasia.[21] Chronic weight loss may be present. Prostatic palpation may reveal enlargement, asymmetry, pain, or increased firmness. Hematologic abnormalities may reveal evidence of acute or chronic inflammation. Azotemia may be present if the neoplastic mass is obstructing both ureters and the urethra. Pyuria, hematuria, and bacteriuria may be present. Neoplastic cells may be present in ultrasound-guided aspirated prostatic fluid, but their absence does not rule out neoplasia. Thoracic and abdominal radiographs should be taken for evidence of asymmetric prostatic enlargement and metastatic disease. Ultrasonography may show focal or multifocal areas of increased echogenicity. A contrast cystourethrogram may show irregularities or obliteration of the prostatic urethra or invasion of the urinary bladder. If radiographic evidence of metastatic disease is not evident, demonstrating the presence of neoplastic cells by needle aspiration or biopsy should make the definitive diagnosis. If an exploratory laparotomy is done to obtain a prostatic biopsy, iliac lymph nodes should be biopsied as well. Prostatic neoplasia has a poor prognosis. Therapeutic options are usually palliative and include prostatectomy or intraoperative radiation.[22] Urinary incontinence is a common complication of prostatectomy in dogs with neoplastic disease.

FELINE PROSTATIC DISEASE

Prostatic disease is uncommon in cats. The feline prostate gland does not undergo spontaneous hyperplasia with age, and bacterial infections within the urinary tract are uncommon. Prostatic neoplasia is usually an adenocarcinoma or results from direct invasion of a transitional cell carcinoma originating from the pelvic urethra or neck of the urinary bladder.[23]

References

1. Krawiec DR, Heflin DH: Study of prostatic disease in dogs: 177 cases (1981-1986), *J Am Vet Med Assoc* 200:1119, 1992.
2. Obradovich J, Walshaw R, Goullaud E: The influence of castration on the development of prostatic carcinoma in the dog: 43 cases (1978-1985), *J Vet Intern Med* 1:183, 1987.
3. Brendler CB, Berry SJ, Ewing LL et al: Spontaneous benign prostatic hyperplasia in the beagle, *J Clin Invest* 71:1114, 1983.
4. Berry SJ, Coffey DS, Strandberg JD et al: Effect of age, castration, and testosterone replacement on the development and restoration of canine benign prostatic hyperplasia, *Prostate* 9:295, 1986.
5. Isaacs JT, Coffey DS: Changes in dihydrotestosterone metabolism associated with the development of canine benign prostatic hyperplasia, *Endocrinology* 108:445, 1981.
6. Borthwick R, Mackenzie CP: The signs and results of treatment of prostatic disease in dogs, *Vet Rec* 89:374, 1971.
7. Barsanti JA: Urinary tract infections. In Greene CE, ed: *Infectious diseases of the dog and cat,* Philadelphia, 1990, WB Saunders.
8. Pyle RL, Hill BL, Johnson JR: Estrogen toxicity in a dog, *Canine Pract* August:39, 1976.
9. Purswell BJ, Parker NA, Forrester SD: Prostatic diseases in dogs: a review, *Vet Med* 95:315, 2000.
10. Laroque PA, Prahalada S, Gordon LR et al: Effects of chronic oral administration of a selective 5a-reductase inhibitor, finasteride, on the dog prostate, *Prostate* 24:93, 1994.
11. Bruchini H, Schmidt RA: Neurologic control of prostatic secretion in the dog, *Invest Urol* 15:288, 1978.
12. Childs SJ: Ciprofloxacin in treatment of chronic bacterial prostatitis, *Urology* 35:15, 1990.
13. Smith JW: Recurrent urinary tract infections in men: characteristics and response to therapy, *Ann Intern Med* 91:544, 1979.
14. Feeney DA, Johnston GR, Klausner JS et al: Canine prostatic disease—comparison of ultrasonographic appearance with morphologic and microbiologic findings: 30 cases (1981-1985), *J Am Vet Med Assoc* 190:1027, 1987.
15. Barsanti JA: Diseases of the prostate gland. In Osborne CA, Finco DR, eds: *Canine and feline nephrology and urology,* Baltimore, 1995, Williams & Wilkins.
16. Cowan LA, Barsanti JA, Crowell W et al: Effects of castration on chronic bacterial prostatitis in dogs, *J Am Vet Med Assoc* 199:346, 1991.
17. Johnston DI: The prostate. In Slatter D, ed: *Textbook of small animal surgery,* Philadelphia, 1985, WB Saunders.
18. Hardie EM, Barstanti JA, Rawlings CA: Complications of prostatic surgery, *J Am Anim Hosp Assoc* 20:50, 1984.
19. Weaver AD: Discrete prostatic (paraprostatic) cysts in the dog, *Vet Rec* 102:435, 1978.
20. Durham SK, Dietze AE: Prostatic adenocarcinoma with and without metastasis to bone in dogs, *J Am Vet Med Assoc* 188:1432, 1986.
21. Hornbuckle WE, MacCoy DM, Allan GS et al: Prostatic disease in the dog, *Cornell Vet* 68:284, 1978.
22. Turrel JM: Intraoperative radiotherapy of carcinoma of the prostate gland in 10 dogs, *J Am Vet Med Assoc* 190:48, 1987.
23. Hubbard BS, Vulgamott JC, Liska WD: Prostatic adenocarcinoma in a cat, *J Am Vet Med Assoc* 197:1493, 1990.

CHAPTER 21

Neuromuscular Disorders

JANET E. STEISS

Neuromuscular disorders in the older dog and cat tend to target a specific segment of the motor unit. A motor unit consists of (1) a motor neuron, the cell body of which resides in the ventral horn of the spinal cord (or the nuclei of certain cranial nerves in the brainstem); (2) its axon, which exits through the ventral root and travels in a peripheral nerve (or cranial nerve); (3) the neuromuscular junction, formed from the terminal nerve branches of each motor axon terminating on individual muscle fibers; and (4) the muscle fibers (myofibers) innervated by that axon (Figure 21-1).

The Veterinary Medical Data Base receives records from all veterinary colleges in the United States and Canada. A search of the Veterinary Medical Data Base for geriatric dogs and cats (10 years or older, all breeds, from January 1990 to September 2000) indicated that the total number of accessions were 76,773 dogs and 26,493 cats. Myopathies were diagnosed in 1.8% of the dogs (1,358 of 76,773) and 1.1% of the cats (282 of 26,493). The numbers for neuropathies were overestimated because they included diseases of the central nervous system as well as the peripheral nervous system; neurologic diseases were reported in 11% of dogs (8,411 of 76,773) and 5.5% of cats (1,450 of 26,493). In my opinion, neuromuscular diseases are probably underdiagnosed. Neuromuscular diseases can progress to fairly advanced stages before the owners note any functional loss. This is especially true for older dogs and cats, in which muscular weakness may be attributed erroneously to the aging process.

HISTORY AND PHYSICAL EXAMINATION

A thorough medical and surgical history can be of immense help toward forming a differential diagnostic list. One expert on neuromuscular diseases in humans advised physicians, "Please listen to the patient, he's trying to tell you what disease he has."[1] This could be paraphrased for veterinary medicine as, "Please listen to the owners, they are trying to tell you what disease is present." The history provides information concerning:

- Time course (acute or chronic, progressive or stable, constant or intermittent)
- Duration of the problem
- Previous and concurrent medical problems
- Medications
- Exacerbating or relieving factors
- Potential exposure to toxins
- Environmental factors (indoor or outdoor, number of animals in household)
- Diet

In addition, the owner should be questioned about signs that likely will not be obvious during the clinical examination, such as whether there has been a change in a dog's bark or a cat's meow or difficulty with eating. Also, even though inherited neuromuscular diseases tend to appear in younger animals, a few inherited diseases have later onset, and the owners can be questioned about similar disorders in the siblings or parents.

After the history has been taken, the next step is to observe the animal's gait if the animal is

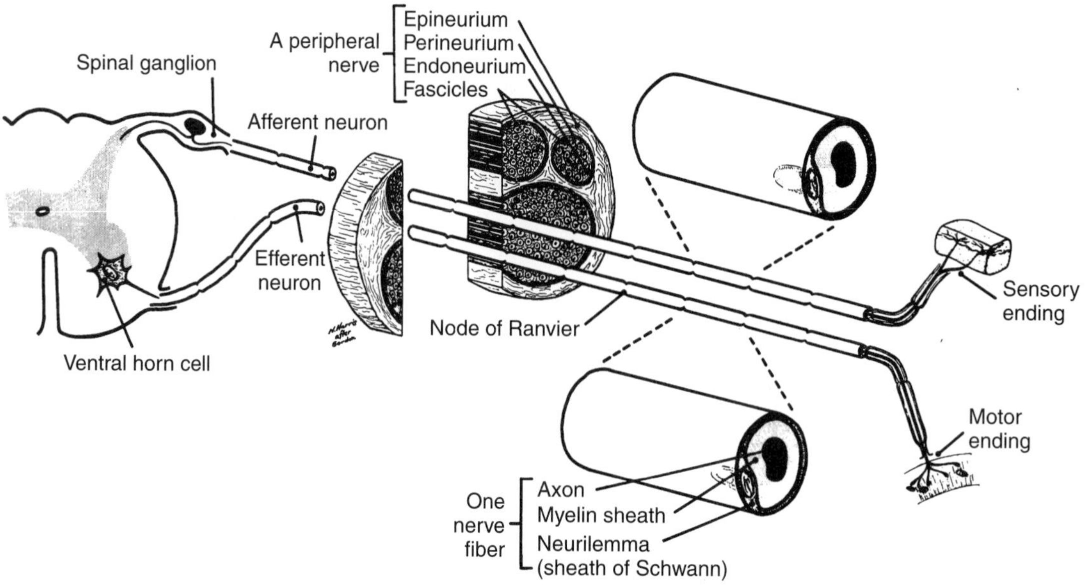

Figure 21-1. This diagram illustrates the motor unit and sensory components of a peripheral nerve. Diseases of the motor unit include those disorders that target the ventral horn cell (neuronopathy), nerve root (radiculopathy), peripheral nerve (neuropathy or axonopathy), neuromuscular junction (junctionopathy), and muscle fiber (myopathy).

ambulatory. In general, neuromuscular diseases are characterized by muscular weakness. The veterinarian can observe the animal walking or trotting and note signs of weakness, such as dropped hocks. If exercise intolerance is suspected because of the history, dogs can be exercised in order to reproduce the condition. At this stage, the veterinarian should have an impression about whether the condition is localized (for example, trauma to a peripheral nerve) or generalized.

After gait analysis, the physical and neurologic examinations are performed. The neurologic examination has been well described in several veterinary textbooks.[2-7] After these examinations have been performed, the veterinarian will have sufficient information to tentatively localize the disorder to a specific part of the motor unit, in addition to having determined whether the disorder is localized or generalized.

MYOPATHIES EVALUATION

Myopathies are broadly classified as inflammatory and noninflammatory.[8] Myopathies are associated with several metabolic and endocrine disorders and are a common cause of muscular weakness in geriatric dogs (Box 21-1). In some cases, the myopathy may be subclinical.[9] The "myopathic syndrome" (Box 21-2) is characterized by generalized weakness, which is bilaterally symmetric, exercise intolerance, or a stiff gait. The gait disturbance is worsened by exercise in most myopathies. Reflexes are usually normal, with the exception of Labrador retriever hereditary myopathy. Pain sensation is intact. Palpation of muscle bellies may suggest muscle pain; this is often seen in dogs with acute polymyositis. Limited joint range of motion can occur if animals have had scarring within the muscles, such as the decreased extension at the stifle in dogs with fibrotic (gracilis) myopathy. Tremors and fasciculations are sometimes seen but are not specific for myopathy. Fasciculations are grossly visible involuntary muscle twitches. Some of these features can be seen with disorders of the neuromuscular junction ("junctionopathies"), such as myasthenia gravis.

Myotonia has different clinical features. In inherited myotonia in chow chows, miniature schnauzers, and several other breeds, the stiffness tends to decrease with exercise. An animal with myotonia tends to appear to have increased muscle mass, whereas other myopathies tend to result in muscle atrophy. However, in inflammatory or immune-mediated myopathies, the muscle mass may appear hypertrophic or swollen during the acute phase. When myotonia is suspected, the veterinarian should try to elicit a dimple contracture. The muscle belly is tapped with a reflex hammer or other instrument or the examiner's

BOX 21-1 Myopathies in Dogs and Cats

Degenerative or Inherited

Bouvier des Flandres myopathy
Congenital myasthenia gravis (Jack Russell terrier, springer spaniel, smooth-haired fox terrier)
Glycogenosis (Swedish Lapland dog, German shepherd, Akita, springer spaniel, toy breeds, Norwegian Forest cat)
Hereditary myopathy of Labrador retrievers
Hypotrophic myopathy (German shepherd)
Muscular dystrophy (Golden retriever, Irish terrier, cat)
Myositis ossificans
Myotonic myopathy (chow chow, Staffordshire terrier, Great Dane, miniature schnauzer)
Nemaline myopathy (cat)

Injury- or Activity-related

Coccygeal muscle injury ("limber tail," "cold tail")
Fibrotic myopathy
Infraspinatus muscle contracture
Myositis ossificans

Immune-mediated

Acquired myasthenia gravis
Dermatomyositis (collie, Shetland sheepdog)
Extraocular myositis
Laryngeal myositis
Masticatory myositis
Paraneoplastic myositis
Polymyositis

Metabolic

Corticosteroid myopathy
Exertional myopathy (rhabdomyolysis)
Hyperadrenocortical myopathy
Hyperkalemic myopathy
Hypernatremic myopathy
Hypokalemic myopathy (cat)
Hypothyroid myopathy
Lipid storage myopathy
Malignant hyperthermia
Mitochondrial myopathy

Nutritional

Vitamin E–selenium responsive myopathy

Inflammatory or Infectious

Clostridium species infection
Hepatozoon americanum infection
Leptospirosis
Microfilariasis
Neospora caninum infection
Toxoplasma gondii infection
Trypanosomiasis

Toxic or Drug-induced

D-Penicillamine
Trimethoprim-sulfadiazine

Vascular

Ischemic neuromyopathy (cat)

Paraneoplastic

Thymoma
Other neoplasms

Modified from Braund KG: *Clinical syndromes in veterinary neurology,* ed 2, St Louis, 1994, Mosby.

BOX 21-2 Clinical Signs Associated with Myopathy-decreased Range of Motion

Exercise intolerance
Muscle atrophy
Muscle dimpling (suggestive of myotonia)
Muscle hypertrophy or swelling
Muscle pain on palpation
Stiff gait
Muscle weakness

Modified from Braund KG: *Clinical syndromes in veterinary neurology,* ed 2, St Louis, 1994, Mosby.

finger. The examiner should try to test the tongue or muscles that are not covered with a lot of hair. Because some muscles seem to show dimpling more so than other muscles, test more than one muscle.

NEUROPATHIES EVALUATION

Neuropathies are defined by the following terms: *mononeuropathy* (affecting one nerve); *polyneuropathy* (a generalized disorder affecting multiple nerves, usually bilaterally symmetric); *motor neuropathy* (limited to motor nerve fibers); *sensory neuropathy* (limited to sensory nerve fibers); and *sensorimotor neuropathy* (affecting both sensory and motor axons—most peripheral nerves contain both sensory and motor fibers).

The basic pathology underlying neuropathies is either primary demyelination (which is rare) or axonal ("Wallerian") degeneration (with secondary demyelination). Characteristics of neuropathies are decreased or absent reflexes, decreased or absent muscle tone, and weakness (paresis) or paralysis (Box 21-3). Within several weeks of onset, neurogenic muscle atrophy becomes

BOX 21-3 Clinical Signs Associated with Disorders of Peripheral Nerves (Neuropathy) and Neuromuscular Junction

Motor*
Decreased range of motion
Denervation atrophy
Flaccid paresis or paralysis
Muscle fasciculations
Reduced or absent reflexes (hyporeflexia or areflexia)
Reduced or absent muscle tone (hypotonia or atonia)
Dysphonia or dyspnea (laryngeal dysfunction)
Dysphagia (pharyngeal dysfunction)
Regurgitation (esophageal dysfunction)

Sensory*
Abnormal sensation (paresthesia)
Decreased pain or sensation (hypalgesia or hypesthesia)
Absent pain or sensation (analgesia or anesthesia)
Proprioceptive deficits, ataxia
Reduced or absent reflexes without muscle atrophy
Self-mutilation

Autonomic
Anisocoria or dilated pupils
Bradycardia
Decreased tear production
Decreased salivation

Modified from Braund KG: *Clinical syndromes in veterinary neurology,* ed 2, St Louis, 1994, Mosby.
*Sensorimotor neuropathies are associated with a combination of motor and sensory signs.

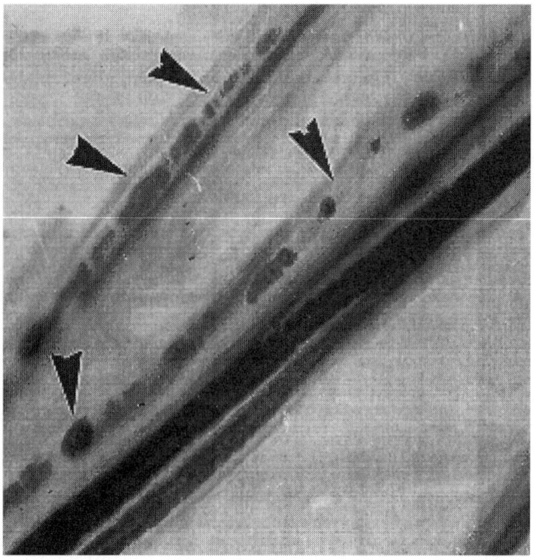

Figure 21-2. Teased nerve fibers showing several smaller caliber fibers *(arrow heads)* undergoing axonal degeneration in a Doberman pinscher with clinical signs of dancing Doberman disease. Caudal cutaneous sural nerve. Osmium tetroxide ×640. (Braund KG and Steiss JE: Unpublished data, 1999)

obvious. In polyneuropathies, pelvic limbs are usually affected first. As a guideline, the onset is acute in traumatic and ischemic neuropathies, subacute in polyradiculoneuritis, and insidious in most polyneuropathies. Self-mutilation may occur because of abnormal sensation. For confirmation of the diagnosis, the animal may undergo needle electromyography and nerve conduction studies and biopsy of nerve (Figure 21-2) and muscle (Figures 21-3 through 21-6).

Cranial nerve dysfunction can be associated with disease of the central nervous system or with an isolated neuropathy. Cranial nerve VII (the facial nerve) can be affected in polyradiculoneuritis or hypothyroid neuropathy. Dysfunction of cranial nerve X (the vagus nerve) results in dysphagia and megaesophagus; this nerve may be affected in giant axonal neuropathy of German shepherds, in laryngeal paralysis and megaesophagus in young dalmatians, or in laryngeal paralysis-polyneuropathy complex in older large-breed dogs.

Neuropathies are frequently associated with trauma. Some of the other neuropathies include idiopathic polyradiculoneuritis (coonhound paralysis), brachial plexus avulsion, idiopathic facial paralysis, ischemic neuromyopathy, peripheral nerve sheath tumors, and tick paralysis, as well as myasthenia gravis, which is a disorder of neuromuscular transmission. Metabolic neuropathies, such as diabetic neuropathy, are now diagnosed more frequently. Paraneoplastic neuropathies are rarely diagnosed but may be more prevalent than currently suspected; these are immune-mediated peripheral nerve disorders, which are associated with the presence of neoplasia, such as carcinoma or adenoma.[10] Nerve sheath tumors are relatively common, frequently causing lameness that initially can be confused with orthopedic problems. Numerous degenerative, breed-specific disorders have been reported but are rare. Other probable causes of peripheral neuropathy in small animals are listed in Box 21-4. As in humans, the specific causes of polyneuropathies in small animals often remain unknown, and therefore the term *idiopathic* is used.

If the underlying cause can be identified, such as diabetes mellitus or hypothyroidism, then treatment of the disorder may result in some improvement of clinical signs. Many dogs with

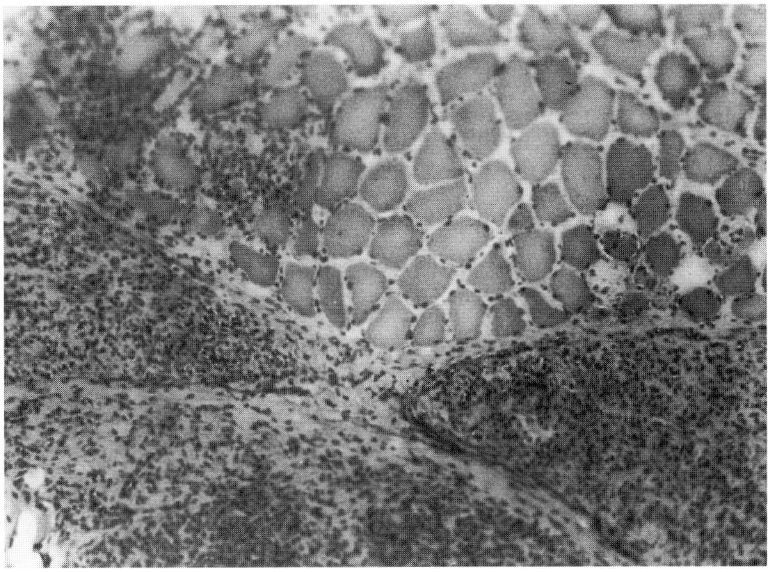

Figure 21-3. Frozen section of a limb muscle biopsy from a dog with polymyositis showing mononuclear cell infiltration. (H & E stain, ×100.)

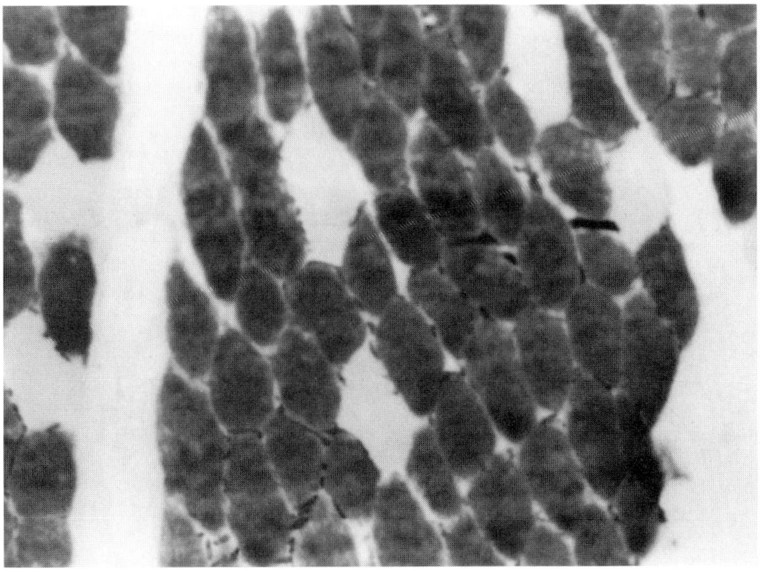

Figure 21-4. Frozen section of a limb muscle biopsy from a dog with confirmed hypothyroidism. There is a marked shift in myofiber types to a type 1 predominance. (Adenosine triphosphatase stain, pH 4.3, ×100.)

polyradiculoneuritis (coonhound paralysis) recover spontaneously, provided that they receive good nursing care, including soft bedding and frequent turning to avoid decubital ulcers. In the presumed immune-mediated neuropathies, such as chronic inflammatory demyelinating polyneuropathy, the majority of dogs and cats have been clinically responsive to corticosteroid therapy, although to varying degrees.[11,12] Unfortunately, for dogs suspected of having dysesthesia and neuropathic pain, there are few recommendations on pharmacologic treatment. Clinical trials to evaluate the response to drugs such as gabapentin would seem to be warranted in future.

DISORDERS OF NEUROMUSCULAR TRANSMISSION EVALUATION

Disorders of neuromuscular transmission may be the result of a defect localized to the presynaptic region (hypocalcemia, botulism, tick paralysis), synaptic cleft (cholinesterase inhibitors), or postsynaptic membrane (acquired myasthenia

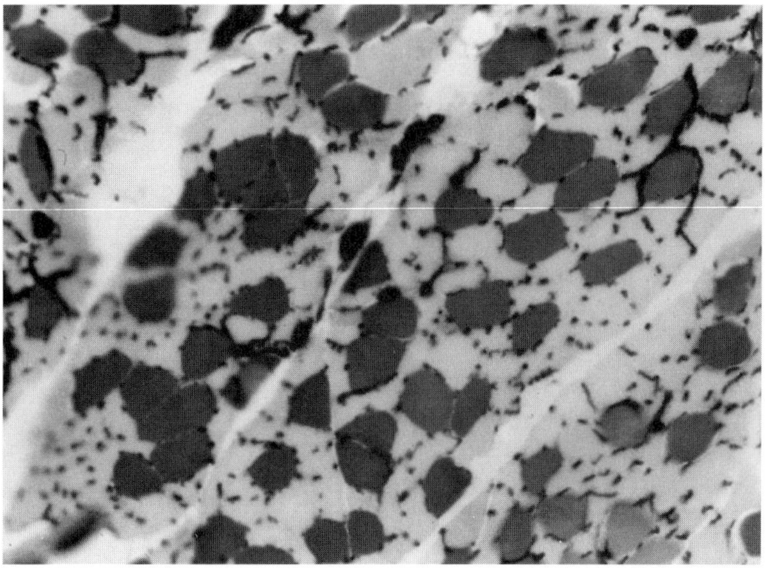

Figure 21-5. Type 2 myofiber atrophy in a muscle biopsy from a dog with hyperadrenocorticism, muscle atrophy, and muscle weakness. (Adenosine triphosphatase stain, pH 4.3, ×100.)

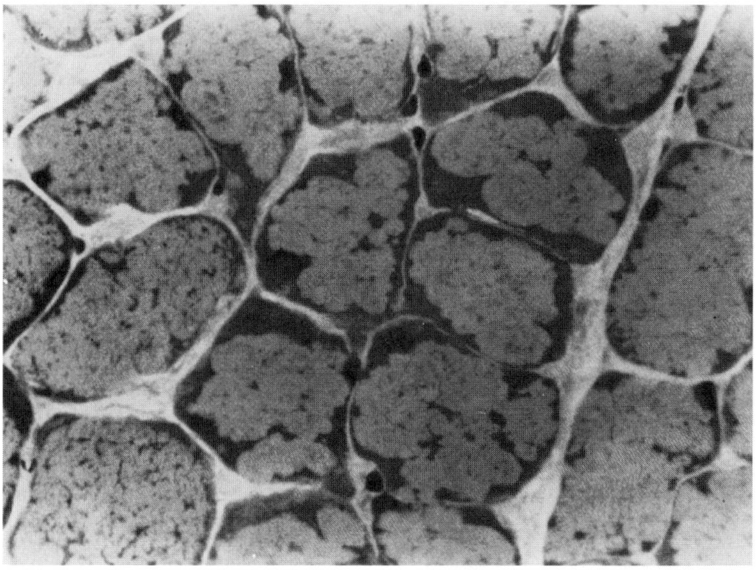

Figure 21-6. Muscle biopsy section from a dog with hyperadrenocorticism and myotonia showing myofibers having a cross between lobulated-like and ragged-red–like cytoarchitectural changes. (H & E stain, ×400.)

gravis). Certain diseases of the neuromuscular junction, such as botulism and tick paralysis, produce signs that mimic a diffuse polyneuropathy.

Ancillary Diagnostic Evaluations

Clinical Pathology. A complete blood count, serum chemistry profile (including serum electrolytes and creatine kinase), and urinalysis should be performed in all cases to evaluate for underlying systemic (e.g., inflammatory or metabolic) disease. In cases in which the lesion localization includes neuronopathy or radiculopathy, cerebrospinal analysis may be included. Metabolic screening is important for potentially treatable causes of neuropathies such as hypoglycemia secondary to an insulinoma,[13] hypothyroidism,[14,15] and hyperglycemia secondary to diabetes mellitus.[16-20]

Serum levels of several enzymes may reflect muscle damage. Serum creatine kinase levels are increased in muscle disorders associated with myonecrosis or increased cell membrane permeability. The half-life of serum creatine kinase is about 12 hours. However, the presence of increased serum creatine kinase levels is not neces-

BOX 21-4 Neuropathies in Dogs and Cats

Degenerative or Inherited

Birman cat polyneuropathy
Congenital deafness (dalmatian, Jack Russell terrier, pointer, and others)
Dancing Doberman disease
Distal denervating disease
Distal symmetric polyneuropathy
Dysautonomia (dog, cat)
Facial paralysis
Giant axonal neuropathy (German shepherd)
Globoid leukodystrophy (cairn and West Highland white terriers)
Glycogenosis (Norwegian Forest cat)
Hereditary ataxia (Jack Russell terrier, smooth-haired fox terrier)
Hypertrophic neuropathy (Tibetan mastiff)*
Hypomyelinating polyneuropathy (golden retriever)
Laryngeal paralysis (Siberian husky, Bouvier des Flandres, dalmatian)
Megaesophagus
Progressive neuronopathy (cairn terrier)
Rottweiler distal sensorimotor polyneuropathy
Sensory ganglioradiculitis
Sensory neuropathy (boxer, English pointer, dachshund, Jack Russell terrier)
Sensory trigeminal neuropathy
Sphingomyelinosis (Siamese cat)*
Spinal muscular atrophy† (Brittany spaniel, Swedish Lapland dog, giant-breed crosses, pointer, German shepherd, rottweiler, cairn terrier)
Vestibular disease

Developmental

Optic nerve hypoplasia

Immune-mediated

Brachial plexus neuropathy
Chronic relapsing polyneuropathy
Chronic relapsing polyradiculoneuritis
Paraneoplastic neuropathy
Polyradiculoneuritis (coonhound paralysis)
Trigeminal neuritis

Metabolic

Diabetic neuropathy
Hyperchylomicronemia
Hyperoxaluria (cat)
Hypoglycemia
Hypothyroid neuropathy

Neoplastic

Peripheral nerve tumors

Nutritional

Hypervitaminosis A (cat)

Inflammatory or Infectious

Labyrinthitis
Optic neuritis
Poliomyelitis† (rabies, postvaccinal rabies, feline polioencephalomyelitis)
Toxoplasmosis
Neosporosis

Traumatic

Brachial plexus avulsion
Spinal trauma†
Traumatic neuropathy

Toxic

Botulism‡
Lead ingestion
Organophosphate and carbamate toxicity
Ingestion of ototoxic drugs
Tick paralysis‡
Vincristine ingestion
Walker hound mononeuropathy

Vascular

Hemorrhagic myelomalacia
Infarction
Ischemic neuromyopathy (cat)

Modified from Braund KG: *Clinical syndromes in veterinary neurology*, ed 2, St Louis, 1994, Mosby.
*The two known examples of spontaneously occurring primary demyelinating neuropathies in dogs and cats.
†Indicates involvement of ventral horn cells within the spinal cord.
‡Indicates a disorder of the neuromuscular junction.

sarily diagnostic of myositis.[8] Serum creatine kinase levels should be interpreted in conjunction with other clinical signs. For instance, a tentative diagnosis of polymyositis would be considered if the animal had increased serum creatine kinase, muscle pain on palpation, and electromyographic abnormalities. Mild elevations in serum creatine kinase activity can be associated with needle electromyographic examination,[16] intramuscular injections, or neuropathies.[21] In addition to serum creatine kinase activity, serum aspartate aminotransferase and serum alanine aminotransferase activities[22] may be increased in muscle diseases, although these serum enzymes are also increased with damage to other tissues such as liver and myocardium.[2]

Evaluation of adrenal and thyroid function should be performed in cases of chronic muscle weakness and atrophy, particularly if other clinical signs suggest an endocrine abnormality. Myopathy associated with hypothyroidism and myopathy or myotonia associated with hyperadrenocorticism have been described.[9,15,23-26] Dogs with hypothyroidism and a concurrent polyneuropathy have improved at least partially in response to thyroid supplementation.[14]

Serum antinuclear antibody titers may be useful in the diagnosis of inflammatory myopathies because immune-mediated diseases are presumed to be an underlying cause of these disorders.[8] Serum electrolyte evaluation should be part of the screening of any animal showing muscle weakness. Cats are particularly sensitive to electrolyte imbalances.[27] Secondary hyperkalemia and muscle weakness may occur in association with numerous clinical conditions including metabolic acidosis, hypoadrenocorticism, renal failure, and hyperaldosteronism. Iatrogenic causes may include intravenous potassium administration and the use of potassium-retaining diuretics. Initial clinical signs are usually referable to cardiovascular abnormalities. Other serum electrolyte abnormalities, including hypernatremia, hypocalcemia or hypercalcemia, hypomagnesemia or hypermagnesemia, and hypophosphatemia or hyperphosphatemia, may result in signs of neuromuscular dysfunction, although specific myopathies associated with these disorders have not been reported. Resolution of clinical signs should occur with normalization of serum electrolyte concentrations. Muscle biopsies of cats and dogs with serum electrolyte abnormalities have not been abnormal.

Plasma lactate levels should be measured before and after exercise in dogs with exercise intolerance and muscle weakness.[8] Lactic acid is the end product of glycolysis. Elevations in plasma lactate levels may occur in hypoxic or ischemic injury. Decreased or increased lactate levels can be seen in healthy field-trial pointers in training consisting of slow speed, long duration ("roading") or high speed, short duration ("running"), respectively.[28] Increased lactate levels have also been documented in Labrador retrievers in training.[29] Alternatively, instead of reflecting physiologic stress, altered lactate levels may be associated with disorders of oxidative metabolism. In several cases, lactic acidemia associated with muscle weakness, atrophy, exercise intolerance, and lipid storage myopathy has been documented as an acquired disorder in older dogs.[30]

Electrodiagnostic Evaluation. The advantage of electromyography is that it is a noninvasive method used to confirm a diagnosis of neuromuscular disease, to localize the disease, and to identify what muscles or nerves should be biopsied. Electromyography can also be used to detect subclinical disease.[31] Electromyography is especially important in the diagnosis of neuromuscular disorders because of the veterinarian's inability to communicate with the animal regarding sensation or to conduct muscle testing to diagnose weakness. One reason to consider referral is for electromyographic testing. Because of the expense of the equipment and the need for additional training, electromyographic testing is mostly restricted to veterinary colleges and board-certified veterinary neurologists in specialty practices.

Electromyographic testing involves two parts—needle electromyography and nerve conduction studies. Needle electromyography involves inserting fine-gauge needle electrodes into specific muscles to determine the presence of abnormal spontaneous electrical activity (fibrillation potentials, positive waves, fasciculation potentials, complex repetitive discharges, and myotonic discharges). This systematic study of individual muscles determines the distribution of the disorder.

Most types of abnormal spontaneous discharges are not specific to either neuropathies or myopathies, but can be found with either. Therefore, the second part of the electromyographic examination is the measurement of nerve conduction velocity of peripheral nerves that are selected based on the distribution of the clinical signs and needle electromyographic examination. Both motor and sensory nerve conduction velocity can be measured. Evaluation of the amplitude of the evoked potentials following repetitive nerve stimulation protocols provides information about the integrity of neuromuscular transmission.[32] Single fiber electromyography is a more sensitive indicator of disorders of neuromuscular transmission, but this technique has seldom been reported in veterinary medicine.[33] Electromyography is usually performed with the animal under anesthesia. However, in cases in which the anesthetic risk is high, needle electromyography (but not nerve conduction velocity testing) can be done with the animal awake, under manual restraint.

Imaging Procedures. Imaging of neuromuscular disorders in humans has been reviewed, in reports comparing ultrasonography, computed tomography, and magnetic resonance techniques.[34]

Ultrasonographic imaging can be used to image muscle and some peripheral nerves.[35-38] The techniques have been extensively reported in human patients.[39-41] Compared with magnetic resonance imaging, the advantages are that ultrasonography is relatively inexpensive and the animal does not need to be under general anesthesia. Although the appropriate transducers are likely available in many facilities, the ultrasonographer does need to have experience in imaging these particular tissues.

Magnetic resonance imaging has also been used in the diagnosis of neuromuscular disorders in humans. Its applications have included athletic injuries such as acute muscle strain and inflammatory myopathies.[42] Magnetic resonance imaging can be used to identify focal muscle structural lesions, to determine their extent, to characterize their composition, to direct invasive procedures, and to monitor therapies.[42] However, the role for magnetic resonance imaging in the diagnosis of neuromuscular disorders in dogs and cats remains to be determined. Major drawbacks are the cost and the requirement for general anesthesia.

Muscle Biopsy. For muscle and peripheral nerve, it is essential to use a laboratory that specializes in handling these tissues. The pathologist should be contacted before biopsies are taken, in order to ensure optimal tissue sampling and handling. Muscle specimens placed in formalin have limited diagnostic value. In contrast, frozen sections can be stained for biochemical and immunochemical reactions that may yield important diagnostic information. Frozen sections may also be used for the biochemical assay of specific enzymes and substrates.[21]

An involved muscle should be sampled. This selection is based on the clinical signs or the electromyographic findings. Severely atrophied muscle should be avoided because it may show only secondary, nonspecific changes. In generalized disorders, muscles routinely sampled include the vastus lateralis, triceps brachii, cranial tibial muscle, and extensor carpi radialis; in focal disorders, specific muscles are biopsied, such as temporalis or masseter in masticatory myositis.

The muscle biopsy should be performed with the animal under general anesthesia, following electromyographic testing if electromyography is done. It is best to avoid sampling from the same muscles that have been tested with electromyography, because inadvertently taking a biopsy sample from a site that includes a needle track from an electromyography needle insertion could lead to an erroneous diagnosis. Using sterile technique, a small skin incision is made overlying the muscle to be biopsied, subcutaneous tissues are separated, and the fascia overlying the muscle is incised and retracted. Using a sharp blade, a cylinder of muscle approximately 1 × 2 × 1 cm is taken parallel to the longitudinal direction of the muscle fibers. The sample is wrapped in saline-dampened gauze (moistened, but not dripping wet), placed in an airtight container, and stored in a refrigerator at 4° C until shipping. The sample should be shipped on wet ice (cold packs) in a well-insulated Styrofoam container and delivered to the laboratory within 24 hours.

Nerve Biopsy. Techniques used for the collection of peripheral nerve biopsies have been described.[43] Fascicular biopsies of the common peroneal, ulnar, tibial, and caudal cutaneous antebrachial nerves are most commonly taken. Sensory and motor nerve fascicles can be sampled. The basic pathologic reactions are axonal (Wallerian) degeneration and demyelination. These histologic changes in many nerve biopsies are nonspecific and do not yield a specific diagnosis. However, in cases in which the veterinarian is unsure of whether nerve or muscle is involved in the disease, sampling both nerve and muscle is advisable.

Tests for Specific Diseases

In cases of inflammatory myopathies, serum titers for *Toxoplasma gondii* and *Neospora caninum* may be useful. Infections in older dogs may result in clinical signs of multifocal central nervous system involvement along with polymyositis.[44] Other infectious agents including *Ehrlichia canis*[45] and *Borrelia burgdorferi* may result in an inflammatory myopathy, and testing can be performed for these agents, particularly in endemic areas. *Hepatozoon americanum* is a protozoan organism that can infect muscle and can be diagnosed by muscle biopsy.

If there is a history or suspicion of exposure to organophosphates, measurement of plasma cholinesterase levels may be indicated. A radioimmunoassay for the detection of serum acetylcholine receptor antibodies is indicated for the diagnosis of acquired myasthenia gravis.[46] An immunocytochemical assay for serum antibodies against type 2M myofibers is indicated for the diagnosis of masticatory muscle myositis.[47] Although the serum assay is highly suggestive of masticatory myositis, a muscle biopsy should also be performed.[8]

SPECIFIC NEUROMUSCULAR DISEASES

The reader is referred to books on veterinary neurology for information on specific neuropathies and myopathies.[2-7] Some of the most frequently diagnosed myopathies in older dogs and cats are described in the following sections.

Specific Neuropathies

The neuropathies diagnosed most frequently in dogs referred to veterinary colleges as indicated by the Veterinary Medical Data Base are Horner's syndrome, facial nerve paralysis, optic nerve blindness or optic neuritis, peripheral nerve sheath tumors, and polyradiculoneuritis. The corresponding results for neuropathies in cats are Horner's syndrome, optic nerve blindness or optic neuritis, facial nerve paralysis, neuropathy due to endocrine disease, and brachial plexus avulsion. Another neuropathy that has been reported more recently is chronic inflammatory demyelinating neuropathy.[11] This disorder affects mature dogs and cats of any age.

Specific Myopathies

For dogs, the most frequently reported myopathies found in the Veterinary Medical Data Base are polymyositis, endocrine myopathies, and myositis associated with trauma. Myasthenia gravis and tick paralysis are also listed in this category, although they are more specifically disorders of neuromuscular transmission. In addition, myopathies associated with storage of neutral lipid within myofibers have been more recently recognized in older dogs,[8,30] but the incidence of such disorders is not yet reliably reflected in the database. For feline myopathies, the most reported conditions were polymyositis, tumors involving muscle (fibrosarcoma, adenocarcinoma, rhabdosarcoma, and squamous cell carcinoma), ischemic muscle necrosis, myasthenia gravis, and myositis ossificans.

Polymyositis. Polymyositis is a generalized inflammatory myopathy. Underlying causes include infectious agents *(T. gondii, N. caninum, E. canis)* and ill-defined immune-mediated mechanisms. Polymyositis may also occur as a paraneoplastic disorder and is described in association with thymoma in dogs and cats.[48-50] Elevations in serum creatine kinase are usually marked, muscle pain may be evident on palpation, and muscle biopsies should be diagnostic (see Figure 21-3).

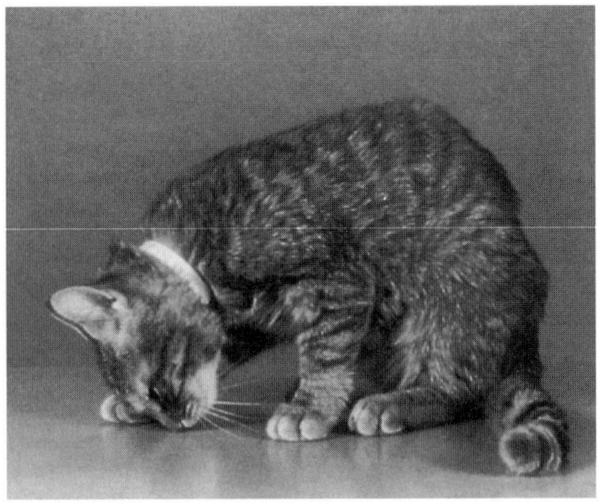

Figure 21-7. Ventroflexion of the neck in a cat with hypokalemic myopathy and generalized muscle weakness. (Photograph courtesy of Mike Podell, DVM, Ohio State University, Columbus, Ohio.)

Hypokalemic Myopathy. Hypokalemic myopathy has been well documented in the cat.[51] It is important to differentiate this disorder from polymyositis in this species, because the clinical presentation may be identical. As in polymyositis, ventroflexion of the neck (Figure 21-7) and generalized muscle weakness with a moderate to markedly elevated serum creatine kinase may be found. Serum potassium concentrations are normal in cases of polymyositis and less than 3.5 mEq/L in cases of hypokalemic myopathy. Muscle biopsies from cats with hypokalemic myopathy are usually normal. In one series of cases, improvement in muscle strength in hypokalemic cats resulted from changing the diet to one with higher potassium content or after dietary supplementation with potassium.[50]

Hypothyroid Myopathy. Myopathies have been reported in dogs in association with hypothyroidism. Clinical signs include weakness, stiffness, and muscle atrophy. Although not fully documented, megaesophagus may also occur in hypothyroid dogs, with possible resolution of the esophageal dilatation following thyroid replacement therapy. Laryngeal paralysis has also been reported in association with hypothyroidism,[52] although the majority of these cases probably are related to a peripheral neuropathy. For a discussion of the clinical diagnosis of hypothyroidism, the reader is referred to Chapter 14. The diagnosis of muscle involvement is dependent on electromyographic examination followed by nerve and muscle biopsies (see Figure 21-4). On electromyography, nonspecific findings such as fibrillation potentials and positive sharp waves may be found in hypothyroid dogs, along with complex repetitive discharges, which are indicative of chronicity. In dogs with prominent weakness and muscle atrophy, selective type 2 fiber atrophy may be the only abnormal finding. In some cases, changes consistent with neuropathy (angular atrophy of both type 1 and type 2 fibers) are observed. The presence of nemaline rods in type 1 fibers or abnormal glycogen inclusions may be observed in some dogs.[8] Thyroid supplementation should be initiated.

Hyperthyroid Myopathy. Clinical signs of neuromuscular dysfunction have been described in hyperthyroid cats. In one study, muscle weakness was relatively frequent.[53] Clinical signs of muscle weakness included ventroflexion of the neck, muscle tremors, muscle atrophy, and collapse. Serum creatine kinase levels were high in some cats. Myotatic reflexes were normal to exaggerated. Diminished reflexes were rarely observed. Myasthenia gravis has not been documented to be associated with hyperthyroidism in cats, although two cats on methimazole treatment with associated muscle weakness tested positive for acetylcholine receptor antibodies.[8] Reestablishment of a euthyroid state can be achieved by the use of antithyroid drugs, radioactive iodine, or thyroidectomy. With correction of hyperthyroidism, neuromuscular signs have resolved.[53]

Glucocorticoid Excess. Muscle weakness and myopathy have been associated with naturally occurring hyperadrenocorticism in dogs and with iatrogenic hyperadrenocorticism in cats and dogs.[54] Dogs appear to be particularly sensitive to exogenous corticosteroids, and muscle atrophy and weakness may develop. Clinical signs consistent with a neuromuscular disorder include a stiff gait, muscle weakness, and atrophy. In some severely affected dogs with hyperadrenocorticism, pelvic limb rigidity and inability to walk have been noted (Figure 21-8). Usually, animals with hyperadrenocorticism show other clinical signs consistent with glucocorticoid excess including polydipsia, polyuria, alopecia, and a pendulous abdomen. A discussion on the laboratory diagnosis of hyperadrenocorticism and iatrogenic hyperadrenocorticism may be found in Chapter 17. Electromyographic examination followed by muscle biopsy is required for confirmation of the neuromuscular disorder.

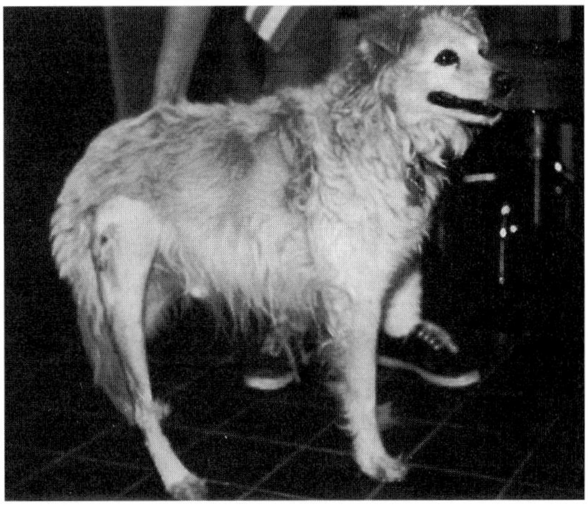

Figure 21-8. Pelvic limb rigidity in a dog with hyperadrenocorticism and myotonia. (Photograph courtesy of Don Levesque, DVM, Veterinary Neurological Center, Phoenix, Ariz.)

Myopathy of Hyperadrenocorticism. Examination of muscle biopsies may show variable changes ranging from selective type 2 fiber atrophy (see Figure 21-5) in dogs with severe muscle weakness to "ragged-red–like" fibers and lipid storage in dogs with pelvic limb rigidity and myotonia of hyperadrenocorticism (see Figure 21-6). Clinical signs have been reported to improve after therapy for hyperadrenocorticism. However, most dogs have a poor prognosis for complete resolution of a myopathy despite control of elevated cortisol levels. In contrast, return of muscle strength should occur in cases of iatrogenic hyperadrenocorticism.

Hypoadrenocorticism. Muscle weakness occurs frequently in association with hypoadrenocorticism in dogs and cats.[55,56] Clinical signs usually respond to treatment of the disorder. Dysphagia and megaesophagus may occur in association with muscle weakness, and these signs should also resolve.

SPECIFIC DISORDER OF NEUROMUSCULAR TRANSMISSION

Acquired Myasthenia Gravis

The most common disorder of neuromuscular transmission in dogs and cats is acquired myasthenia gravis.[8,57] Muscle weakness is caused by antibody-mediated destruction of postsynaptic acetylcholine receptors. Acquired myasthenia gravis affects numerous breeds of dogs with a bimodal age-related incidence with peaks at 1 to 3 years and 9 to 13 years of age.[46] In a retrospective case-control study in cats, Shelton and co-workers (2000)[58] found that the breed with the highest relative risk of acquired myasthenia gravis was the Abyssinian (including Somali). Relative risk increased after cats were 3 years old. Myasthenia gravis can manifest with signs of focal muscle weakness affecting the esophageal, pharyngeal and facial muscles, with generalized weakness, or in an acute, fulminating form. One study indicated that one fourth of dogs with idiopathic megaesophagus had focal myasthenia gravis.[59]

Generalized muscle weakness ranges from exercise intolerance that improves with rest to acute tetraplegia with hyporeflexia. Dogs with either focal or generalized signs and megaesophagus often present with aspiration pneumonia. In the geriatric age group, thoracic radiography may reveal a cranial mediastinal mass. Intravenous administration of edrophonium chloride (0.1 mg/kg) should result in transient improvement in muscle strength, although some dogs that are severely affected may not show a positive response. Some degree of improvement in muscle strength also may occur in dogs with other neuromuscular disorders. On electrodiagnostic testing, when repetitive nerve stimulation is used, a decline in the amplitude of successive potentials ("decrementing response") that reverses with edrophonium chloride is highly suggestive of myasthenia gravis. False-negative results can occur with this testing procedure, and false-positive results may occur because of technical error. Single fiber electromyography may provide a more sensitive technique for evaluating neuromuscular synaptic function[33] but has not been widely adopted in veterinary practice at this time.

Quantitation of the acetylcholine receptor antibody titer using antigen specific immunoprecipitation radioimmunoassay is sensitive and specific and documents an immune response against acetylcholine receptor antibody titers. False-positive results do not occur, but false-negative values may be found in the rare seronegative case.[59] Anticholinesterase drugs remain the primary treatment for acquired myasthenia gravis.[46] Pyridostigmine bromide, 1 to 3 mg/kg orally twice daily, is preferred over neostigmine, because fewer cholinergic side effects are described. Pyridostigmine bromide is available in tablet, elixir, and injectable forms. The elixir form is preferred for dogs with megaesophagus because delivery to the stomach may be more reliable than with the tablet form. The elixir should be diluted with equal parts of water to avoid irritation. For cases in which regurgitation is severe and treatment cannot be given orally, injectable pyridostigmine ($^1/_{30}$ of the oral dose) should be used. A gastric feeding tube should be placed in severe cases in which nothing can be taken orally. The gastric tube facilitates maintenance of nutrition and drug therapy. Addition of corticosteroids is recommended for animals that do not respond optimally to anticholinesterase drugs alone. Dewey and co-workers (1999) reported on the response to treatment with an immunosuppressive drug, azathioprine, in five dogs.[60] They concluded that there is a potential role for azathioprine in the treatment of acquired myasthenia gravis in dogs.

REFERENCES

1. Brooke MH: *A clinician's view of neuromuscular diseases,* Baltimore, 1977, Williams & Wilkins.
2. Braund KG: *Clinical syndromes in veterinary neurology,* ed 2, St. Louis, 1994, Mosby.
3. Chrisman CL: *Problems in small animal neurology,* ed 2, Philadelphia, 1991, Lea & Febiger.
4. de Lahunta A: *Veterinary neuroanatomy and clinical neurology,* Philadelphia, 1977, WB Saunders.
5. Oliver JE, Hoerlein BF, Mayhew IG: *Veterinary neurology,* Philadelphia, 1987, WB Saunders.
6. Oliver JE, Lorenz MD, Kornegay JN: *Handbook of veterinary neurology,* ed 3, Philadelphia, 1997, WB Saunders.
7. Wheeler SJ, ed: *BSAVA manual of small animal neurology,* ed 2, Cheltenham, UK, 1995, British Small Animal Veterinary Association.
8. Shelton GD: Neuromuscular disorders. In Goldston RT, Hoskins JD, eds: *Geriatrics and gerontology of the dog and cat,* Philadelphia, 1995, WB Saunders.
9. Braund KG, Dillon AR, Mikeal RL et al: Subclinical myopathy associated with hyperadrenocorticism in the dog, *Vet Pathol* 17:134, 1980.
10. Mariani CL, Shelton SB, Alsup JC: Paraneoplastic polyneuropathy and subsequent recovery following tumor removal in a dog, *J Am Anim Hosp Assoc* 35:302, 1999.
11. Braund KG, Vallat JM, Steiss JE et al: Chronic inflammatory demyelinating polyneuropathy in dogs and cats, *J Peripher Nerv Syst* 1:149, 1996.
12. Braund KG: Chronic inflammatory demyelinating polyneuropathy in dogs. In Bonagura JD, ed: *Kirk's current veterinary therapy XII: small animal practice,* Philadelphia, 2000, WB Saunders.
13. Shahar R, Rousseaux C, Steiss J: Peripheral polyneuropathy in a dog with functional islet B-cell tumor and widespread metastasis, *J Am Vet Med Assoc* 187:175, 1985.
14. Bichsel P, Jacobs G, Oliver JE: Neurologic manifestations associated with hypothyroidism in four dogs, *J Am Vet Med Assoc* 192:1745, 1988.
15. Jaggy A: Neurologic manifestations of canine hypothyroidism. In Bonagura JD, ed: *Kirk's current veterinary therapy XIII,* Philadelphia, 2000, WB Saunders.
16. Steiss JE, Forsyth G: Effect of electromyography on

serum creatine kinase values in clinically normal dogs and horses, *Am J Vet Res* 45:1199, 1984.
17. Braund KG, Steiss JE: Distal neuropathy in spontaneous diabetes mellitus in the dog, *Acta Neuropathol* 57:263, 1982.
18. Johnson CA, Kittleson MD, Indrieri RJ: Peripheral neuropathy and hypotension in a diabetic dog, *J Am Vet Med Assoc* 183:1007, 1983.
19. Katherman AE, Braund KG: Polyneuropathy associated with diabetes mellitus in a dog, *J Am Vet Med Assoc* 182:522, 1983.
20. Kramek BA, Moise NS, Cooper B et al: Neuropathy associated with diabetes mellitus in the cat, *J Am Vet Med Assoc* 184:42, 1984.
21. Cardinet III GH: Skeletal muscle function. In Kaneko JJ, ed: *Clinical biochemistry of domestic animals,* San Diego, 1989, Academic Press.
22. Valentine BA, Blue JT, Shelley SM et al: Increased serum alanine aminotransferase activity associated with muscle necrosis in the dog, *J Vet Intern Med* 4:140, 1990.
23. Duncan ID, Griffiths IR, Nash AS: Myotonia in canine Cushing's disease, *Vet Rec* 100:30, 1977.
24. Greene CE, Lorenz MD, Munnell JF et al: Myopathy associated with hyperadrenocorticism in the dog, *J Am Vet Med Assoc* 174:1310, 1979.
25. Hoskins JD, Nafe LA, Cho DY: Myopathy associated with hyperadrenocorticism in a dog: a case report, *Vet Med Small Anim Clin* 77:760, 1980.
26. Braund KG, Dillon AR, August JR et al: Hypothyroid myopathy in two dogs, *Vet Pathol* 18:589, 1981.
27. Jones BR: Hypokalemic myopathy in cats. In Bonagura JD, ed: *Kirk's current veterinary therapy XIII,* Philadelphia, 2000, WB Saunders.
28. Steiss JE, Spano J: Roading versus running: what's the difference? *American Field* 246:17, 1996.
29. Matwichuk CL, Taylor SM, Shmon CL et al: Changes in rectal temperature and hematologic, biochemical, blood gas, and acid-base values in healthy Labrador retrievers before and after strenuous exercise, *Am J Vet Res* 60:88, 1999.
30. Shelton GD: Canine lipid storage myopathies, *Proc Am Coll Vet Intern Med Forum* 11:707, 1993.
31. Steiss JE, Orsher AN, Bowen JM: Electrodiagnostic analysis of a peripheral neuropathy in dogs with diabetes mellitus, *Am J Vet Res* 42:2061, 1981.
32. Sims MH, McLean RA: Use of repetitive nerve stimulation to assess neuromuscular function in dogs. A test protocol for suspected myasthenia gravis, *Prog Vet Neurol* 1:311, 1990.
33. Hopkins AL: Single fiber electromyography in the dog, *Proc Am Coll Vet Intern Med Forum* 10:768, 1992.
34. Clague JE, Roberts N, Gibson H et al: Muscle imaging in health and disease, *Neuromuscul Disord* 5:171, 1995.
35. Breur GJ, Blevins WE: Traumatic injury of the iliopsoas muscle in three dogs, *J Am Vet Med Assoc* 210:1631, 1997.
36. Hudson JA, Steiss JE, Braund KG et al: Ultrasonography of peripheral nerves during Wallerian degeneration and regeneration following transection, *Vet Radiol Ultrasound* 37:302, 1996.
37. Hudson JA, Finn-Bodner ST, Steiss JE: Neurosonography, *Vet Clin North Am Small Anim Pract* 28:943, 1998.
38. Kramer M, Gerwing M, Hach V et al: Sonography of the musculoskeletal system in dogs and cats, *Vet Radiol Ultrasound* 38:139, 1997.
39. Adler RS: Future and new developments in musculoskeletal ultrasound, *Radiol Clin North Am* 37:623, 1999.
40. Fornage BD, ed: Musculoskeletal ultrasound. In *Clinics in diagnostic ultrasound,* vol 30, New York, 1995, Churchill Livingstone.
41. Van Holsbeeck M, Introcaso JH: Sonography of muscle. In: *Musculoskeletal ultrasound,* St Louis, 1991, Mosby.
42. Fleckenstein JL, Reimers CD: Inflammatory myopathies: radiologic evaluation, *Radiol Clin North Am* 34:427, 1996.
43. Braund KG: Nerve and muscle biopsy techniques, *Prog Vet Neurol* 2:35, 1991.
44. Dubey JP: *Neospora caninum* infections. In Kirk RW, Bonagura JD, eds: *Current veterinary therapy XI,* Philadelphia, 1992, WB Saunders.
45. Buoro IBJ, Kanui TI, Atwell RB et al: Polymyositis associated with *Ehrlichia canis* infection in two dogs, *J Small Anim Pract* 31:624, 1990.
46. Shelton GD: Canine myasthenia gravis. In Kirk RW, Bonagura JD, eds: *Current veterinary therapy XI,* Philadelphia, 1992, WB Saunders.
47. Shelton GD, Cardinet III GH: Canine masticatory muscle disorders. In Kirk RW, ed: *Current veterinary therapy X,* Philadelphia, 1989, WB Saunders.
48. Carpenter JL, Holzworth J: Thymoma in 11 cats, *J Am Vet Med Assoc* 181:248, 1982.
49. Aronsohn MG, Schunk KL, Carpenter JL et al: Clinical and pathologic features of thymoma in 15 dogs, *J Am Vet Med Assoc* 184:1355, 1984.
50. Klebanow ER: Thymoma and acquired myasthenia gravis in the dog: A case report and review of 13 additional cases, *J Am Anim Hosp Assoc* 28:63, 1992.
51. Dow SW, LeCouteur RA, Fettman MJ et al: Potassium depletion in cats: hypokalemic polymyopathy, *J Am Vet Med Assoc* 191:1563, 1987.
52. Harvey HJ, Irby NL, Watrous BJ: Laryngeal paralysis in hypothyroid dogs. In Kirk RW, ed: *Current veterinary therapy VIII,* Philadelphia, 1983, WB Saunders.
53. Joseph RJ, Peterson ME: Review and comparison of neuromuscular and central nervous system manifestations of hyperthyroidism in cats and humans, *Prog Vet Neurol* 3:114, 1992.
54. LeCouteur RA, Dow SW, Sisson AF: Metabolic and endocrine myopathies of dogs and cats, *Semin Vet Med Surg* 4:146, 1989.
55. Greco DS, Peterson ME: Feline hypoadrenocorticism. In Kirk RW, ed: *Current veterinary therapy X,* Philadelphia, 1989, WB Saunders.
56. Schrader LA: Hypoadrenocorticism. In Kirk RW, ed: *Current veterinary therapy IX,* Philadelphia, 1986, WB Saunders.
57. Shelton GD: Acquired myasthenia gravis: what we have learned from experimental and spontaneous animal models, *Vet Immunol Immunopathol* 69:239, 1999.
58. Shelton GD, Ho M, Kass PH: Risk factors for acquired myasthenia gravis in cats: 105 cases (1986-1998), *J Am Vet Med Assoc* 216:55, 2000.
59. Shelton GD, Willard MD, Cardinet III GH et al: Acquired myasthenia gravis. Selective involvement of esophageal, pharyngeal and facial muscles, *J Vet Intern Med* 4:281, 1990.
60. Dewey CW, Coates JR, Ducote JM et al: Azathioprine therapy for acquired myasthenia gravis in five dogs, *J Am Anim Hosp Assoc* 35:396, 1999.

CHAPTER 22

The Nervous System

JOHNNY D. HOSKINS

Many neurologic diseases occur primarily or exclusively in older dogs and cats. Age of onset of clinical signs and the duration and course of the disease process are important considerations in the formulation of differential diagnoses in affected animals. There are some minor differences between young and old animals with regard to the neurologic examination, and it is important for the veterinarian to recognize these differences so that a normal variance is not interpreted as a significant problem.

As dogs and cats mature to old age, several processes decrease the senses of sight and hearing; as a result, reactions to response tests may be altered. Obviously, reflexes or reactions directly involving hearing and vision are affected, but in addition to these, the animal may be hypersensitive to external stimuli (i.e., sensitive to noise if the animal is blind and sensitive to touch if it is deaf). It is important to initially work slowly with a geriatric animal that has diminished senses and to handle the animal for a few minutes before beginning the neurologic examination. This will allow the patient to become acclimated to the environment and the examiner. Animals that are blind may appear to be slightly hypermetric in their gait and during postural testing. In addition, they may have brisk myotatic tendon reflexes as a result of increased sensitivity to touch. Therefore, even if both gait and postural test reactions are normal, the veterinarian should not overinterpret hyperreflexia of the myotatic tendon reflexes.

Iris atrophy is a common aging change in older dogs and cats (Figure 22-1). It is a common cause of incomplete pupillary light reflexes and therefore should always be ruled out before optic or oculomotor nerve deficits are considered as the cause of pupillary light reflex abnormalities. Clues that iris atrophy may exist include irregular pupil margins, strands of iris that span across portions of the pupil, and the presence of large holes in the iris stroma or iris dilator muscle that resemble multiple pupillary openings.[1] In some breeds of dogs, especially cocker spaniels, the palpebral

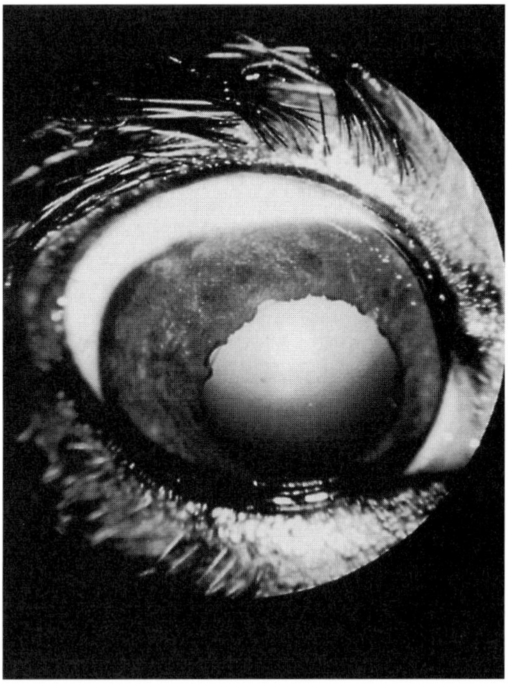

Figure 22-1. Iris atrophy in an 11-year-old mixed breed dog with a dilated pupil.

reflex may be less complete when compared with that in younger dogs of the same breed. This appears to be a result of motor weakness to eyelid closure and not sensory loss, because sensation to the head and face is normal. These animals usually have had no history of a previous episode of facial nerve paralysis, either idiopathic or secondary to otitis media. It is uncertain whether this finding represents a partial palsy or is just an age-related change.

The older dog and cat may not be as alert and responsive to external stimuli as a younger animal. When assessing functions such as following, menace reflex, and response to auditory stimuli, the veterinarian should not always overinterpret a depressed response as indicating neurologic deficits. A depressed response could represent nothing more than a change in the animal's general interest in these external stimuli. The older dog with degenerative disease of the coxofemoral joints may have what appears to be slow tarsal replacement (proprioceptive testing). This response may result from the reluctance of the dog to flex the hip because of pain. Therefore, mild slowing of tarsal replacement should not be assumed to have a neurologic cause. Certainly, however, prolonged "knuckling over" of the foot will not be caused by orthopedic disease.

BOX 22-1 Signs Associated with Intracranial Disease

Supratentorial Lesions

Seizures
Blindness and menace deficits with normal pupillary light reflex and cranial nerve VII function (contralateral to an ipsilateral lesion)
Postural reaction deficits (contralateral to a unilateral lesion)
Consciousness abnormalities
Abnormal behavior (head pressing, wandering, bellowing)
Hemiinattention
Circling (usually toward the side of the lesion)
Head turn (usually toward the side of the lesion)

Infratentorial or Brain-stem Lesions

Cranial nerve deficits (cranial nerves III through XII)
Paresis (ipsilateral to unilateral lesion)
Sensorium abnormalities
Cardiac and respiratory abnormalities
Sleep abnormalities (narcolepsy or cataplexy)

Cerebellar Lesions

Ataxia and dysmetria
Intention tremor
Vestibular signs
Menace deficits with normal vision and normal cranial nerve VII function
Decerebellate rigidity
Pupillary abnormalities
Increased frequency of urination

Bagley RS: Common neurologic diseases of older animals, *Vet Clin North Am* 27:1451, 1997.

NEUROLOGIC DISEASES

Major areas affected within the nervous system include the intracranial space, cranial nerves, spinal cord, and peripheral neuromuscular apparatus.[2] The intracranial nervous system includes the supratentorial structures (cerebral hemispheres, basal nuclei, diencephalon, mesencephalon); the infratentorial structures (pons, medulla oblongata); and the cerebellum (Box 22-1). Cranial nerves can be affected both within and outside of the intracranial space as they course to areas of the head. The spinal cord contains pathways coursing to and from the intracranial nervous system and the cell bodies that form the peripheral nerves. The peripheral neuromuscular apparatus contains the peripheral nerves, neuromuscular junction, and muscles (see Chapter 21).

SUPRATENTORIAL STRUCTURAL DISEASES

Diseases that are likely to cause clinical signs (see Box 22-1) related to changes in supratentorial structures in the older dog or cat include neoplasia, inflammatory disease, vascular disease, senile degeneration, and metabolic disorders.

METABOLIC DISEASES

An animal's cortical and brain-stem function may be altered by metabolic diseases, such as liver, renal, and pancreatic disease; hyperglycemia or hypoglycemia; serum electrolyte disturbances (altered serum sodium, potassium, chloride, calcium, and magnesium concentrations); and acid base abnormalities.[2,3]

In addition to common signs of liver disease, older dogs or cats presented with hepatic encephalopathic signs may show seizures, ptyalism, and behavioral changes. The diagnosis of hepatic encephalopathy is supported by clinical signs and abnormal liver function tests such as measurement of serum bile acids. Ultrasonography and liver biopsies are needed to confirm the type of liver disease present.

Hypoglycemia can occur secondary to insulinoma, extrapancreatic neoplasia, liver disease, hypoadrenocorticism, and insulin overdose. Clinical signs often attributed to the neuroglycopenia include depression, weakness, and intermittent twitches of limb or head muscles. Diagnosis is based on the presence of resting hypoglycemia (repeated blood glucose concentrations <40 mg/dl) and associated clinical signs. Ultrasonography of the pancreas may show large insulinomas or evidence of metastasis to lymph node or liver. Extrapancreatic neoplasms are usually relatively large and palpable or found by survey abdominal radiography. Excision of an insulinoma or extrapancreatic neoplasia will usually result in increased serum glucose concentrations. In nonexcisional lesions, medical treatments including increased number of feedings daily, corticosteroids, and diazoxide may be helpful.

Dogs with diabetic ketoacidosis may have cerebral signs, such as depression and altered behavior, but whether these changes are related to the hyperglycemia or other physiologic derangements is unknown. Cats with hyperglycemia that require large doses of insulin to control blood glucose should be evaluated for acquired acromegaly, which is commonly associated with a primary pituitary tumor. Enlargement of facial features and body organs is usually caused by an excess of growth hormone.

Hypernatremia in older dogs and cats commonly results from decreased water intake. This may occur because of alterations in awareness of thirst or physical inability to drink water. Hypernatremia and adipsia in an older animal, if not associated with decreased water intake, should warrant an evaluation for structural brain disease.

Hyperthyroidism of cats may be associated with clinical signs and include restlessness, hyperexcitability, irritability, aggression, wandering, pacing, circling, insomnia, and seizures. Apathy, lethargy, and depression occur infrequently. Focal neurologic deficits may result from associated cerebrovascular accidents and secondary to hypertension. Diagnosis is supported by increased serum thyroxine concentrations. Treatment of the hyperthyroidism often will improve clinical signs if a structural problem such as a cerebrovascular hemorrhage is not concurrently present.

Hypothyroidism has been associated with a variety of intracranial and cranial nerve abnormalities in dogs.[4] Whether these signs reflect a primary metabolic disturbance or secondary structural abnormalities associated with underlying vascular disease is not always known. Atherosclerosis has been found in association with hypothyroidism in some dogs. Diagnosis based on a single low serum thyroxine concentration can be misleading in older animals with other systemic disorders (euthyroid sick syndrome). Response of the neurologic signs to thyroid supplementation is variable.

Hypercalcemia induced by malignancy may result in generalized central nervous system depression through metabolic alterations. Hypercalcemia causes cerebral vasoconstriction that is similar to the effect it has on renal blood flow, resulting in intracranial ischemia, infarction, and hemorrhage.

Cardiopulmonary diseases that predispose to poor cerebral blood flow may result in apparent neurologic signs. Poor perfusion to the brain may result in syncope; however, seizures are possible if the brain perfusion abnormality is severe or prolonged. The associated muscular weakness may be mistaken for peripheral nerve or muscle disease. Bradyarrhythmias such as third-degree heart block are frequently associated with syncope and seizures. Conversely, intracranial disease resulting in increases in intracranial pressure and cerebral ischemia may predispose to bradycardia, ventricular arrhythmias (brain-heart syndrome), and pulmonary edema.

NEOPLASTIC DISEASES

Brain tumors may be primary (arising from tissue inherent to the brain and its coverings) or secondary (reaching the brain by local extension or hematogenous metastasis).[5] The most common primary tumors of dogs are neuroepithelial (gliomas) (Figure 22-2), meningeal (meningiomas) (Figure 22-3), and lymphoid (reticulosis, lymphosarcoma) in origin. Glial cell neoplasms and pituitary gland tumors (Figure 22-4) occur most commonly in brachycephalic breeds,[6] whereas meningiomas are recognized most often in dolichocephalic breeds.[7] The brain is the most common site for metastasis of systemic neoplasms.[8] Secondary tumors that are commonly associated with metastatic brain disease include nasal adenocarcinoma with its direct extension (Figure 22-5) and distant metastasis from melanoma, hemangiosarcoma, mammary gland adenocarcinoma, pancreatic adenocarcinoma, undifferentiated carcinomas, and adenocarcinoma of multiple origins.

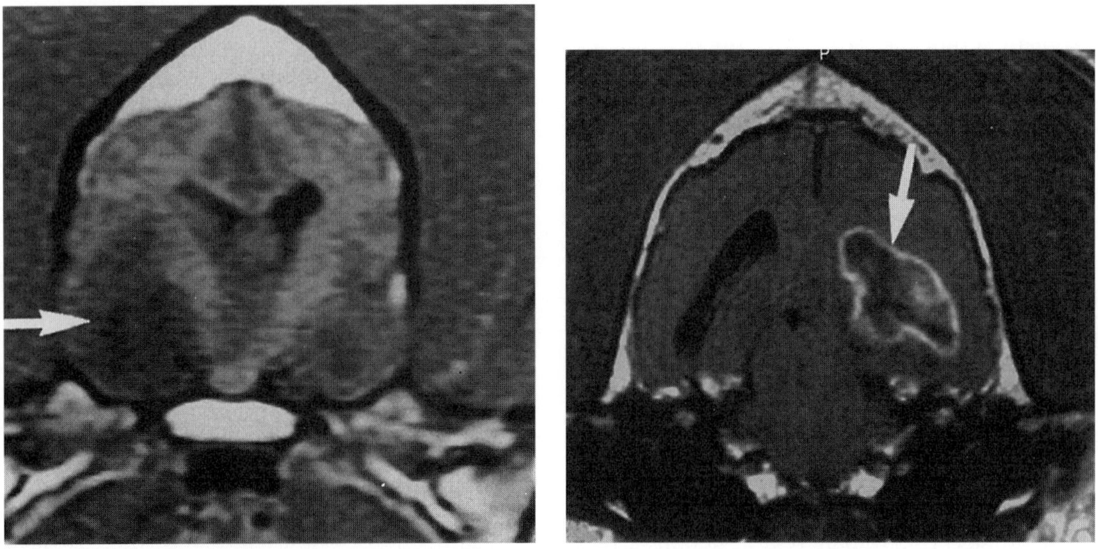

A B

Figure 22-2. A, Transaxial, T1-weighted, contrast-enhanced magnetic resonance image from a dog with seizures. A hypointense lesion is present in left temporal lobe *(arrow)*. Histopathologic diagnosis was an astrocytoma. **B,** Transaxial, T1-weighted, contrast-enhanced magnetic resonance image from a dog with circling and hemiparesis. A ring-enhanced lesion is present in the right medial cerebral hemisphere *(arrow)*. Histopathologic diagnosis was an oligodendroglioma. (From Bagley RS: Common neurologic diseases of older animals, *Vet Clin North Am* 27:1451, 1997.)

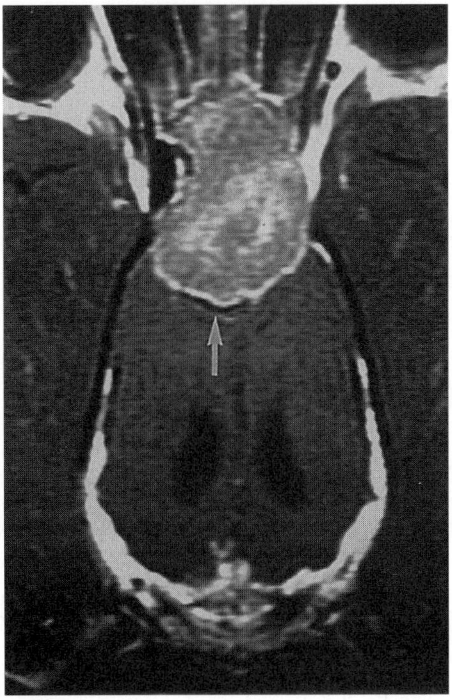

A

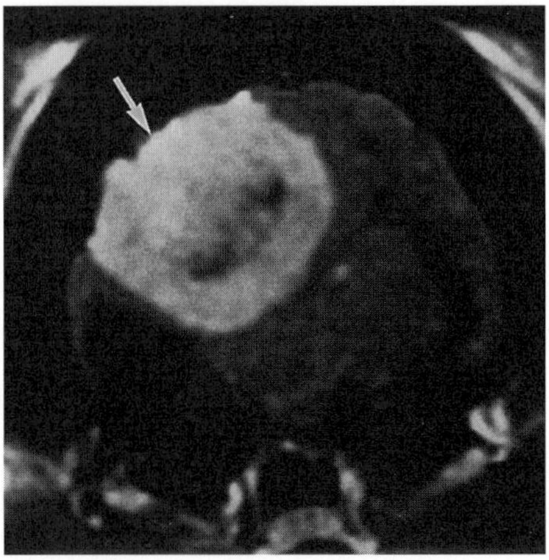

B

Figure 22-3. A, Dorsal, T1-weighted, contrast-enhanced magnetic resonance image from a dog with a meningioma *(arrow)*. **B,** Transaxial, T1-weighted, contrast-enhanced magnetic resonance image from a cat with a meningioma *(arrow)*. (From Bagley RS: Recognition and localization of intracranial disease, *Vet Clin North Am Small Anim Pract* 26:673, 1996.)

Clinical Signs

Regardless of whether the brain tumor is primary or metastatic, clinical signs are usually slowly progressive over several weeks to months or may be rapid in onset and have a short clinical course.[8] The factors responsible for the clinical signs and progression are tumor location, size, and type and the tendency of these tumors to result in hemorrhage (Box 22-2). Most dogs with brain tumors have long histories of vague signs that may be overlooked until signs of brain

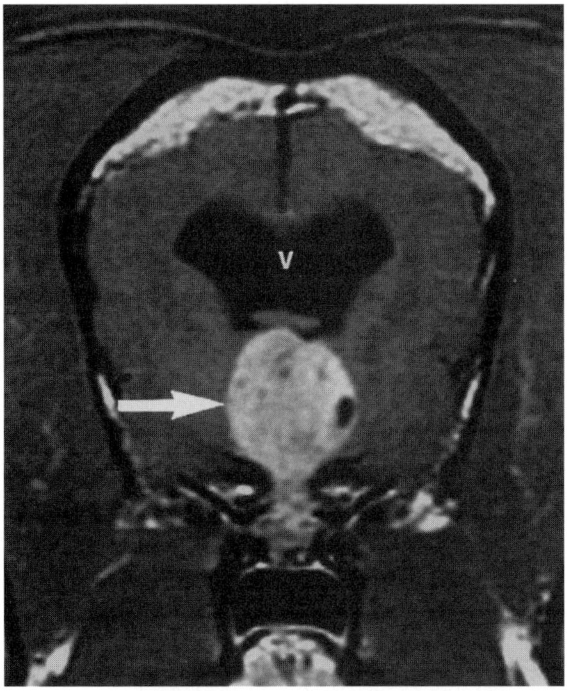

Figure 22-4. Transaxial, T1-weighted, contrast-enhanced magnetic resonance image from a dog with seizures and depression. A contrast-enhancing lesion *(arrow)* extends dorsally from the pituitary region. Associated enlargement of the lateral ventricles *(V)* can be seen. Diagnosis was a pituitary macroadenoma. (From Bagley RS: Common neurologic diseases of older animals, *Vet Clin North Am* 27:1451, 1997.)

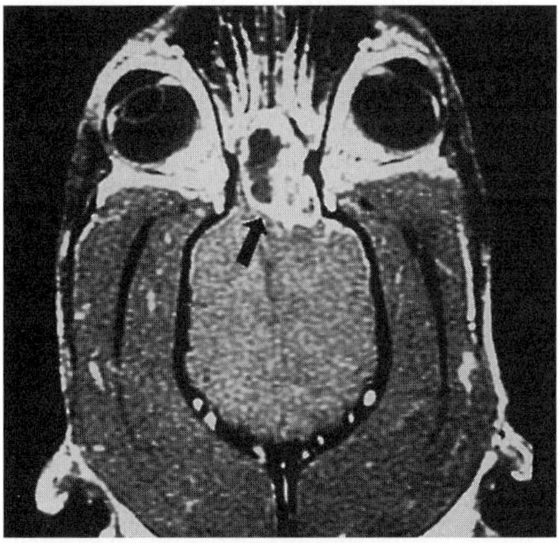

A

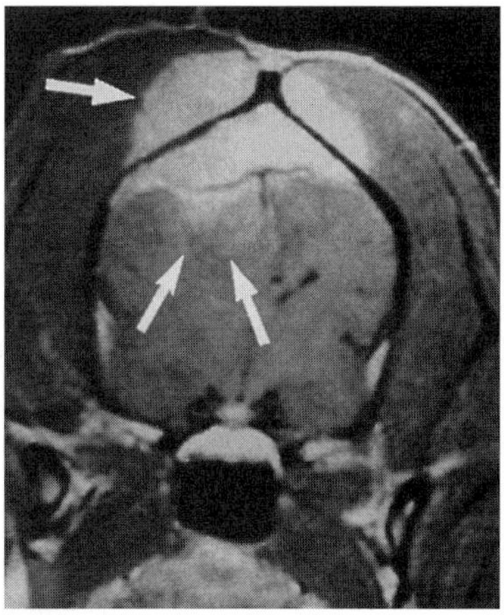

B

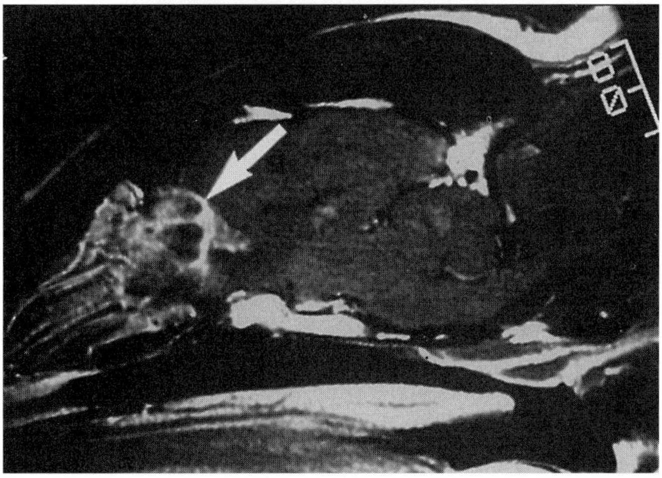

Figure 22-5. A, Dorsal and **C,** sagittal T1-weighted, contrast-enhanced magnetic resonance images from a dog with a nasal adenocarcinoma *(arrows)* extending caudally into the brain. **B,** Transaxial, T1-weighted, contrast-enhanced magnetic resonance image from a dog with osteosarcoma of the dorsal skull extending ventrally into the brain *(arrows)*. (From Bagley RS: Common neurologic diseases of older animals, *Vet Clin North Am* 27:1451, 1997.)

BOX 22-2 Effects of Brain Tumors

Primary Effects
Infiltration of nervous tissue
Compression of adjacent anatomic structures

Secondary Effects
Hydrocephalus
Disruption of cerebral circulation
Local necrosis
Hemorrhage
Disturbance of cerebrospinal fluid flow
Elevated intracranial pressure
Cerebral edema
Brain herniation

dysfunction are well advanced. The clinical signs of brain neoplasms may include anorexia, seizures, altered behavior, circling, head pressing, compulsive walking, altered consciousness, and locomotor disturbances. Cerebral tumors typically cause behavior changes, seizures, visual deficits, and circling. Brain-stem tumors typically cause depression, head tilt, cranial nerve deficits, weakness, and ataxia. Cerebellar tumors typically cause ataxia, head tilt, circling, and tremor. Choroid plexus tumors may also include signs of vomiting and bradycardia.[9] Acute-onset blindness and dilated, nonresponsive pupils may be the only clinical signs of an intracranial tumor, which usually is located in the chiasmal region.[10]

Diagnosis

Survey skull radiographs, cerebrospinal fluid analysis, or special imaging techniques such as computed tomography or magnetic resonance imaging are commonly incorporated into the clinical evaluation of an animal suspected to have neoplasia of the central nervous system. Survey skull radiographs are of limited value in the diagnosis of a primary brain tumor; however, they may be helpful in the detection of neoplasms of the skull or nasal cavity that have affected the brain by local extension. Radiographs of the skull may occasionally reveal erosion or hyperostosis of the calvarium in association with a primary brain tumor or document areas of mineralization within a neoplasm.

Cerebrospinal fluid analysis is often helpful in the evaluation of animals suspected of having an intracranial tumor, especially if the tumor communicates with the ventricles or subarachnoid space. Although cerebrospinal fluid changes are often nonspecific, when they are considered in combination with the animal's history and the results of the neurologic examination, they may permit an accurate diagnosis. Cerebrospinal fluid analysis may reveal a definitive diagnosis if neoplastic cells are visualized, but this is unusual except in cases of lymphosarcoma. Unless neoplastic cells are present, the cerebrospinal fluid analysis will provide only indirect evidence that a tumor exists. In general, increased cerebrospinal fluid protein content and normal to increased cerebrospinal fluid white blood cell counts are considered the typical changes seen with brain tumors. Meningiomas are more commonly associated with a neutrophilic pleocytosis; however, pleocytosis can be seen with other tumors as well. Choroid plexus papillomas may cause dramatic increases in cerebrospinal fluid protein concentration. Primary intracranial neoplasia is usually associated with a cerebrospinal fluid white blood cell count of fewer than 50 cells/μL with variable elevations of cerebrospinal fluid protein. In contrast, metastatic or invasive neoplasia is associated with higher white blood cell counts and protein concentrations in the cerebrospinal fluid.[11]

Because most intracranial tumors are not visible on survey radiographs, computed tomography and magnetic resonance imaging allow localization of tumors, facilitate brain biopsy, help in determining the feasibility of surgical removal of a tumor, allow for a high degree of certainty about tumor type and for localization before radiation therapy, improve the owner's ability to make decisions regarding care, and enable the veterinarian to more accurately advise owners regarding therapy and prognosis.

Computed tomographic findings for various brain tumors are as follows. Meningiomas are usually broad-based, peripherally located masses that were enhanced homogeneously with contrast material. Among the brain parenchymal tumors, astrocytomas are not distinguished easily from oligodendrogliomas because both tumors have similar tomographic features of ringlike and nonuniform enhancement and poorly defined tumor margins. Choroid plexus tumors are seen as well-defined, hyperdense masses that have marked uniform contrast enhancement. Pituitary tumors are distinguished readily by their location, minimal peritumoral edema, uniform contrast enhancement, and well-defined margins. In addition to defining primary brain tumors, computed tomography may be helpful in identifying nasal tumors that have extended into the rostral cerebrum.[12,13] Affected dogs may have no clinical signs of nasal disease. Magnetic resonance imaging is optimal for demonstrating the amount of nasal or cerebral involvement and shows detailed anatomic features of these brain tumors.

Although imaging techniques can help to localize tumors, tumor biopsy and histopathologic examination still remain the definitive methods for diagnosis of brain tumor type. Ideally, an intracranial lesion should undergo biopsy before therapy of any type. However, biopsy is not always attempted because of the risks involved. Attempting to perform a biopsy of a brain stem neoplasm may cause significant morbidity. The advantages of a histopathologic diagnosis are that a more accurate prognosis and determination of potential response to therapy can be given to the owner based on the biologic behavior of the neoplasm, and that it can be used to differentiate some inflammatory and nonneoplastic masses that may be confused with neoplasia when seen with the imaging techniques.[14]

Treatment

Control of secondary tumor effects, such as increased intracranial pressure or cerebral edema, and tumor eradication (or reduction) are the primary therapy for an intracranial tumor. Palliative therapy for dogs with brain tumors consists of the administration of glucocorticoids for reducing edema and, in some cases, for retarding tumor growth. Some animals with brain tumors demonstrate dramatic improvement in clinical signs for weeks or months with sustained glucocorticoid therapy. Should seizure control be needed, phenobarbital is the drug best suited for control of generalized seizures. Eradication or reduction of a brain tumor is the primary consideration for the long-term survival of a dog with a brain tumor. Therapy for a brain tumor may include surgery, irradiation, chemotherapy, and immunotherapy.[15-17]

Palliative therapy for brain tumors is administration of glucocorticoids. Glucocorticoids readily penetrate the blood-brain barrier and have some direct antitumor activity. Dexamethasone is preferred in acute and severe cases, whereas prednisone or prednisolone may be used for maintenance. Brain tumors of any histopathologic type or location always carry a poor prognosis. Most dogs with brain tumors eventually die or are euthanized as a direct result of the tumor.

INFLAMMATORY DISEASES

Granulomatous Meningoencephalitis

Granulomatous meningoencephalitis occurs primarily in adult female dogs, most often purebred and members of small breeds. Disseminated granulomatous lesions primarily affect the white matter of the cerebrum, caudal brain stem, cerebellum, and cervical spinal cord and cause multifocal forebrain signs, whereas seizures may be the primary sign if a focal granulomatous lesion is present in the cerebrum.[18] Animals with the disseminated granulomatous disease often show an acute and fulminating clinical course, whereas those with focal granulomatous disease tend to have subtle signs at the beginning and a more prolonged clinical course. Although initially glucocorticoids may improve the neurologic status of most affected dogs, granulomatous meningoencephalitis is a progressive disease.

The cerebrospinal fluid collected from a dog suspected to be affected typically shows an elevated protein content (40 to 1,000 mg/dl) and increased white blood cell count (primarily of mononuclear cells, both lymphocytes and macrophages). The most consistent diagnostic findings from the cerebrospinal fluid analysis are obtained before any glucocorticoids are administered. In addition, imaging techniques may help in defining focal lesions of granulomatous meningoencephalitis.[14,19]

Treatment. Symptomatic therapy with glucocorticosteroids has proved successful in temporarily alleviating clinical signs or slowing disease progression. Prednisone has been the most frequently used glucocorticoid; doses ranging from 2 to 4 mg/kg daily appear to be adequate. Dexamethasone and methylprednisolone also are useful. Cessation of glucocorticoid therapy is invariably associated with rapid and dramatic clinical deterioration, and, therefore, glucocorticosteroids should not be discontinued. Radiation therapy may prove to be very beneficial for the treatment of focal granulomatous meningoencephalitis.

Pug, Maltese, and Yorkshire Terrier Encephalitis

Pugs, Maltese, and Yorkshire terriers with the acute nonsuppurative meningoencephalitis (and associated with extensive cerebral necrosis) are presented with a sudden onset of seizure activity and neurologic deficits referable to involvement of the cerebrum, brain stem, and meninges.[20-23] Dogs may have difficulty walking, be weak or uncoordinated, circle, have a head tilt, head press, exhibit blindness with normal pupillary light reflexes, or show signs of cervical rigidity and pain. These neurologic signs progress rapidly, and within 5 to 7 days the dogs develop uncontrollable seizures, become recumbent, and drift into a comatose state. Dogs with slowly progressive disease are presented because of generalized or partial motor seizures but are usually neurologically normal after the seizures. Diagnosis should be suspected on the basis of the signalment and characteristic clinical and laboratory features. Cerebrospinal fluid analysis is characterized by an increased nucleated cell count, with the predominant cell type being the small lymphocyte. Definitive diagnosis requires necropsy or brain biopsy. There is no specific treatment for this disease, although treatment with phenobarbital may decrease the severity and frequency of the seizures for a short period of time.

VASCULAR DISEASES

Vascular disease involving the supratentorial structures is assumed to be uncommon in older dogs and cats. Thrombosis, infarction, and hemorrhage can occur spontaneously; secondary to drug therapy (L-asparaginase, anticoagulants); thrombocytopenia and other bleeding disorders; trauma; hypertension (hyperthyroidism, hyperadrenocorticism); atherosclerosis from hypothyroidism; and infection (septic emboli). Sudden onset of neurologic signs may be initially progressive as the vascular event results in secondary brain disease and edema.[24] Cerebrospinal fluid analysis may be normal or may show increased protein content, xanthochromia, or dull-brown coloration. Hemorrhage and infarction may be seen with brain imaging techniques. Diagnosis is supported by cerebral angiography; however, this is uncommonly performed in dogs and cats. Many animals show a dramatic improvement over the first 3 to 10 days after the onset of signs, although some animals never return to a normal functional status.[25] In general, if no improvement is seen within 7 to 10 days after the onset of signs, the animal most likely will not have a complete recovery.

Feline ischemic encephalopathy is an ischemic necrosis of the cerebral hemisphere of cats.[26] The distribution of the infarction is usually in the area supplied by the middle cerebral artery. Cerebrospinal fluid often contains elevations in protein content. Prognosis for life is good after the first 48 hours, as this is a nonprogressive disorder. Residual neurologic deficits, most notably seizures, may persist throughout life.

SENILE DEGENERATION

Primary age-related degenerative brain disease of older dogs and cats usually manifests as abnormal behavioral activity that demonstrates progressive deterioration of sensory integration and motor capabilities. Loss of cognitive function or sensory input with age results in somnolence, alterations in sleep-wake cycles, and inappropriate urination. Aimless wandering, pacing, aggression, and apparent irritability are also possible. Onset of behavioral abnormalities in older animals can result from structural brain disease such as tumor and should warrant intracranial imaging. Loss of cortical parenchyma with age contributes to the enlargement of intracranial ventricles as seen with advanced imaging studies. Treatment of senility and cerebral dysfunction in geriatric dogs and cats is currently in its infancy. Current treatment involves the daily administration of selegiline at 0.5 mg/kg orally once daily for dogs and 0.25 mg/kg orally once daily for cats.

DISEASES OF THE CEREBELLUM

Cerebellar dysfunction is characterized by truncal ataxia, a broad-based stance, dysmetria in which the limbs either overstep (hypermetria) or understep (hypometria), and tremor that is most pronounced when the animal attempts a goal-oriented movement (i.e., intention tremor) (see Box 22-1). Supratentorial diseases, such as cerebellar infarction, focal granulomatous meningoencephalitis, and neoplasia, may also localize to the cerebellum. An idiopathic cerebellar degeneration of Brittany spaniels, usually spayed females, first occurs between 7 and 13 years of age.[27] Initial clinical signs begin as thoracic limb spasticity and hypermetria that progresses to obvious ataxia, head tremor, nystagmus, and extension of head. The head is also carried closer to the ground. Slow progression of signs is seen until the animal is unable to stand and walk. Decreased numbers of Purkinje cells and cerebellar necrosis are found on histopathologic examination.

BRAIN-STEM DISEASE

When cranial nerve dysfunction is associated with paresis of two limbs on one side (hemiparesis or hemiplegia) or all four limbs (tetraparesis or tetraplegia), focal brain-stem disease or multifocal disease should be suspected (see Box 22-1). Common diseases of the older dog or cat that may localize to the infratentorial or brain stem region include neoplasia, inflammatory disease, and vascular disease (infarction).

SPECIFIC CRANIAL NERVE DISEASES

Cavernous Sinus Syndrome

Primary and metastatic neoplasia and inflammatory disease affecting the venous cavernous sinus, which lies on the floor of the skull and encircles the pituitary gland, may cause abnormalities of cranial nerves III, IV, and VI, the ophthalmic branch of cranial nerve V, and sympathetic input to the eye.

Trigeminal Nerve Diseases

Idiopathic trigeminal neuritis, or mandibular paralysis, can affect any dog breed, and there is no sex or age predilection. The dog's history is repeatable and consists of acute-onset dropping of the lower jaw, which progresses rapidly (within 24 hours) to inability to close the mouth. If the dog's history indicates a progressive lower jaw weakness that occurs over days to weeks, then the dog does not have idiopathic trigeminal neuritis.

The neurologic examination shows bilateral dysfunction of the mandibular nerve (also referred to as the *motor branch of the trigeminal nerve).* Unilateral mandibular nerve damage does not result in a dropped lower jaw. Dogs affected with idiopathic trigeminal neuritis are usually alert, very responsive, and have no problem swallowing food if it is placed over base of the tongue. In addition, there are no sensory deficits to the head and face, no gait or postural test deficits, and no other cranial nerve deficits.

Treatment consists of supportive therapy during the first 7 to 10 days. The reason that limited therapy is needed is because most dogs are much improved in 7 days, and all dogs will be recovered in 3 to 4 weeks. Corticosteroids can be used such as prednisone at 1 mg/kg daily for 7 to 10 days, but clinically they do not appear to shorten the dog's recovery time.

Trigeminal nerve abnormalities can occur with infiltrating neoplasia, such as lymphosarcoma, that involves a branch or the entire nerve. Cranial nerve VII and the sympathetic system may also be involved. Nerve sheath tumors that arise within the trigeminal nerve and cause unilateral temporalis and masseter muscle atrophy ipsilateral to the nerve sheath tumor are common.[28] Surgical excision can result in long-term resolution.

Facial Nerve Diseases

Idiopathic facial nerve paralysis is acute in onset, but because the deficits may not be alarming to the owner, facial nerve paralysis may not be recognized as an acute problem. Idiopathic facial nerve paralysis is seen primarily in adults, and cocker spaniels are affected more often than other breeds. The owner may complain that the dog is unable to blink, has a drooping lip or ear, drools from one side of the mouth, or has excessive tearing or a dry eye. Neurologic examination shows deficits related only to cranial nerve VII dysfunction, such as wide palpebral fissure, lack of menace and palpebral reflexes, drooping lip or ear, drooling on affected side, and, in some dogs, decreased tear production. Sensation to the face is normal. In long-standing cases in which resolution has not occurred, facial muscle contractures may develop. The primary differential causes include otitis media, neoplasia of peripheral cranial nerve VII (nerve sheath tumor, lymphosarcoma, or meningioma), brain-stem disease (other cranial nerve deficits, motor deficits, or postural test reaction deficits should be noted in this situation), and cranial nerve VII deficits, which may occasionally be seen as part of the manifestation of myasthenia gravis, hyperinsulinism (islet cell tumor), coonhound paralysis, or granulomatous meningoencephalitis. Diagnostically, tympanic bullae radiographs should be obtained to assess for possible middle ear disease, especially in the dog that has had a history of chronic external ear disease. The Schirmer tear test should be done to assess the need for tear supplementation. Although a definitive cause-and-effect relationship between hypothyroidism and facial nerve paralysis has not been proved, thyroid function testing should be done, because some dogs will be hypothyroid and need thyroid supplementation. The good news is that in most cases of facial nerve paralysis, dogs can function well with facial nerve deficits and may need only long-term artificial tear supplementation.

Vestibulocochlear Nerve Diseases

Peripheral vestibular disease occurs in both dogs and cats.[29] Older dogs and young to middle-

TABLE 22-1. PERIPHERAL VERSUS CENTRAL VESTIBULAR SIGNS

SIGNS	CENTRAL DISEASE	PERIPHERAL DISEASE
Head tilt	Present	Present
Falling, rolling	Present	Present
Nystagmus		
Horizontal	Present	Present
Rotary	Present	Present
Vertical	Present	Absent
May change with position of head	Yes	No
Cranial nerve deficits	Cranial nerves V, VI, VII	Cranial nerve VII may be involved
Horner's syndrome	No	May be present
Gait dysfunction	Severe ataxia, ipsilateral hemiparesis	Mild ataxia
Cerebellar signs	Possible	No

aged cats are most commonly affected.[30] Cats in the northeast United States are commonly affected in late summer and early fall. The animal's history is characterized by a sudden onset (over a course of hours) of head tilt, incoordination, and nystagmus (Table 22-1). The incoordination may be so severe that the animal is nonambulatory. Vomiting that is secondary to vertigo may be seen during the first 24 to 48 hours. The neurologic examination shows a head tilt, falling or rolling toward the head tilt, and horizontal to rotary nystagmus (spontaneous nystagmus with the fast phase away from the head tilt). The type of nystagmus does not change. A generalized incoordination and a wide base stance are present. Other cranial nerve deficits are not seen, and no weakness or postural test deficits exist. If weakness, vertical nystagmus, or postural test deficits are seen, then a brain-stem lesion involving the central vestibular system is most likely (see Table 22-1). On the initial day of presentation, the animal's incoordination and disorientation may be too severe to allow adequate assessment of strength and postural test reactions. Therefore, 48 hours may elapse before any assessment may be effectively done to separate central vestibular disease from peripheral vestibular disease. Once the signs have been localized to the peripheral vestibular system, the primary differential considerations are otitis media or interna and head trauma with resultant fracture of the petrous temporal bone. If facial nerve paralysis and Horner's syndrome are present on the same side of the head tilt, an otitis media or interna may coexist. Therefore, a thorough external ear examination and skull and tympanic bullae radiographs may be needed to rule out otitis media or interna and head trauma with resultant fracture of the petrous temporal bone.

Treatment for peripheral vestibular disease is supportive care. Most peripheral vestibular signs in dogs will resolve on their own. The timetable for this is usually consistent, and if the dog does not follow this timetable, there should be concern that the initial diagnosis was not correct. The nystagmus should disappear within 4 days; within 7 days the dog should be able to ambulate fairly well; and by 3 weeks the gait should be normal. A few dogs may have a residual head tilt or some incoordination when performing quick movements that require a lot of agility. Treatment that may be helpful during the initial days include fluid therapy for euhydration, diazepam (5 to 15 mg three times daily) for sedation if severe disorientation exists, meclizine (25 mg once daily in dogs) for vertigo, and diphenhydramine (4 to 8 mg per dog) for vertigo. Treatment is usually unnecessary after the initial 72 to 96 hours.

Toxicity may affect the peripheral or central vestibular and cochlear receptors. Parenterally or topically administered aminoglycosides may cause deafness and vestibular signs. Streptomycin and gentamicin usually damage the vestibular receptors, whereas neomycin, kanamycin, tobramycin, and amikacin damage the auditory receptors. Topical antiseptic ear flushes such as concentrated chlorhexidine solutions may also damage the vestibular and cochlear receptors in the middle and inner ear.[31] Toxicity with metronidazole may result in central vestibular signs in dogs and cats of all ages.[32] Clinical signs of metronidazole toxicity are usually associated with high doses; however, because the liver metabolizes metronidazole, toxicity may occur even at recommended dosages in animals with underlying liver dysfunction. Ataxia is usually the initial clinical sign and may progress to nystagmus and severe vestibular dysfunction. Serum concentrations of metronidazole will be in the toxic range if measured soon after the clinical signs begin. If there is any delay in collecting blood for drug concentration measurement after the initiation of clinical signs, serum concentrations of metronidazole may be decreased into the normal range even as the clinical signs persist. There is no specific treatment for metronidazole toxicity. Discontinuation of the drug is imperative. If clinical signs are initially severe, dogs may die. Other dogs recover completely, usually requiring up to 2 weeks for recovery.

Tumors of the caudal fossa, such as choroid plexus tumors and meningiomas, may cause vestibular signs. Older animals with persistent vestibular signs, even if these signs are consistent with peripheral vestibular disease, should undergo advanced imaging procedures for assessment of both the central and the peripheral vestibular areas.

Diseases of Cranial Nerves IX and X

Diseases of cranial nerves IX and X result primarily in dysphagia and laryngeal or pharyngeal problems.[33] Dysphagia may be seen with myopathy, peripheral neuropathy, and neuromuscular junctional disease. Central disease involving these cranial nerve nuclei may result in dysphagia or pain on swallowing. Hydrocephalus, neoplasia, and inflammatory diseases may occur. Laryngeal paralysis occurs without obvious cause in older dogs and, rarely, older cats (see Chapter 9 for additional details).

SPINAL CORD AND VERTEBRAL COLUMN DISEASES

Spinal cord (Table 22-2) and vertebral column diseases seen more commonly in older dogs include intervertebral disk disease, cervical vertebral instability (wobbler disease), degenerative myelopathy (in German shepherd dogs), spondylosis deformans, and spinal cord neoplasia. Other disorders, such as inflammation, infections (canine distemper and fungal, bacterial, or protozoal infections), trauma, and vascular disease (fibrocartilaginous embolic myelopathy) also occur.

Intervertebral Disk Disease

Middle-aged dogs are most commonly affected with the typical intervertebral disk disease condition; however, intervertebral disk extrusion or protrusion often occurs in older dogs. Intervertebral disk disease in cats of all ages is uncommon and when present is usually related to traumatic insult. Clinical signs of intervertebral disk disease include spinal pain and varying degrees of limb dysfunction. Spinal pain without paresis may result in agitation, aggression, and increased activities such as walking or pacing. Spinal pain may be the only clinical sign noted in older dogs. Abnormalities, such as collapse of the intervertebral disk space, deformities of the intervertebral foramina, radiopaque material in or around the spinal cord, and decrease in the size of the dorsal articular joint space, may be noted on

TABLE 22-2. GENERAL SYNDROMES RESULTING FROM LESIONS OF THE FUNCTIONAL AREAS OF THE SPINAL CORD

SPINAL SEGMENTS	CLINICAL SIGNS
C1-C5	Tetraparesis or tetraplegia, ± neck pain Normal to exaggerated spinal reflexes
C6-T2	Tetraparesis or tetraplegia, ± neck pain Decreased to absent spinal reflexes—thoracic limbs Normal to exaggerated spinal reflexes—pelvic limbs
T3-L3	Paraparesis or paraplegia, ± back pain Normal spinal reflexes—thoracic limbs Normal to exaggerated spinal reflexes—pelvic limbs Upper motor neuron bladder (large urinary bladder, good tone, difficult to manually express)
L4-S3	Paraparesis or paraplegia, ± lower back pain Normal spinal reflexes—thoracic limbs Decreased to absent spinal reflexes—pelvic limbs Upper motor neuron bladder (large urinary bladder, poor tone, easy to manually express)
Caudal	Paresis of tail Decreased tail tone Decreased tail sensation

survey radiographs of the spine. Although these abnormalities are suggestive of intervertebral disk disease, these changes do not always correlate with clinical significant spinal or nerve compression. Accurate assessment for spinal compression requires performing myelography or advanced imaging studies.

Mildly affected dogs with only pain or mild paresis may be managed with cage confinement for at least 2 weeks. If after 2 weeks signs are not improved, further diagnostic evaluation of the spine and surgery should be considered. More severely affected dogs—those that are unable to support weight—are surgical candidates and require timely diagnosis and surgical treatment. Animals that retain deep pain sensation have an 80% to 90% chance of being able to walk at some time after surgery. When deep pain is absent, the prognosis for walking decreases to 50%. If deep pain perception is absent for longer than 48 hours, the prognosis for return to walking decreases below 5%. Corticosteroid therapy for pain relief and muscle relaxation may initially be helpful. Long-term treatment of dogs with corticosteroids for signs of intervertebral disk disease may result in side effects, such as iatrogenic hyperadrenocorticism, deterioration of renal function, and gastrointestinal ulceration.

Cervical Vertebral Instability (Wobbler Syndrome)

Canine wobbler syndrome is a major cause of cervical spinal cord compression in large-breed dogs (e.g., Doberman pinscher).[34] The cervical spinal cord compression may be characterized as being either static or dynamic compression. Static compression occurs secondary to stenosis of the vertebral canal, malformation of the articular processes, degenerative changes of the articular facets, cervical disc protrusion, and hypertrophy of the ligamentum flavum and joint capsule. Dynamic compression produces intermittent pressure on the spinal cord that is dependent on the neck posture. Causes of dynamic compression include instability and excessive motion of the cervical vertebrae and hypertrophy of the dorsal longitudinal ligament that results in spinal cord compression when the neck is extended.

The history is usually characterized by an insidious onset of paresis or ataxia of all four limbs, particularly of the hindquarters. When evaluating the gait, the thoracic limbs may appear normal at first, although the owner may report dragging of the toenails or a stiff gait in the forelimbs. On presentation, neurologic deficits related to a cervical lesion are evident. Deficits vary in severity from mild ataxia and hindlimb proprioceptive deficits to nonambulatory tetraparesis. Additional thoracic limb abnormalities may include extensor spasticity and marked scapular muscle atrophy if C6 to C7 cord segments are involved. Sensory perception to the limbs is rarely, if ever, attenuated, and most dogs do not have overt pain.

Radiography, both survey radiography and myelography, provides the definitive diagnosis and facilitates exclusion of those conditions that have similar presenting signs.[35] The changes recognized with survey radiography (Figures 22-6 and 22-7) include the following: tipping of the craniodorsal aspect of the vertebral body into the spinal canal (the site of vertebral tipping does not always correlate with the site of myelographic compression), stenosis of the vertebral canal, especially at the cranial aspect of the vertebrae, malformations of the vertebral bodies, with rounding of the cranioventral aspect, collapsed disc spaces, or spondylosis, and degenerative changes of the articular facets. Despite these changes, myelography is essential for accurate localization of spinal cord compression. Myelography (Figures 22-8 and 22-9) demonstrates extradural spinal cord compression by dorsal cord compression resulting from hypertrophied

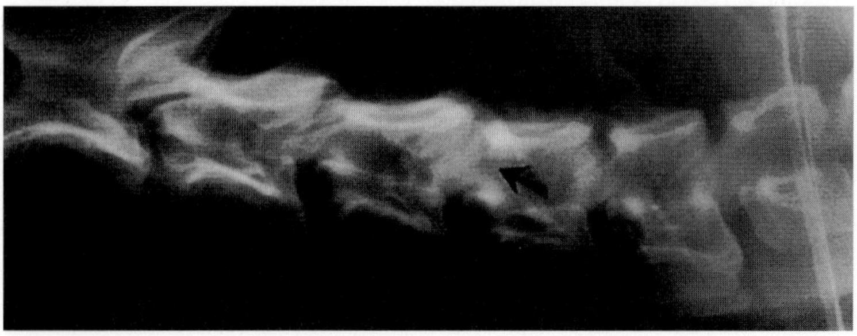

Figure 22-6. Lateral cervical spinal radiograph of a 10-year-old Doberman pinscher with wobbler syndrome. Note the degenerative changes in the articular facets *(arrow)* and slight narrowing of C4 to C5 disk space.

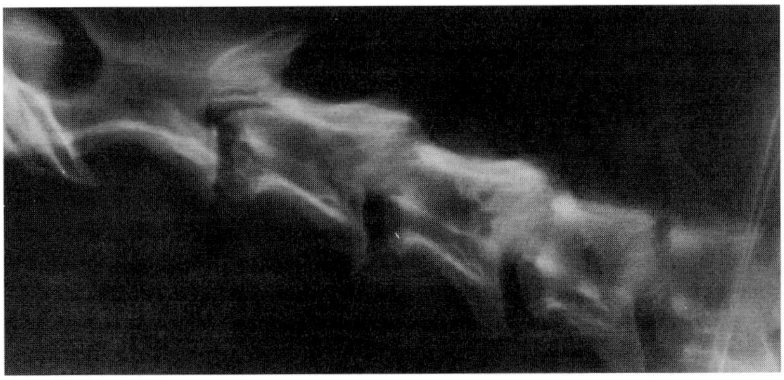

Figure 22-7. Lateral cervical spinal radiograph of an 8-year-old Doberman pinscher with wobbler syndrome. Note the degenerative changes of the articular facets and narrowed disk space at C4 to C5 and the rounding of the cranioventral aspect of C5 vertebral body.

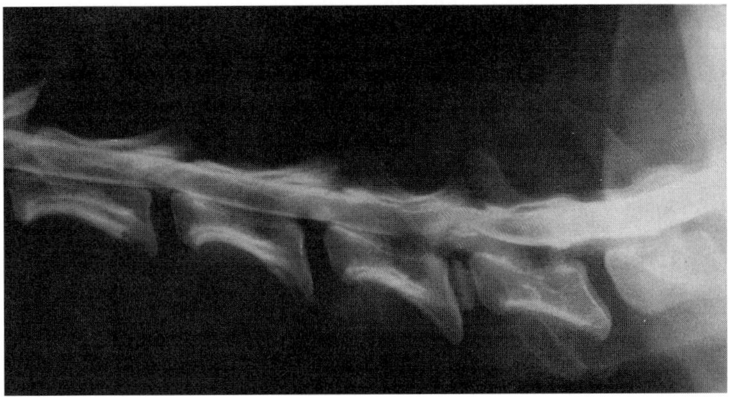

Figure 22-8. Lateral view of a cervical myelogram. Dorsal to the mineralized disc at C5 to C6. Note the dorsal deviation of the ventral dye column that is typical of compression seen secondary to hypertrophy of the dorsal annulus.

ligamentum flavum (lateral view), ventral cord compression resulting from hypertrophied dorsal annulus fibrosis (lateral view), lateral cord compression resulting from articular facet malformation (ventrodorsal view), and compression resulting from a stenotic vertebral canal or instability manifested by vertebral tipping. In addition to standard myelography, stress myelography (flexion, extension, traction) (Figure 22-10) may be useful in determining the nature of the compressive lesion. Sites of compression vary in position and number. The highest incidence is at C5 to C6. Incidence appears to decrease with increased distance from C5 to C6. About 70% of the intervertebral disc–associated lesions are localized at C6 to C7.

The clinical course of untreated wobbler syndrome is variable but usually is chronically progressive. Medical or surgical treatment attempts may relieve clinical signs temporarily or permanently. Medical therapy consists of glucocorticosteroids, rest, and/or a neck brace. Static compressive lesions, such as malarticulations, malformed vertebrae, and disk disease cannot be alleviated with medical therapy alone. At best, dynamic lesions are ameliorated, but the underlying instability or malformation is still present. A neck brace, if used, should incorporate the cranial thorax as well as the entire cervical area to immobilize the caudal cervical region. Cage rest can also provide enough restriction to produce short-term relief, particularly when used in conjunction with glucocorticosteroids. Medical therapy can be used to improve neurologic function before surgery, for the old dog in which the risk of surgery negates the surgical option, and for the dog whose owner cannot afford surgical treatment.

Surgical therapy is the only method by which an existing cervical lesion, whether static or dynamic, can be decompressed. Goals of neurosurgery are to decompress a compressive lesion and to stabilize an unstable dog.[36] A static compressive lesion will require a surgical approach that is different from that used for a dynamic lesion. In the former, a ventral decompressive surgery is needed, whereas in the latter, a distraction surgery at the site of instability is needed to keep the dorsal longitudinal ligament "stretched out" so that during neck movement

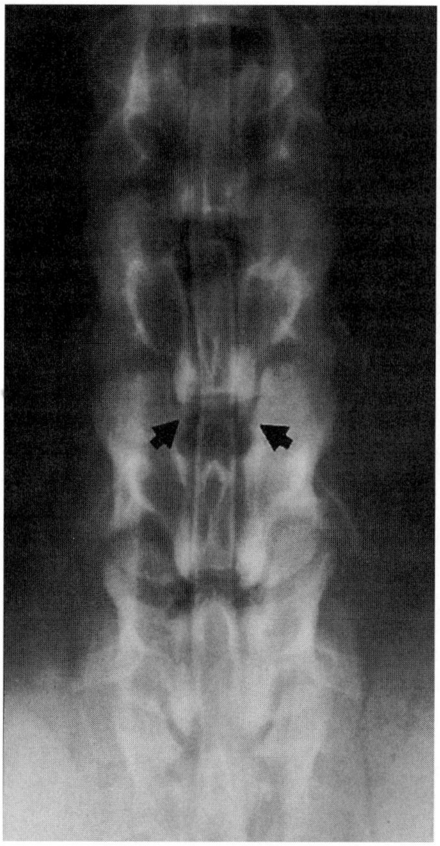

Figure 22-9. Ventrodorsal view of a cervical myelogram revealing narrowing of the spinal cord *(arrows)*, resulting from articular facet malformation.

(primarily neck extension), the redundant dorsal longitudinal ligament does not compress the spinal cord. Because of the different compressive lesions that may exist in the dog with wobbler syndrome, the importance of myelographic examination, including traction views, becomes apparent.

Degenerative Myelopathy

Degenerative myelopathy, primarily a thoracolumbar spinal cord condition, has been diagnosed primarily in aged German shepherd dogs.[37,38] Other purebred and large mixed-breed dogs of older age may also experience this condition, but the incidence in the German shepherd dog is far higher than that in other breeds. The condition is uncommon in older cats. The cause of this disease is unknown. The history and clinical signs of affected dogs reveal a slowly progressive hindlimb dysfunction that begins with ataxia. The dysfunction is secondary to loss of proprioceptive function. Knuckling of the toes, wearing of the nails of the inner digits of the rear paws, and stumbling initially characterize the ataxia. Later, signs of hypermetria develop. As the disease progresses, signs of upper motor neuronal dysfunction become evident and include hyperreflexia of myotatic hindlimb reflexes, presence of crossed extensor reflexes, and development of Babinski's sign. Throughout this progression, weakness in the hindlimbs continues to develop. In the latter stages of the disease, urinary and fecal incontinence may develop. The course of the disease is reported to be 6 months to 1 year from the first appearance of clinical signs. If the owner decides to maintain the dog past the point of severe hindlimb dysfunction, foreleg dysfunction and finally brain-stem involvement can eventually develop.

Spinal myelography is the preferred diagnostic test to rule out intervertebral disk herniation and spinal neoplasia, which are the two primary differential diagnoses that may resemble degenerative myelopathy. The myelography results should be normal in dogs with only degenerative myelopathy. Cerebrospinal fluid analysis is usually normal. Although nonsteroidal antiinflammatory drugs appear to slow the progression of degenerative myelopathy, the excessive levels required invariably lead to gastrointestinal irritation. The only treatment for degenerative myelopathy that potentially alters the course of the disease is epsilon-aminocaproic acid. The suggested dose of epsilon-aminocaproic acid is 500 mg orally every 8 hours. Side effects appear to be limited to gastrointestinal irritation. Epsilon-aminocaproic acid does not cure degenerative myelopathy but presumably controls the degenerative process.

Fibrocartilagenous Embolic Myelopathy

Ischemic myelopathy or fibrocartilagenous embolic myelopathy results secondary to vascular thrombosis and infarction of the spinal cord.[39] Although ischemic myelopathy is often the result of fibrocartilagenous embolization of spinal vessels, other primary vascular thrombi may also result in spinal ischemia. Intraspinal hemorrhage or edema may result in similar clinical signs. Additionally, spinal cord trauma from a variety of causes often results in spinal ischemia. Therefore, evaluation for underlying hemorrhagic tendencies with coagulation profiles, platelet counts, and bleeding times are useful for this purpose. Non-

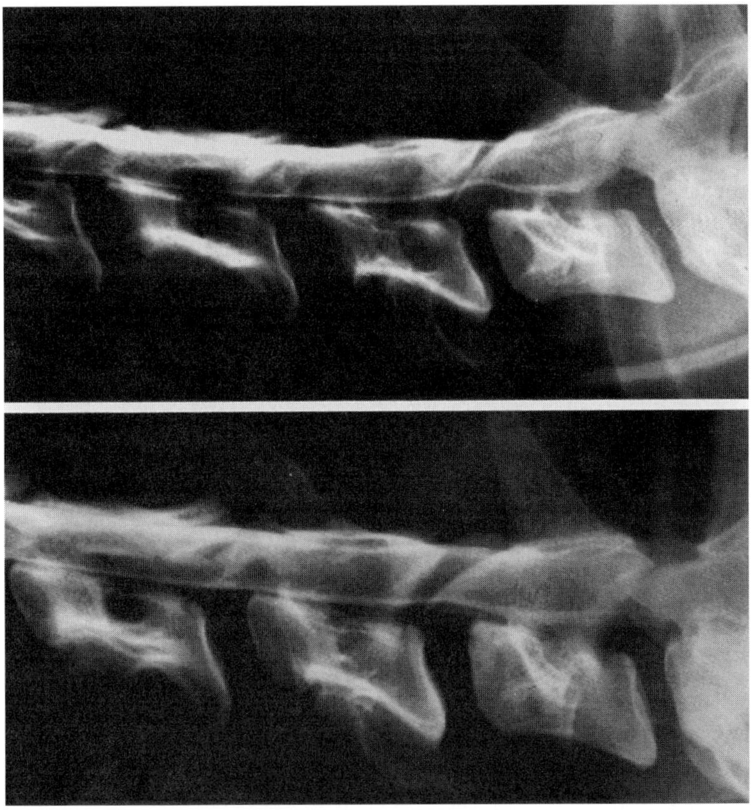

Figure 22-10. Lateral cervical myelography in an 8-year-old Doberman pinscher with wobbler syndrome. **A,** Note the dorsal deviation of the dye column at C6 to C7 in the lateral view (nontraction position). **B,** The lateral traction view reveals dissipation of the compressive lesion when forward traction was applied to the neck. This is most indicative of a dynamic compressive lesion from hypertrophy of the dorsal longitudinal ligament.

chondrodystrophoid dogs are affected. Clinical signs of spinal cord dysfunction occur acutely. These dogs usually have no spinal hyperesthesia when examined; however, they may seem to be in pain initially (within the first 24 hours after onset). Spinal cord involvement is usually asymmetric, and the infarction commonly involves a spinal intumescence. Therefore, reduced motor neuron signs in one or more limbs are frequently seen. The signs are usually not progressive after the first 24 hours.

Diagnosis is supported by exclusion of other disease processes. Definitive diagnosis can only be made at necropsy. Myelography is normal or may show spinal cord swelling during the acute phases of the disease. Spinal cord swelling and intramedullary increases in signal intensity may be noted with advanced imaging studies. Cerebrospinal fluid collected caudal to the lesion may be normal or may contain increased nucleated cells and protein. A predisposition to formation of thrombi should be investigated with platelet counts, bleeding times, coagulation profiles, and antithrombin III measurements. There is no specific treatment for this disease. The prognosis depends on the severity of clinical signs and, possibly, cerebrospinal fluid analysis findings. Loss of deep pain sensation is a poor prognostic sign for return to function. If deep pain sensation remains, many animals will recover useful spinal function.

Diskospondylitis

Diskospondylitis is infection in the intervertebral disk space and surrounding vertebral bodies that can occur focally in any area of the vertebral column or in multiple sites.[40] The most common organisms associated with diskospondylitis are bacteria, specifically, *Staphylococcus intermedius, Brucella canis,* and *Escherichia coli.* Rarely, fungal infections such as paecilomycosis and aspergillosis may be causative. Larger breeds of dogs are more commonly affected. Spinal pain is the most consistent clinical sign. Paresis is usually mild unless the infectious process extends into the spinal canal. Paraspinal muscle atrophy, most likely caused by local denervation or associated myositis, around the affected area may be severe. Diagnosis is supported by the radiographic findings of lytic vertebral end plates on either side of the affected disk space(s). Radionucleotide scanning may reveal lesions of bone inflammation before changes are notable on survey radiography. Treatment includes prolonged antimicrobial administration specific for the organism present. The antimicrobial agent chosen depends on the sensitivity spectrum of the organism cultured. Prior to definitive culture results, or when cultures are negative but radiographic signs are suggestive of this disease, enrofloxacin should be used. If blood or urine cultures are negative, and clinical improvement is not seen on antimicrobial therapy, surgical exploration and direct disk space culture should be performed.

Spondylosis Deformans

Spondylosis deformans is commonly found in middle-aged to older dogs and cats. The cause of spondylosis deformans in older animals is not always known; however, chronic, mild vertebral instability and associated intervertebral disk damage, specifically of the annulus fibrosis, are probable causes. In many older animals, spondylosis deformans is found incidentally. Although this bony change does not often cause obvious clinical disease, if the proliferative bone extends dorsally and laterally to compress exiting peripheral nerves, pain and limb dysfunction may result (Figure 22-11). Survey radiographs show the bony proliferation (Figure 22-12); however, transaxial viewing such as that afforded with advanced imaging techniques is preferred to show lateral peripheral nerve compression. If nerve impingement is found, surgical removal may bring about improvement in clinical signs.

Spinal Cord Tumors

Spinal cord tumors can be either primary or secondary (metastatic). The typical history is one of a slowly progressive loss of neurologic function

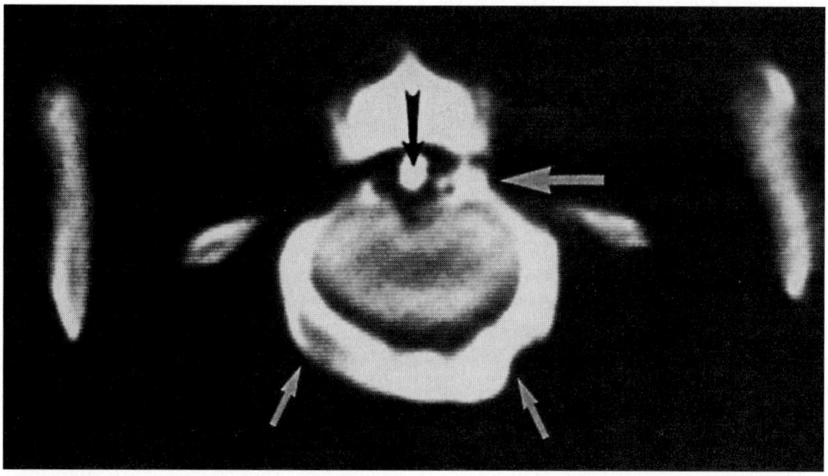

Figure 22-11. Transaxial scan of the lumbar spine after subarachnoid injection of contrast medium *(black arrow)*. The associated spondylosis deformans *(small arrows)* impinges on the right exiting peripheral nerve *(larger arrow)*. (From Bagley RS, Tucker RL: Specialty board review, neuroradiology, *Prog Vet Neurol* 7:62, 1996.)

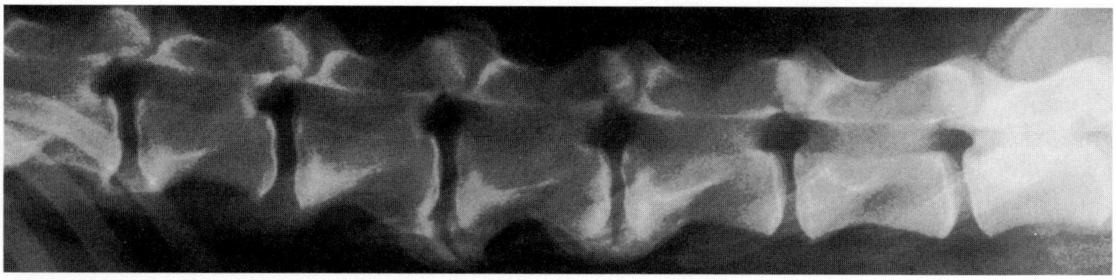

Figure 22-12. Lateral spinal thoracolumbar radiograph in a 12-year-old German shepherd dog showing bony spurs, ventral bridging at L3 to L4 and L4 to L5, and beginning of ventral bridging at L1 to L2.

in the limbs without periods of improvement. Occasionally, acute onset of signs may be seen when hemorrhage is associated with the tumor or when the spinal cord is affected by metastatic neoplasia. The signs of spinal cord dysfunction—spinal hyperesthesia, proprioceptive and motor deficits, and compromised deep pain sensation—vary in severity depending on the tumor location, extent of involvement, and type. Neck pain is a common sign of intradural-extramedullary and extradural tumors of the cervical spinal cord but is uncommon with intramedullary tumors. As with brain tumors, cerebrospinal fluid analysis seldom provides specific information to diagnose a spinal tumor. Spinal cord lymphosarcoma is the only tumor type likely to release malignant cells into the cerebrospinal fluid.

Radiography remains the primary diagnostic tool in the diagnosis of spinal cord tumors. Survey radiographs (Figure 22-13) may show proliferation (e.g., with vertebral osteosarcoma); lysis of the bone (e.g., with multiple myeloma or nerve root or sheath tumors); or scalloped lamina, giving an expansible appearance to the spinal canal secondary to "pressure atrophy."[41] Myelography (Figure 22-14) is needed to clearly define the location of primary spinal cord neoplasia or other soft-tissue neoplasms such as hemangiosarcoma or lymphosarcoma. Computed tomography and magnetic resonance imaging can provide additional information. Once the tumor has been localized with these imaging techniques, surgical exploration and acquisition of tissue for histopathologic examination are required for a definitive diagnosis.[42]

LUMBOSACRAL DISEASES

Lumbosacral diseases may be acquired as a result of malarticulation, malformation, or intervertebral disk protrusion in older dogs.[43] The associated spinal compression usually affects the L7, sacral, and caudal nerve roots, as these

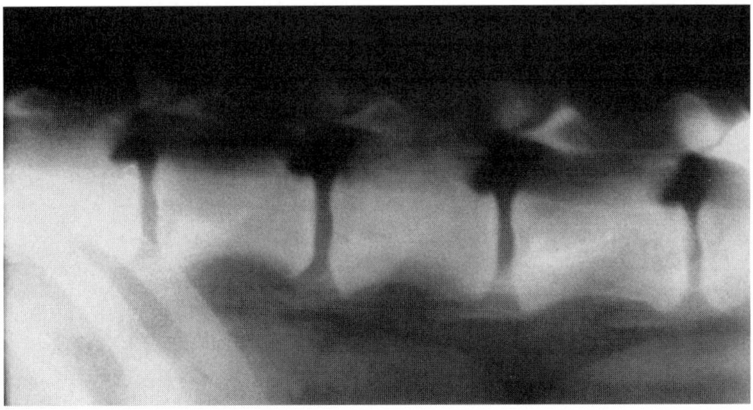

Figure 22-13. Radiograph of the lumbar spine from a 10-year-old Labrador retriever revealing a proliferative lesion involving the lamina of L3 vertebrae. Histopathologic examination revealed this lesion to be osteosarcoma. Clinical signs consisted of focal vertebral pain and paraparesis.

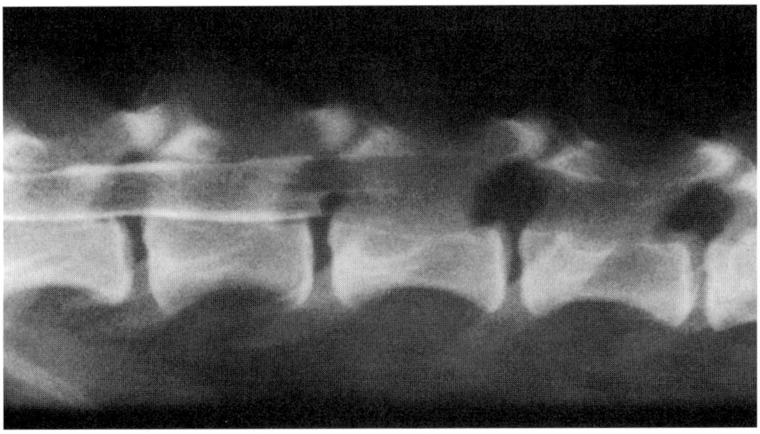

Figure 22-14. Lateral view from an iohexol myelogram showing obstruction to flow of contrast material at L2 to L3 vertebral level. Survey lumbar spinal radiographs were normal. At surgery a proliferative compressive soft-tissue extradural mass was found, and histopathologic examination revealed an anaplastic meningioma. Clinical signs consisted of a slowly progressive spastic paraparesis.

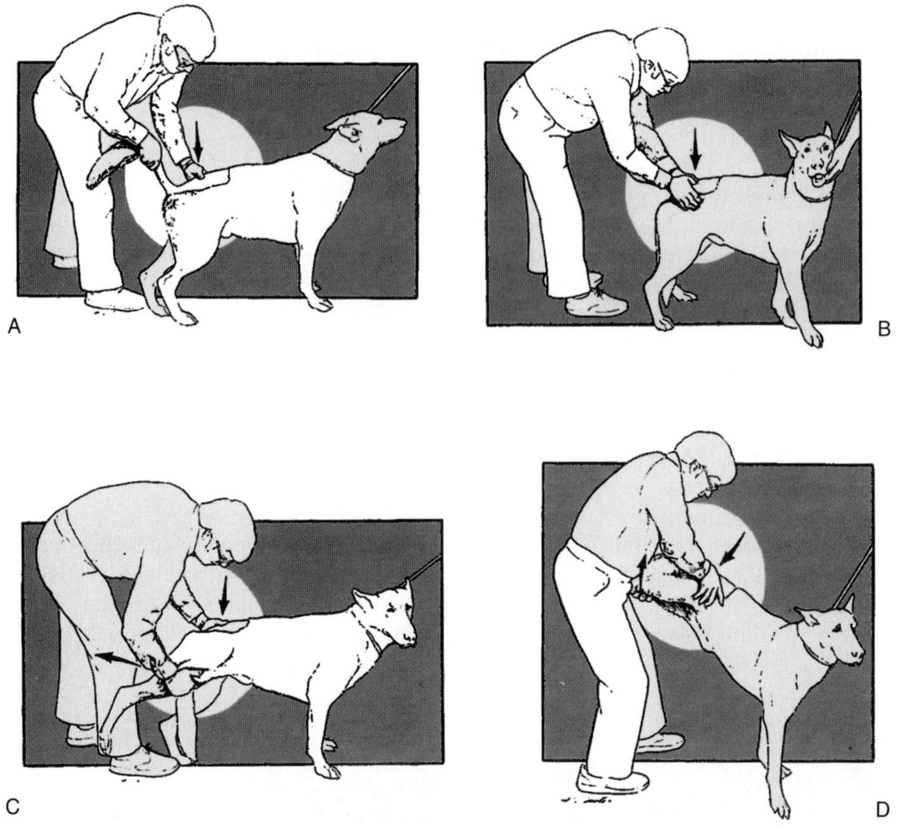

Figure 22-15. Physical examination to detect lumbosacral diseases. Arrows indicate the direction of pressure application. **A,** The tail is manipulated to check for tone and hyperesthesia. **B,** In the lumbosacral push test, pressure is applied at the lumbosacral junction. **C,** The hips are individually extended with and without pressure over the lumbosacral region. **D,** In the lordosis test, both hindlimbs are elevated and extended while pressure is applied at the lumbosacral junction. (From Chambers JN: Degenerative lumbosacral stenosis in dogs, *Vet Med Rep* 1:166, 1989.)

traverse through the lumbosacral area. Compression can result dorsally from the interarcuate ligament or ventrally from the bulging annulus fibrosis. The L7 nerve roots are often also compressed from a ventral direction as they exit the vertebral canal at the foramen. Occasionally, neoplasia or diskospondylitis can result in lumbosacral compression. Primary inflammation of the cauda equina is rare.

Lumbosacral diseases most often occur in large-breed dogs such as the German shepherd and Labrador retriever. Clinical signs include pain on palpation dorsal to the lumbosacral area, fecal or urinary incontinence, and lower motor neuron signs in the pelvic limbs (Figure 22-15). Pelvic limb tremor may reflect weakness or pain. A painful response may be seen with dorsal extension of the lumbosacral joint; however, it can also be seen with hip dysplasia. Diagnosis is based on showing nerve compression via myelography, epidurography, diskography, or advanced imaging studies (Figures 22-16 to 22-18).[44-46] The dural sac sometimes terminates caudal to the lumbosacral joint in large dogs, and compression in this area may be seen with myelography. Myelography is also helpful to exclude spinal lesions of the lumbosacral intumescence. Because often only nerve root compression exists with this disease, myelographic studies of this area do not adequately show this compression. Advanced imaging studies have the advantage of providing a transaxial view of the lumbosacral joint, allowing an assessment of the foraminal areas, where exiting nerves are often compressed. Cerebrospinal fluid analysis is usually not helpful, as the spinal cord proper has terminated cranial to the level of this compression. Electromyographic and nerve conduction velocity studies of the pelvic limbs and tail may reveal spontaneous activity consistent with denervation or slowed conduction velocities. Although these changes are not specific for nerve compression, abnormal results of these studies

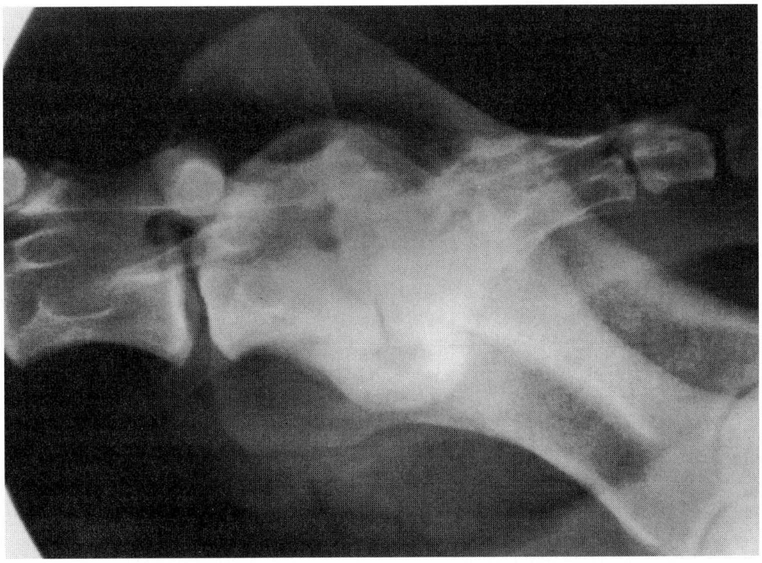

Figure 22-16. Lateral spinal radiograph in a dog with degenerative lumbosacral stenosis revealing collapse of L7-S1 disk space and excessive ventral spondylosis. This dog was presented for evaluation of pain in the tailhead region.

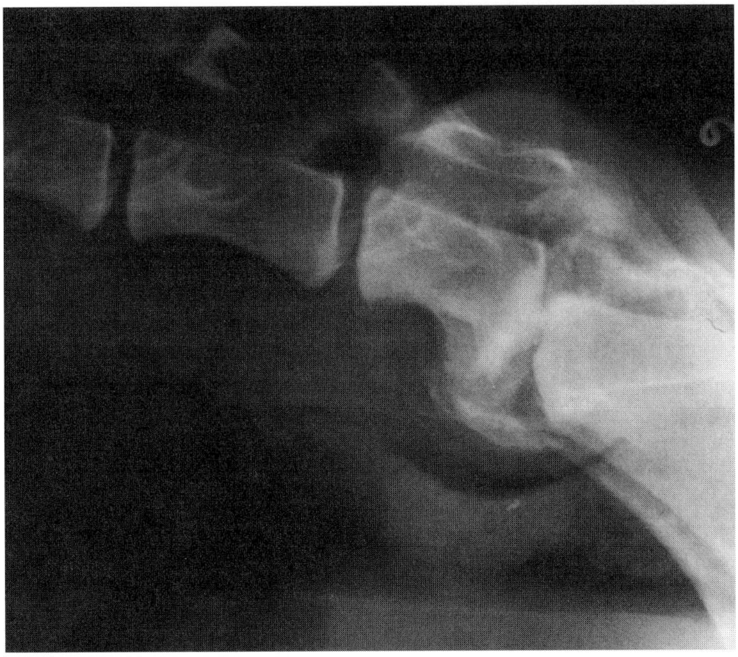

Figure 22-17. Lateral spinal radiograph of a 15-year-old female whippet showing ventral deviation of the sacrum, collapse of L7-S1 disk space, and ventral spondylosis. This dog had severe pain in the tailhead region, painful defecation, and urinary and fecal incontinence.

tend to incriminate lower motor neuron disease as a cause of the clinical signs. Treatment involves surgical decompression or stabilization of the lumbosacral area. When surgical decompression is not chosen, rest and analgesic agents are used with varying degrees of success. Mild clinical signs are more likely to respond to medical therapies. Once fecal or urinary incontinence occurs, improvement in clinical signs even with surgical decompression is less likely.

TREMORS

An idiopathic tremor may occur in older dogs, primarily in wirehaired fox terriers, Airedale terriers, and other terrier breeds.[47,48] As affected dogs get older, a progressive tremor of the pelvic limbs may begin and progress to involve the thoracic limbs. These animals never display weakness and have normal neurologic examinations, and tremors are accentuated during the excite-

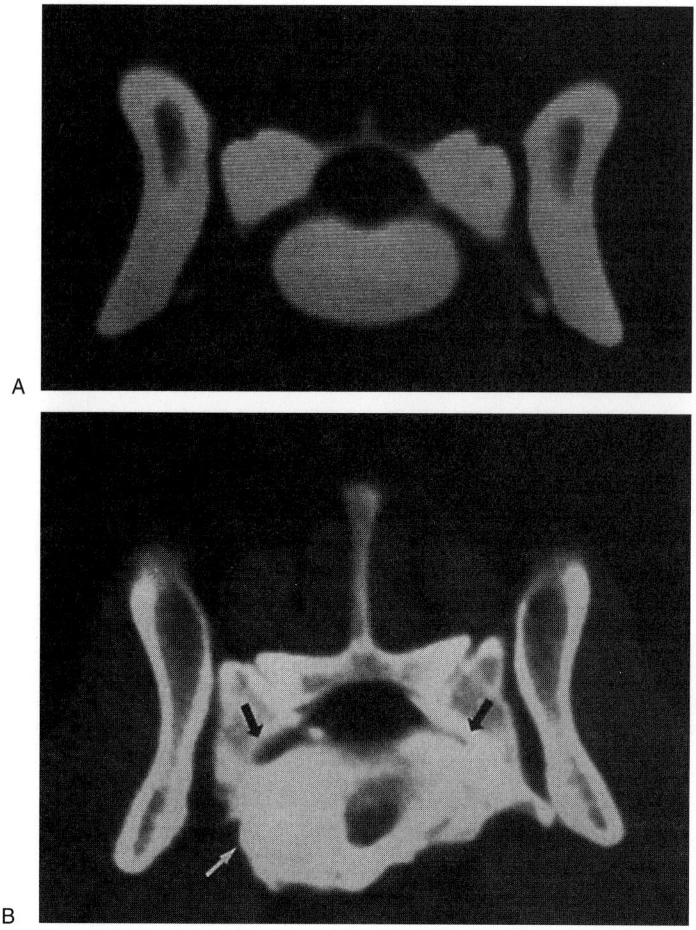

Figure 22-18. Transaxial scan views of a normal dog **(A)** and a dog with lumbosacral disease **(B)**. Note the ventral spondylosis *(white arrow)* and the narrowing of the intervertebral foramen *(black arrows)*.

ment that accompanies physical examination. They are primarily seen when the animal is standing and disappear when running or walking, making it unlikely that the tremors are of cerebellar origin. These tremors may be a form of benign essential tremor or an accentuation of physiologic tremor. This benign condition should be differentiated from tremors caused by aflatoxicosis, "white dog shaker syndrome," cerebellar neoplasia, and hypocalcemia. The current recommendation is not to treat this condition, but rather to counsel the owner that the disorder is benign and rarely debilitating.

REFRACTORY SEIZURES

Refractory seizure activity occurs when an anticonvulsant has been used as monotherapy, the high end of the therapeutic blood level has been obtained for the anticonvulsant, and the dog continues to have the same or an increased number of seizures; when a dog has developed side effects from an anticonvulsant that now preclude its use; or when a dog that has been well controlled for months or years has a significant increase in seizure frequency.[49-51] The following therapeutic rules often assist in the clinical management of refractory seizures in older dogs.

RULE ONE: At least the following should be obtained for all dogs with refractory seizures: a complete blood count, serum chemistry panel, urinalysis, measurement of serum bile acids, and measurement of blood level of the specific anticonvulsant that is being used.

RULE TWO: Regardless of the anticonvulsant used, any dog with seizures that have been well controlled for years that become poorly controlled despite a therapeutic blood level for the anticonvulsant in use deserves an aggressive work-up to investigate the possibility that the dog has now acquired a new problem that also causes seizures (e.g., brain tumor, insulinoma, or hepatic disease).

Case Study 1

The dog is receiving phenobarbital (PB) or primidone (PM) monotherapy twice daily and is having poor seizure control:

Step 1. Measure a trough PB blood level. If the level is below 30 μg/ml, then increase dose to attain a level of 40 μg/ml, using the following formula:

$$\text{New dose} = \text{Old dose} \times \frac{\text{Desired serum concentration}}{\text{Measured serum concentration}}$$

If a trough level of 40 μg/ml is reached and the seizures are still poorly controlled, then Step 2 can be tried before abandoning the monotherapy. Remember that it takes 11 to 14 days to attain steady state levels with PB and PM; therefore, trough level must be rechecked after that time has elapsed.

Step 2. Switch to thrice-daily therapy with PB, or add potassium bromide (BR) to PB (see Step 3). If thrice-daily therapy with PB is used, use the same dosage for each treatment as for the twice-daily dosage for the first few weeks, and then try to decrease dosage. A dose of 18 to 30 mg/kg divided three times daily is as much as most dogs will tolerate without continued drowsiness or ataxia.

Step 3. Add BR at 30 mg/kg/day divided into twice daily doses, and if dog becomes sedated decrease PB dosage by 20%. Thereafter, increase the BR dosage every 2 weeks by 10 mg/kg daily until a dosage of 50 mg/kg daily is reached. The goal for BR is to attain a blood level of 1 to 1.5 mg/ml before decreasing the PB dosage. Once this level is attained, PB can be further decreased. The ultimate goal is to attain levels in the range of 10 to 25 μg/ml for PB and 1.5 to 2.5 mg/ml for BR. The dog's response will indicate whether the low or high end of the dosage range is needed. Keep in mind that each dog can be different and that some dogs may tolerate a higher blood level of BR in combination with PB; therefore, if there are no signs of toxicity at 2.5 mg/ml of BR, the dose of BR can continue to be increased if needed.

Case Study 2

The dog is receiving PB or PM, and drug levels are being maintained in the therapeutic range. Seizure frequency is increasing rapidly, and therapeutic levels of BR are needed faster than in the situation in Case Study 1.

In this instance, the veterinarian can use a total loading dosage of 600 mg/kg of BR. This should achieve a serum level of 1 to 1.5 mg/ml. This dosage is divided into four daily doses during the next 24 to 36 hours to reduce the risk of vomiting and induction of severe sedation. If sedation is severe, then stop the loading and go to maintenance dosage. Once the loading dosage is finished, go to the beginning maintenance dosage of 20 to 30 mg/kg daily. It is helpful to measure the BR serum level after loading to see if the 1- to 1.5-mg/ml target level has been attained. Tapering of PB dosage is then done as in Case Study 1. Some veterinarians prefer to give the loading dosage of BR by administering 120 mg/kg daily for 5 days to attain the total dose of 600 mg/kg.

Case Study 3

The dog is receiving PB or PM and has now developed evidence of hepatotoxicity, which necessitates stoppage of PB or PM therapy. The PB or PM should be stopped immediately, because the hepatotoxicity may not always be simply dose related, and PB or PM administration at any dosage could continue to be detrimental to the dog's liver function.

Step 1. Stop PB or PM completely and obtain a PB blood level. This will help with further decisions about BR maintenance dosage.

Step 2. Immediately start the loading dosage of BR (600 mg/kg daily) divided into four daily doses during the next 24 to 36 hours.

Step 3. Begin maintenance dosage of BR at 40 mg/kg daily and increase to 60 to 70 mg/kg daily during the next 4 weeks. Perform BR blood level at beginning of maintenance dosage. If PB level in Step 1 is high (30 μg/ml) then BR will certainly cause depression, and a lower starting maintenance dose may be needed. In addition, these dogs have liver disease, and the blood levels of PB may remain higher for a longer period of time owing to slower metabolism of the PB. This is why the initial PB level in Step 1 can aid in making decisions about the initial maintenance dosage of BR.

Step 4. Perform BR blood level 6 weeks after initiating maintenance therapy. The goal is to attain a BR level of 2.5 to 3.5 mg/ml. Because this is monotherapy, steady state levels of BR may not be attained for 8 to 9 weeks, but these initial blood levels can give some guidance.

Case Study 4

The dog is receiving BR monotherapy, maintenance and steady state blood levels are in therapeutic range, and seizure frequency has not changed.

Step 1. Begin PB at 1 mg/kg twice daily.

Step 2. Perform blood PB level in 2 weeks.

Step 3. The goal is to improve seizure control with the smallest dose of PB possible. When used with BR, response may be seen when the PB level is 5 to 10 μg/ml, as opposed to the 25 to 40 μg/ml levels when PB is used alone.

Case Study 5

The dog is receiving PB and BR, levels of both are in the therapeutic range, and seizure activity is unchanged (see Step 2), or the dog is experiencing intolerable side affects of PB and BR combination therapy (see Step 1).

Step 1. For the dog with intolerable side affects, perform blood levels for PB and BR and decrease dosage of whichever one is in the high end of the therapeutic range.

Step 2. Add felbamate at a dosage range of 5 to 20 mg/kg three times daily. This drug reaches steady state levels after the fourth or fifth oral dose, and it is not a sedative.

Step 3. If felbamate is not effective in decreasing frequency of the seizures, this presents a very difficult situation. Fortunately, this occurs in only 5% to 7% or less of dogs with seizures. If it does occur, then two other recently marketed anticonvulsants can be tried (see steps 4 and 5)

Step 4. Try gabapentin at 300 mg daily up to 1,800 mg daily and divide into three times daily doses or four times daily doses or a dosage range of 25 to 50 mg/kg daily divided three times daily or four times daily.

Step 5. If gabapentin is found to be ineffective, then lamotrigine at 1.5 to 7.5 mg/kg given four times daily can be tried.

Management of Cluster Seizures

When the dog is experiencing multiple seizures within a 24- to 48-hour time period, the following management may be followed:

1. Immediately after the first seizure, administer clorazepate 0.5 to 2 mg/kg twice to three times daily for the next 48 to 96 hours. Then, stop the clorazepate. Clorazepate may be used in addition to the existing anticonvulsant maintenance therapy. Clorazepate is not used as maintenance therapy; it is used only to help during the time of seizure activity, or
2. Administer diazepam (2 mg/kg/dose) rectally immediately after the first seizure via a plastic teat cannula and syringe. This can be done three to four times during a 24-hour period. Additional rectal administration of diazepam is done only if other seizures occur during the next 24 hours. Rectal diazepam should not be used and the owner should be instructed to seek veterinary attention if the dog has had four or more seizures during a 24-hour period, the dog is excessively depressed, or the dog has rectal bleeding.

References

1. Smedes SL: Geriatric ophthalmic disorders. In Kirk RW, Bonagura JD, eds: *Current veterinary therapy XI*, Philadelphia, 1992, WB Saunders.
2. Bagley RS: Common neurologic diseases of older animals, *Vet Clin North Am* 27:1451, 1997.
3. Cuddon PA: Metabolic encephalopathies, *Vet Clin North Am* 26:893, 1996.
4. Jaggy A, Oliver JE, Ferguson DC et al: Neurological manifestations of hypothyroidism: a retrospective study of 29 dogs, *J Vet Intern Med* 8:328, 1994.
5. Gavin PR, Fike JR, Hoopes PJ: Central nervous system tumors, *Semin Vet Med Surg* 10:180, 1995.
6. Kipperman BS, Feldman EC, Dybdal NO et al: Pituitary tumor size, neurologic signs, and relation to endocrine test results in dogs with pituitary-dependent hyperadrenocorticism: 43 cases (1980-1990), *J Am Vet Med Assoc* 201:762, 1992.
7. Kornegay JN: Central nervous system neoplasia. In Kornegay JN, ed: *Contemporary issues in small animal practice: neurologic disorders*, New York, 1986, Churchill Livingstone.
8. Fenner WR: Metastatic neoplasms of the central nervous system, *Semin Vet Med Surg* 5: 253, 1990.
9. Hammer AS, Couto CG, Getzy D et al: Magnetic resonance imaging in a dog with a choroid plexus carcinoma, *J Small Anim Pract* 31:341, 1990.
10. Davidson MG, Nasisse MP, Breitschwerdt EB et al: Acute blindness associated with intracranial tumors in dogs and cats: eight cases (1984-1989), *J Am Vet Med Assoc* 199:755, 1991.
11. Nafe LA: The clinical presentation and diagnosis of intracranial neoplasia, *Semin Vet Med Surg* 5:223, 1990.
12. Moore MP, Gavin PR, Kraft SL et al: MR, CT, and clinical features from four dogs with nasal tumors involving the rostral cerebrum, *Vet Radiol* 32:19, 1991.
13. Moore MP, Bagley RS, Harrington ML et al: Intracranial tumors, *Vet Clin North Am* 26:759, 1996.
14. Plummer SB, Wheeler SJ, Kornegay JN et al: Computed tomography of nonneoplastic brain disorders, *Proc Am Coll Vet Intern Med* 9:891, 1991.
15. Gallagher JG, Berg J, Knowles KE et al: Prognosis after surgical excision of cerebral meningiomas in cats: 17 cases (1986-1992), *J Am Vet Med Assoc* 203:1437, 1993.
16. Gordon LE, Thacher C, Matthiesen DT et al: Results of craniotomy for treatment of cerebral meningioma in 42 cats, *Vet Surg* 23:94, 1994.
17. LeCouteur RA: Brain tumors of dogs and cats, *Vet Med Rep* 2:332, 1990.
18. Pumarola M: Canine granulomatous meningoencephalitis (CGME), *J Vet Intern Med* 4:25, 1992.
19. Speciale J, Van Winkle TJ, Skinberg SA et al: Computed tomography in the diagnosis of focal granulomatous meningoencephalitis: retrospective evaluation of three cases, *J Am Anim Hosp Assoc* 28:327, 1992.
20. Bradley GA: Myocardial necrosis in a Pug dog with necrotizing meningoencephalitis, *Vet Pathol* 28:91, 1991.
21. Jull B, Merryman J, Thomas W et al: Necrotizing encephalitis in a Yorkshire terrier, *J Am Vet Med Assoc* 211:1005, 1997.
22. Stalis I, Chadwick B, Dayrell-Hart B et al: Necrotizing meningoencephalitis of Maltese dogs, *Vet Pathol* 32:230, 1995.
23. Van Winkle T, Stalis I, Summers B: Necrotizing meningoencephalitis in Maltese dogs: a comparison with pug encephalitis, *Vet Pathol* 29:446, 1992.

24. Thomas WB: Cerebrovascular disease, *Vet Clin North Am* 26:925, 1996.
25. Meric SM: Seizures. In Nelson RW, Couto CG, eds.: *Essentials of small animal internal medicine,* St Louis, 1992, Mosby.
26. Shell L: Feline ischemic encephalopathy (cerebral infarct), *Feline Pract* 24:32, 1996.
27. LeCouteur RA, Kornegay JN, Higgins RJ: Late onset progressive cerebellar degeneration of Brittany spaniel dogs, *Proc Ann Vet Med Forum* 6:657, 1988.
28. Bagley RS, Tucker RL: Specialty board review, neuroradiology, *Prog Vet Neurol* 7:62, 1996.
29. Schunk KL: Disease of the vestibular system, *Prog Vet Neurol* 1:247, 1990.
30. Shell LG: Idiopathic vestibular disease, *Feline Pract* 23:27, 1995.
31. Merchant SR, Neer TM, Tedford BL et al: Ototoxicity assessment of a chlorhexidine otic preparation in dogs, *Prog Vet Neurol* 4:72, 1993.
32. Dow SW, LeCouteur RA, Poss ML et al: Central nervous system toxicosis associated with metronidazole treatment of dogs: five cases (1984-1987), *J Am Vet Med Assoc* 3:365, 1989.
33. Shores A, Vaughn DM, Holland M et al: Glossopharyngeal neuralgia syndrome in a dog, *J Am Anim Hosp Assoc* 27:101, 1991.
34. Burbidge HM: A review of wobbler syndrome in the Doberman pinscher, *Aust Vet Pract* 25:147, 1995.
35. Sharp NJH, Wheeler SJ, Cofone M: Radiological evaluation of 'Wobbler' syndrome—caudal cervical spondylomyelopathy, *J Small Anim Pract* 33:491, 1992.
36. Dixon BC, Tomblinson JL, Kraus KH: A modified distraction-stabilization technique for canine caudal cervical spondylomyelopathy using an interbody polymethyl methacrylate plug, *Vet Surg* 24:425, 1995.
37. Clemmons RM: Degenerative myelopathy. In Bojrab MJ, ed: *Disease mechanisms in small animal surgery,* Philadelphia, 1993, Lea & Febiger.
38. Toenniessen JG, Morin DE: Degenerative myelopathy: a comparative review, *Compend Contin Educ Pract Vet* 17:271, 1995.
39. Cauzinille L, Kornegay JN: Fibrocartilaginous embolism of the spinal cord in dogs: review of 36 histologically confirmed cases and retrospective study of 26 suspected cases, *J Vet Intern Med* 10:241, 1996.
40. Moore MP: Discospondylitis, *Vet Clin North Am* 22:1027, 1992.
41. Fingeroth JM, Prata RG, Patnaik AK: Spinal meningioma in dogs: 13 cases (1972-1987), *J Am Vet Med Assoc* 191:720, 1987.
42. Seppälä MT, Haltia MJJ, Sankila RJ et al: Long-term outcome after removal of spinal schwannoma: a clinicopathological study of 187 cases, *J Neurosurg* 83:621, 1995.
43. Ferguson HR: Conditions of the lumbosacral spinal cord and cauda equina, *Semin Vet Med Surg* 11:254, 1996.
44. De Haan JJ, Shelton SB, Ackerman N: Magnetic resonance imaging in the diagnosis of degenerative lumbosacral stenosis in four dogs, *Vet Surg* 22:1, 1993.
45. Chambers JN, Selcer BA, Butler TW et al: A comparison of computed tomography to epidurography for the diagnosis of suspected compressive lesions at the lumbosacral junction in dogs, *Prog Vet Neurol* 5:30, 1994.
46. Sisson AF, LeCouteur RA, Ingram JT et al: Diagnosis of cauda equina abnormalities by using electromyography, discography, and epidurography in dogs, *J Vet Intern Med* 6:253, 1992.
47. Bagley RS: Tremor syndromes in dogs: diagnosis and treatment, *J Small Anim Pract* 33:485, 1993.
48. Bagley RS, Kornegay JN, Wheeler SW et al: Generalized tremors in Maltese: clinical findings in seven cases, *J Am Anim Hosp Assoc* 29:141, 1993.
49. Neer TM: Personal communication, Louisiana State University, 2001.
50. Podell M: Seizure management in dogs. In Bonagura JD, ed: *Kirk's current veterinary therapy XIII,* Philadelphia, 2000, WB Saunders.
51. Lane SB, Bunch SE: Medical management of recurrent seizures in dogs and cats, *J Vet Intern Med* 4:26, 1990.

Supplemental Reading

Bagley RS, Klopp L, Wheeler SW et al: Trigeminal nerve sheath tumor in dogs, *J Vet Intern Med* 10:177, 1996.
Chambers JN: Degenerative lumbosacral stenosis in dogs, *Vet Med Rep* 1:166, 1989.

CHAPTER 23

Health Care Programs

JOHNNY D. HOSKINS

Geriatric dogs and cats make up a large portion of the animals seen in most veterinary practices. The veterinarian's responsibility to older dogs and cats is to delay, or at least minimize, the progressive deterioration of the body systems from the natural aging process and provide an improved quality of life for the weeks or months ahead.[1,2] Delivery of improved health care to the geriatric dog and cat through the use of state-of-the-art medical and surgical therapy and competent nutritional management are the primary goals for comprehensive health care.[3]

ESTABLISH THE HEALTH STATUS

Physical Evaluation

Clinical evaluation of the older dog or cat always begins with a complete medical, behavioral, and surgical history and performance of a thorough physical examination. The signalment, such as breed, age, and sex, current or past medications, and owner concerns are obtained from the animal's history. A variety of questions regarding the animal's behavior should be asked, such as whether any of the following are present: house-soiling, incontinence, altered ability to recognize commands or people, muscle weakness or disorientation, disruption of the sleep-wake cycle, repetitive and compulsive disorders, persistent vocalization, intolerance of being left alone, and tremors or shaking.

After the history is collected, a thorough physical examination is performed in a systematic manner. The examination of body systems should be complete and should address specific physical concerns about the animal that the owner may indicate (Box 23-1). Because cancer is an important owner concern for the older dog or cat, generalized or irregular enlargement of any organ should be considered serious, and ancillary diagnostic procedures should be recommended. Organ enlargement often indicates an infiltrative disease, inflammation, or cancer. Thorough inspection of the mouth and teeth is especially important because of the increased incidence of orodental disease and oral tumors in older dogs and cats.

Because many older dogs or cats are presented with heart murmurs and breathing problems, thoracic auscultation should be done in a quiet room to determine the severity of the heart murmur and whether arrhythmias or conduction

BOX 23-1 Problems That May Affect Geriatric Dogs and Cats

Obesity
Cancer
Halitosis (may signify orodental disease)
Lusterless haircoat and skin changes
Changes in behavior
Altered ability to rise or walk
Anesthesia risk
Altered vision and hearing
Heart murmur or heart failure
Abnormal urine production or kidney failure
Coughing (may signify chronic bronchial disease)
Urinary or fecal incontinence

disturbances are present. Detecting abnormal heart or lung sounds may prompt thoracic radiography and electrocardiography, and possibly echocardiography and indirect blood pressure measurements.

Detailed inspection of the skin, coat, nails, ear canals, and eyes[4] may identify ongoing problems of infection, immune-mediated disease, degenerative disease, or cancer. Owners of older dogs and cats often complain of abnormal odors or discharges, so the body openings should be inspected and palpated.

The examination of the musculoskeletal system begins by observing the dog or cat standing. The animal is observed at rest for unequal weight bearing and abnormal conformation of the bones, joints, and muscles. Next, the animal is observed while it is walking and trotting to detect lameness and, if lameness is present, which limb is affected. Hypermetria, shortened stride, and any other gait abnormalities are noted. In cases of subtle musculoskeletal problems, it may be necessary to walk the animal in tight circles or up and down stairs to detect the abnormality.

Some neurologic disorders may cause signs suggestive of musculoskeletal problems. As the examiner watches the movement of an animal, it is necessary to distinguish between neurologic-induced ataxia and musculoskeletal-induced lameness. Conscious proprioception should be tested in both the front and rear legs. A complete neurologic examination should be performed in those cases in which neurologic disease is suspected.

The animal's limbs and joints should be individually examined for any asymmetry in size, shape, temperature, and sensitivity. The hind limbs are evaluated with the examiner behind the animal, and the forelimbs are evaluated with the examiner in front of the animal. Attention is then directed to the neck and back, after which a thorough examination of each leg is conducted. Individual leg examination is started proximally and slowly progresses in the distal direction. Joint effusion and periarticular changes resulting in increased joint size should be recorded. After the limbs are examined, attention is directed to the neck and back.

Manipulation of each joint is performed with the animal in lateral recumbency. Joint manipulation includes assessment of the normal range of motion, response to hyperextension or hyperflexion, and stability of the ligaments supporting the joint. Crepitus, "clicks," and any pain response should be noted. Examination of each stifle joint includes evaluation for cranial and caudal cruciate ligament rupture and for patellar luxation. The hip joints are evaluated for laxity in the joint capsule and for pain. Comparison with the opposite unaffected limb is helpful.

Laboratory Evaluation

Geriatric health care incorporates the use of blood and urine screening tests. Regularly performed laboratory tests of seemingly healthy or unhealthy animals allow for recognition of a spectrum of diseases that previously were thought to be uncommon but are actually common (Box 23-2). Abnormal laboratory values should be investigated fully, and ancillary diagnostic procedures added as needed.

Educating the owners about the benefits of obtaining baseline and regularly scheduled laboratory information sets the stage for continual monitoring during the animal's life. Thorough owner education allows a higher quality of services to be provided with a higher level of success and satisfaction for the older animal. When a veterinarian waits until disease is suspected to recommend blood and urine tests, it is difficult for the owner to understand the value of preventive medicine. The owners of the older dog or cat should be encouraged to have their animal examined at least annually. Regularly scheduled vaccinations and internal and external parasite controls should be recommended and enforced. Which vaccinations and how often should be recommended based on the individual animal's risk assessment for exposure to infectious agents and the possibility of developing an immune-mediated disease.

Even in the older animal, fecal examinations should be done. If the animal has suggestive clinical signs, skin scrapings should be done as well. The most common parasites seen in older dogs and cats are fleas, ticks, ear mites, and tapeworms. Other parasites, such as hookworms, whipworms, *Giardia* species, and *Demodex* species, can also occur in older animals because of diminishing function of the immune system. Most animals should receive heartworm, flea, and tick preventive medication. These preventive products are safe to use even in older animals and also in animals of breeding age, as long as the instructions on the label are followed. Annual retesting for canine and possibly feline heartworm disease is recommended.

Another important facet of preventive medicine is education of owners, especially in the areas of nutrition, proper exercise, natural aging process, cancer and its effects, and bereavement and hos-

BOX 23-2 Commonly Encountered Geriatric Diseases

Geriatric Dog	Geriatric Cat
Chronic pain	Chronic pain
Diabetes mellitus	Inflammatory bowel disease
Hyperadrenocorticism	Diabetes mellitus
Hypothyroidism	Secondary hepatic lipidosis
Prostatic disease	Chronic renal disease
Obesity	Pancreatic disease
Cardiovascular disease	Feline triad disease complex
Chronic airway disease or pneumonia	Obesity
Degenerative joint disease	Cancer
Cataracts and glaucoma	Orodental disease
Keratoconjunctivitis sicca	Cataracts and glaucoma
Cancer	Keratoconjunctivitis sicca
Orodental disease	Degenerative joint disease
Urolithiasis	Hyperthyroidism
Anemia	Urolithiasis
Urinary and fecal incontinence	Anemia
Hepatopathies	Hepatopathies
Chronic renal disease	Cardiovascular disease
Hypertension	Hypertension
Lumbosacral instability	Water imbalance problems

pice counseling services. Such consultative advice provides owners with quality educational information. The veterinarian and hospital staff serve a vital role in educating people of all ages in the local community about proper humane health care.

LIFE-STAGES GUIDELINES

A lifetime incorporates the sum of the various life stages of dogs and cats. Age by itself is not a disease. The following life stages apply to most dogs and cats:

- Pediatric life stage—between birth and 6 months of age for both dogs and cats.
- Young-adult life stage—6 months through 2 to 5 years of age for dogs; age ranges for this life stage vary according to the specific dog breed, because the large- and giant-dog breeds spend less time as a young adults. For cats, the young adult life stage lasts from 6 months to 4 years of age.
- Mature adult life stage—2 years through 5 to 12 years of age for dogs. The age ranges for this life stage vary according to the specific dog breed, because the large- and giant-dog breeds spend less time as mature adults. Mature adult life stage for cats lasts from 4 years to 12 years of age.
- Senior life stage—follows mature adulthood. May be defined as *the geriatric years,* but many owners prefer to think of their pets as "senior citizens." The oldest dog on record was 29 years old. The oldest cat on record was 34 years old.

HEALTH CARE PROGRAMS

A comprehensive geriatric health care program can provide a way to target key geriatric-related health problems and detect disorders early enough for medical and surgical management (Box 23-3). The acceptance of an older dog or cat into the health care program depends on its general health status, which may be determined from the case history, physical examination, and other diagnostic procedures, and not on actual age. The health care program may include different levels of health evaluation (e.g., Program One for the apparently healthy animal, Program Two for the animal with minor health concerns, and Program Three for the animal with major health concerns) (Box 23-4).

Implementation of Health Care Program

The first step in the initiation of a geriatric health care program is for the veterinarian to understand the full scope and need for geriatric health care services in the daily routine of the veterinary hospital. Next, the program should then be explained completely to the hospital staff, including how it fits into their daily activities.

BOX 23-3 Annual Health Evaluation for Geriatric Dogs and Cats

Geriatric Dog

- Perform complete physical examination and record accurate body weight. During the mature adult years, dogs have the tendency to steadily gain excessive body weight. The extreme importance of dietary management and regularly performed exercise for the prevention of obesity should be emphasized to the owner. On the other hand, unexpected or inappropriate weight loss is a definitive indication that a complete clinical and laboratory evaluation should be recommended.
- Check for external parasites, such as fleas, ticks, mange mites, and ear mites, and institute treatment for specific parasites identified.
- Perform fecal examination for intestinal parasites, specifically *Giardia* species, and deworm with broad-spectrum product.
- Screen for canine heartworm infection, canine ehrlichiosis, and Lyme borreliosis.
- Prescribe medications and canine heartworm- and flea-prevention products.
- Perform blood and urine screening tests for organ dysfunction.
- Check the heart for rhythm disturbances using electrocardiographic unit.
- Examine the eyes for evidence of cataracts, glaucoma, and "dry eyes."
- Administer vaccinations according to risk assessment of infectious agent(s) exposure.
- Adjust nutrition according to health needs, and institute regular grooming procedures.
- Encourage owner to trim the dog's nails and clean its ear canals monthly.
- Discuss with the owner the natural age-related changes that are occurring and the tendency of dogs to show clinical signs of prexisting medical conditions, such as heart, liver, kidney, and gastrointestinal tract dysfunctions, diabetes mellitus, systemic hypertension, and recurrent eye, ear, and skin disease. Most geriatric dogs will be receiving daily medications for existing medical conditions; therefore discuss the administration and follow-up procedures for the medications being administered and possible drug interactions.
- Fill in the dog's medical health record for each visit and provide a readable copy to the owner.

Geriatric Cat

- Perform complete physical examination and record accurate body weight.
- During the mature adult years, cats have the tendency to steadily gain excessive body weight. The extreme importance of dietary management for the prevention of obesity should be emphasized to the owner. On the other hand, unexpected or inappropriate weight loss is a definitive indication that a complete clinical and laboratory evaluation should be recommended.
- Check for external parasites, such as fleas, ticks, mange mites, and ear mites, and institute treatment for specific parasites identified.
- Perform fecal examination for intestinal parasites, specifically *Giardia* species, and deworm with broad-spectrum product.
- Prescribe medications and feline heartworm- and flea-prevention products.
- Perform blood and urine screening tests for organ dysfunction.
- Check the heart for rhythm disturbances using electrocardiographic unit.
- Examine the eyes for evidence of cataracts, glaucoma,* and "dry eyes."
- Administer vaccinations according to risk assessment of infectious agent(s) exposure.
- Adjust nutrition according to health needs, and institute regular grooming procedures.
- Encourage owner to trim cat's nails and clean its ear canals monthly.
- Discuss with the owner the age-related changes that are occurring and the tendency of cats to show clinical signs of preexisting medical conditions, such as heart, liver, kidney, and gastrointestinal tract dysfunctions, diabetes mellitus, hyperthyroidism, systemic hypertension, and recurrent eye, ear, and skin disease. Most geriatric cats will be receiving daily medications for existing medical conditions; therefore discuss the administration and follow-up procedures for the medications being administered and possible drug interactions.
- Fill in the cat's medical health record for each visit and provide a readable copy to the owner.

*Kroll MM, Miller PE, Rodan I: Intraocular pressure measurements obtained as part of a comprehensive geriatric health examination from cats seven years of age and older, *J Am Vet Med Assoc* 219:1406, 2001.

Ideas and changes should be solicited from the hospital staff, as these may improve the implementation of the program. Because the receptionist is the first person with whom the owner has contact, it is important that the receptionist fully understand the health care program so that he or she can explain the program in common terms to the owner. The technician also has an important and very visible role in this program; the technician can do many in-hospital procedures on the geriatric animal, as well as laboratory procedures, radiographs, and electrocardiograms.

BOX 23-4 Health Screening Levels for a Geriatric Dog and Cat

Program One

Medical, behavioral, and surgical history
Physical examination, including ocular and thyroid gland examination
Complete blood cell count and comprehensive serum chemistry profile
Complete urinalysis, including urine sediment examination
Consultation regarding nutrition, teeth, ears, nails, and skin care
Weight control program

Program Two

All components of Program One
Electrocardiography
Thoracic radiography

Program Three

All components of Program One and Program Two
Abdominal radiography

Ancillary Diagnostic Procedures

Echocardiography for cardiac failure or thoracic disease
Abdominal ultrasonography for any organ enlargement or organ dysfunction
Thyroid gland function tests for hypothyroidism and hyperthyroidism
Indirect blood pressure determination for heart, kidney, or endocrine disease
Liver (serum bile acids), pancreas (serum trypsin-like immunoreactivity test), and small intestinal (serum folate and cobalamin) function assays for hepatic, gastrointestinal, or pancreatic disease
Schirmer tear test for keratoconjunctivitis sicca
Ocular tonometry for secondary glaucoma and uveitis
Urine protein-to-creatinine ratio for proteinuria
Endoscopic examination and biopsy for chronic vomiting or diarrhea
Urine cortisol-to-creatinine ratio screening for hyperadrenocorticism

The daily activities of the health care program should be worked out to include appointment schedules, office and examination room procedures, maintenance of health records, provision of laboratory support, and an owner consultation period to discuss all findings, recommendations, and subsequent examinations. When geriatric animals are scheduled, appointments should be made during the slower time periods, if possible. Scheduling these animals during less busy periods during the day, week, or year and encouraging owners to use these time periods can provide additional services with minimal additional overhead.

Adequate time is set aside for owner consultation so that a complete case review is possible. The consultation should start with a private discussion between the hospital staff and the owner, without the animal, regarding various test results or other important items such as revisits or recommendations. The veterinarian should always participate in a portion of the consultation period. Specific recommendations to the owner should be provided in writing. Next, the owner makes payment for the services and schedules another appointment, if necessary. Finally, the animal is reunited with the owner and any final items are discussed or demonstrations using the animal are done.

References

1. Goldston RT: Geriatrics and gerontology, *Vet Clin North Am Small Anim Pract* 19:ix-x, 1, 1989.
2. Mosier J: How aging affects body systems in the dog. In *Geriatric medicine: contemporary clinical medicine and practice management approaches,* Lenexa, Kan, 1987, Veterinary Medicine Publishing.
3. Hoskins JD: Geriatric preventive medicine. In *Geriatric medicine,* St Louis, 1993, Ralston Purina.
4. Kroll MM, Miller PE, Rodan I: Intraocular pressure measurements obtained as part of a comprehensive geriatric health examination from cats seven years of age and older, *J Am Vet Med Assoc* 219:1406, 2001.

Index

Page references followed by b indicate a box; references followed by f indicate a figure, references followed by t indicate a table.